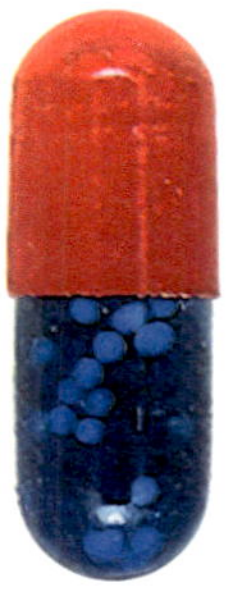

← Hans Hollein, “Non-physical Environment,” 1967 (detail). Pill and typewriter on paper, 8¼ × 6¾ inches. Private archive Hollein.

SICK ARCHITECTURE

EDITED BY
BEATRIZ
COLOMINA;
WITH
NICK AXEL,
GUILLERMO
S. ARSUAGA,
AND E-FLUX
ARCHITECTURE

THE MIT PRESS

CAMBRIDGE,
MASSACHUSETTS
LONDON,
ENGLAND

PREFACE

Sick Architecture began as a series of interdisciplinary PhD seminars at Princeton University's School of Architecture, running from 2017 to 2021. With a title that evolved from "The Illnesses of Modern Architecture" to "Architecture in the Age of Pandemics," the series explored an ever-expanding range of diseases and their impact on architecture and the city: Black Death, Cholera, Typhoid Fever, Malaria, Sick Building Syndrome, HIV/AIDS, Ebola, Population Control, Disability, Allergies, ADD, Alzheimer's, Autism, Addiction, and Burnout, among others. Despite the presence in our discussions of AIDS, Ebola, SARS, and H1N1, pandemics seemed, even to us, distant in time and space. The uncanny arrival of Covid-19 in 2020 made the research immediate and urgent.

In 2020, and again in 2022, in partnership with e-flux Architecture, papers coming out of the seminar were published along with invited texts by transdisciplinary scholars. The idea was to contribute to the ongoing discourse on the current pandemic not by talking about it directly, but by offering a look back and out. In 2022, in partnership with Nikolaus Hirsch and Silvia Franceschini, *Sick Architecture* was exhibited at CIVA, Brussels, with work by additional scholars, architects, and artists. This book develops the contributions from this extended collaborative process, adding even more new authors and topics in the hope of continuing to think together about the intimate relationship between sickness and architecture.

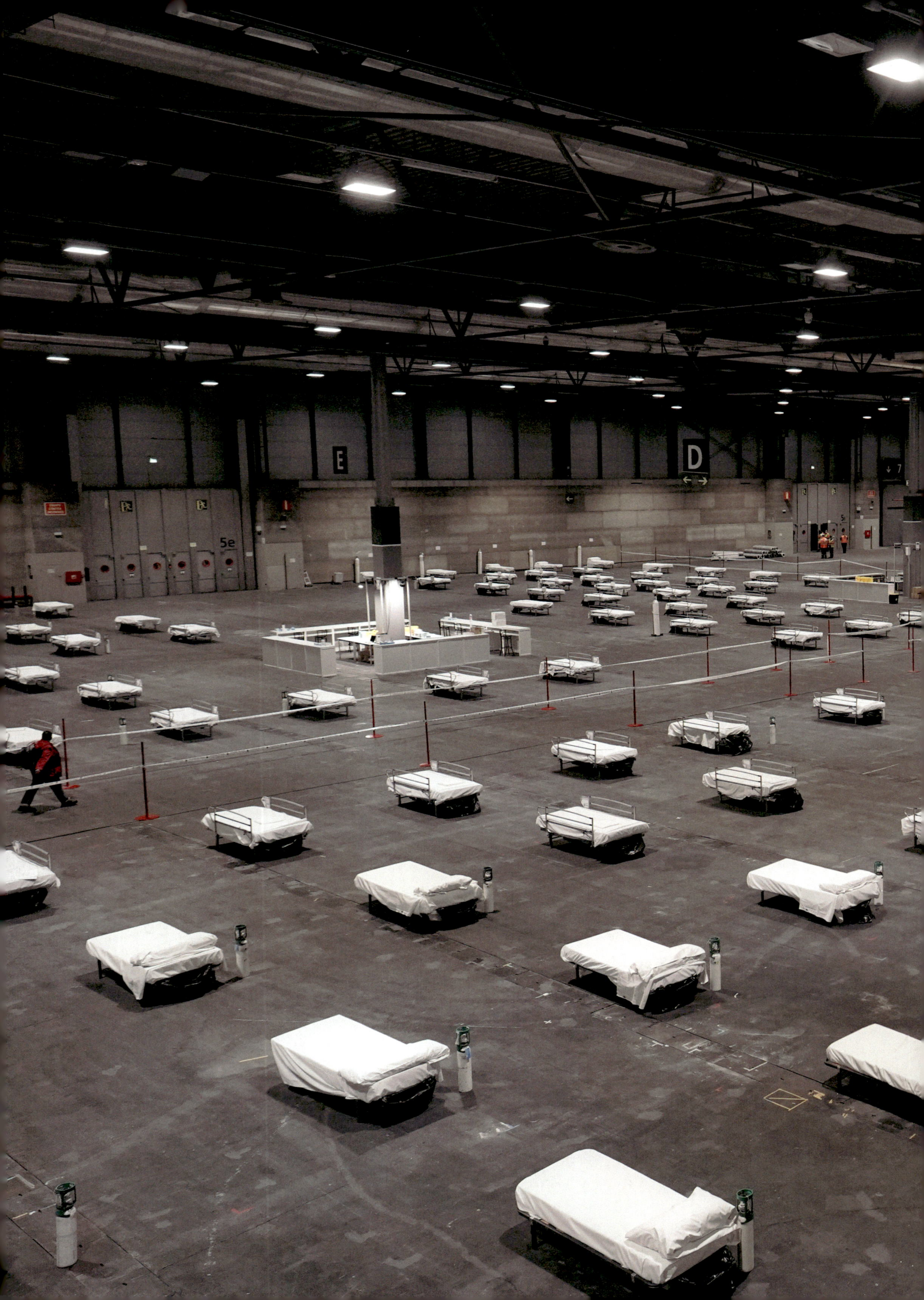
E
D
5e

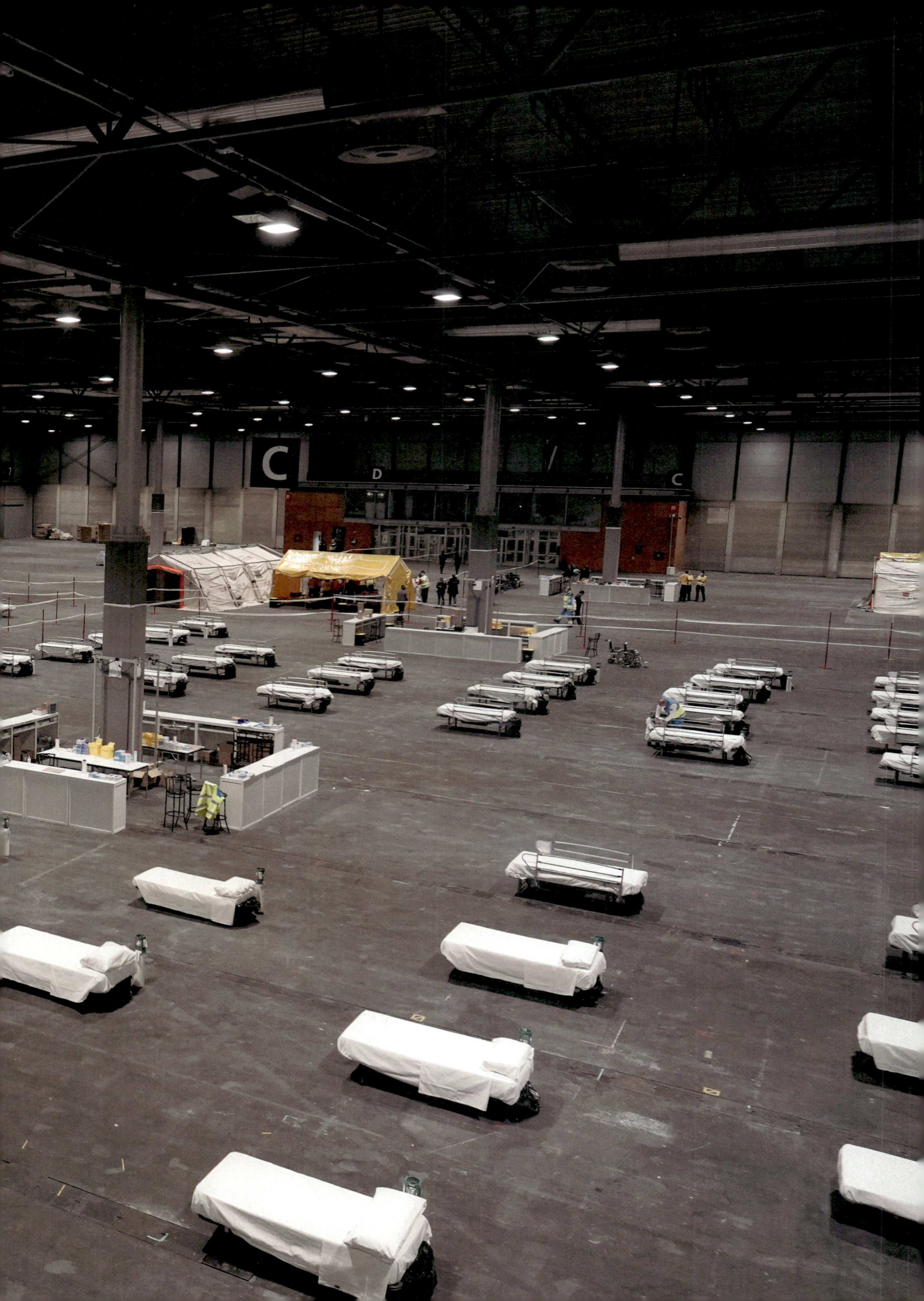
C
D
C

← A field hospital with 5,500 beds and an intensive care unit for patients with COVID-19, IFEMA exhibition complex, Madrid, March 22, 2020.

→ Influenza patients at Camp Funston in Fort Riley, Kansas, at the beginning of the 1918–1919 flu epidemic.

INTRODUCTION

BEATRIZ COLOMINA

A grid of empty white beds in a dark cavernous space, waiting for bodies. One architecture inside another. A field hospital set up within days to accommodate 5,500 patients in the exhibition halls of Madrid's IFEMA convention center. Buildings designed for temporary events hosting an emergency medical architecture, a space for disease. The scene was repeated all over the world, from Belgrade to Lahore, Wuhan, Kuala Lumpur, São Paulo, Mexico City, New York, and countless other cities during the early days of the Covid-19 pandemic. Vast halls, centers, stadia, armories, and urban parks were turned into field hospitals. It was not the first time. During the 1918 flu epidemic that killed more people than the two world wars combined, huge empty spaces were filled with beds. A photograph of a field hospital in a US army training camp in Camp Funston, Kansas, where the 1918 virus first emerged, shows hundreds of ill soldiers in a grid of beds—an uncanny foretelling of what would happen a century later.

In health emergencies, all buildings are medicalized. Large spaces become hospitals, and houses become quarantine spaces. Every detail and every use of every building is scrutinized in terms of sickness. Public discourse becomes architectural. Medical crises bring architecture to the foreground.

Yet sick architecture is not simply the architecture of emergency. On the contrary, it is the architecture of normality. Past health crises are inscribed into the everyday. Each architecture not only carries the traces of prior diseases but has been completely shaped by them. Every new disease is hosted within an architecture formed by previous diseases in a kind of archaeological nesting of disease. Every medical event activates deep histories of architecture, along with all the associated fears, misunderstandings, prejudices, inequities, and innovations.

Architecture and illnesses have always been entangled, from the very first Neolithic structures to Covid-19. It could even be argued that the beginning of architecture is the beginning of disease. As the physician Benjamin Ward Richardson put it when introducing *Our Homes and How to Make them Healthy*, a compendium of texts by doctors and architects published for the 1884 International Health Exhibition in London: "Man, in constructing protection from exposure has constructed the conditions for disease." All architecture is sick, permanently suspended between resisting and producing disease.

Doctors and architects have long been partners in a kind of dance, often exchanging roles, collaborating and influencing each other, even if not always in synchrony. Furniture, rooms, buildings, cities, parks, and infrastructures are produced by medical emergencies that layer one on top of another over the centuries. We tend to forget very quickly what produces these layers. Collective amnesia forms as soon as the emergency passes. We act as if each pandemic is the first, as if trying to bury the pain and uncertainty of the past.

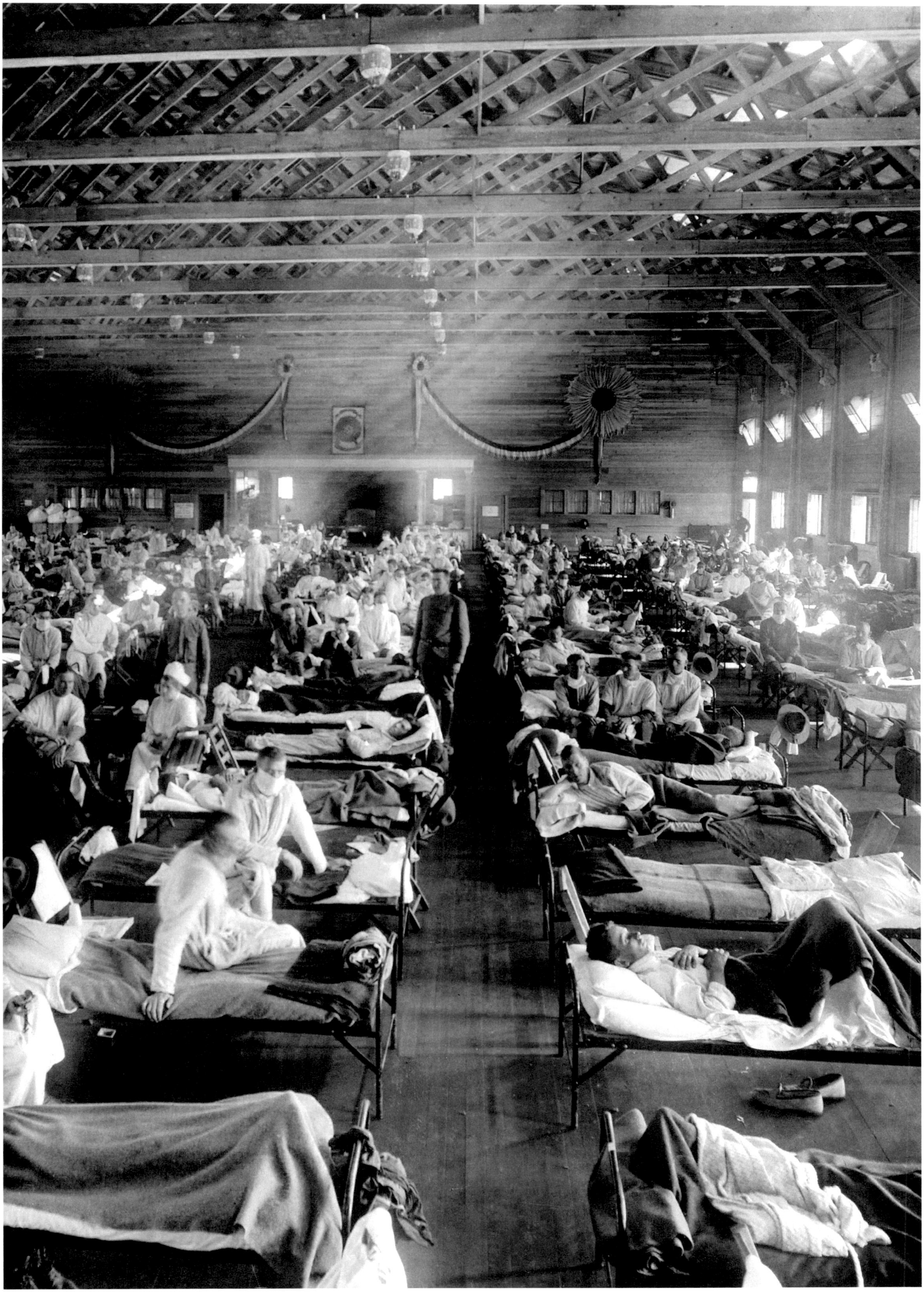

The relationship between architecture and health is ancient. Imhotep, the Egyptian architect of the stepped pyramid of Djoser at Saqqara, built around 2680 BCE, was also a doctor and the author of many medical treatises more than two millennia before Hippocrates, who is usually considered the "father of medicine." Vitruvius, in the first century BCE, established Western architectural theory by insisting that all architects study medicine: "Healthfulness being their chief object." A large part of the *Ten Books on Architecture* is devoted to the question of health. Vitruvius gives detailed instructions on how to determine the healthiness of a proposed site for a city by returning to the ancient method of sacrificing an animal native to the area and inspecting its liver to make sure it is "sound and firm." Likewise, for the health of individual buildings, the text applies the theory of the four humors, the dominant medical paradigm of the time, to organize the orientation and ventilation of buildings. More striking, it argues that those who are deeply unwell can be cured through design, rebuilding the balance of those "whose strength has been sapped by disease" (including *phthisis,* the ancient Greek term for tuberculosis).

Already in Vitruvius there is the idea that architecture can both prevent and cure disease. This idea has persisted through time. Every subsequent architectural theory has added something to it. Cities represent a kind of accumulation of theories of disease from ancient times to the present. The history of architecture and the history of the city are the history of disease: the history of a series of structures and infrastructures put in place to counter the previous epidemic, always one step behind. From new building types such as lazarettos in fifteenth-century Italy, designed to contain those infected or suspected to be infected by the plague, to the great infrastructure works of the nineteenth century—sewage systems, clean water, urban grids, and parks—cities have been completely reshaped in the name of health.

Modern architecture was also produced under emergency conditions. Throughout the late nineteenth and the first half of the twentieth century, millions died of tuberculosis every year all over the world. Modern buildings offered a prophylactic defense against this invisible microorganism, the *tuberculosis bacilli* that was only definitively identified in 1882. All the defining features of modern architecture—white walls, terraces, big windows, detachment from the ground—were presented as both prevention and cure. Yet the medicinal nature of modern architecture and the unimaginable horror it was responding to have been largely forgotten.

To produce the sense of modern architecture as healthy, nineteenth-century architecture was demonized as nervous, unhealthy, and literally filled with disease, especially the bacilli of tuberculosis. Decorative excess was itself treated as an infection. Modernizing architecture was firstly a form of disinfection, a purification of buildings that would lead to a health-giving environment of light, air, cleanliness, and smooth white surfaces, without cracks or crevices where contagion might lurk.

It was not until 1928 that the first modern antibiotic, penicillin, was accidentally discovered by Alexander Fleming when he observed that mold stopped the growth of bacteria—an unwitting reactivation of the knowledge in Imhotep's practice of applying moldy bread to skin infections. Plants with antibacterial properties have been central to the health practices of many Indigenous communities all over the world for millennia and are now closely studied in universities and medical research centers in the age of antibiotic-resistant bacteria.

While streptomycin, the first antibiotic effective against tuberculosis, was discovered in 1943 and only became widely available a decade later, there was already an antibiotic philosophy of architecture. Modern architecture was the antibiotic. In that sense, modern architecture saved lives. In an age when the life expectancy was forty, with most people dying from bacterial diseases, modern architecture helped create a healthier environment. Yet like all antibiotics, it eventually created its own monsters.

Modern architecture produces sickness, most obviously sick building syndrome. The air-conditioning systems that architects like Le Corbusier celebrated for isolating inside air from the contaminated outside air turned out to be reservoirs and vectors of disease. As in a science fiction horror film, the architecture that was supposed to inoculate its occupants against disease turned against them. Many of the diseases of our time, including obesity, diabetes, numerous cancers, autoimmune disorders, allergies, and autism, are now understood as the consequence of the diminishing diversity of bacteria. Buildings have their own microbiomes, and the diversity of bacteria in buildings is just as important as the bacterial diversity in bodies. The bacteria of buildings continuously enter human bodies and the bacteria of these bodies—along with those of other animals, insects, and plants—are spread out across buildings. But there is a crisis of diversity in this ecology. Just as modern architecture polemically reconfigured the nineteenth-century architectures that preceded it on health grounds, architecture today needs to be dramatically reconfigured in the name of newer paradigms of health and actively engaged in the production of alternative paradigms.

All the archaeological layers of sick architecture are inherently political. Models of health paradoxically produce vulnerabilities to illness. They inevitably draw and maintain lines that privilege and shelter a normalized subject from threatening others. In reverse, to think in terms of sick architecture is to recognize that all borders, whether that of a room or a nation, are medical. Reinforced by countless protocols and policing, these borders are typically not a single line but a nesting of lines at multiple scales, each with their own architecture. Sick architecture is always multiscalar, traversing and defining territory, nation, ethnicity, race, class, and domesticities. It creates models of normality, which are also models of exclusion, disadvantage, and prejudice.

As many of the essays in this collection show, the violent exercise of colonial power, whether external or internal, is inseparable from the architecture of health and is never simply about humans but transspecies relationships. In the Belgian Congo, for example, a 400-meter-wide band—the distance it was thought that no mosquito could fly—separated the Indigenous city from the European city to supposedly prevent yellow fever. The medical border acted as a mechanism of racialization. The mosquito dimensioned the city. The construction of the Panama Canal was also predicated on the conquest of the mosquito. It involved both large- and small-scale interventions, from the clearing of forests and draining of swamps to the installation of screened verandas and other architectural devices deployed along, and reinforcing, racialized lines. Much if not most of the sick architecture in this collection is the state control of bodies, from slavery to eugenics to menstrual cycles. Even the planet is now both sick and a medical instrument to detect illnesses.

Health is not just physical. Already in ancient Greece, a variety of mental illnesses were identified and spatialized inasmuch as sufferers were forced to remain indoors or roam the outdoors without an address. Eventually, specialized buildings offered both isolation and care. The Muslim philosopher and physician Ibn Sina treated the "head sick" with calming gardens and fountains in the first mental hospital, set up in the heart of Baghdad in the eighth century. His *Canon of Medicine* considered psychology to be essential and was the most influential medical text in Europe up until the seventeenth century. The Hospital of the Innocents, considered to be the first psychiatric hospital in the Western world and the model throughout Europe and the Americas, was founded in Valencia in 1410 after observing the Islamic institutions. Eventually, the whole architecture of mental illness was undone by the anti-psychiatric movement in the 1960s, but experimentation continues today in developing architectures that allow those on an expanded mental spectrum to be at once sheltered and engaged in city life.

In fact, the question of mental health has always been part of architectural discourse. Architects act as if their designs will produce a sense of well-being, and each mental condition needs to be countered by architecture. At the turn of the twentieth century in Vienna, Camillo Sitte diagnosed the modern city as producing agoraphobia, in the very moment and place the disorder was being actively discussed. Sitte presented his urban design, inspired by the eccentric narrow streets and small plazas of medieval cities, as a psychological counter. In the late 1940s and 1950s, Richard Neutra fashioned himself as a shrink to his clients, understood as patients. Likewise, when the concept of stress was identified in the 1960s as the predominant reaction to modern life, experimental architects such as Coop Himmelblau worked with psychiatrists to produce prototypes of relaxation architectures. Hans Hollein replaced buildings altogether with an "architecture pill" providing the desired mental state. In reverse, some mental states such as autism are now seen as inherently spatial, implying an alternative architecture in their own right.

In addition to architectures for an expanded mental spectrum, there is the need to embrace an expanded understanding of the physical spectrum. Architecture that normalizes can itself be treated as a form of sickness. The diverse abilities of children, older people, those with limb differences, deafness, or blindness, and/or the chronically ill call for greater hospitality, opportunity, and pleasure from architecture, redefining the very concept of care and transforming the role of buildings in a way that impacts much more than those being treated. Aino and Alvar Aalto offered a crucial paradigm shift when they argued that architects should always design for the person in the "weakest position." The radicality of this is to rethink architecture from vulnerability itself. Sickness is not an exception but the norm, and different degrees of sickness define the human condition.

This dense array of essays engages with a multiplicity of topics, places, scales, and concepts that are loosely gathered into the overlapping categories of Bodies, Borders, Atmospheres, and Landscapes, each understood as architectural categories in their own right. The book is a nonhierarchical, kaleidoscopic almanac with many quirky entries that acts as a resource to think more widely and differently about sick architecture. It is a kind of minimum dose, with so many topics and angles waiting to be added. It is an invitation to collaboratively reconsider the ancient and always urgent question of the relationship of health and architecture.

p8–9 Photo: Borja Sanchez-Trillo/Comunidad de Madrid via Getty Images.
p11 National Museum of Health and Medicine.

BOR

ERS

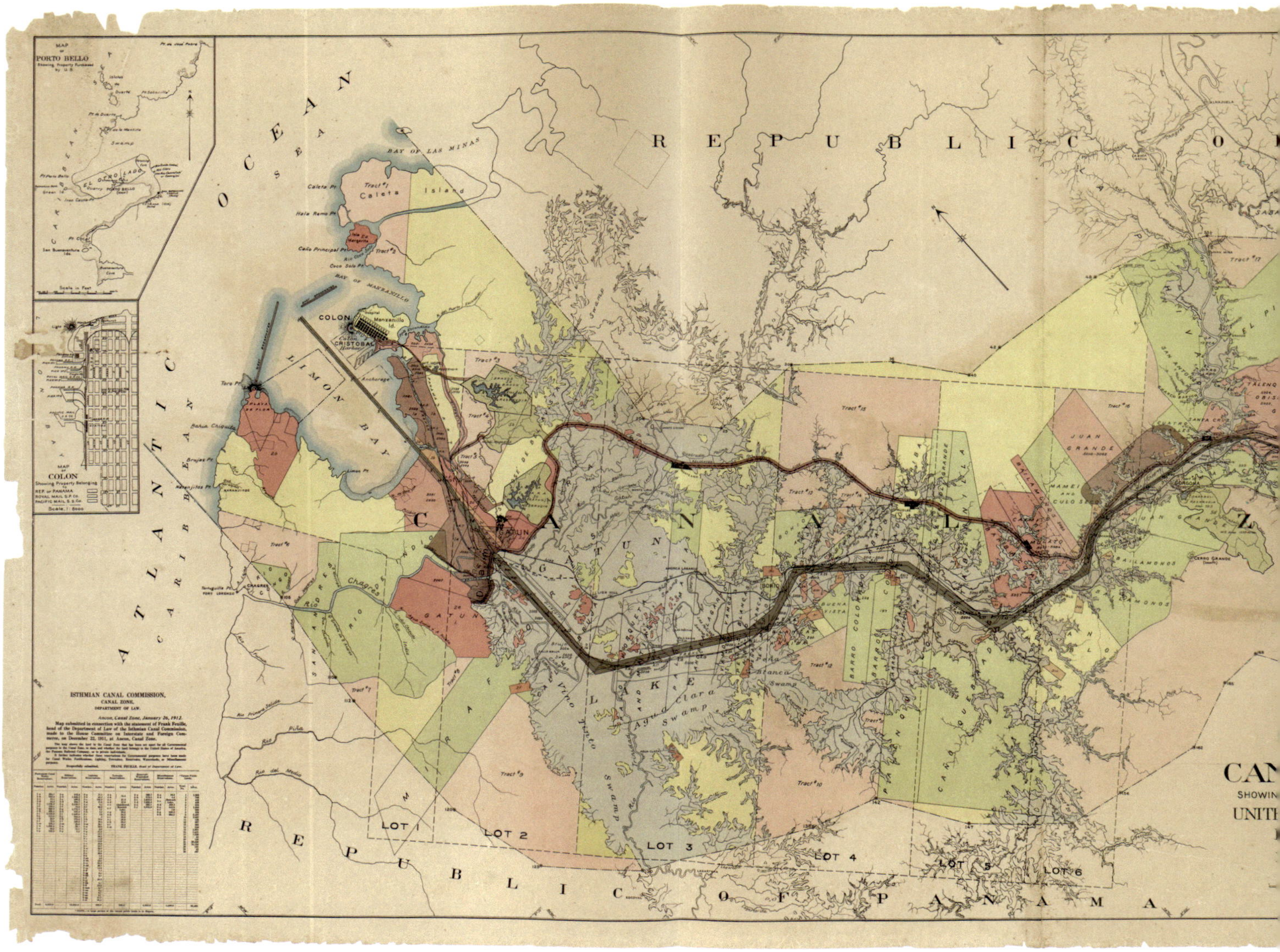

SANITARY IMPERIALISM

DANTE FURIOSO

In 1913, a year before the Panama Canal was completed, the journalist Frederic J. Haskin wrote that "the conquest of the Isthmian barrier *was the conquest of the mosquito.*"[1] This was a period when America's westward expansion was eclipsed by overseas military conquest—the US had gone to war in 1898 with Spain and by 1902 taken control of Cuba, Puerto Rico, the Philippines, and Guam. President Theodore Roosevelt intensified this ongoing project of US interference in Central America and the Caribbean, supporting a coup d'état in the Colombian province of Panama by US-friendly businessmen in 1903.[2] The newly independent nation granted the US outsized political and military influence in the region, in large part due to the creation of the US Panama Canal Zone, a ten-mile-wide strip of US territory that cut through the area. As the site of the construction and subsequent operation of the transisthmian canal that continues to operate today, the territory was a testing ground for a unique kind of architecture that reconfigured the relationship between humans and mosquitoes.[3]

↑ Isthmian Canal Commission, map of the Canal Zone showing property belonging to the United States of America, Panama R. R. Co., and lands claimed by private persons, 1912.

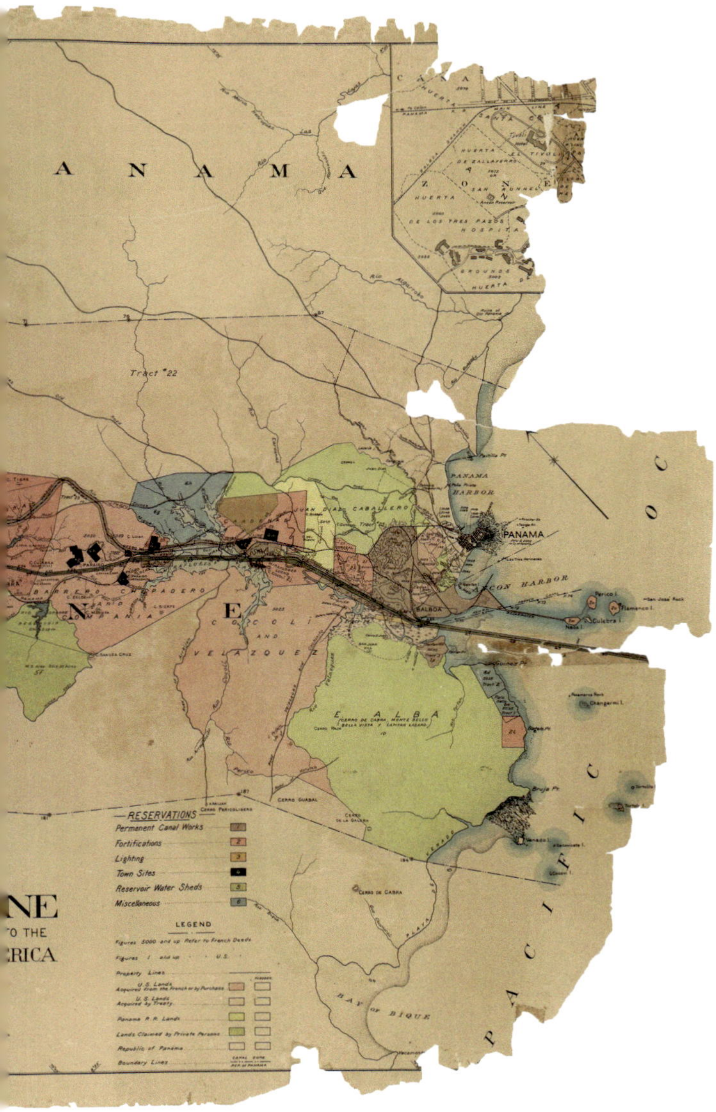

The connection between mosquito control and the imperial ambitions of the United States can be seen in the work of William C. Gorgas, the Alabama-born Army surgeon who led efforts to eradicate yellow fever and malaria—both mosquito-borne diseases—during the first US occupation of Cuba (1898–1902), and was subsequently appointed Chief Sanitary Officer in Panama. For Gorgas, controlling yellow fever and malaria took on historic dimensions. Reflecting on his work, Gorgas claimed that he had "made sanitary discoveries that will enable man to return from the temperate regions to which he was forced to migrate long ages ago, and again live and develop in his natural home, the tropics."[4] Nevertheless, mosquito control efforts were not simply about making work in hot climates tolerable for white US employees from more temperate zones. How workers lived and the way housing was designed demonstrated overlapping US policies, prevailing perceptions of the tropical environment, and the conflicts between engineers and workers of various social classes, races, and ethnicities. In particular, the dwellings erected for the Isthmian Canal Commission (ICC) conjoined the management of mosquitoes with the manipulation of interactions between people of different races and social classes.

Groundwork

The geography of Central America, with its relatively short distance between the world's two largest oceans and abundance of rivers and lakes, made the amphibious transport of goods across the Isthmus of Panama a viable industry throughout the colonial period. In the nineteenth century, entrepreneurs, explorers, and engineers began to propose numerous plans and designs for a canal to connect the Atlantic and Pacific Oceans in Nicaragua and Panama.[5] Chief among them was the French project undertaken by the Compagnie Universelle du Canal Interocéanique, which began work in 1879 under Ferdinand de Lesseps, who had previously completed the Suez Canal in 1869. Although the sea level canal succeeded in Egypt, it failed in Panama, due in large part to its mountainous topography, as well as high death rates from yellow fever and malaria, which was popularly understood to be a serious threat to any renewed efforts.[6]

As part of the US Government, in 1904 the ICC began building a canal that would traverse the varied topography of the isthmus with a series of locks. This would allow ships to move upward in elevation until they reached the man-made Lake Gatún, which was created during construction by damming adjacent rivers. In light of the French failure, efforts to curb yellow fever and malaria began promptly with the creation of twenty-five sanitary districts corresponding to existing cities, including the larger terminal port cities of Panama City and Colón; smaller towns along the proposed canal route, like Ancón and Gorgona; and work camps near major canal excavation, like Culebra.[7] The kind of sanitary work varied considerably between the port cites, inland towns, and work camps.

When Gorgas arrived in Panama in 1904, he brought more than knowledge of anti-mosquito techniques. He arrived with anxious determination. In his last two months in eastern Cuba, the Army surgeon estimated that his troops had "a constant sick rate of over six hundred per thousand," almost entirely due to yellow fever.[8] The end of the French effort and the beginning of the US canal construction came on the heels of a trio of discoveries related to the transmission of malaria in 1897. Research performed in colonial contexts from British India to US-occupied Cuba debunked the long-held miasma theory that malaria was the product of the bad air (*mal'aria* in Italian). Thus, precisely as the US began planning the construction of the canal, Gorgas understood that his sanitation work had a clear target and enemy:

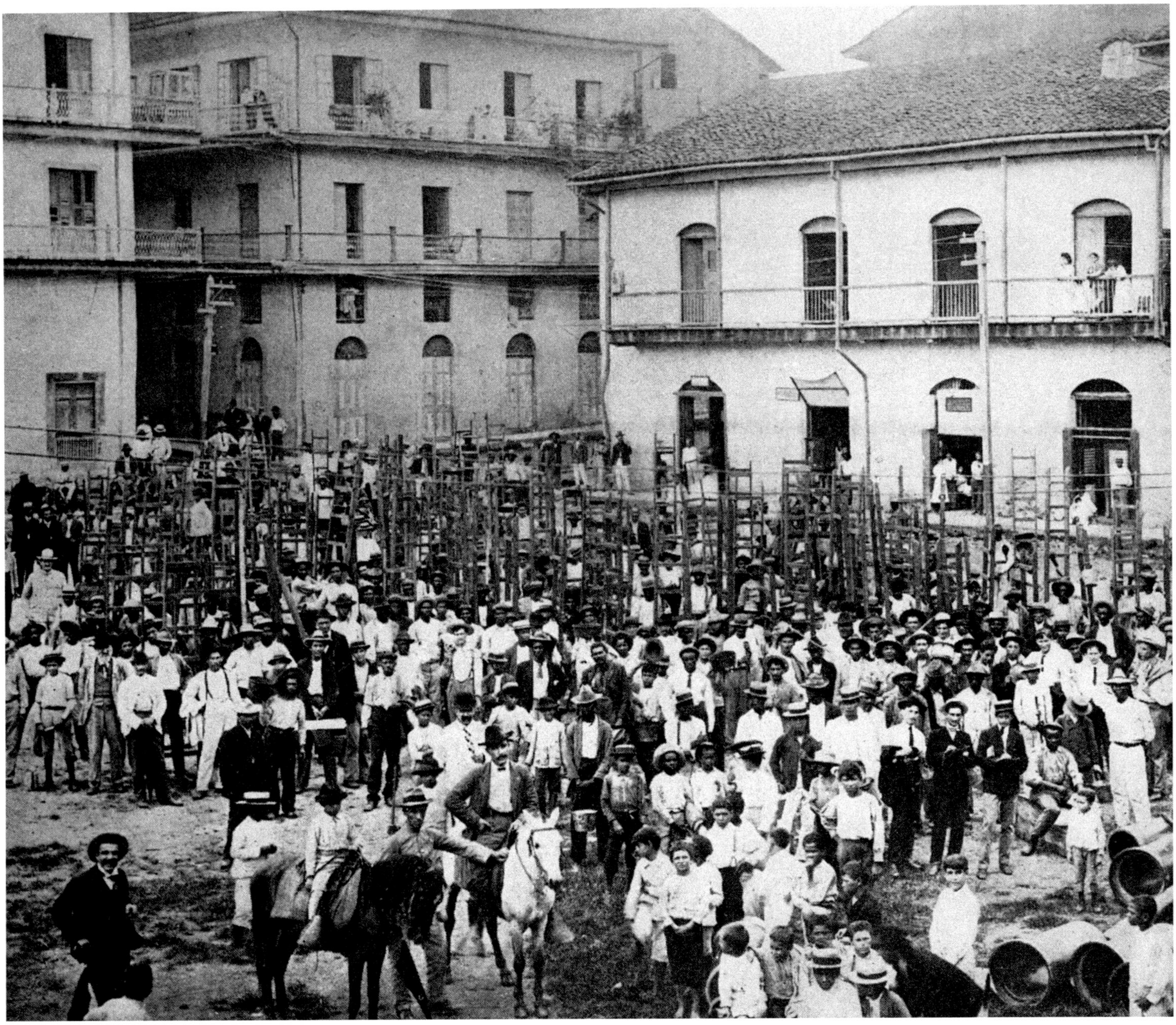

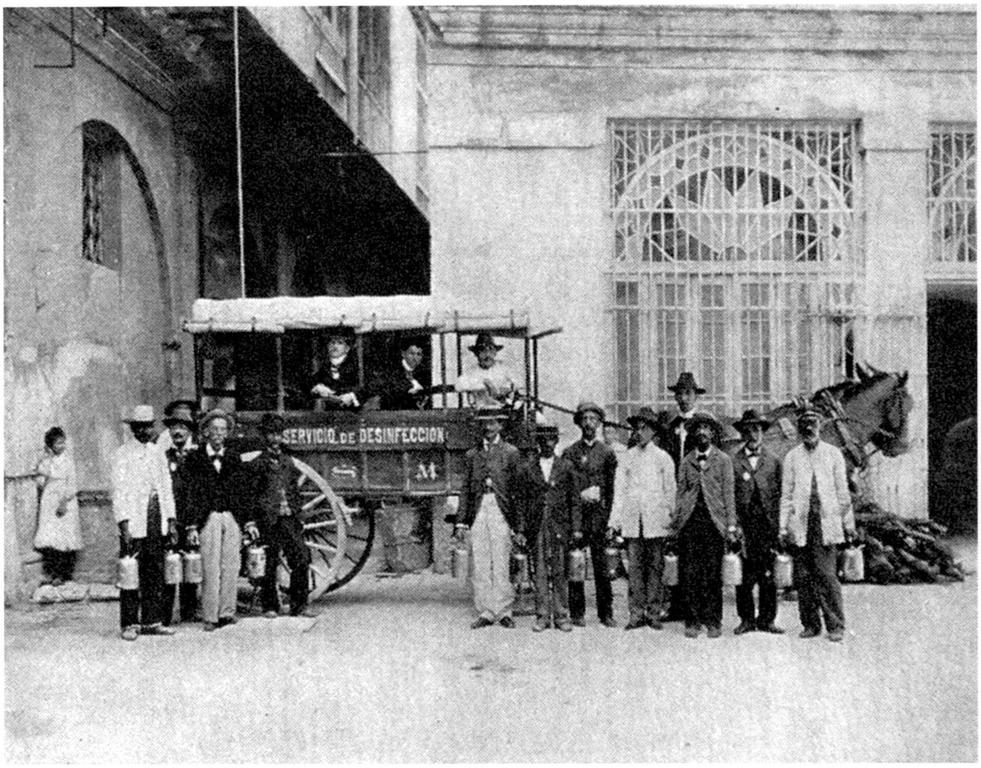

↑ Mosquito brigade in Panama displaying the tools of sanitary inspection, fumigation, and oil spraying. Ladders in hand, the group stands next to the underground water pipes that would be installed to improve the removal of waste water. Undated.

→ Anti-mosquito brigade directed by William C. Gorgas in US-occupied Cuba, ca. 1903.

the mosquito.[9] Assuming that canal workers would experience a similar sick rate to the US soldiers who occupied Cuba during the Spanish-American War, Gorgas estimated after ten years in Panama that measures taken against yellow fever saved no less than thirty-nine million days of sickness for the entire labor force, or $39,420,000.[10] Gorgas and others saw sanitation work as indistinguishable from the military occupation in Cuba and the success of the canal construction in Panama.

Gorgas's sanitary efforts involved different strategies for different geographies and diseases, as yellow fever primarily affects urbanized, tropical areas and malaria tends to affect more rural areas.[11] Short-term yellow fever eradication was a relatively attainable goal in smaller urban areas like Panama City and Colón, but the measures taken were extreme. In 1904 and in Panama City alone, a city of 20,000 inhabitants, Gorgas reports his team used 120 tons of insect powder—the entire annual supply of the United States.[12] Spraying was largely carried out by mosquito brigades, which inspected households for compliance with the newly mandated sanitary measures, checked sick people to be quarantined, and made repairs and modifications to the existing urban housing stock. Given that many locals were not only indifferent to the new authority's demands but resistant to yellow fever itself, these brigades also policed the activity of local residents.[13]

The more protracted battle was with malaria, a disease caused by parasites that were widespread among the mosquito populations in the hilly forests of the Darien region. This effort quickly became inseparable from broader efforts to manage and divide the diverse labor force needed to construct the canal. Excavation and other building activities for the project took place along railroad lines that snaked across the isthmus connecting Panamanian towns, rural settlements, and a constantly shifting set of work camps. Because of the scale and speed of construction, a massive labor force was needed. While indentured Chinese laborers had been used to build US railroads, officials were aware of the dubious optics of the coup and acquisition of the Canal Zone. This made them reluctant to use indentured labor for fear of public outcry in a postemancipation environment.[14]

There was much debate not only about who to enlist to build the canal, but also how to prevent workers from organizing unions. As one official testified to the US Congress in 1906, "there must be on the Isthmus a surplusage of labor. Otherwise, we will have interminable strikes."[15] That is, by ensuring there were always more workers than available work, the ICC could keep a pool of eager wage earners and potential strike breakers if needed. Furthermore, rather than one vulnerable workforce, Chief Engineer John Stevens believed that having several different nationalities and ethnicities would make them

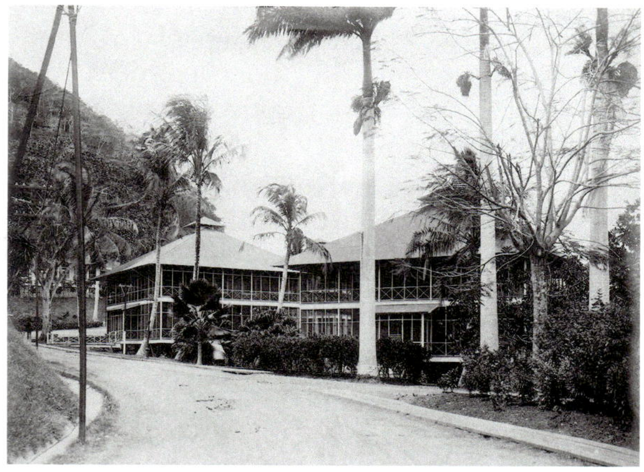

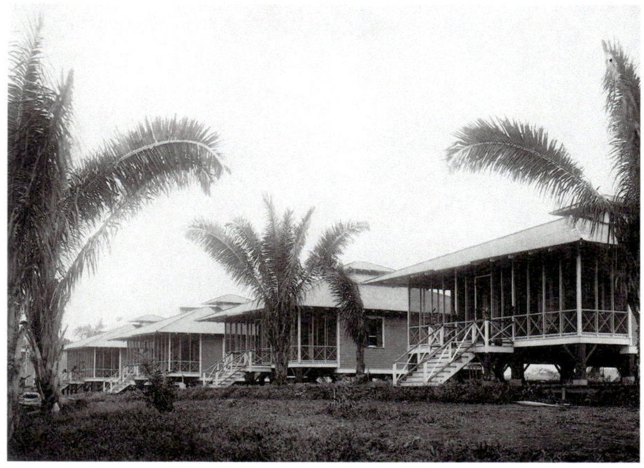

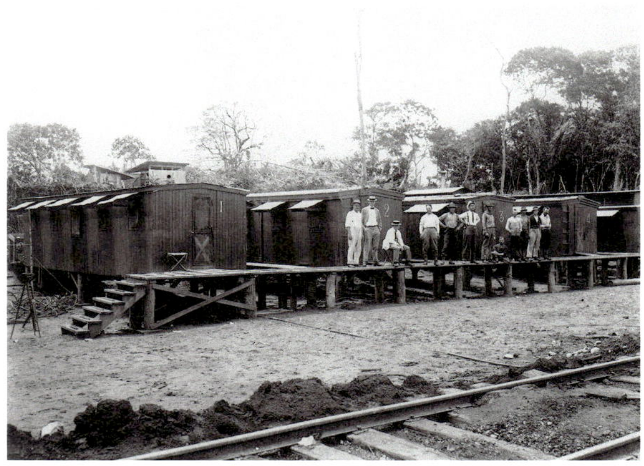

↑ Parker O. Wright Jr., ICC Type 13, two-story, single-family house, Ancón, Panama Canal Zone, ca. 1907.

– Parker O. Wright Jr., ICC Type 17 single-family house, Empire, United States Canal Zone (Panama), ca. 1907.

↓ Old boxcars used as barracks, 1910.

easier to divide and create competition, compelling everyone to work harder.[16] In order to do this, the ICC created a segregated, dual payment system: the gold and silver rolls.

While the system had many exceptions due to the challenges of getting consistent work for all the positions needed, white workers from the US were mostly hired for skilled positions and received payment in gold. These "gold roll" employees could spend leisure time in segregated clubs and spend their earnings at special segregated commissaries. "Silver roll" employees were paid at a lower rate and in a less valuable metal, with limited access to Canal Zone amenities. West Indians and Black workers from the United States were mostly assigned to the silver roll. European laborers like Spaniards and Italians occupied a liminal racial category at the time, with some attaining gold roll status, but most were also on the silver roll. As a system of segregated payment, commissaries, and housing, the gold and silver roll system constituted an apartheid society, a perverse reincarnation of the contemporary Jim Crow system that was already in full effect in the United States.[17]

Typologies of Segregation and Separation

From the very beginning, the ICC, the US Government under Roosevelt, and the canal construction project faced constant critique within the US Congress, from the general public, and by journalists. While accusations of graft were perhaps the most common, suggestions of inefficient construction efforts and worker mistreatment—often connected to sickness—were leveled by progressive reformers.[18] The ICC purportedly offered free housing to all its gold and silver roll employees, but it was never in sufficient supply. The quality of these accommodations, especially at the start of the project, was the subject of prominent criticism.[19] Gold and silver roll employees were also provided separate and unequal housing: in the early years, many silver roll laborers lived in tents completely open to the elements. As late as 1910, Galician workers on the silver roll were living in boxcars ventilated only by a few small, punched openings. Black laborers, also paid in silver, lived in conditions that "ranged from difficult to appalling."[20] When West Indians requested basic amenities like blankets and shelter to keep their clothes from being soaked in the rain, the US government responded that they didn't even need sheds.[21]

In late 1907, the *Canal Record*, a publication distributed for free to gold roll employees and sold to silver roll employees, featured a series of articles by Parker O. Wright Jr., the supervising architect for the ICC's Department of Buildings in charge of the design and construction of worker and staff housing, mess halls, hospitals, offices, social spaces, and industrial buildings for the canal project. In the first article, Wright states that "for the accommodation of white employees, 24 types of buildings have been designed and built."[22] He also reassures readers that new housing can "meet all the requirements of necessity and comfort in a tropical, insect infested country," describing his new designs as rational solutions to the problem of providing decent accommodation while keeping out mosquitoes.[23] Proclaimed as the creation of "the American type" in tropical Panama, his designs can be understood as part of an ongoing project of linking types and typology to national identity and race.[24]

Although abundant passive air ventilation and insect screens are widespread in warm climates today, extensive screened building exteriors were not common amenities in Panama before the beginning of the twentieth century.[25] According to Wright, the design of new housing types was driven by cost, mosquito-proofing, and suitability for the different ranks of ICC workers.[26] For white workers on the gold roll, he developed designs that ranged from single-family homes for married couples featuring wraparound porches on all sides, to more compact eight-bedroom quarters for bachelors. The amount of screened space provided was proportional to the ICC employees' ranks. For example, Type 13 not only features a wraparound screened porch as a circulation space, but also a prominent band of empty space surrounding the enclosed bedrooms and living rooms at the houses' interiors. For Black employees on the silver roll, Wright designed "Standard 1 Colored Barracks," which features minimal screen space and one large, undifferentiated interior. In a second article,

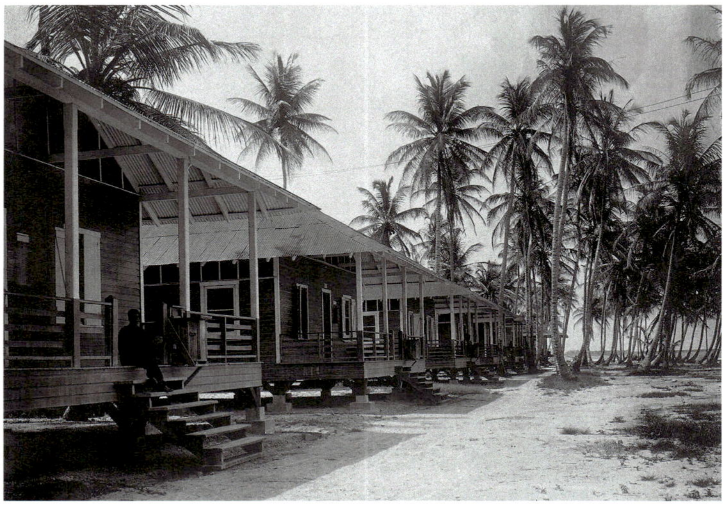

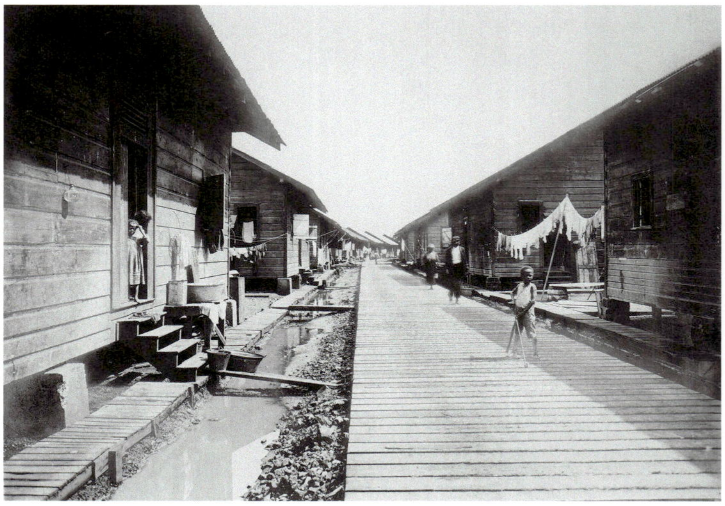

← ICC houses with self-closing garbage cans, Toro Point, Panama Canal Zone, 1911.

↙ Old French buildings used as housing for Black laborers, Cristóbal, Panama Canal Zone, 1905.

→ Parker O. Wright Jr., ICC Type 17 single-family house, Empire, United States Canal Zone (Panama), ca. 1907.

↘ Ground-floor plan of ICC housing for Black employees, ca. 1907.

Wright touts the ability for housing to accommodate a workforce that was intentionally broken up into ethnic and racial subgroups:

> In providing building for the use of laborers or "silver" employees engaged in the construction of the Canal, special consideration has been given to their design with a view of meeting the requirements of the different nationalities and their habits of living.[27]

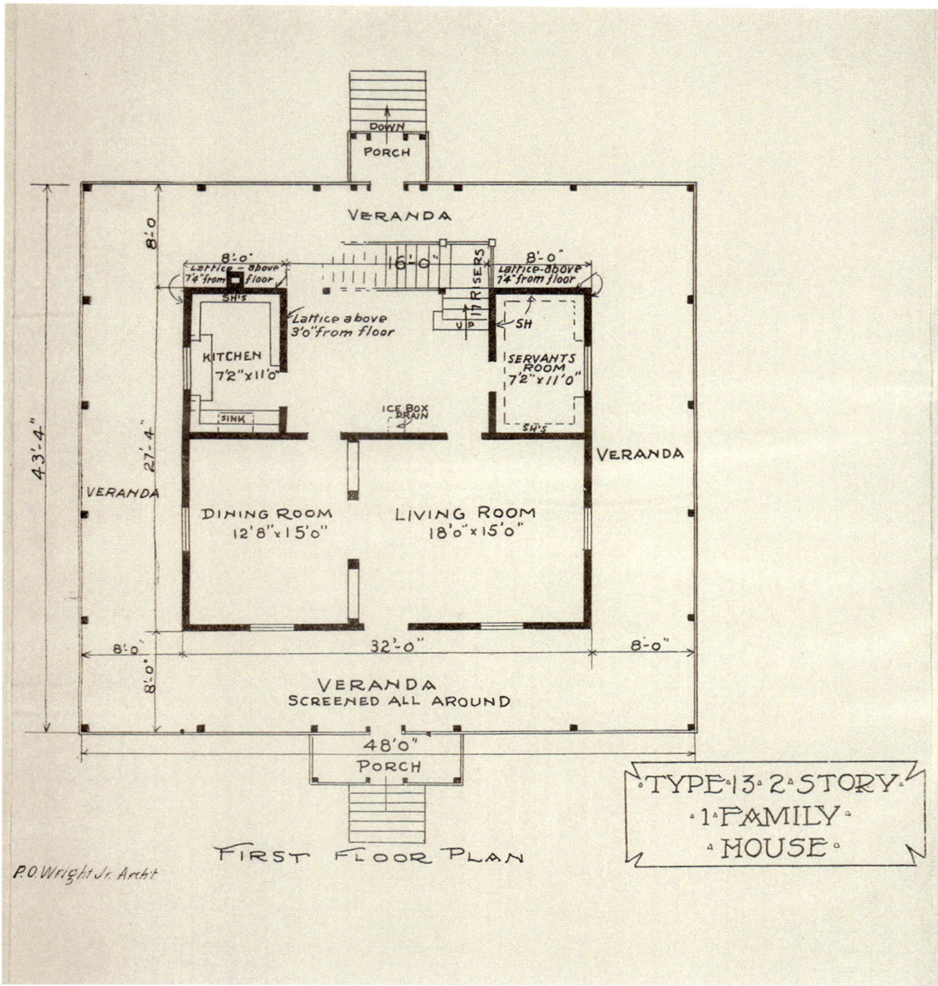

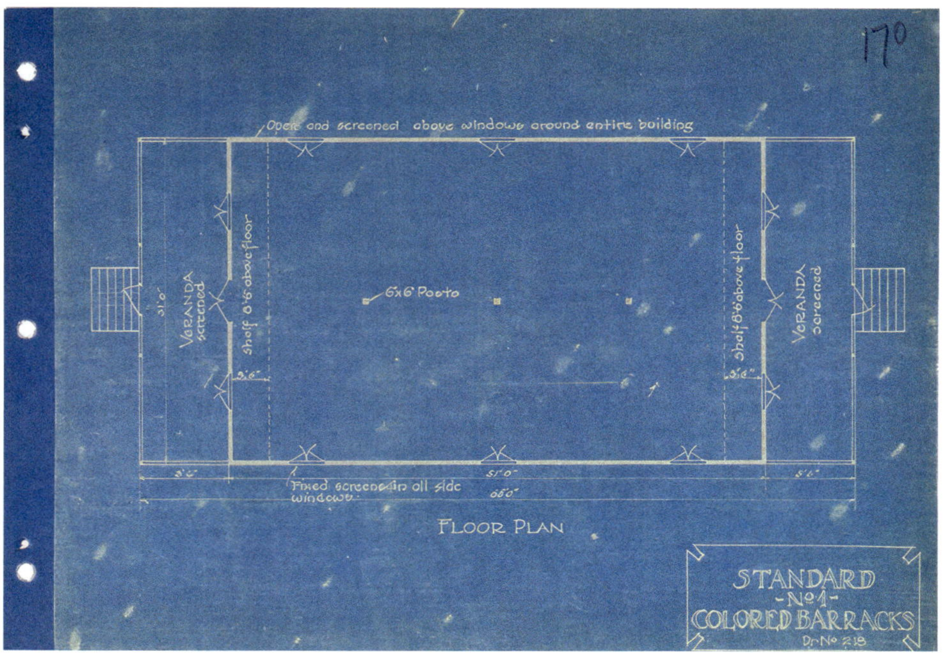

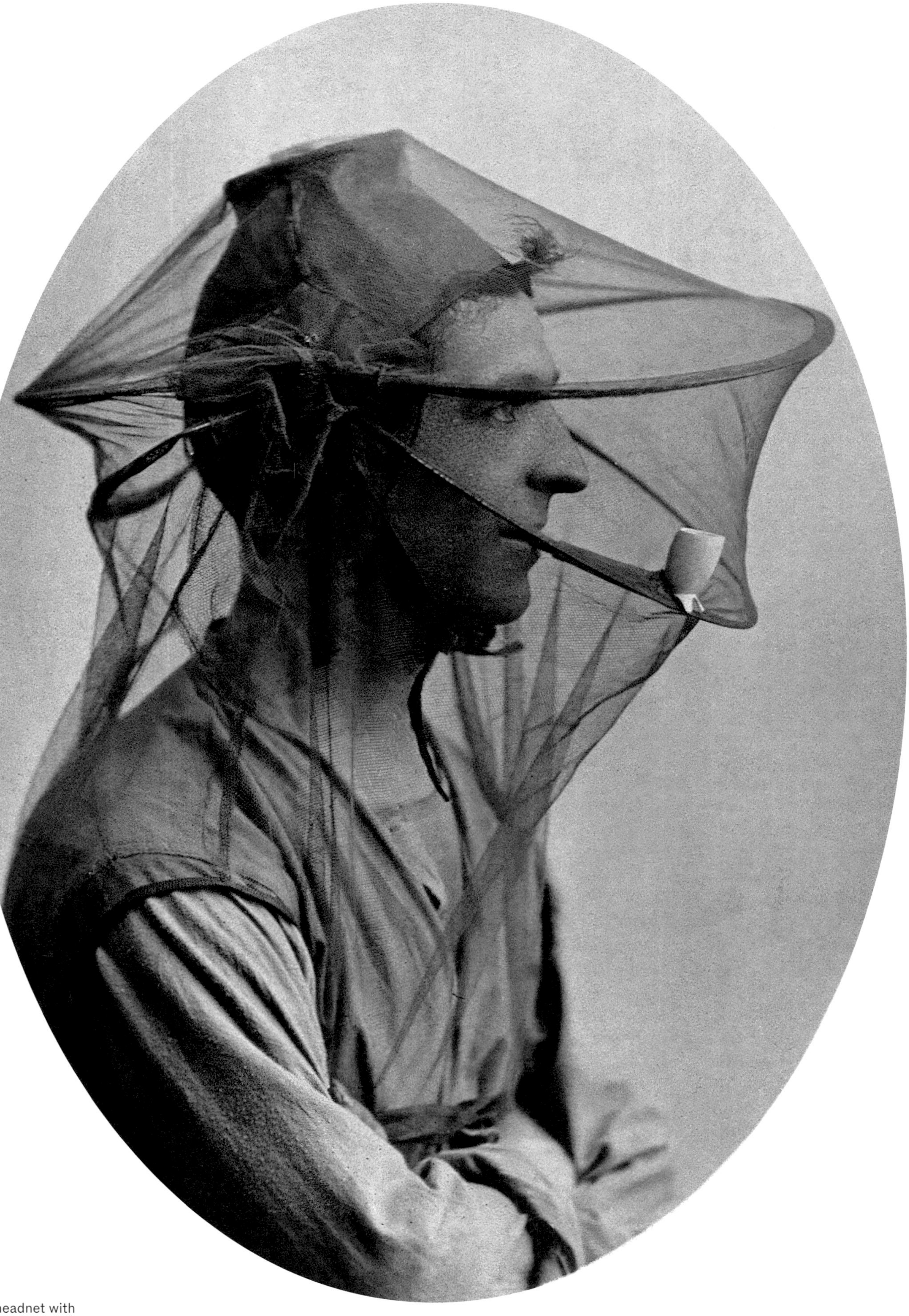

↑ Mosquito headnet with a cap, modeled by a man in profile smoking a pipe, ca. 1902–1918.

Wright's second article focuses on dividing men into married and unmarried quarters, and the arrangement of the kitchens and mess halls. Screening for mosquitoes is only mentioned for its ability to make the buildings capable of accommodating larger masses of laborers:

> These barracks are provided to accommodate 40 to 80 men, allowing an average of 560 cubic feet of air per man. In case it should become necessary to increase the number of men, there is always a sufficient supply of air on account of the circulation provided by the openings at the top of the walls, the end verandas, no matter what the crowding might be, the air could not become foul.[28]

Housing types for gold roll employees and standard barracks for silver roll employees used screens in different ways. For the former, they structured a large band of protective space in the verandas, which served as an attractive amenity for white employees. For the latter, screens allowed the ICC to maximize the number of largely nonwhite workers crammed into the barracks while armoring the agency against any complaints of unhealthy living conditions.

Dwellings for gold roll employees also used insect screens to structure interactions between inhabitants and domestic servants. Wright explains that the possibility of mosquitoes entering these houses has been reduced by minimizing the number of doors through the screened exterior, and ensuring that doors from kitchens or servants' quarters never led directly to the exterior. "In general, all screening should be so arranged that it will present the least temptation to servants or other *careless persons* to leave open the doors or windows, and the least opportunity to the ever-watchful mosquito to make its entry," he writes.[29] And in describing housing designed for silver roll employees, Wright states: "Special consideration has also been given to the sanitary features of these buildings as well as to the location of them, also to methods of protecting the mosquito screening, the doors and windows, against careless and especially against willful injury."[30] Wright's words reveal the patronizing and paternalistic attitudes typical of colonialism and its architecture.

The history of typology in architecture has been linked to criminology and closely associated with scientific racism, social Darwinism, and the quest to categorize and rank people and buildings according to race.[31] This is particularly evident in Wright's designs of dining areas. For example, Type 13, a house for married gold roll employees with families, came supplied with a kitchen, bedroom furniture, a fully equipped dining room, and storage space. In addition, it featured "a mosquito bar," an area designated for the concoction and serving of anti-malaria tonics with quinine and gin (or perhaps just gin).[32]

No such conveniences were provided for silver roll employees. Galicians eventually moved out of box cars, receiving standard barracks and a free-standing dining hall that allowed communal eating, and West Indians received some segregated barracks but were served food from an open-air counter.[33] Worst off were convicts, most of them Black, who were relegated to a fenced-off corral with abysmal food and shelter and forced to build roads and dig ditches without pay.[34]

The vast difference in the quality of housing was often explained and justified in terms of an incorrect correlation between race and disease immunity. George W. Goethals, who took over from Stevens as chief engineer of the project in 1907, responded to requests from West Indian workers for mosquito nets and screens by repeating a common and racist misunderstanding: "It is generally admitted ... [that] the colored people are immune."[35] Yet in 1912, "as many as two-thirds of all West Indians reported sick or required medical attention ... [most] of them catching malaria several times and confronting injury more than once."[36] By concentrating their anti-malarial efforts on gold roll employee dwellings, US government officials allowed disease to spread.[37]

Rendering Nature Tropical

During the construction of the Panama Canal, work carried out by Gorgas's sanitation teams paralleled (and often misinterpreted) research by entomological workers who were also stationed in the new US Canal Zone. While studying insects like mosquitoes, these scientists discovered a landscape that was highly influenced by human activity. That is, as rivers were dammed to create the canal, engineers were unwittingly expanding and improving the habitats for mosquitoes faster than concurrent sanitary efforts could counteract these environmental transformations.[38] The use of the screen, a porous material, not only brought the design of low-cost housing in line with some of this epidemiological research but calibrated the entire building skin to the scale of the mosquito. Wright also took into account the interaction between different metal alloys and the humid air. His designs specified the wire used for the screening as No. 18 mesh—its opening size calibrated to the millimeter to prevent the passage of the anopheles mosquito—and comprised of at least ninety-five percent bronze or brass, to prevent corrosion in the humid air of the Darien region.[39]

Similar attention is depicted in popular engineering handbooks disseminated in the decades following the Panama Canal's completion, like Henry Home's *The Engineer and the Prevention of Malaria* (1926). Geared toward industrialists and businessowners to explain the science of malaria control, the book scrutinizes enlarged photos of the warp, weft, and hole count of cotton netting to determine how to

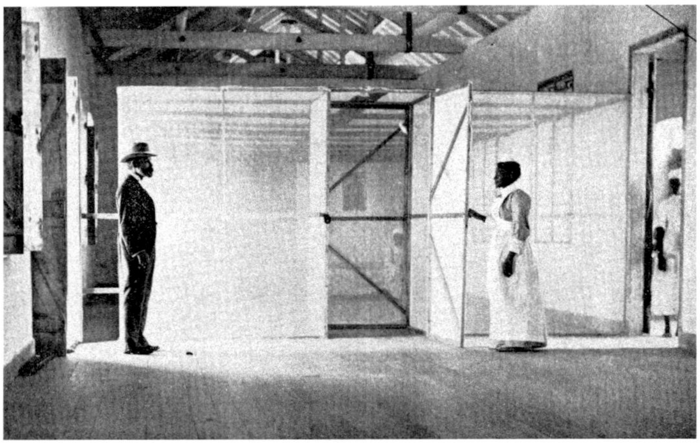

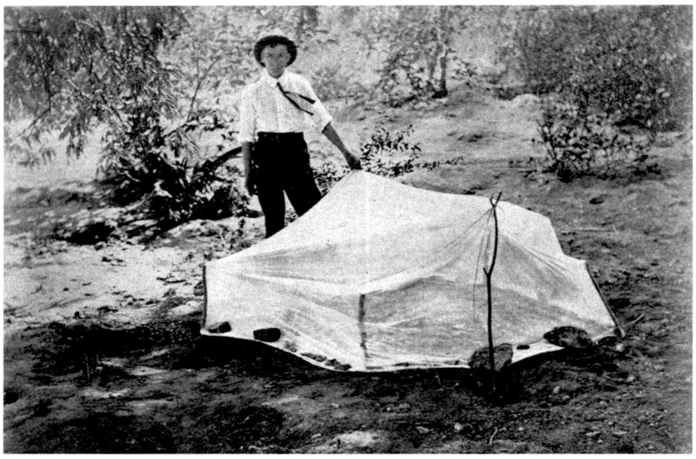

specify and approve the correct fabric for preventing mosquito intrusion. Home also provides detailed information on the percentage of ferrous metals in copper alloys and the correct method for calculating wire gauge and mesh density for mosquito screens.[40] Stressing the importance of this technical information, he offers a familiar reference:

> In the case of the Panama Canal, anti-malarial works are said to have cost 5.5 percent of the cost of construction, and without this expenditure it is improbable that the large body of white and black labor employed on the canal could have been kept together.[41]

If Home believed screens and other antimalarial work helped control an otherwise unmanageable workforce, prevailing views on race structured the very use of these antimalarial tactics. Just as entomological workers realized that the canal construction project was itself exacerbating disease, antimosquito architecture allowed malaria to spread while reinforcing racial hierarchies.

The fact that different types of housing reinforced ethnic and racial divisions cannot be separated from concepts about the tropics as a place. As David Arnold has argued, disease was associated with "a deep sense of alienation and danger," and "was thus one of the defining characteristics of the tropics well before the 1890s, one of the factors that divided the civilized, temperate North from the heat, humidity and backwardness of the tropics."[42] Similarly, for Nancy Stepan, "the 'tropical' came to constitute more than a geographical concept; it signified a place of radical otherness to the temperate world, with which it contrasted and which it helped to constitute."[43] Gorgas's belief that sanitation work in Panama proved that "the white man can live and thrive in the tropics" contains the familiar assumption that the tropics are fundamentally distinct, a place unto itself that can only be made suitable for civilization through the effort of engineering and science.[44]

In using deep-screened verandas and roof ventilation to solve the problem of disease and heat, Wright and the ICC effectively adapted to the architectural scale the mosquito houses, nets, and traps that were widely disseminated among entomological workers in colonial contexts at the time. While these devices were often used to catch mosquitoes, the ICC types enclose the inhabitants. But despite Gorgas's posturing of a "return" to the tropics, President William Howard Taft initiated a policy of "depopulation" in 1912 that would begin after the completion of the canal, abandoning work camps and minimizing permanent settlement as much as possible.[45]

Throughout the Caribbean region at the beginning of the twentieth century, the use of screen and net-covered structures mediated the relationship between people and mosquitoes, and between people of different races and social classes. The domestic types in the Canal Zone figured the tropical landscape as constantly dangerous, in need of a buffer zone of protection. By managing laborers through their relationship to insects—and each other—this low-cost architecture was crucial in the broader effort to turn the isthmus into an imperial outpost and render the landscape tropical.

← A temporary screened ward with screened double doors, St. Lucy's Almshouse, Barbados, ca. 1909.

↙ Screen used for collecting crab-hole mosquitoes, Bridgetown, Barbados, ca. 1909.

An earlier version of this essay was originally published by e-flux Architecture in 2022.

p16–17 Courtesy of the Library of Congress.
p18 (top), p19 (top and middle), p20 (right), p21 Courtesy of Linda Hall Library of Science, Engineering & Technology, Kansas City, Missouri.
p18 (bottom) Reproduced from William Crawford Gorgas, *Sanitation in Panama* (New York: D. Appleton and Co., 1915).
p19 (bottom) Courtesy of Panama Canal Museum Collection (University of Florida), Seminole, Florida.
p20 (left), p22 Courtesy of the Wellcome Collection, London.
p24 Reproduced from Rubert W. Boyce, *Mosquito or Man? The Conquest of the Tropical World* (London: J. Murray, 1909).

1. Frederic J. Haskin, *The Panama Canal* (Garden City, NY: Doubleday, Page & Company, 1913), 105; my emphasis. Haskin was a prolific journalist in his day. The title of this essay comes from Nancy Stepan, "Imperialism and Sanitation," in *The Cuba Reader: History, Culture, and Politics*, ed. Aviva Chomsky, Barry Carr, Alfredo Prieto, and Pamela Maria Smorkaloff (Durham: Duke University Press, 2019), 147.
2. Tulio Halperín Donghi, *Historia contemporánea de América Latina* (Buenos Aires: Alianza Editorial, 2005), 298–299. Originally published in Italian by Giulio Einaudi Editore, 1967.
3. The Panama Canal Zone continued to be legally part of the United States until October 1, 1979. There is an extensive bibliography on conditions in the US territory. See Marixa Lasso, *Erased: The Untold Story of the Panama Canal* (Cambridge, MA: Harvard University Press, 2019); Julie Greene, *The Canal Builders: Making America's Empire at the Panama Canal* (New York: Penguin Press, 2009); and Michael L. Conniff, *Black Labor on a White Canal: Panama, 1904–1981* (Pittsburgh: University of Pittsburgh Press, 1985).
4. William Crawford Gorgas, *Sanitation in Panama* (New York: Appleton, 1915), 288–289.
5. Lasso, *Erased*, 17.
6. Alexander Missal, *Seaway to the Future* (Madison: University of Wisconsin Press, 2008), 23–24.
7. Missal, *Seaway to the Future*, 26.
8. Gorgas, *Sanitation in Panama*, 279.
9. For a discussion of the European context see Andrea Bagnato, "Microscopic Colonialism," e-flux Architecture, December, 2017, https://www.e-flux.com/architecture/positions/153900/microscopic-colonialism/.
10. Gorgas's estimate was based on the approximate cost of one dollar a day for hospital care at that time. Gorgas, *Sanitation in Panama*, 281.
11. Paul S. Sutter, "'The First Mountain to Be Removed': Yellow Fever Control and the Construction of the Panama Canal," *Environmental History* 21, no. 2 (2016): 253.
12. Gorgas, *Sanitation in Panama*, 151.
13. Sutter, "'The First Mountain to Be Removed,'" 253.
14. Conniff, *Black Labor on a White Canal*, 25.
15. Greene, *The Canal Builders*, 48. See "Hearings before the Committee on Interstate and Foreign Commerce of the House of Representatives, on the Isthmian Canal" (Washington, DC, GPO, 1906), 33–35.
16. Greene, *The Canal Builders*, 47.
17. For an in-depth analysis of the racialized labor policies used during the construction of the canal, see Conniff, *Black Labor on a White Canal*, 31–36.
18. Conniff, *Black Labor on a White Canal*, 191–225.
19. Greene, *The Canal Builders*, 135.
20. Conniff, *Black Labor on a White Canal*, 29.
21. Greene, *The Canal Builders*, 135.
22. Parker O. Wright Jr., "Commission Buildings, I," *Canal Record*, December 11, 1907, 117.
23. Wright, "Commission Buildings, I," 117.
24. For example, Charles Davis has demonstrated that in early twentieth-century architectural discourse, prominent designers such as Louis Sullivan were also highly concerned with the relationship between architectural and national types. Charles L. Davis, *Building Character: The Racial Politics of Modern Architectural Style* (Pittsburgh: University of Pittsburgh Press, 2019), 167.
25. Photographs of the housing built by the French canal company show little to no use of screened windows.
26. Wright emphasizes materials, and construction details had to be considered to suit the "official status of employees, the cheapest methods of construction, and an effective method of screening." Wright, "Commission Buildings, I," 117.
27. Parker O. Wright Jr., "Commission Buildings, II," *Canal Record*, December 25, 1907, 134.
28. Wright, "Commission Buildings, I," 134.
29. Wright, "Commission Buildings, I," 147; my emphasis.
30. Wright, "Commission Buildings, II," 134.
31. Georges Teyssot, *A Topology of Everyday Constellations* (Cambridge, MA: MIT Press, 2013), 69.
32. "Dwelling Houses in the Panama Canal Zone," *Carpentry and Building* 30 (July 1908): 234.
33. As Alexander Missal argues, to "cover up this discrimination, malaria's persistence was blamed on the West Indians' presumed preference to live in the bush." Missal, *Seaway to the Future*, 61.
34. The arduous work involved in initial sanitary engineering efforts, which were inseparable from the creation of basic infrastructure of the Canal Zone, such as clearing brush, cutting trees, leveling the ground, draining swamps and marshes, and filling ditches, was accomplished through the forced labor of convict gangs. Benjamin D. Weber, "The Strange Career of the Convict Clause: US Prison Imperialism in the Panamá Canal Zone," *International Labor and Working Class History* 96 (Fall 2019): 84.
35. Greene, *The Canal Builders*, 135
36. Greene, *The Canal Builders*, 133.
37. Paul S. Sutter, "Nature's Agents or Agents of Empire? Entomological Workers and Environmental Change during the Construction of the Panama Canal," *Isis* 98, no. 4 (2007): 750–751.
38. Sutter, "Nature's Agents or Agents of Empire?," 730.
39. Parker O. Wright, Jr., "Commission Buildings, III," *Canal Record*, January 8, 1908, 147.
40. Henry Home, *The Engineer and the Prevention of Malaria* (London: Chapman & Hall, 1926), 136, 137–138.
41. Home, *The Engineer and the Prevention of Malaria*, 3.
42. David Arnold, "The Place of 'The Tropics' in Western Medical Ideas since 1750," *Tropical Medicine and International Health* 2, no. 4 (April 1997): 309.
43. Nancy Stepan, *Picturing Tropical Nature* (London: Reaktion, 2006), 17.
44. Gorgas, *Sanitation in Panama*, 289.
45. Lasso, *Erased*, 2.

SMALL FAMILY–HOUSED NATION

SHIVANI SHEDDE

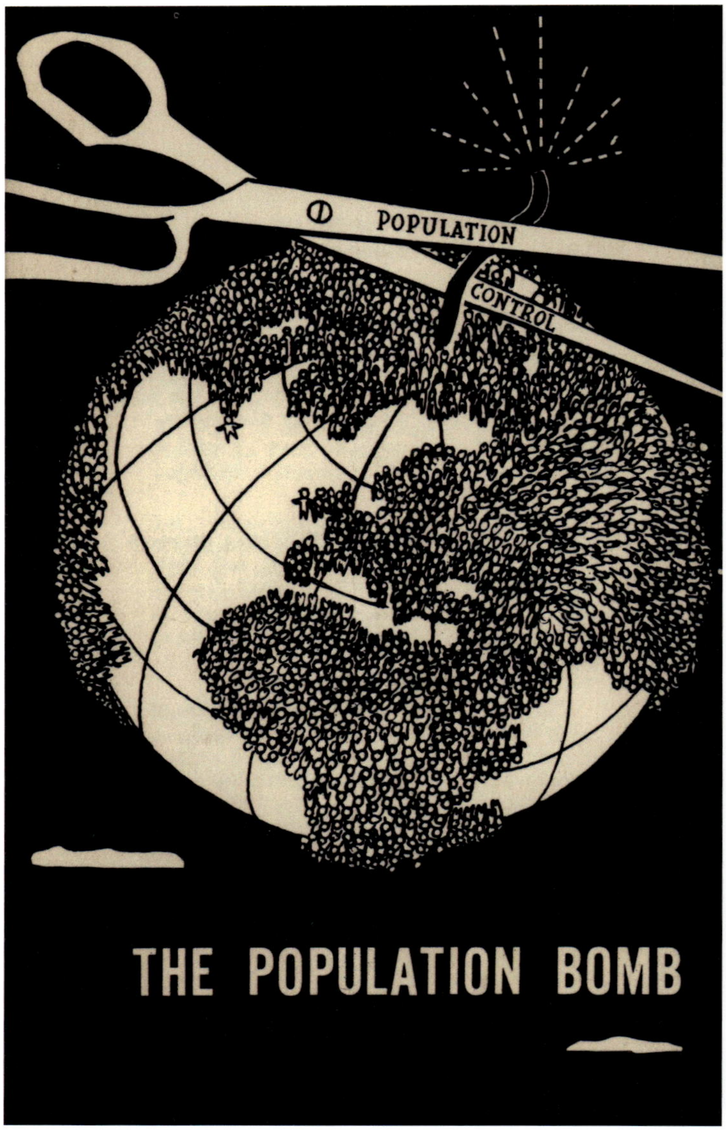

"I heard Annie is not doing the submission" is one of the first lines of the Indian cult classic by Arundhati Roy and Pradip Krishen, *In Which Annie Gives It Those Ones* (1989). The film follows a cast of characters as they navigate the expectations of an architecture school in the postcolonial capital city in 1974: "*Pata nahin yaar Annie ka kuch. I asked him* ... and he started giving those ones ... *wo hi apne* rural-urban nexus *wale*" ("I don't know much about Annie, I asked him and he gave his usual spiel on the rural-urban nexus"). The dialogue continues, referencing development rhetoric which saw the problems of town and country as reciprocally linked.[1] Annie, an architecture student, is burdened with the supposed responsibility of solving the "poor problem." The proposal he arrives at speaks to a technocratic vision that responded to India's migration "crisis" of the 1970s, as more people moved from rural areas to urban ones: "You know how many miles of railway track there are in India?" he asks, "Sixty thousand ... so I got a freaked out idea ... it's bloody revolutionary ... it could reverse the whole process of urbanization. Persuade *buggers* to stay in the villages instead of screwing themselves up in the cities."[2]

Annie's sentiment can be read as symptomatic of the architectural dilemmas encountered when large Indian cities became a battleground leading up to, during, and in the aftermath of a nationwide state of emergency declared by Prime Minister Indira Gandhi in 1975. Tired of the country's reputation being blemished by charges of corruption, security threats, student and labor unrest, not least the uncontrolled poverty within a rapidly growing population, Gandhi's turn to authoritarianism resulted in the suspension of citizens' democratic and institutional rights. Alongside this, she laid forth a new, paternalistic vision for the Indian nation, one that claimed to act in the people's best interests, even if it acted alone. Within the built environment of large Indian cities, recent migrants and the urban poor were subjugated to rampant housing demolitions to make way for new structures that would relocate them to governmentally sanctioned and publicly funded living quarters. For Gandhi, these measures and others—the eradication of poverty, pollution, and overpopulation—were necessary in order to gain true independence from colonial rule. Through modernization, those who had been "oppressed for centuries" would finally be uplifted.[3] Overpopulation and poverty were intertwined and broadcast through government media, as was the prime minister's slogan, *garibi hatao* (remove poverty), which further imbricated population control as a prerequisite for social mobility and economic development. Architects were recruited to respond to a fraught political situation, and housing emerged as one of many solutions to a problem with no clear resolution.

The 1970s was also a time when Euro-American environmental consciousness focused on the threat of overpopulation. Publications such as Stewart Brand's *Whole Earth Catalog* (1968–1971) and Paul Ehrlich's *The Population Bomb* (1968) had moved the ideas of "overpopulation" and "population control" into the remit of state politics as well as quotidian parlance. Succumbing to racial and neo-Malthusian discourse that described much of the poverty-stricken third world as a threat to "planetary" health with its "unsustainable" fertility rates, these

← Cover of the "Experimental Issue" of *The Population Bomb*, 1954.

↓ Planned urban settlements, from *The Problem of Housing in India* (Ministry of Works, Housing & Supply, 1957).

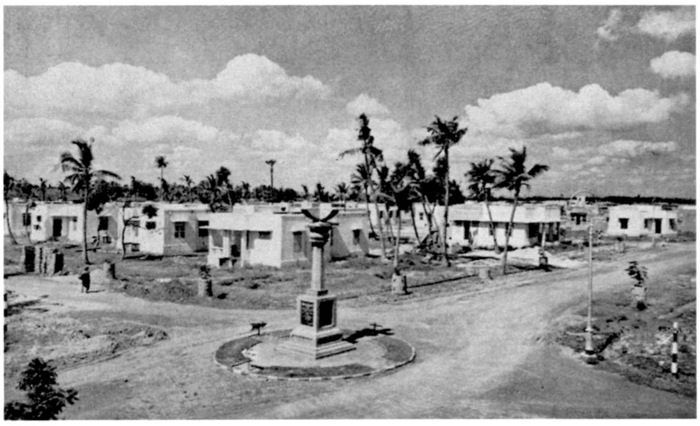

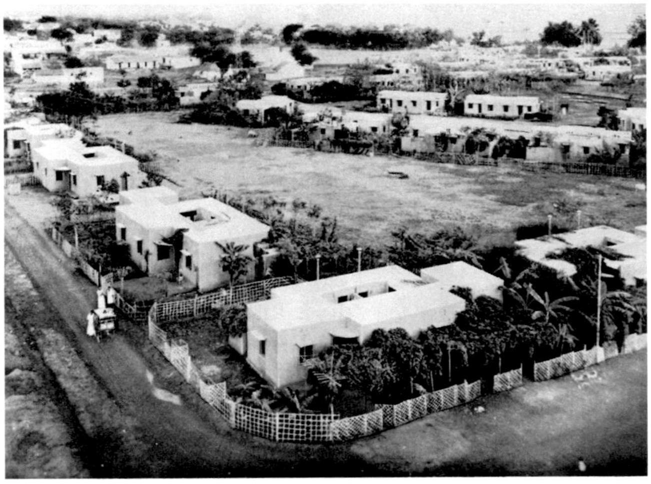

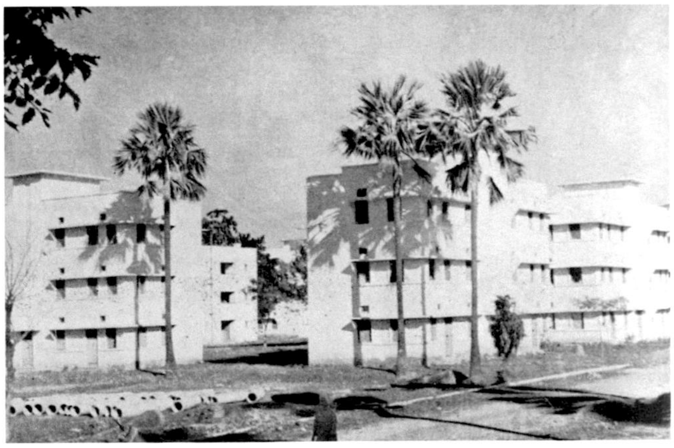

environmental movements focused on the fragility of life on "Spaceship Earth" and its imminent prospects of resource scarcity and limited "carrying capacity."[4] The 1970 UN Conference on Human Survival, for instance, attended by the architect Buckminster Fuller, was one of many gatherings organized to "examine the human condition in a world which has become a single geographic community and in which the principal problems have to do with the survival of the human species itself."[5] The conference identified the "problem of the environment" as being compounded by the "population problem," and set the stage for environmentally conscious, yet morally suspect, architectural practices.

Although not sealed from Western environmentalism, population discourse in India was nothing new, nor was it politically sidelined. Gaining speed and accruing significance in the postindependence era of the 1950s, the development of policies for family planning was seen as crucial to the state's project of modernization, which included poverty alleviation and economic growth. Guided by the sustained efforts of American and British birth control activists, the Ford Foundation, the United Nations advisory missions for demography, the International Planned Parenthood Federation (IPPF), the Rockefeller Foundation, and USAID, by the early 1970s Indian family planning efforts had provided a gamut of contraceptive services to over ninety million people aged fifteen to forty-four, who were in the reproductive age group.

Family planning was originally marketed and rolled out on a voluntary basis. In rural areas, mobile health and education services traveled from village to village to preach an optimum family size. Extensive mass media campaigns flashed positive, easily understandable messages about contraception through the press, radio, television, films, folk songs, drama parties, puppets, exhibitions. In larger cities, birth control propaganda took hold of the built environment, marked by an inverted vermillion equilateral triangle with the slogan *Do Ya Teen Bacche, Bus* (Two or three children ... enough). Influenced by the aims of the growing global environmental movement, however, family planning in India soon became linked to a question of who was allowed to have children, which culminated in a set of coercive tactics to keep people from reproducing. From April to December of 1976, over seven million sterilization surgeries were performed involuntarily on both poor men and women.[6]

If overpopulation as a "disruption of the functioning environment" was identified as a serious concern for the continuation of life on earth, family planning services could only be part of the "solution."[7] Technical aid deemed national planning and development as a necessary tool to determine and implement the constraints that would most effectively govern unwanted reproduction, while

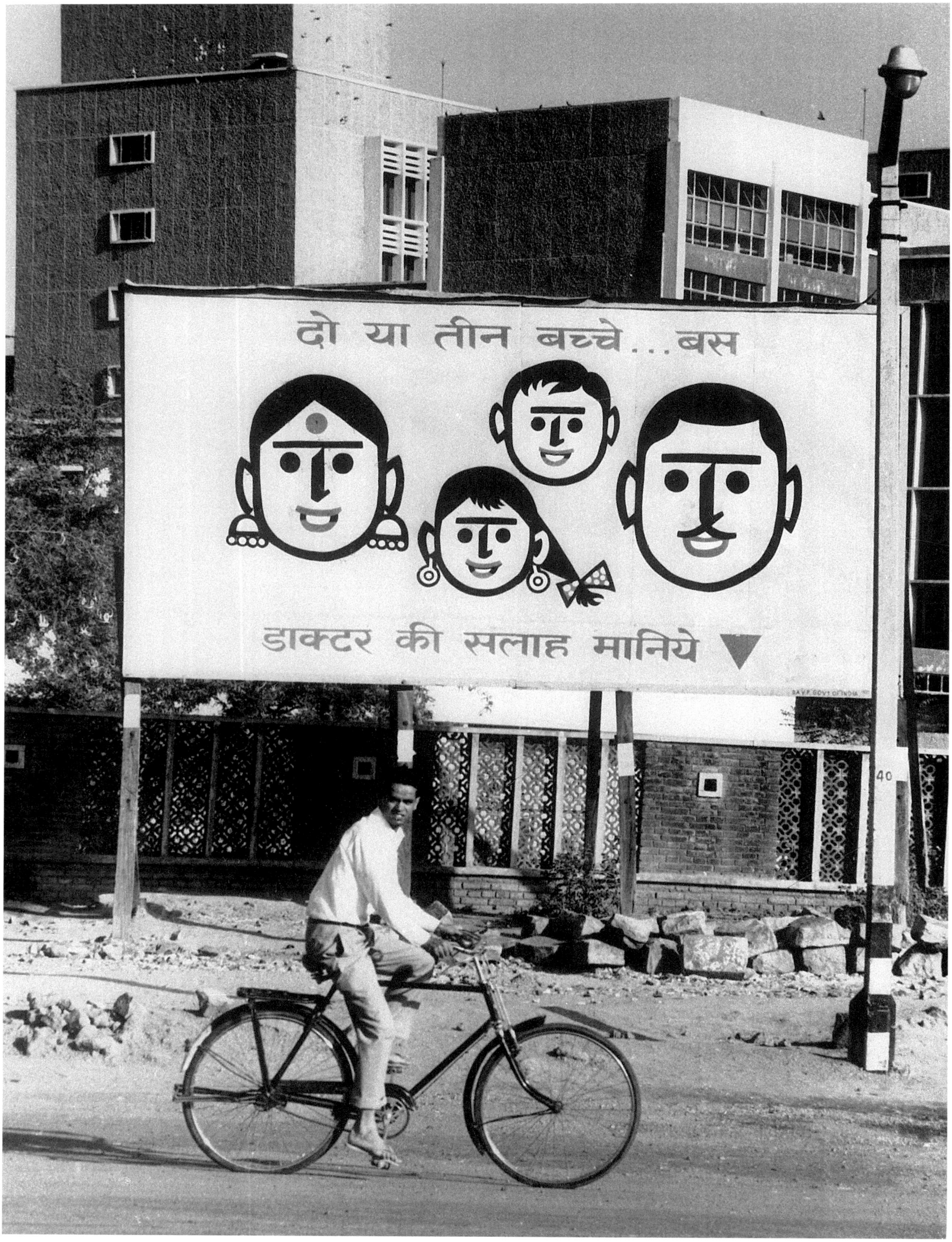

↑ Family planning posters taking over the built environment, New Delhi, 1969.

→ Rural house, Chandigarh, 1951–1955.

discourses of population and poverty were taken up in the field of planning and architecture. Architects like Charles Abrams, C. A. Doxiadis, and Buckminster Fuller developed theories about the relationship between rapid population growth and urbanization that were generally attributed to rural-urban migration patterns. Their attempts were acknowledged in nation-building programs across the decolonizing world through an adoption of policies for lowering population growth in an effort to prevent urban sprawl and create "planned" cities. In India, as the government's nation-building mandate highlighted the need to bring lower income populations into a middle class, national planning and its consequent architectural directives addressed housing through a hierarchical servicing of society corresponding to inhabitants' salaries and earning capacities.

Modernization, poverty alleviation, and the provision of shelter to the masses were some of the essential concerns of postwar reconstruction programs across the postcolonial world. Keeping with the nation's socialist ethos, questions of planning and housing for an expanding swell of Indians occupied leadership, crystallizing with the 1956 Slum Clearances Act. Pamphlets released by the government argued, "The problem of housing and slum-clearance in India is a challenge to the entire philosophy of democratic planning which inspires our efforts today. On how we solve it, will depend, to a great extent, the success or failure of the great experiment [i.e., independence and nation building] which is now underway."[8] Over the course of twenty years, family planning programs and the enactment of housing policy became entangled with the Indian government's skirmishes with democracy. The demolition of a settlement around the Turkman gate in New Delhi in 1976, for example, erupted in public anger and condemnation and eventually contributed to Gandhi's reelection loss once the emergency was suspended. As such, the modernization of housing and all that it entailed—the development of unit "types," rigorous town planning, demolitions, and forced relocations—cannot be understood without the involvement of family planning.

Modernity, Environmentalism, and the Nation

Over the course of the 1970s, housing figured on Gandhi's agenda to complete "the unfinished revolution."[9] Her father—the first prime minister of India, Jawaharlal Nehru—had also placed great emphasis on housing. At the opening of the UN International Exhibition on Low-Cost Housing and Community Improvement, held in New Delhi in 1954, Nehru noted, "The house is not merely a place to take shelter from the rain or the cold or the sun. It should be an enlargement of one's personality, and if human welfare is our objective, this is bound up with the house."[10] Nehru's ruminations captured the blind hope of the first few years of independence, as he laid out a promise that the Indian state would eliminate shelter scarcity. While the figure of the modern house represented social health and vitality, and an acceptance into the modernity of many new nation-states, it posed a challenge. Under his tenure, and within a growing bureaucracy of the young country, national policies were formulated that increasingly rendered housing as something technical, managed by experts for its planning, design, and construction, and addressed to the nation as a whole.[11] Unsurprisingly, a technical approach that focused on planning and top-down intervention did little to alleviate the causes of poverty. Addressing the Seventh Housing Ministers' Conference in 1962, Nehru was less optimistic as he deliberated on the "problem of housing." His humanistic conviction that the house was an essential component for the betterment of "man" nonetheless remained, as he noted: "Now, take slums. ... It pains me to see them, because they reduce the human being living there to a slightly sub-human level. ... So I think that we should concentrate on the removal of slums."[12]

When Indira Gandhi was elected, the question of the house was reinvigorated but this time approached more sociologically. Treading an urban-rural divide, housing in 1970s India was at the crux of overlapping discourses of development, habitation, and environment. The provision of housing came to be seen as a marker of democracy, where the imagination of multistory structures in urban areas made of either prefabricated or poured concrete stood in stark contrast to mud, straw, bamboo, or wooden rural houses that were subject to self-build policies. While such an urban-rural divide was conceptually grounded in competing visions of modernity articulated by M. K. Gandhi and Nehru—the former's timeless past of the

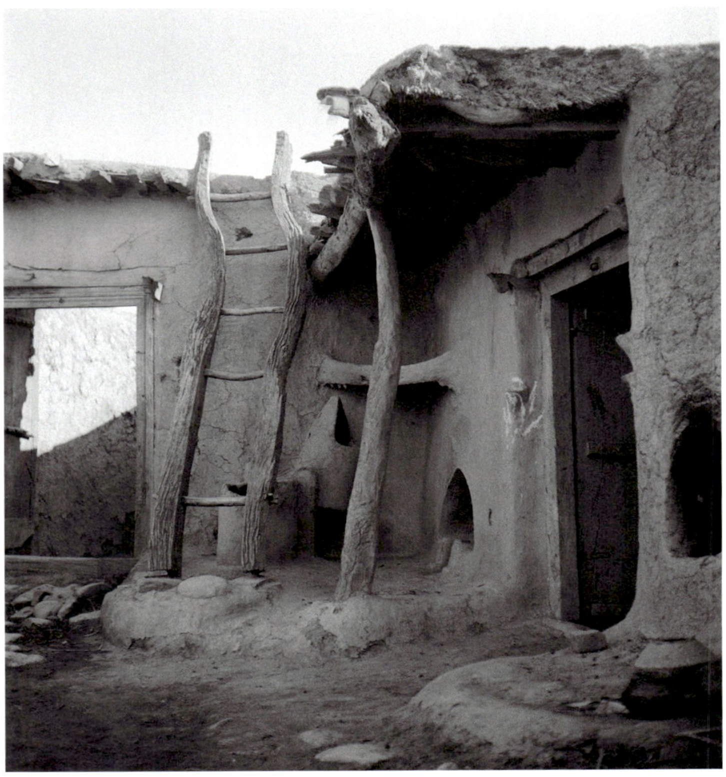

village versus the latter's modern future of the city, which ultimately became part of the government's postcolonial agenda—it also allowed very different battles of housing governance to be waged, even if the subjects of such governance moved between village and city.[13]

To spread a message of new, modern ways of living in cities, the Ministry of Broadcasting and Information released a series of educational documentary films. Biren Dass's *Solving the Problem*, released in 1960, for instance, echoed Nehru's concerns, claiming that "eradication of slums is vital to India's progress." The film focused on considerations undertaken by municipal and town planning authorities to "remove this blight from the fair face of India" and provide housing for lower-income groups.[14] On the other hand, Balkrishna Kulkarni's 1963 *Layouts for Living*, released one year before Nehru's death, was explicit in framing inequality and housing issues as colonial problems. Tracing the urban influx of migrants to the centralization and industrialization of factories, the film argued that during the colonial period "men lived as they could and where they could, in congested buildings and slums. In this squalid environment, men's lives lacked all traces of beauty and serenity." The proposed remedy was a "plan for living" that would take into consideration the "population explosion" that was plaguing the urban environments through "congestion and haphazard growth" in cities like Calcutta, Bombay, and Delhi. Panning over chawls, "native towns," and slum settlements, the film's subtext can be understood as the intertwining of population growth with poverty, which perpetuated a liberal gaze that stressed the improvement of conditions for "oppressed classes."

By the late 1960s, however, the message had changed, with focus shifting from rural-to-urban migration (widely seen as the main contributor to slum growth) to overpopulation. The narrator of Prem Prakash's 1969 film *Struggle for Space*, for instance, declared: "Tens of thousands of houses are being built every year, but they are not enough. Almost overnight the new housing colonies become slums. The reason? Our population is growing faster than we can build."[15] The stigmatization of slums was not a new phenomenon in the subcontinent. As Sheetal Chhabria has shown, the slum was already positioned as a city's "internal other" by the early twentieth century.[16] Painted as vectors of disease, by midcentury slums were also a constant reminder of agrarian crises-fueled migration, if not ideas of "impurity" inherent to a caste-based society.[17] These concerns were captured by Pratap Parmar's 1970 film *Housing for the People*, which declared:

> Shanty towns spring up from mud and asphalt alike, with what seems to be an unnatural abandon. Grimy *mohallas* and tumbled-down one-room tenements, and in them, families of men packed in like sardines, sharing squalor and apathy with each other. These things make for neither dignity nor convenience. Yet people must live somewhere, one must have a roof over one's head, even if it has to be shared with a crowd.[18]

Denoting slums as distinct spaces opposed to the modernity that was expected of the postcolonial nation, these educational and informational films partook in a colonial project that problematized shelter through metrics of hygiene, sanitation, and poverty. Moreover, both films, with voiceovers in English, were targeted at a middle-class urban population in an effort to cultivate public "dignity," an oft-repeated feature of the Indian anticolonial project. *Struggle for Space* and *Housing for the People* warned against the flood of villagers and migrants to the city, recasting the bodies and houses of slum dwellers as thorns to a project of modernization. *Housing for the People* made this clear: "A nation is known by the way its people live. A people living in clean, neat houses are a clean, neat people." The visual and discursive problematization of certain forms of shelter was a process of describing and cataloguing what would be fit and unfit for the postcolonial nation.

The depiction of a modern India with planned townships and modernist living quarters can be understood as the attempt to apply an architectural solution to a social problem. Such a rationale was aided by a combination of bureaucrats, urban planners, architects, and family planning proponents who leveled the rhetoric of modernization against the "unmodern" elements: migrants, slum dwellers, beggars, construction site laborers, and generally the urban poor. *Struggle for Space* was the most forthright:

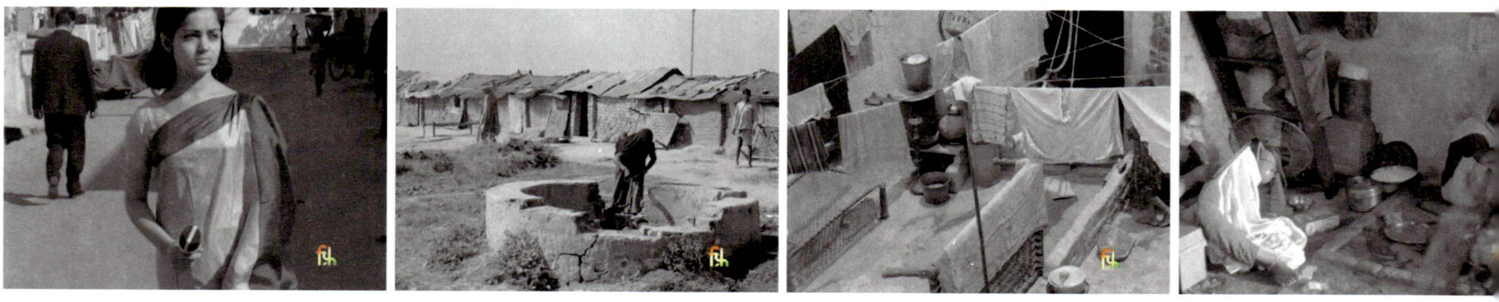

↑ Scenes from *Housing for the People*, 1970.

> To meet the demands for adequate accommodation for all our people, we will need to double the number of houses in the next twenty years. This demand will mean the scarcity of construction materials and rising costs, which most of us are unable to bear. This construction is gradually encroaching upon the rural areas, once again eating up agricultural lands. As the population increases, we will face increasing scarcities: lack of space for children's education, lack of food, lack of all other amenities, transport, hospitals, water, electricity. ... But our hope for tomorrow depends on the right decision today.[19]

Cutting to the symbol of family planning, the red triangle, the film ended with a clear prescription: small, nuclear families would ease the burden of housing provision, which in turn would benefit the health, infrastructure, and economy of the nation.

Here, it is important to consider how family planning was also part and parcel of Indira Gandhi's anticolonial environmental strategy. Apart from initiating policies for wildlife and forest conservation, setting up task forces, and initiating seminars for environmental planning, Gandhi famously disputed the arguments of Western environmentalists at the 1972 Stockholm Conference on the Human Environment, where she retorted, "Are not poverty and need the greatest polluters?" Arguing that "the environment cannot be improved in conditions of poverty; nor can poverty be eradicated without the use of science and technology," Gandhi emphasized discrepancies in the environmental ethics of the Global North vis-à-vis the South and claimed that "better planning and better action" were of primary concern for India's postcolonial condition.[20] She continued:

> The extreme forms in which questions of population or environmental pollution are posed obscure the total view of political, economic and social situations. ... It is an over-simplification to blame all the world's problems on increasing population. Countries with a small fraction of the world population consume the bulk of the world's production of minerals, fossil fuels and so on. Thus, we see that when it comes to the depletion of natural resources and environmental pollution, the increase of one inhabitant in an affluent country, at his level of living, is equivalent to an increase of many Asians, Africans or Latin Americans at their current material levels of being.[21]

For Gandhi, narrowing global power disparities could only be achieved through a nation's self-reliance. Recognizing that a well-implemented family planning program was necessary "for a healthier and more conscious population," one that was responsive to the needs of the environment, Gandhi also argued that "no method of population control can be effective without education and without a visible rise in the standard of living."[22]

The Stockholm speech highlighted an ongoing program, "Design for Living," which had been conceived as a joint proposal between India, Mexico, Finland, Czechoslovakia, Japan, Poland, and Yugoslavia. Originally presented in 1966 at the 14th General Conference of UNESCO, the program encouraged a design rationale that brought to the fore the importance of mankind's natural habitat and saw a need for inculcating "new principles of civilized living," as well as the engineering of "basic materials" to promote a "design for survival."[23] The conjuncture of built and natural habitats as legacies that needed to be bestowed on "all" rather than "some" was, in this instance, a fundamental reinterpretation of Western environmentalist doctrine. Gandhi went on to claim that the program grasped the full implications and impact of technical advance: "It will not be easy for large societies to change their style of living. They cannot be coerced to do so, nor can governmental action suffice. People can be motivated and urged to participate in better alternatives."[24] These alternatives, at least in India, were based in a belief that economic mobility was directly linked to modern housing.

Seen through the distinct efforts of government media, the modernization program can be understood as a confluence of different anxieties. The argument of a lack of space was indebted to debates about resource scarcity from an impending population bomb and was not unrelated to discourses of dignity and anticolonial nation building, as well as conversations about modern housing and sanitation. By the 1970s, as slums and other lower-class tenements continued to be the target of modernization, a peculiar typology emerged to house, or rather rehouse, the poor through rehabilitation schemes. If the 1954 UN

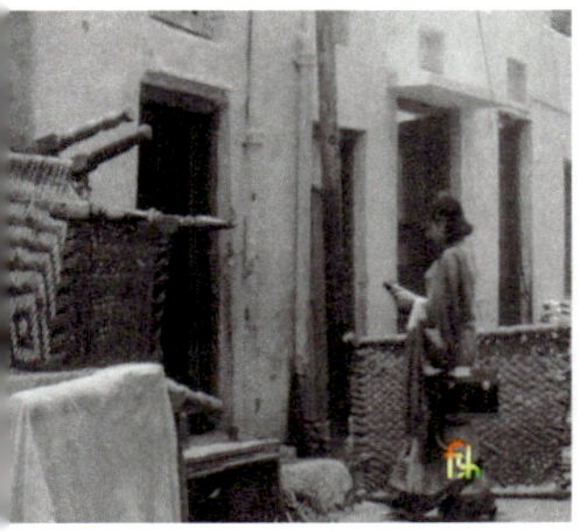
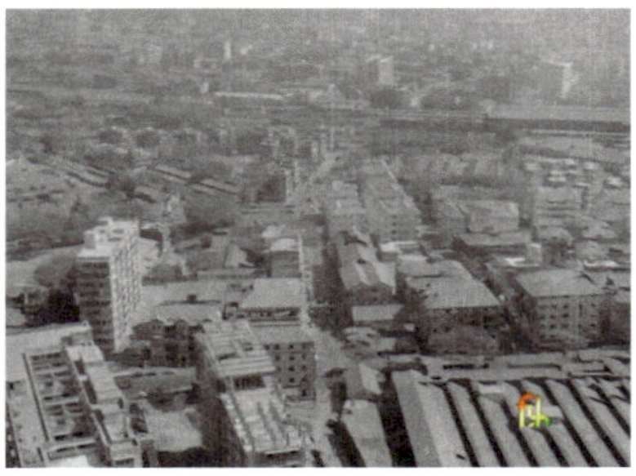
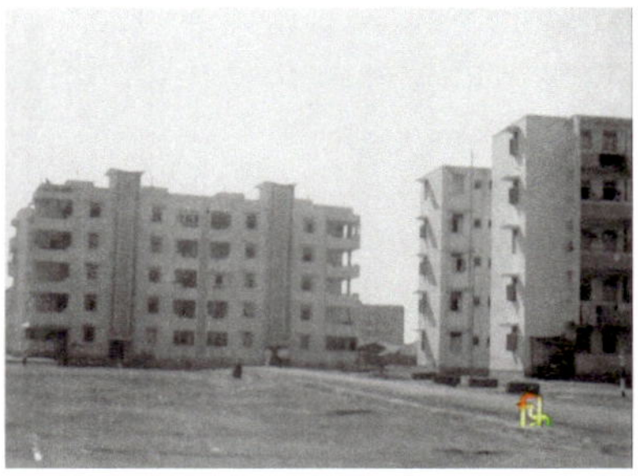
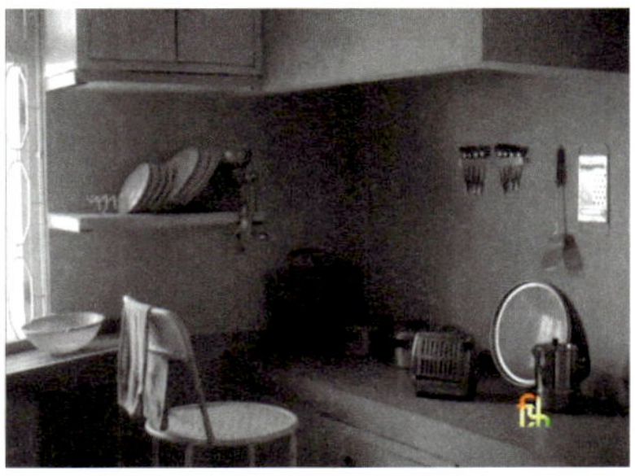

Exhibition under Nehru focused on the cost of materials and quick assembly of model homes especially for those displaced by the violence of partition, by the 1970s under Gandhi, housing design focused on the merits of the small, hygienic, single-family home for the urban poor.

Economizing the Home

While ideas of environmental conservation spearheaded by postcolonial leaders like Gandhi highlighted better standards of living, population management and resource scarcity (whether food, water, or land) were the horizons by which many new nations planned their development programs as they decolonized. Housing was therefore a key concern of India's five-year plans. Nevertheless, environmental anxieties about the "population bomb" were anchored within developmental aspirations. Government documents were littered with this duality, as they claimed that "vast developments by way of large increases in agricultural and industrial production have [already] been neutralized by population growth," and argued for a "manifold expansion of employment, housing, educational and other facilities."[25] Yet ever-increasing housing shortages reached a crescendo in 1968. As a result, India's Ministry of Health and Family Planning lamented the lack of funding allocated to address the question of housing and began to lobby the Planning Commission to divert its attention to the need for—and the construction of—low-income housing.

Throughout the 1960s, the Indian state partnered with the Ford Foundation to conduct studies on urban housing and urbanization taking place across the country and advised the government on ways to "engineer" communities to develop modern values and embrace a development process. Such an impulse—to eradicate the problems of overcrowding and overpopulation through interventions at the community level—was a simultaneous process of diagnosis and remedy, where the pathologization and elimination of unwanted behaviors that characterized rural migrants to the city would successfully create a good urban environment conducive to maintaining social order. Under the Foundation's influence, by 1966 the Ministry of Health and Family Planning produced a report that linked urban community development with the health of the nation, noting:

> It is generally agreed that Community Development seeks to mobilize people and to create [in] them an urge to change and improve their conditions of living by their own efforts and resources. ... This concept of Community Development is of prime importance to the building of a healthy democratic base for our welfare state, which far from being a purely paternal benevolent entity, must depend for its subsistence and growth on the active participation of the people who must be stimulated to think, decide and act for themselves and utilize fully the opportunities offered by the national plans.[26]

The failure to cope with the "crisis" of rapid urbanization was largely seen by the Foundation as the result of "administrative inertia" rather than a scarcity of resources.[27] In response, recognizing the growing deficit of housing numbers, the government deftly repositioned the conversation from one that centered on shelter scarcity to security, amending and expanding the various housing "schemes" that, since the 1950s, had targeted different income and labor populations. These included a low-income group scheme, an industrial housing scheme, a slum clearance and improvement scheme, a plantation labor housing scheme, and a village housing scheme, to name a few. Such a shift focused the deficit away from the government's supposed fiscal incapacity to provide housing for a growing population, and toward personal improvement and responsibility to ensure that population numbers, at least at the family level, could be brought within reasonable limits.

Accordingly, Indian planners and policymakers conceived of a multilayered system to solve the housing question that involved the division of powers between the central and state governments as well as regional town planning centers and municipal housing boards, private developers, and builders' associations. While not a uniquely Indian story, such a heavy bureaucratization—the "development raj"—was also seen in the country's Family Planning Program, which took into consideration "the total man in the total environment" and executed its initiatives through an "interdisciplinary team working in co-operation with the representative institutions of the people," or across various government departments.[28] By 1969, the Ministry of Health and Family Planning was merged with the Ministry of Works, Housing, and Urban Development to form a single consolidated entity called Health, Family Planning, Works, Housing, and Urban Development.

That same year, a working group was set up within the Ministry to "ameliorate the unsatisfactory housing conditions in the country" and alleviate poverty with the introduction of "higher standards of living" and strict population control.[29] Consisting of a team that included engineers, bureaucrats, and architects (including the president of the Indian Institute of Architects, J. R. Bhalla, and the famed modernist architect Achyut Kanvinde), the working group attempted to highlight the design of housing across different regions, climates, and other "local conditions." Their work resulted in the publication of over 5000 architectural designs for houses that could be implemented anywhere in the country. By the early 1970s, the National Buildings Organization

(NBO) in New Delhi selected fifty-six designs, of which thirty-six were distributed to different housing boards, municipal corporations, improvement trusts, central public works departments, and other state and local government authorities for implementation.[30] Each was designed for one of four different socioeconomic groups: houses with a "plinth area" less than 350 square feet were for slum dwellers and contained only a kitchen and multipurpose room; those between 350 and 400 square feet were for low-income groups, and those between 400 and 650 square feet for lower-middle-income groups, both of which had one bedroom; and those between 650 and 900 square feet were for middle-income groups and had two bedrooms.

The emphasis on standardization—a feature introduced to India through colonial public works—continued to be relevant to the government throughout the 1970s, even as architects began to advocate for a regionalist approach in terms of form and space. To this point, 1969 was also the year a national convention on housing was held in New Delhi, organized by the NBO and the Indian Institute of Architects (IIA), where the problems inherent to standardization across the nation crystallized, even if such a technique was not discarded. The convention was opened by the president of India, V. V. Giri, who noted that slums "grown" in the cities were an affront to human dignity. His address to the delegates captured the dire housing situation: a shortage of twelve million units in urban areas and the incredible task of rehabilitating fifty million homes in the hinterlands.[31] Invoking assessments made by the Ford Foundation, he called on architects and engineers to devise quicker and cheaper methods of building along with technical innovation.[32] Taking a multipronged approach to housing at various scales—city, community, and unit—the convention was spread across three days and consisted of delegates presenting papers and formulating resolutions that would be submitted to the Ministry. The outcomes included long-term programs for the financialization of housing through insurance schemes and providence funds, the adoption of newer, cheaper building

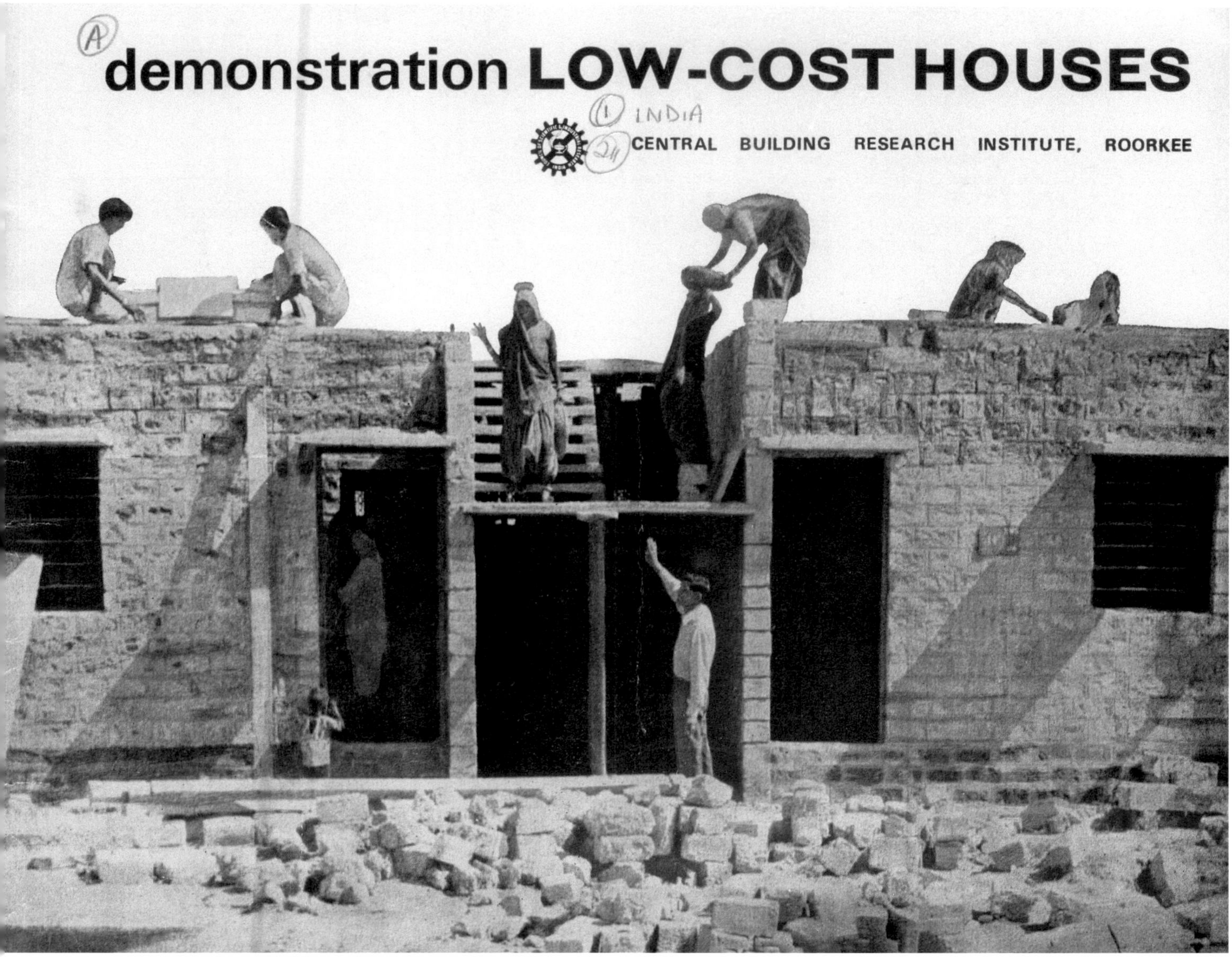

↑ *Demonstration Low-Cost Houses*, published by the Central Building Research Institute, 1975.

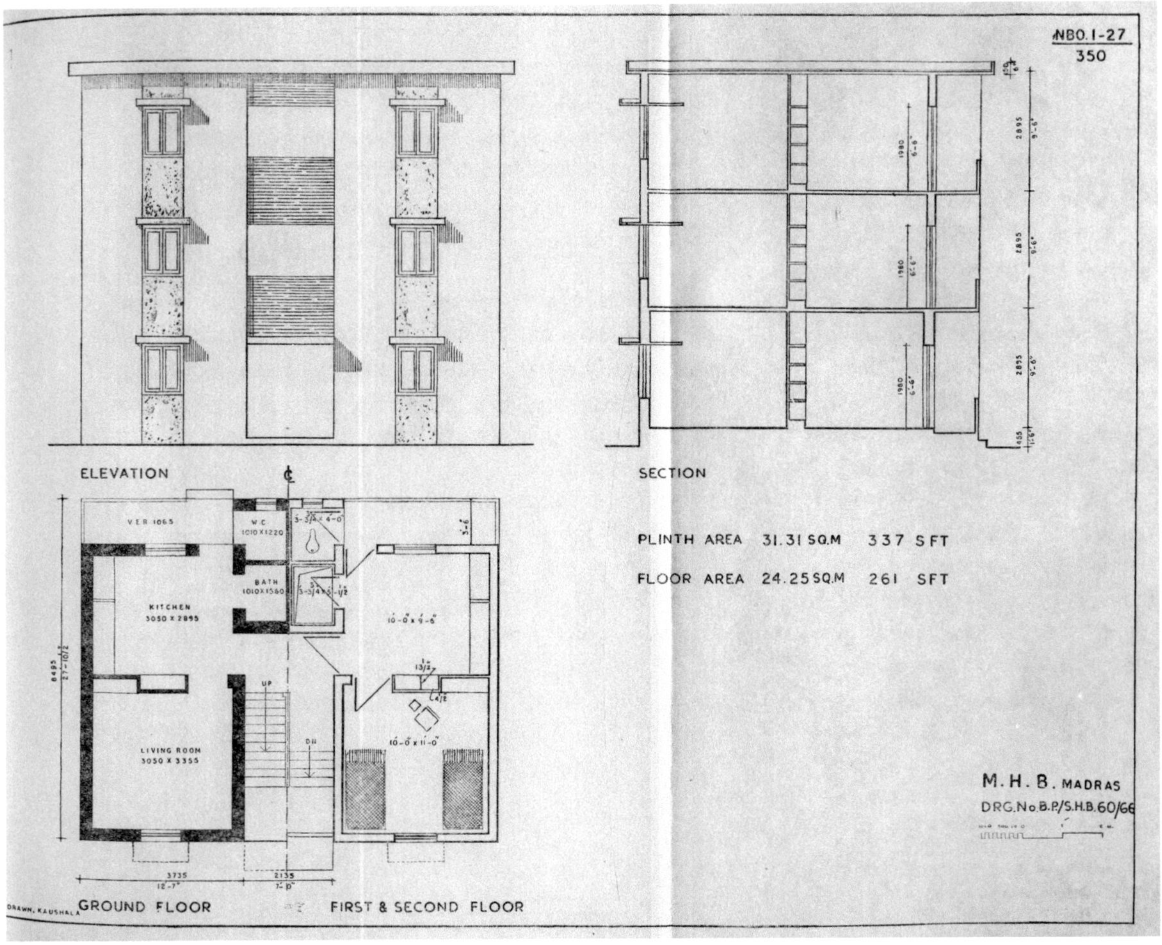

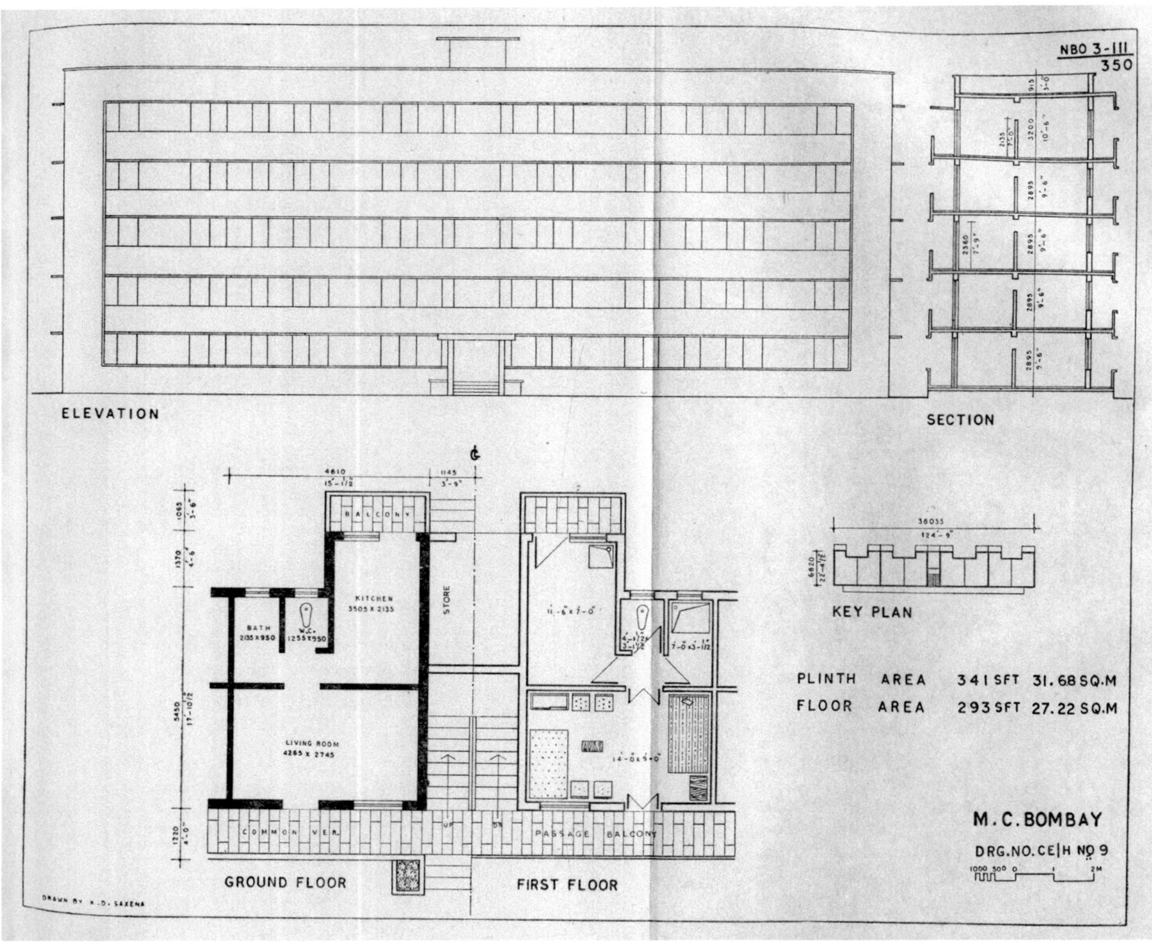

↑ Plans submitted to the Madras Housing Board and Municipal Corporation Bombay of houses for low-income groups, 1966.

materials, and the standardization of construction techniques, technologies, and unit size for government-sponsored projects.

The published resolutions reflect a certain amount of disagreement on the best way to tangibly address the urgent challenges outlined by Giri. Notwithstanding the demand for dignified housing from below—by industrial and municipal workers, "backward classes," or Dalits—technocrats addressed the housing question and targeted dismal urban conditions as a process of getting people off the streets. Some argued that bare, single-room housing units should be provided to the masses, which could eventually, with additional public-sector financial assistance, be improved over time. Others argued that "significant improvement in the housing of the low and very low-income families must be recognized instead of leaving the problem to be solved at a later date when resources become available."[33] A third faction argued for a sites-and-services approach, where "improvement of housing conditions of families in squatter settlements, majority of whom are recent migrants, may not be possible except through planned areas of semi-permanent structures along with the basic infrastructure for hygiene and communal facilities ... which are capable of progressive improvement."[34]

The convention also stressed the need for further research to be undertaken into the question of "materials, construction techniques and other policy and organization matters which could continuously throw light on ways and means by which housing can be improved both quantitatively and qualitatively," giving insight into the unease regarding the state's distressed economy, as ministries and different federal governments fought over the allocation of funds.[35] Amidst a chronic cement shortage, the convention made clear that the form any type of low-income housing took was bound to its economic implications.[36] While concern over housing cost was certainly not novel, and indeed a key feature of the 1954 exhibition, the urgency of low-cost housing to reduce the threat of overpopulation and slum growth supplanted these earlier conversations. Over the next few years, government conferences focused on the significance of construction costs—such as the 1971 seminar on Cost Reduction in Housing in Bombay—while private research departments, the NBO, and the Central Building Research Institute (CBRI) released pamphlets detailing various aspects of construction.

Economic primacy allowed government reports to continue justifying smaller housing for lower-income groups throughout the 1970s, claiming that standards such as those determined by the American Public Health Association (which were referenced and used by the Ministry of Housing, Works, and Supply in its construction projects) for "healthy" housing were "far-fetched" for a growing population.[37] Nearly a decade after the 1969 convention, a 1977 report reiterated that "it is not possible at present to meet the need-based requirement of every family."[38] Based on the recommendations of Public Works Department bureaucrats, and architects B. V. Doshi and Kulbir Singh, the report stated: "The cost of a house is disproportionately large with reference to the paying capacity of the low-income householders. Also it is not possible to provide reasonable accommodation for which these householders may be able to pay economic rent."[39]

While strategies to manage the nation's economic future featured high on the 1969 convention's agenda, far less attention was devoted to social and cultural questions of housing. Resolutions simply stated that "a deeper study" would be required to deal with regional diversity within the nation. Indeed, while delegates noted that the implementation of standards was at odds with the traditions and customs of a disparate population, the solutions they considered fell within a logic of austerity, where proleptic assessments made sure that the "reduced provision of spaces could be effectively used without impairing the living efficiency."[40] Additionally, the convention stressed the need for stricter centralization of authority, reducing the autonomy of federal states to intervene in matters of housing and flattening, to some extent, typological and material differences inherent to traditional building.[41] National housing conversations such as those at the convention thus cultivated a discourse in which the question of low-income housing was rendered answerable as an economic question rather than a social one. What this suggests is that housing, from the outset, was a physiocratic endeavor that targeted different populations through conceptions of what the economy could and could not sustain.

Here it is important to revisit the relationship between family planning and low-income housing. As many historians have remarked, the use of brute force to drive people to vasectomy camps and compulsory sterilization theaters marked the era when fertility control was used as a technocratic solution to poverty induced by overpopulation.[42] Housing, too, was a technocratic tool to house the poor who were subjected to sterilization programs. But such an analysis precludes a discussion on the conception of difference that was essential to the implementation of these schemes. While concerns about the national economy were cited as the reason for housing and space standards, amenity provision was also bound to determinations of illiberality that poorer sections of society represented, especially at a time leading to a national emergency, when unrest, disorder, unemployment, internal migration, and uncontrolled population growth posed a threat to the same economy. Further, the fictionalized enemy of slum growth legitimated the government's calibration of the small home. Subjecting low-income populations to family planning and rehousing, rehabilitation or resettlement schemes were an occasion that invited architectural design as a prophylactic to the problem. The poorest sections of society receiving the smallest homes signaled the pressure that such families would face if they were to be rehoused, often away from their spaces of work, or if they were to expand, having neither the land, the space, nor the means to do so.

Next was the question of form. While the provision of housing and whether it was multistory, high-density, or low-density differed between cities like Delhi, Bombay, Calcutta, or Madras (which were catered to by their individual housing boards), the designs were largely regulated by the central government and distributed by the NBO. In a techno-rationalist vein, these designs were a marked departure from the tenements that were the subject of clearance and rehabilitation. Debating the benefits of multistory construction, delegates from the 1969 convention ambivalently noted that its success "would depend very much upon the understanding of the social aspects of families and communities and therefore, detailed studies of sociological aspects of housing related to specific housing development should be undertaken."[43] Indeed, modernized housing was acknowledged to contribute to the disruption of social life, and while architects sought to integrate the dwelling "with the total housing environment," their approach ultimately cast a blind eye on the reinforcement of precarity.[44] The relocation of populations into multistory units advanced a low-cost solution to the restitution of "dignity," and yet families housed in this way remained inadequately provided for in a more humanistic sense, one that accounted for tradition and culture.[45] The artificial separation of housing as a service and the complexity of traditional, communal existence enforced spatial chasms, if not ghettoized housing developments.

Finally, there was the question of coercion. The tactics leveled by family planning schemes against the poor were mirrored by large-scale slum clearances. As already discussed, slums were seen as the epitome of poverty, moral denigration, crime, and disease, but by the 1970s they also came to be delimited through their "illegality," making them a target of state impunity and reform.[46] Despite the celebratory rhetoric of housing proponents, dwellers were neither consulted nor given an option to refuse either the demolition of their surroundings or their rehousing. If housing was to transform social behavior and create a "desirable sociological and physical environment necessary for the healthy growth of individuals," slum clearance and forced resettlements were seen as imperative for the government to achieve its goals.[47] Ultimately, even as housing was promoted as an amenity for the poor, its architecture became an elaborate plan targeted at them.

Coda

By 1975, the year of Gandhi's state of emergency, a group of young architects including H. D. Chhaya, Satish Dabral, Vinod Gupta, Romi Khosla, Narendra Dengle, M. N. Ashish Ganju, and Vasant Kamath submitted a memorandum to the prime minister and proposed "new ways of solving the problems of the poor in the modern process of urbanization."[48] Just as Annie does in the opening scenes of *In Which Annie Gives It Those Ones*, architects lamented the "deteriorating physical and social environments caused by the insensitive handling of massive housing projects for the poor," and suggested a vastly different approach to housing: one that was based on dialogue with the people being housed, and a shift in design responsibility from government bureaucrats to the private architect. The memorandum, while supported by Gandhi, was ineffective in bringing about systemic change. From June 1975 to March 1977, 150,105 demolitions were undertaken in Delhi alone, an eighty-two percent increase from the previous two years.[49]

In the context of Indian family planning, measures to quell a global population crisis crystalized alongside a national emergency that reinforced the need to target poor people who consistently had larger families. Within this context, the governance of reproduction was not simply a product of medicalized discourse, but a social good to ensure the health and dignity of the nation.[50] The resulting national housing programs were created against a backdrop of an aspirational modernity, where poorer populations needed to be taught—through demonstration—how to live. Housing thus emerged as a political instrument that wielded evidence of the government's benevolence, if not legitimacy. And yet the implementation of these programs was beset by contradictions. While housing programs were conceived within a social contract, they maintained insecurity rather than dispensing with it.

An earlier version of this essay was originally published by e-flux Architecture in 2020.

p26 Hugh Moore Fund Collection, Department of Rare Books and Special Collections, Princeton University Library.
p28 AP Newsfeatures Photo.
p29 Pierre Jeanneret fonds, Canadian Centre for Architecture. Gift of Jaqueline Jeanneret.
p30-31 Ministry of Information and Broadcasting, Films Division, India.
p33 CBRI, India.
p34 National Buildings Organisation and UN Regional Housing Centre ECAFE, India.

1. For a discussion on this nexus, see Edward Soja, "Rural-Urban Interaction," *Canadian Journal of African Studies* 3, no. 1 (Winter 1969): 284–290. The concept of a "folk-urban continuum" was introduced by Robert Redfield, a University of Chicago anthropologist. Robert Redfield, "The Folk Society," *American Journal of Sociology* 52 (January 1947).
2. *In Which Annie Gives It Those Ones*, directed by Pradip Krishen, screenplay by Arundhati Roy (1989). For a discussion on migration and urbanization, see Donald J. Bogue and Zachariah, "Urbanization and Migration in India," in *India's Urban Frontier*, ed. Roy Turner (Berkeley: University of California Press, 1962). Also see Saghir Ahmad, "Urbanization in India: An Annotated Bibliography" (M. Lib Sc. Thesis, Aligarh Muslim University, 1979–1980).
3. Indira Gandhi, *Selected Speeches and Writings of Indira Gandhi*, vol. 3: *September 1972–March 1977* (New Delhi: Publications Division, Ministry of Information and Broadcasting, Government of India, 1984), quoted in Asha Nadkarni, *Eugenic Feminism: Reproductive Nationalism in the United States and India* (Minneapolis: University of Minnesota Press, 2014), 173.
4. Donella Meadows et al., *The Limits to Growth: A Report for the Club of Rome's Project on the Predicament of Mankind* (Falls Church, VA: Potomac Associates, 1972).
5. U Thant, "S-0885-0001-42-00001," in "Items in Conference on Human Survival, 25 May 197," United Nations Archives Container S-0885-0001: Operational Files of the Secretary General U. Thant: Speeches, Messages, Statements and Addresses.
6. Matthew Connelly notes that no other country attempted to control its fertility over such a long period. India was the first country to adopt policies to reduce rather than improve fertility, and together with other South Asian countries was the testing ground for new contraceptive techniques. See Matthew Connelly, *Fatal Misconception: The Struggle to Control World Population* (Cambridge, MA: Harvard University Press, 2008).
7. John P. Holdren and Paul R. Ehrlich, "Human Population and the Global Environment: Population Growth, Rising per capita Material Consumption, and Disruptive Technologies have made Civilization a Global Ecological Force," *American Scientist* 62, no. 3 (May-June 1974): 282.
8. *The Problem of Housing in India* (Government of India, Ministry of Works, Housing & Supply, 1957).
9. *The Problem of Housing in India*, 198. "Unfinished Revolution" was also the title of Gandhi's speech at the 1970 Non-Aligned Meeting in Lusaka.
10. Jawaharlal Nehru, "Opening Remarks at the International Exhibition on Low-Cost Housing by the Prime Minister, 25 October 1953," New Delhi.
11. For a discourse on planning in India and its political contradictions, see Partha Chatterjee, "Development Planning and the Indian State," in *Empire and Nation* (New York: Columbia University Press, 2010).
12. File no. 2/22/62-HI, National Archives of India.
13. For a discussion of these two competing visions see Farhan Karim, *Of Greater Dignity than Riches* (Pittsburgh: University of Pittsburgh Press, 2018); Peter Scriver and Amit Srivastava, "Nation Building: Architecture in the Service of the Postcolonial State," in *India: Modern Architectures in History* (London: Reaktion, 2016). Also see William Glover's discussion on the troubled category of "villager in the city" that was the demographic focus in the building of new towns: William Glover, "The Troubled Passage from 'Village Communities' to Planned New Town Development in Mid-Twentieth-Century South Asia," *Urban History* 39, no. 1 (2012).
14. *Solving the Problem*, directed by Biren Dass (Films Division, Government of India, 1960).
15. *Struggle for Space*, directed by Prem Prakash (Films Division, Government of India, 1969).
16. Sheetal Chhabria, *Making the Modern Slum: The Power of Capital in Colonial Bombay* (Seattle: University of Washington Press, 2019).
17. For an account on the entanglements of caste struggles, sanitation, and urban planning in Bombay, see Juned Shaikh, *Outcaste Bombay: City Making and the Politics of the Poor* (Seattle: University of Washington Press, 2021).
18. *Housing for the People*, directed by Pratap Parmar (Films Division, Government of India, 1970).
19. *Struggle for Space*, directed by Prem Prakash.
20. Indira Gandhi, "Human Environment: Address to the Plenary Session of the United Nations Conference on Human Environment at Stockholm, June 14, 1972," in *Indira Gandhi Speeches and Writings* (New York: Harper Row, 1975), 193.
21. Gandhi, "Human Environment," 195.
22. Gandhi, "Human Environment," 193.
23. "A Design for Living: A Project for UNESCO Action Sponsored by Consensus at the Nehru Round Table, New Delhi, September, 1966," *MARG* 20, no. 3 (June 1967): 5.
24. Gandhi, "Human Environment," 199.
25. *India: Family Planning Programme since 1965* (Government of India, Ministry of Health, Family Planning and Urban Development, Department of Family Planning, 1968), 1.
26. *Report of the Rural-Urban Relationship Committee* (Government of India, Ministry of Health & Family Planning, 1966), quoted in Karim, *Of Greater Dignity than Riches*, 168–169. For a discussion on the Ford Foundation in India, see Sam Collings-Wells, "Developing Communities: The Ford Foundation and the Global Urban Crisis, 1958–1966," *Journal of Global History* 16, no. 3 (Cambridge: Cambridge University Press, 2021), 336–354.
27. Colin Rosser, *Urbanization in India: An International Urbanization Survey Report to the Ford Foundation* (New York: Ford Foundation, 1972),7.
28. On "development raj" see David Ludden, "India's Development Regime," in *Colonialism and Culture*, ed. Nicholas Dirks (Ann Arbor: University of Michigan Press, 2000), 245–287. See also *India: Family Planning Programme since 1965*, 7.
29. See *Annual Report 1968–1969* (New Delhi: Ministry of Health, Family Planning, Works, Housing and Urban Development, 1969), 31. Also see *Report of the Development Group on Low Cost Housing* (New Delhi: Ministry of Works and Housing, National Buildings Organisation and UN Regional Housing Centre ESCAP, September 1977), 1.
30. *A Collection of Designs of Houses for Low Income Groups* (New Delhi: Government of India National Buildings Organisation and UN Regional Housing Centre ECAFE, 1969), iii.
31. *Report on "Housing Convention" Organised Jointly by National Buildings Organisation and the Indian Institute of Architects* (New Delhi: Government of India National Buildings Organisation and UN Regional Housing Centre ECAFE, 1969).
32. "The failure to make reasonable provision for housing wants robs the economic system of one of the principal rewards of economic growth and breeds restlessness, discontent and instability." *Report on 'Housing Convention' Organised Jointly by National Buildings Organisation and the Indian Institute of Architects* (New Delhi: Government of India National Buildings Organisation and UN Regional Housing Centre ECAFE, 1969), 3.
33. *Report on "Housing Convention,"* 7.
34. *Report on "Housing Convention,"* 8.
35. *Report on "Housing Convention,"* 12.
36. "The standards of space and other facilities are linked up with costs." *Report on "Housing Convention,"* 7.
37. *Report of the Development Group on Low Cost Housing*, 8.
38. *Report of the Development Group on Low Cost Housing*, 8.
39. *Report of the Development Group on Low Cost Housing*, 9.
40. *Report on "Housing Convention,"* 13.
41. Whether such an approach was successfully implemented is debatable. See Curt Gambetta, "Substitutions of Modernity: The Materiality of House-Making in Postcolonial India" (PhD diss., Princeton University, November 2023). On the other hand, the centralization of housing finance was adopted the year after, in 1970, through HUDCO (Housing and Urban Development Corporation).
42. Marika Vicziany, "Coercion in a Soft State: The Family-Planning Program of India: Part I: The Myth of Voluntarism," *Pacific Affairs* 55, no. 3 (Autumn 1982): 373–402.
43. *Report on "Housing Convention,"* 6.
44. *Report on "Housing Convention,"* 7. "Housing concepts dealing with such minimum standards of dwelling must integrate the dwelling with the total housing environment within which the families should be able to derive a fair degree of satisfaction by using not only the dwelling but other environmental facilities."
45. Additionally, delegates noted that multistory structures and high-density designs would eliminate the need to worry about rising land values.
46. For a discussion on the differences between illegal and legal informal settlements or "slums," see Ayona Datta, *The Illegal City: Space, Law and Gender in a Delhi Squatter Settlement* (London: Routledge, 2012).
47. *Report of the Development Group on Low Cost Housing*, 8. On the other hand, Gyan Prakash notes that slum clearance in a city like Delhi came to be promoted as an aesthetic ideal, one in which "urban beautification" was an essential component of the modernization project. See Gyan Prakash, *Emergency Chronicles: Indira Gandhi and Democracy's Turning Point* (Princeton: Princeton University Press, 2019), 281.
48. "Memorandum Submitted by Young Architects: To the Prime Minister Smt. Indra Gandhi on 12th August, 1975," GREHA, Delhi, India, https://architexturez.net/doc/az-cf-21707.
49. *Shah Commission of Inquiry, Interim Report II* (Ministry of Home Affairs, 1978), quoted in Prakash, *Emergency Chronicles*.
50. Savina Balasubramanian, "Motivating Men: Social Science and the Regulation of Men's Reproduction in Postwar India," *Gender and Society* 32, no. 1 (February 2018): 37.

ALCOHOL AFTER THE APOCALYPSE

ANGELIKA ELLEN JOSEPH

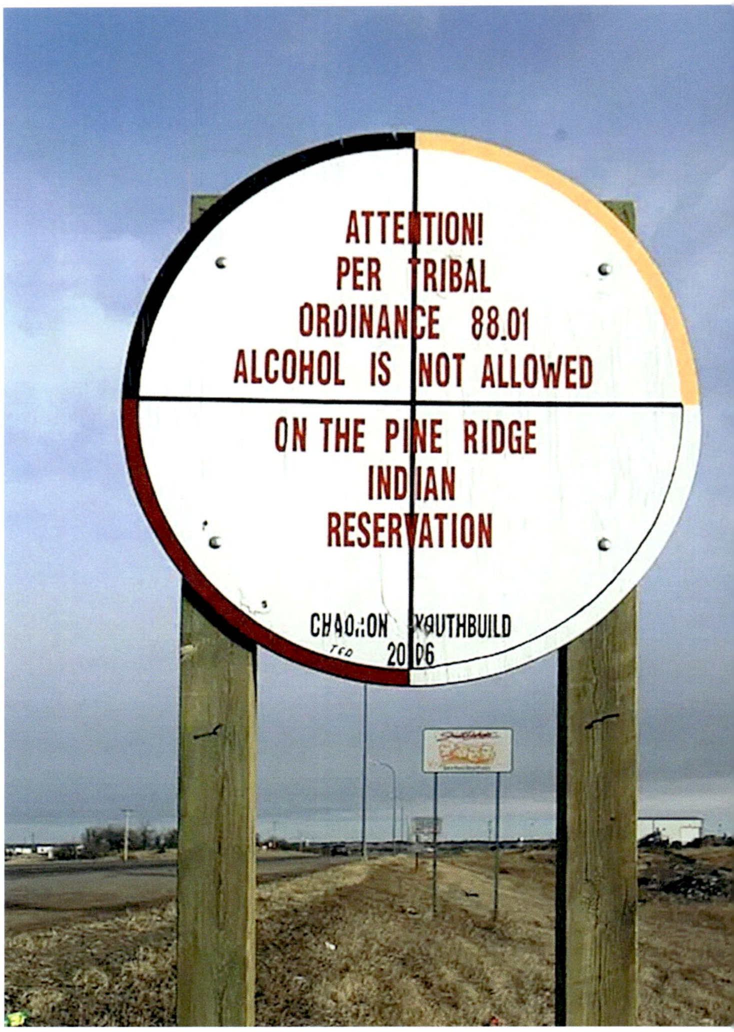

↗ Signs at the border between Whiteclay, Nebraska, and Pine Ridge, South Dakota.

Take Nebraska state highway 87 as far as you can north until it becomes South Dakota state highway 407. Where these two highways meet, you'll see a tipi on the left-hand side of the two-lane highway, standing next to a flagpole. At the top of that flagpole, you'll see a flag you probably don't recognize, and below it, you'll see one you do: the US flag flying upside down. On the right-hand side of the road, you'll see a painted wood sign, which you might recognize as a medicine wheel.[1] It reads: "Attention! Per tribal ordinance 88.01 alcohol is not allowed on the Pine Ridge Indian Reservation." Just past that, you'll see a darker wood sign that reads "Now entering P.O.W. Camp #344 established by the B.I.A. [Bureau of Indian Affairs] March 3rd 1871 a.k.a. Pine Ridge Indian Reservation."[2] Finally, a shiny white metal sign towers high. "South Dakota," it says, with a bright yellow image of the presidential faces which desecrated the sacred and stolen Black Hills. Welcome to the Oglala Lakota Nation.

The line in the ground just crossed, separating the land of the Oglala Lakota Nation from the state of Nebraska, is a particularly contentious one. From the 1940s to 2017, this line was marked by alcohol. Pine Ridge Indian Reservation does not allow alcohol within its boundaries, but on the other side

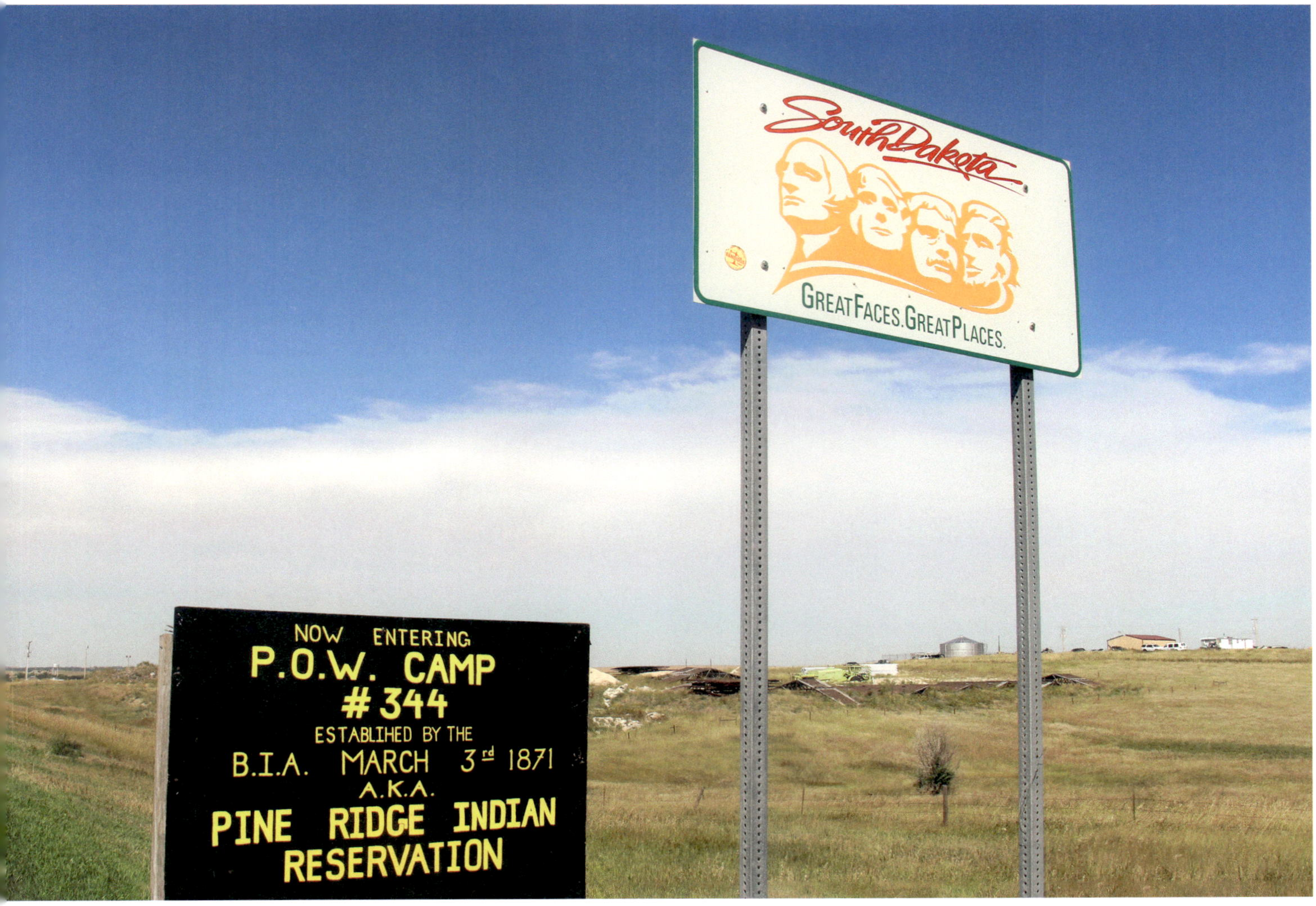
South Dakota
Great Faces. Great Places.
NOW ENTERING
P.O.W. CAMP
#344
ESTABLIHED BY THE
B.I.A. MARCH 3rd 1871
A.K.A.
PINE RIDGE INDIAN
RESERVATION

of this line sits the unincorporated area of Whiteclay, Nebraska. In 2011, the four liquor stores in Whiteclay sold the equivalent of 4.3 million twelve-ounce cans of beer—a rate of 841 cans of beer per Whiteclay resident per day, if the beer was being sold to the residents.[3] But it wasn't. Instead, it was being sold to residents of Pine Ridge Indian Reservation, a dry reservation marked by high rates of alcoholism, alcohol-related illness, and alcohol-related deaths.

Mapping Pine Ridge

The territoriality of alcohol has been an active force in shaping and defining the spatial boundaries of Indian Country for more than two hundred years. In 1802, President Thomas Jefferson sought the overall restriction of alcohol on tribal lands, and Congress proceeded to pass a law granting the president the right to "to prevent or restrain the vending or distributing of spirituous liquors among all or any of the said Indian tribes."[4] This catalyzed one of the first quests to try to legally define Indian Country.[5] It also led to the creation of the Commissioner of Indian Affairs in 1832, with associated legislation stating: "No ardent spirits shall be hereafter introduced, under any pretense, into the Indian country."[6] This law was expanded in 1834 to introduce penalties for the sale or distribution of alcohol into reservations, except when it was distributed to the US military occupying these lands. These laws continued beyond the passage of the Twenty-first Amendment and the end of Prohibition. After Native American veterans returned from World War II, they petitioned for their right to drink. In 1953, Native Americans were finally given the right to be served alcohol anywhere in the US, and reservations were allowed to determine whether they would permit alcohol on their land or not.[7] About two-thirds of reservations currently allow alcohol. Pine Ridge Indian Reservation does not.

The first time Pine Ridge appears on a map as a reservation or sectioned-off territory is in "Map Showing the Position of Nebraska State Troops in Indian Campaigns of the Winter of 1890–91," which was included in report Senate No. 352 from the Committee on Military Affairs, printed on March 10, 1892. This map depicts reservation boundaries along with the settlement patterns of the Oglala Lakota, Nebraska National Guard, and United States troops. At the top of the map, an Oglala Lakota settlement is marked within the reservation boundary with small X's and labeled "Hostile Indians." US troops are also settled within the reservation along White Clay Creek and Wolf Creek and are depicted with detailed tent symbols almost three times the size of the X's meant to depict tipis. Yet photographs of the two settlements look more similar than different, so much so that when I first saw the photograph of the US troops' encampment, I mistook the tents for exceptionally clean and standardized tipis.

Below these settlements is a rectangular sectioned-off portion of land labeled "Friendly Indian Reservation in Nebraska," which meets Pine Ridge Indian Reservation at the South Dakota/Nebraska border.[8] The upper portion of this reservation is covered in the same X's that marked the tipi settlements of the "Hostile Indians." While the reservation's borders are straight and definite, the "Friendly" Oglala Lakota settlement appears to spill over them without disruption, coming all the way up to the creeks directly below Pine Ridge Agency.

The territory the US designated as a "Friendly Indian Reservation in Nebraska" during the Indian Wars has persisted, under various guises, into the twenty-first century. After the US Army ended its so-called "Pine Ridge Campaign" in 1891, the "Friendly Indian Reservation in Nebraska" was held as a "buffer," meaning that neither white settlers nor Oglala Lakota were allowed to live within its boundaries. The purpose of this land reserve, at least officially, was to protect people and property by keeping the white settlers away from the Oglala Lakota and vice versa. In 1904, President Theodore Roosevelt declared the buffer zone to be unnecessary, and without consulting with the tribe, reduced it to one square mile.[9] Settlers quickly rushed in and formed the unincorporated area of Whiteclay. The earliest archival image of Whiteclay is a 1910 photograph of a newly established post office. Nebraska route 87, which ends in Whiteclay

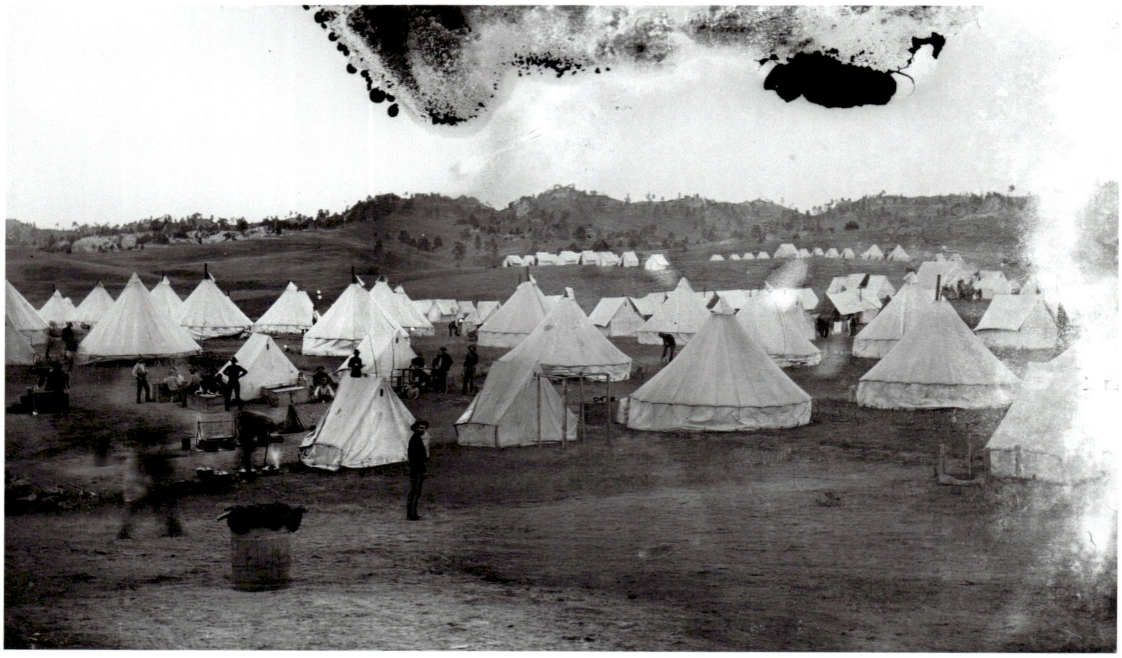

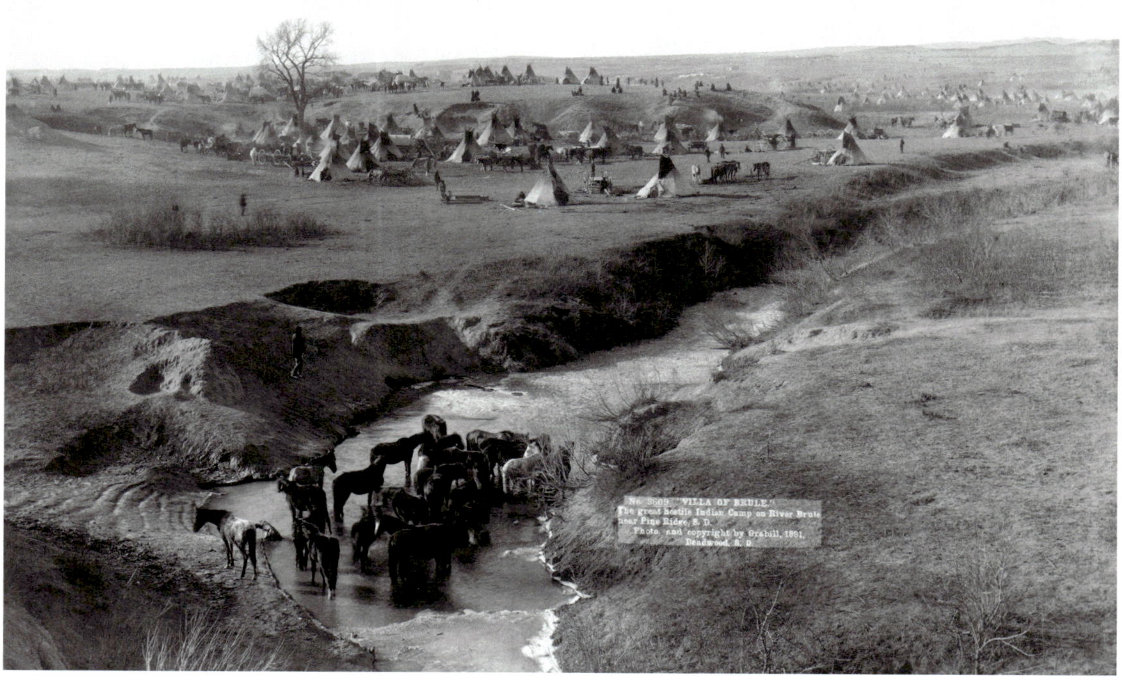

↖ Pine Ridge Agency, South Dakota, 1890 or 1891.

← John C. H. Grabill, Villa of Brule, Great Hostile Indian Camp on River Brule, near Pine Ridge, South Dakota, 1891.

↗ Map showing positions of state troops in Indian campaigns of the winter of 1890–1891.

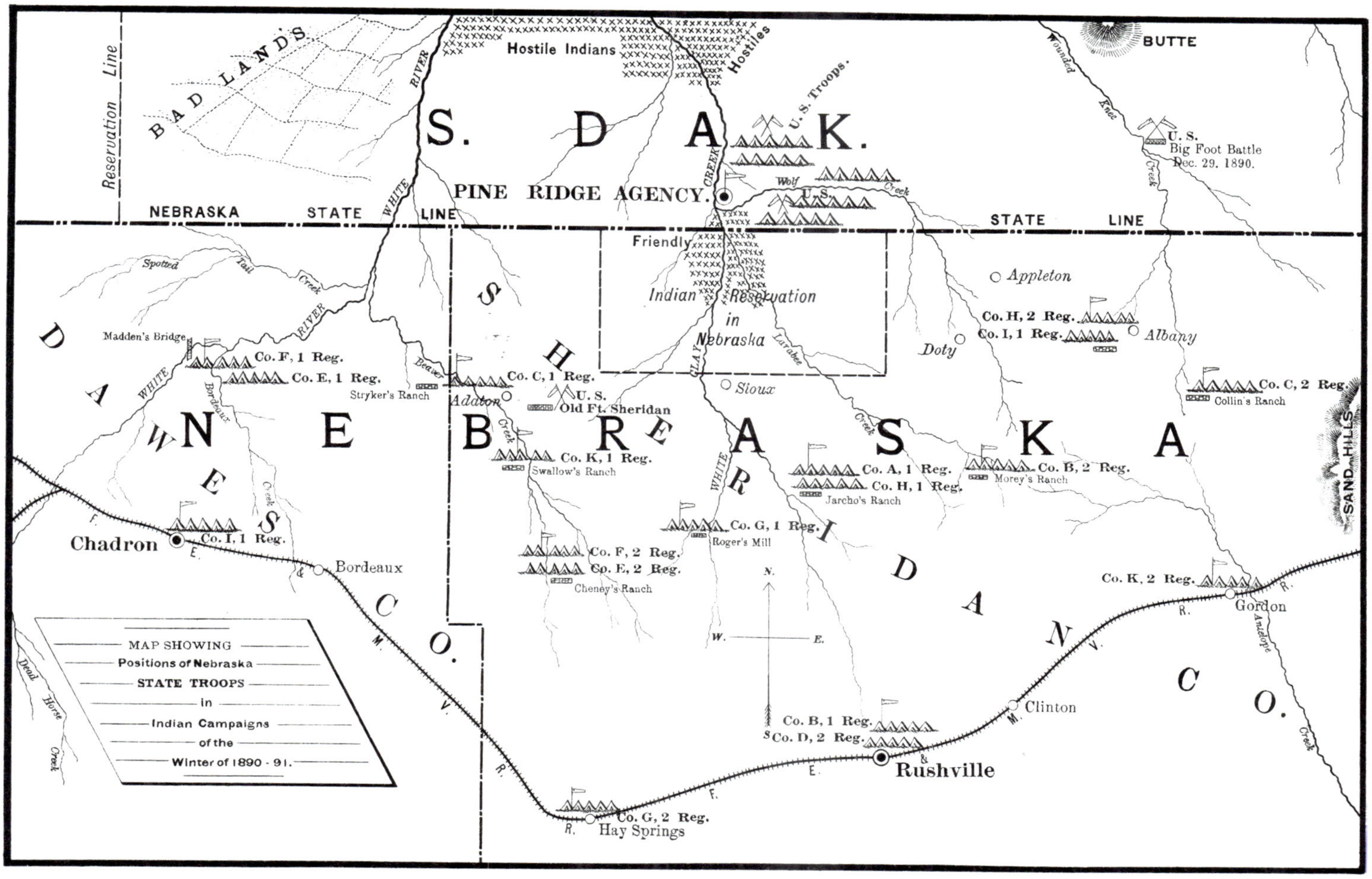

right outside the reduced buffer zone, was completed in 1935, and the first photographs of bars and taverns appeared in 1940. From this point onward, Whiteclay sold alcohol.

In the 2010s, generations of alcohol-related conflicts and deaths in and around Pine Ridge Reservation culminated in legal disputes. Lawyers argued that Whiteclay's liquor stores sold alcohol without there being any legal place for customers to consume it. Liquor consumption is illegal on the premises of these stores, it's illegal on the highway, and it's illegal on the reservation. In 2017, the Nebraska State Liquor Control Commission voted not to renew any of the liquor licenses in Whiteclay, citing the areas' insufficient law enforcement, and the associated public health impacts and sexual abuse of young girls.[10] The liquor licenses expired on April 30, 2017.[11] But allowing existing liquor licenses to lapse without renewal is not outright prohibition, and store owners have continued to pursue liquor licenses. To consider the level of Oglala Lakota pain and death in Whiteclay only within the legality of alcohol sales would be to miss the point. It's not unreasonable to state that an unincorporated area associated with such high levels of pain and death among white Americans would not continue unchecked for generations and generations.

Camp Embodied, Camp in Bodies

Statistics show that Native Americans get less life, liberty, and pursuit of happiness than all other Americans. Native Americans as a whole have the highest rate of poverty, the highest rate of unemployment, the lowest median income, the lowest rate of educational attainment, and lowest life expectancy of any racial or ethnic group in the United States.[12] On Pine Ridge Indian Reservation, these disparities are present at their extreme. Oglala Lakota County is the most populous county within the reservation and one of the poorest counties in the United States.[13] In 2012, more than ninety percent of the residents lived below the poverty line, according to federal statistics.[14] The unemployment rate was last reported at more than eighty percent in 2005. The Department of the Interior subsequently stopped recording unemployment—the rate was so high that the particular number had no meaning. One in four children on the reservation is born with fetal alcohol syndrome or the less severe fetal alcohol spectrum disorder (FASD).[15] Nationally, the rate is one in one hundred. In South Dakota, Native American boys and men ages fifteen through twenty-four die from suicide at four to five times the national rate.[16]

Life expectancy is one of the most cited metrics in articles discussing the reservation. In 2014, a study from the University of Washington's Institute for Health Metrics and Evaluation found that the life expectancy for residents of Oglala Lakota County was 66.8 years—the lowest of any county in the United States.[17] This position has held constant since the study was first begun in 1980. Summit County, Colorado, a mere 420 miles away, boasts the highest in the country, with a life expectancy twenty years longer. The life expectancy of Oglala Lakota County is below that of India, Sudan, and Iraq. Other data from the Indian Health Services hospital on the reservation puts the life expectancy at less than fifty years, which would give Pine Ridge Indian Reservation the lowest life expectancy of any place in the Western Hemisphere besides Haiti.[18]

With all this in mind, statistical data regarding the residents of Pine Ridge Indian Reservation is notoriously incomplete. Native Americans are the most undercounted demographic by the United States Census.[19] The Oglala Lakota Housing Officer estimates the reservation's population to be more than twice the number reported by the census. And it is reasonable to assume that Native Americans who are not counted on the census are disproportionately struggling with poverty, homelessness, and addiction.

When conducting this research, I did not set out looking for statistics that paint a bleak picture of life on the reservation. Yet nearly every article—from legal studies, public health, history, Native American studies, and more—makes a point of drawing from a statistical arsenal to paint Pine Ridge Indian Reservation as a place where there's a fair chance you'll be drunk before you're born and drunk when you die, and that the time between these two events will be short, poor, and painful. There is a certain rationale behind this type of presentation. In legal studies, it can help quantify impact or damages, and in public health, it is essential to quantify the environment and the health outcomes. It runs the risk, however, of falling into the tradition of presenting Native Americans as the mere "pawns and victims" of misguided government policies, as the fallen, constrained, or diminished remains of once-great warriors, or as existing in a world so unimaginable and unlike anyone else that Native Americans continue to exist on the margins or outside.

These "social" realities of the reservation manifest themselves clearly in the geographic identification of Pine Ridge Indian Reservation as a place. It's possible to identify Oglala Lakota County instantaneously on almost any map of the country. It's a fairly regularly shaped county in the middle of the country, but invariably, on any map showing county-by-county data, from obesity to diabetes to life expectancy, Oglala Lakota County pops out. Rates in Oglala Lakota County are always anomalous and extreme. More often than not, the rates recorded in Oglala Lakota County set the high or low point of the scale. Oglala Lakota bodies and life mark the reservation as a place because they embody and express the cumulative pain and trauma of this land.

Intergenerational Trauma, Intergenerational Camp

The perpetual concentration of Oglala Lakota pain and death localized on this specific section of land is not simply coincidental, a "social" problem, or indicative of some moral failure or absolute lack of willpower. In the legal proceedings, town hall meetings, and news coverage regarding Whiteclay's liquor sales, white benefactors of those sales continually framed the situation as the simple result of the invisible hand. As Sheridan County Commissioner Loren L. Paul put it, alcohol sales in Whiteclay had nothing to do with race. Whiteclay is just what happens when you have free enterprise, and "If you have a demand, somebody is probably gonna step in and fill that." According to this logic, the Oglala Lakota were the only ones responsible for the liquor sales, alcoholism, murders, accidental deaths, and fetal alcohol spectrum disorder. The liquor stores were there only because the Oglala Lakota kept buying liquor. Nobody was forcing them to buy it, and theoretically, they could stop doing so any time they wished.

The idea of the "drunk Indian" is ubiquitous in both Native and non-Native thought. For some, it's indicative of a genetic or biological predisposition due to the lack of alcohol in Native American life before contact. For anthropologist Ruth Benedict, alcohol and drug use is explained by the fact that Indigenous Americans "valued all violent experience, all means by which human beings may break through the usual sensory routine, and to all such experiences they attributed the highest value."[20] Vine Deloria Jr. posits that Native American youth drink in order to be the "real Indian" anthropologists lead them to believe they should be.[21] Oglala Lakota activist Russell Means hypothesized that Native Americans are predisposed to alcoholism because commodity foods distributed on reservations make people accustomed to a high-sugar diet in utero, and alcohol is the most efficient way to satisfy the resulting sugar craving.

For Anishinaabe anthropologist Lawrence Gross, however, alcoholism is one of the many symptoms of post-apocalypse stress syndrome (PASS), a culturally specific form of historical or intergenerational experienced by Native Americans today. For Gross, colonization was the apocalypse. The resulting syndrome explains the "personal trauma, social dysfunction, and crisis in worldview" that Native Americans experience as a result of continued "imposed cultural destruction."[22] Post-apocalypse stress syndrome is similar to post-traumatic stress disorder (PTSD) except that the causal trauma, resulting symptoms (alcoholism, substance abuse,

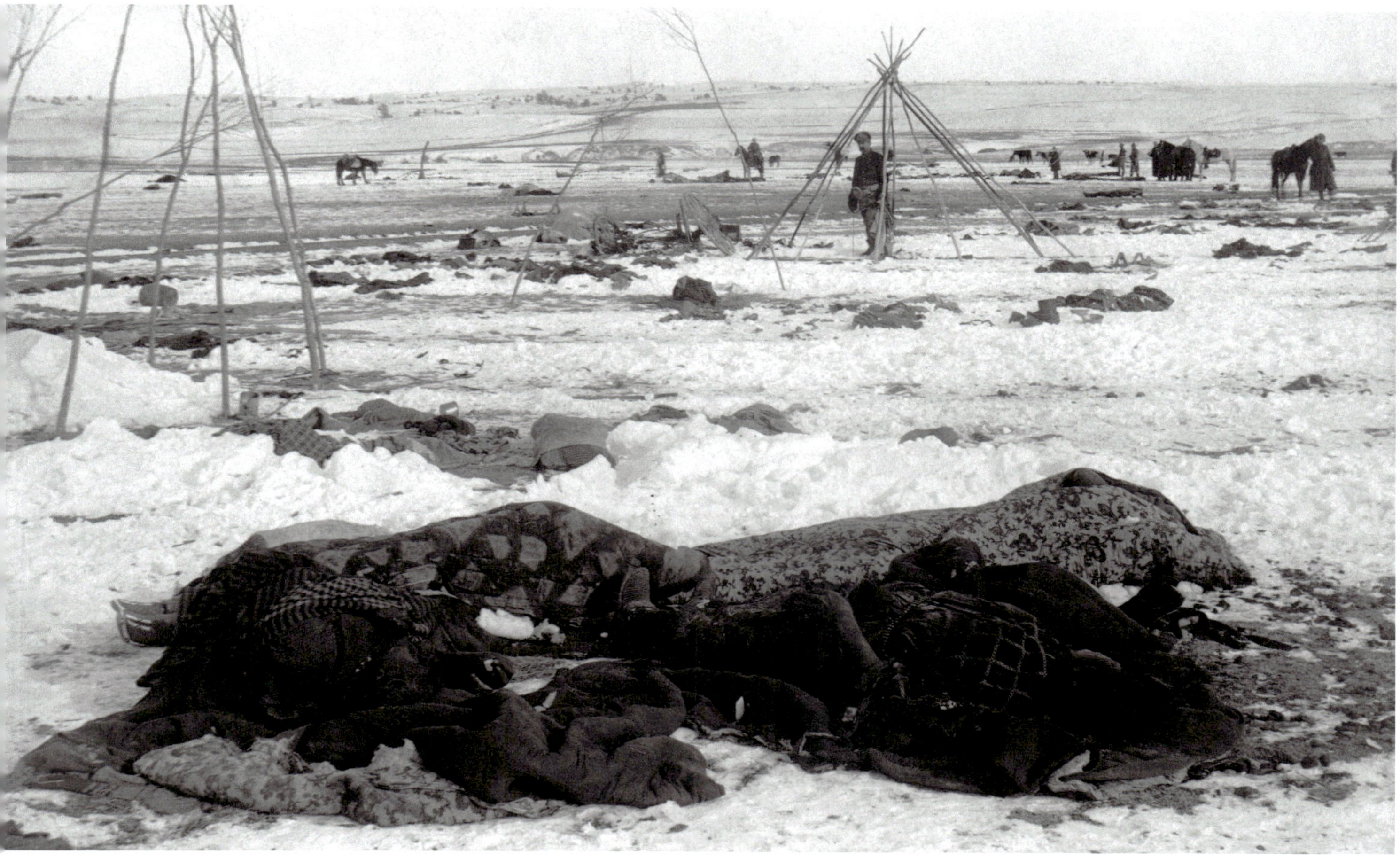

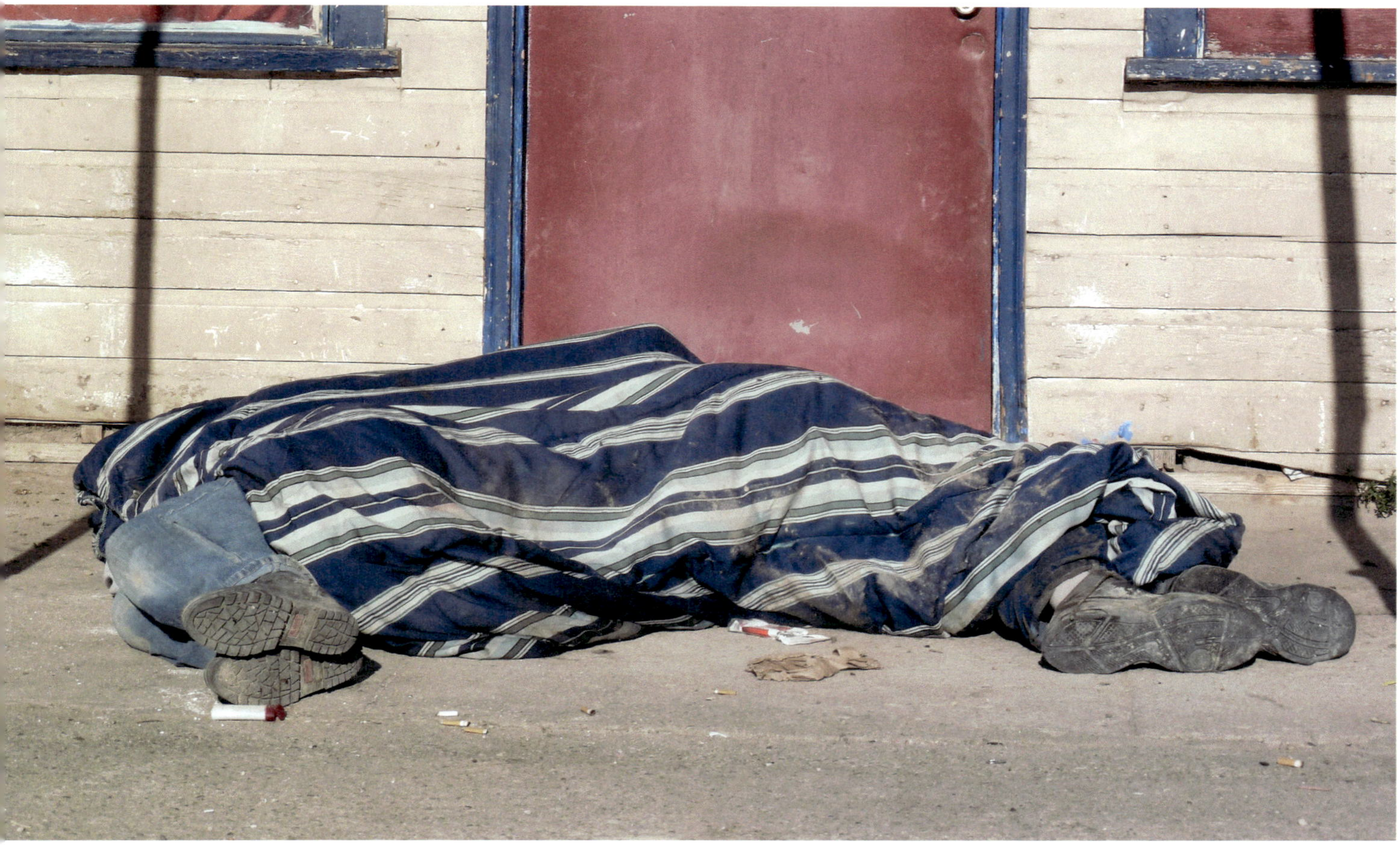

↑ Chief Spotted Elk's camp three weeks after the Wounded Knee Massacre by the US Army, including bodies of several Lakota Sioux people wrapped in blankets in the foreground and US soldiers in the background, 1891.

↓ People covering themselves with a blanket on a street in Whiteclay, 2013.

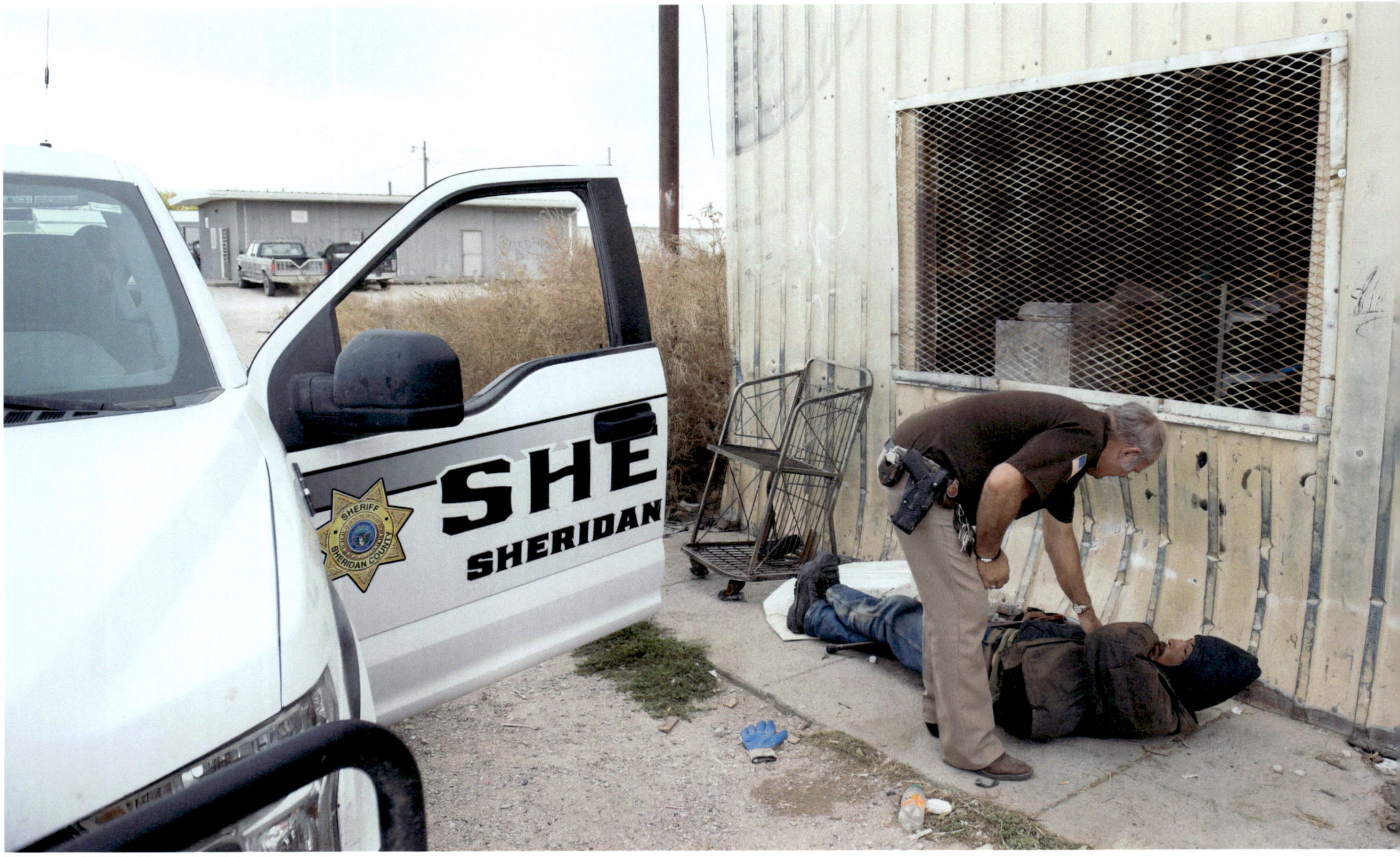
SHE
SHERIDAN
SHERIFF
SHERIDAN COUNTY

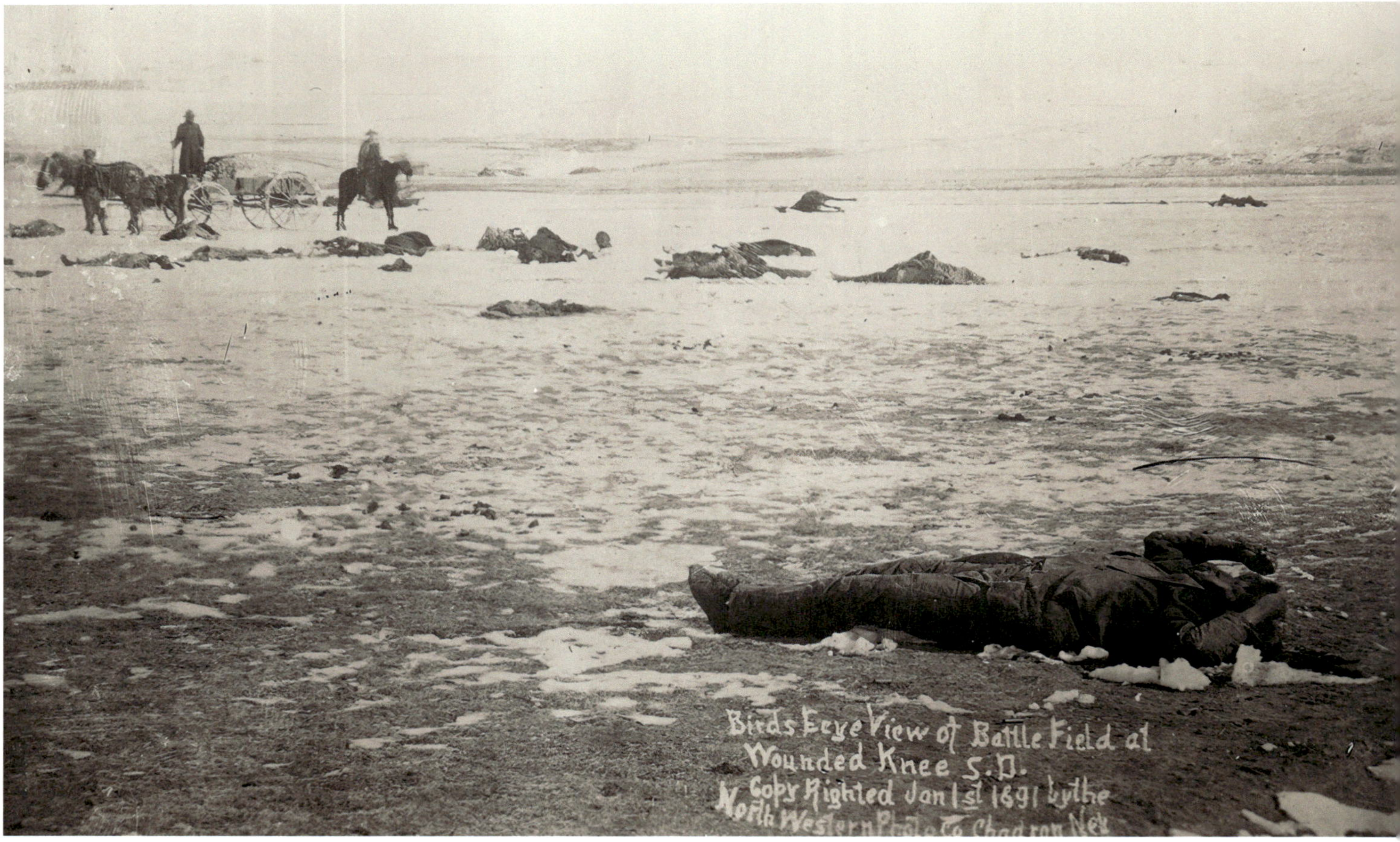
Birds Eeye View of Battle Field at
Wounded Knee S.D.
Copy Righted Jan 1st 1891 by the

↑ Sheridan County Sheriff Terry Robbins checks on a drunk man lying in front of an abandoned building in Whiteclay on Friday, October 14, 2016.

↓ Battlefield at Wounded Knee, South Dakota, 1890.

interpersonal violence, joblessness, suicide, and more), and ultimate healing do not occur at the level of the individual but the community. In this sense, historians Roy Rosenzweig and David Paul Thelen have demonstrated that Native Americans are the only cultural or racial group in the United States to both explain alcoholism within national history and hold the belief that telling the truth about history will solve community problems such as poverty and alcoholism.[23]

As a town, Whiteclay appears quite innocuous; a few buildings on the side of a single road, just as in so many other places in the country. But it's impossible to examine the town's architecture alone. Bare life and Oglala Lakota death predominate in the landscape. The buildings are scarred with artifacts of pain like writing on prison walls, detention centers, or scratches on the inside of a coffin. There are people on the ground out front. The road is lined with crosses for the dead. Pine Ridge Indian Reservation and the adjacent Whiteclay have existed continually for more than a hundred years. It is, in many senses, an intergenerational camp. Indeed, the Pine Ridge Indian Reservation is extraterritorial in a legal sense, and is openly refer to as Prisoner of War Camp #344 by the Oglala Lakota. But the dissonance between the physical and legal nature of Whiteclay and its actualized human impact make it unclear exactly how to define the boundaries of the camp. Is it Pine Ridge Indian Reservation? Is it Whiteclay, Nebraska? Is it both?

Constraining the boundaries of the camp to Pine Ridge Indian Reservation is incongruent with the way the Oglala Lakota have—through interviews, political campaigns, graffiti, and signage—consistently marked Whiteclay as the source of death and pain for their people. The Oglala Lakota Nation utilized the reservation's extraterritorial sovereignty as a protective force by maintaining culturally and historically informed laws such as the complete alcohol ban. While Whiteclay wasn't officially extraterritorial like the reservation, Nebraska did not enforce its own laws, despite the illegal alcohol sales and consumption, rampant sexual violence, and drunk driving, and the Oglala Lakota were not legally able to enforce laws on land outside of their sovereign jurisdiction. The territoriality of alcohol in Whiteclay thus functioned as a mechanism to keep the Oglala Lakota people in an unending and intergenerational camp; a camp that can be seen and defined in the bodies of the people; a camp that flowed without resistance across the state line, just as the little X's marking the "Friendly Indian" settlement did back in 1890–1891.

There are no fences with barbed wire keeping the Oglala Lakota there. There are no police, troops, or armed militia forcing people to drink. The reports coming out of the Indian Health Services hospital on the reservation are incomprehensibly grim, but there are no gallows for hangings, no "death walls" for firing squads, no gas chambers for mass executions. Instead, it's the everyday architecture that perpetuates the elimination of the Oglala Lakota. The absence of police is the infrastructure of this camp. The dogma of free-market capitalism is the infrastructure of this camp. Oglala Lakota bodies lie on Oglala Lakota land in Whiteclay just as they did after the Wounded Knee Massacre on December 29, 1890. Back then, white settlers were rewarded with twenty medals of honor for the courageous massacre.[24] In 2010, the official reward was $414,000 through state

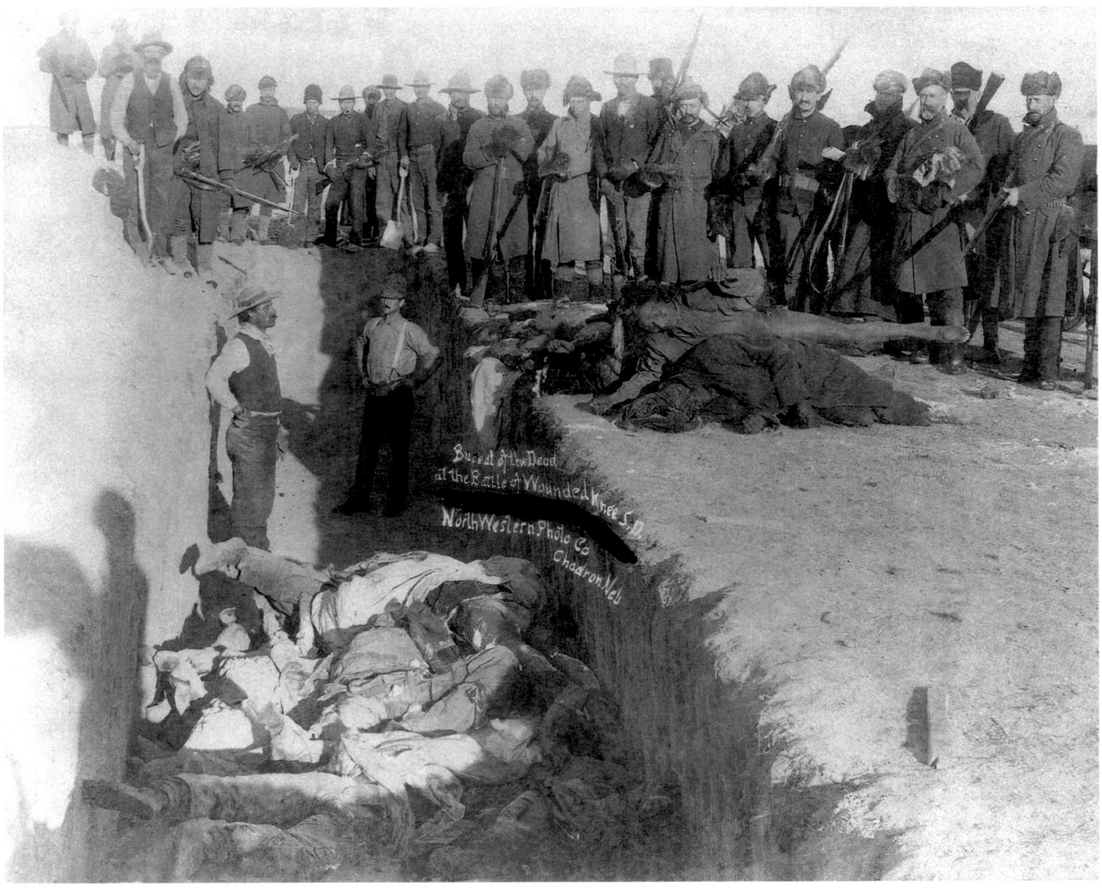

→ Burial of the dead at the Battle of Wounded Knee, South Dakota, 1890.

and federal excise taxes, according to the state's Liquor Control Commission.[25]

The land that was once the "Friendly Indian Reservation in Nebraska" continues to do what it was designed to do back when the reservation was first created. The territoriality of alcohol weaponizes the Oglala Lakotas' post-apocalypse stress syndrome to keep them in an intergenerational camp. In 1890, it mattered little to US troops that the Lakota resistance and theft which supposedly necessitated military intervention was a direct result of the US policy of killing all the buffalo. In the same way, the off-reservation liquor stores marked by Lakota addiction and death are the Oglala Lakotas' own fault. It doesn't matter that they've lived through the apocalypse and survived. And it's absolutely not even worth thinking about who ended their world in the first place.

Postscript In August of 2022, I visited the border between Pine Ridge Indian Reservation and Whiteclay, Nebraska. Architecturally, Whiteclay looked about the same as it did when I first encountered it, walking the streets of Google Earth years prior. Most of the buildings were the same, including the liquor stores. But the border between Whiteclay and Pine Ridge felt entirely different. Whiteclay was fairly empty. The two people who happened to be outside that day were standing, and sober—in stark contrast to the more than twenty people who happened to be sitting or lying on the ground along the highway when the Google Street View car rolled through in 2014. Without liquor licenses, Whiteclay resembled a ghost town; with liquor licenses, it had been the land of the living dead. And now, the drive from Pine Ridge to Whiteclay was just a drive.

It worked. Banning the sale of liquor seems to have disrupted the way the territory currently called Whiteclay had functioned for more than a hundred years. For the first time in a long time, Oglala Lakota people did not appear to be contained there. This wasn't a place for pacification, or a place for people who were drawn away from their families, as it had been when it was the "Friendly Indian Camp" in 1890, or when "Whiteclay" still had liquor licenses. Leaving Whiteclay, I felt confident that the place I was standing was not a camp, at least not on that day. But I couldn't say that was the end of camp in Whiteclay, or that the Friendly Indian Reservation in Nebraska had finally been obliterated. For now, at least, Whiteclay was not the epicenter of Oglala Lakota death.

One legal intervention had effectively rendered the liquor stores powerless. What previously were the epicenter of Oglala death less than five years earlier were now just boarded-up buildings. Regular buildings, displaying signs they no longer needed. It was remarkable how normal they looked. They were not crumbling or destroyed. They looked like they could have been closed for an hour, not years. After I left, however, the shuttered liquor stores started to feel like a threat in my mind's eye. Someone owned those buildings. They didn't sell them, remodel them, or run a different type of store. Instead, they kept them—architectural weapons ready to go. The liquor signs that still hang from their walls were signs of settler hope and a threatening, not at all insincere promise that as soon as liquor licenses are issued again, they will be back.

An earlier version of this essay was originally published by e-flux Architecture in 2022.

1. For a succinct introduction to Lakota medicine wheels, see Black Hill State University's introduction to their on-campus medicine wheel: https://www.bhsu.edu/president/sustainability/Medicine-Wheel.
2. The date on the sign corresponds with the passage of the Indian Appropriations Act of March 3, 1971, which stated that Native American Nations would not be recognized "as an independent nation, tribe, or power with whom the United States may contract by treaty."
3. Timothy Williams, "Indian Beer Bill Stalls; Industry Money Flows," *New York Times*, April 11, 2012.
4. *US Statutes at Large* 2 (1802): 139, 146. *Trade and Intercourse Act of 1802,* Section 21. As cited in "A Review of Research on Alcohol and Drug…"
5. Jill E. Martin, "'The Greatest Evil' Interpretations of Indian Prohibition Laws, 1832–1953," *Great Plains Quarterly* (Winter 2003): 37–38.
6. *US Statutes at Large* 4 (1832): 564. Also see "Native American Nations & State Alcohol Policies: An Analysis," white paper, NABCA Research, August 2017, nabca.org/native-american-nations-state-alcohol-policies-analysis.
7. William Douglas Back, "The Ineffectiveness of Alcohol Prohibition on the Navajo Indian Reservation," *Arizona State Law Journal* 1981, no. 4 (1981): 927–928.
8. The "Friendly Indians" referred to were Oglala Lakota people who had been disarmed, pacified, and held in a densely packed settlement under constant outside supervision. They did not fight with the US troops against the "Hostile Indians" as other tribes had done in the past.
9. Chris Bowing, "A Day in the Life (and Death) of Whiteclay," *Nebraska Quarterly* (2017): 43, https://www.case.org/system/files/media/file/NebQuarter%20Fall%202017.pdf.
10. Bowing, "A Day in the Life (and Death) of Whiteclay."
11. Bowing, "A Day in the Life (and Death) of Whiteclay."
12. Dedrick Asante Muhammad, Rogelio Tec, and Kathy Ramirez, "Racial Wealth Snapshot: American Indians/Native Americans," National Community Reinvestment Coalition, November 18, 2019; "Disparities," Indian Health Services, October 2019.
13. "The Reservation," *Red Cloud Indian School*, https://www.redcloudschool.org/reservation.
14. Timothy Williams, "Indian Beer Bill Stalls; Industry Money Flows," *New York Times*, April 11, 2012.
15. "Future Campaign: Former Lakota Hope Center," *Sober Indian / Dangerous Indian*, accessed December 20, 2020; Nicholas Kristof, "A Battle with the Brewers," *New York Times*, May 5, 2012.
16. "Oglala Sioux Tribe," Suicide Prevention Resource Center, 2012, https://sprc.org/grantee/oglala-sioux-tribe/.
17. Laura Dwyer-Lindgren, Amelia Bertozzi-Villa, Rebecca W. Stubbs, Chloe Morozoff, Johan P. Mackenbach, Frank J. van Lenthe, Ali H. Mokdad, et al., "Inequalities in Life Expectancy among US Counties, 1980 to 2014: Temporal Trends and Key Drivers," *JAMA Internal Medicine* 177, no. 7 (2017):1003–1011, doi:10.1001/jamainternmed.2017.0918. Pine Ridge Indian Reservation is the darkest county on the map, located toward the southwest corner of South Dakota.
18. Jonathan Eig, "Sadly, Sioux Funeral Home Thrives on Chronic Ills of Local Reservation," *Wall Street Journal*, March 5, 2002; Timothy Williams, "Indian Beer Bill Stalls; Industry Money Flows," *New York Times*, April 11, 2012.
19. "Making Indian Country Count: Native Americans and the 2020 Census," NCAI Written Testimony for the Senate Committee on Indian Affairs, National Congress of American Indians, February 14, 2018.
20. Ruth Benedict, *Patterns of Culture* (Boston: Houghton Mifflin, 1989), 80.
21. Vine Deloria Jr., *Custer Died for Your Sins: An Indian Manifesto* (Norman: University of Oklahoma Press, 1988).
22. Lawrence William Gross, *Anishinaabe Ways of Knowing and Being* (Farnham, UK: Ashgate, 2014), 33.
23. White Americans, in contrast, explain alcoholism through personal and family histories. Roy Rosenzweig and David P. Thelen, *The Presence of the Past: Popular Uses of History in American Life* (New York: Columbia University Press, 1998), 173.
24. Dana Lone Hill, "The Wounded Knee Medals of Honor Should be Rescinded," *Guardian*, February 18, 2013.
25. Williams, "Indian Beer Bill Stalls; Industry Money Flows."

p38 Nicole Bengiveno/The New York Times.
p39 Image by uneditedmedia is licensed under CC BY-NC-ND 2.0. uneditedmedia.com.
p40 (top) Western History and Genealogy Department, Denver Public Library, X-31316.
p40 (bottom) John C. H. Grabill Collection, Library of the Congress, Prints and Photographs Division.
p41 ProQuest Congressional.
p43 (top), p45 Library of the Congress, Prints and Photographs Division.
p44 (top) Photo Jake Crandall.
p44 (bottom) Brigham Young University, Lee Library, L. Tom Perry Special Collections.

THE *CORDON SANITAIRE* IN BELGIAN CONGO: BETWEEN PLAN AND REALITY

SIMON DE NYS-KETELS
JOHAN LAGAE
KAREL PROOT

→ Celebrating helicopters as flying *machines à guérir* and technological marvels of Western postwar modernity, these photographs circulated widely, featuring for instance on the cover of the 1958 Expo edition of the periodical *Belgique d'Outremer*. Taken by C. Lamote, who worked for the Centre of Information and Documentation of Belgian Congo and Ruanda-Urundi, the backdrop of the photographs of the *flight sanitaire* is anything but coincidental. With the Sabena Towers of Belgian architect Claude Laurens in the background, colonial propaganda deployed iconic, postwar architecture to underline the victory of Western medicine over tropical disease.

On May 16, 1955, King Baudouin of Belgium arrived by plane in Leopoldville (today Kinshasa), for what would become a highly mediatized trip through Belgian Congo.[1] Colonial authorities had meticulously prepared the event. In the two days before the king's arrival, helicopters poured fourteen tons of DDT over Congo's capital city to reduce the risk of malaria, adding another 3.6 tons the day the king set foot for the first time on Congolese soil.[2] This torrent of DDT, however, was only the culmination of a much broader insecticide campaign that had started after World War II, with rural pesticide experiments, chemical spraying of river banks, and widespread disinfection of stagnant waters in the largest urban centers.

Propaganda from these campaigns was abundant, yet reached its apogee in photographs of the *flight sanitaire*, which featured the medical service's newly purchased helicopter in front of the Sabena building, an icon of the emerging tropical modernist style. These illustrations were part of a longstanding tradition of colonial state propaganda on healthcare that, by the 1950s, sought to convey the image that "the indefatigable ammunition of science" had finally won the "war in the jungle ... against an enemy that buzzes and crawls."[3] Yet as historian Nancy Hunt points out, the "glossy semiotics" that presented Belgian Congo as a "medical model colony," staffed with potent "engineers of happy land," was also meant to mask a "nervous" and often impotent administration deploying "forced labor, chains, the *chicotte* [whip], [and] the color bar" to compensate for its own weaknesses.[4]

Nervous sanitization efforts marked the entire colonial period in Belgian Congo, which often manifested as spatial and urban design. Already during the mid- and late nineteenth century, particular design solutions such as the tropical helmet or bungalow were developed to medically protect Europeans in a continent that was feared at the time as a "White man's grave."[5] By the 1910s, the African body was increasingly being portrayed as the main culprit of contagion, and African urban neighborhoods, or so-called *cités indigènes*, became feared as breeding grounds for malaria-carrying mosquitoes and other insects. Urban planning solutions emerged to respond to these new medical beliefs, and tropical medicine served as a scientific legitimation of urban segregation along racial lines, a process historian Maynard W. Swanson termed the "sanitation syndrome."[6]

Two years after the 1931 Paris conference on "Urban Planning in Colonies and Tropical Countries," organized in the context of the Exposition Coloniale Internationale and attended by delegations of doctors, urbanists, administrators, and architects from several colonial powers, René Schoentjes, a

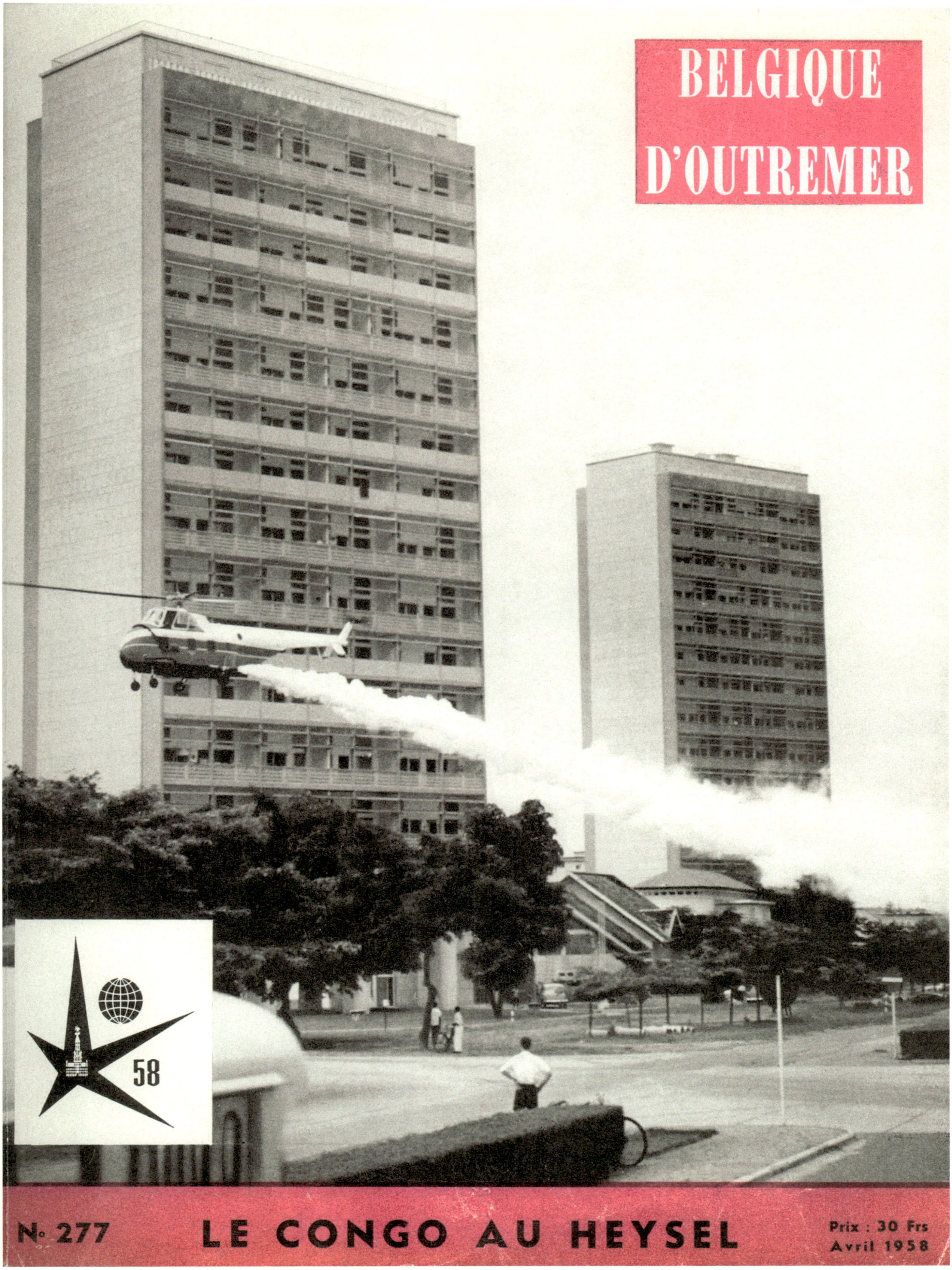
BELGIQUE
D'OUTREMER
58
N° 277
LE CONGO AU HEYSEL
Prix : 30 Frs
Avril 1958

1921

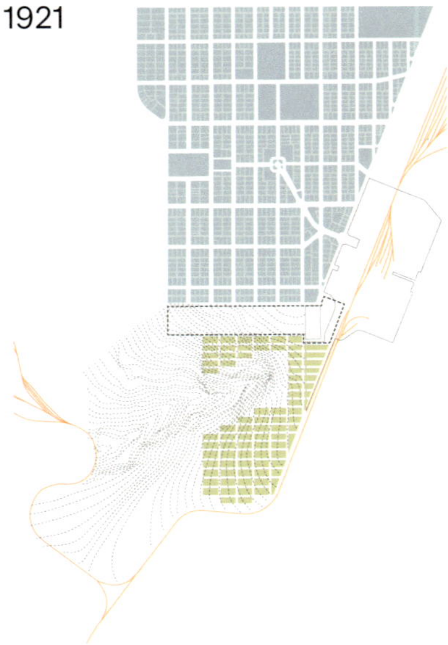

1929

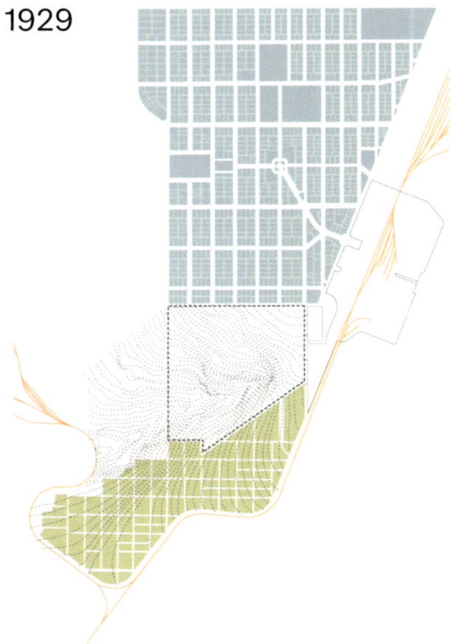

European city
---- *Cordon Sanitaire*
Cité Indigène

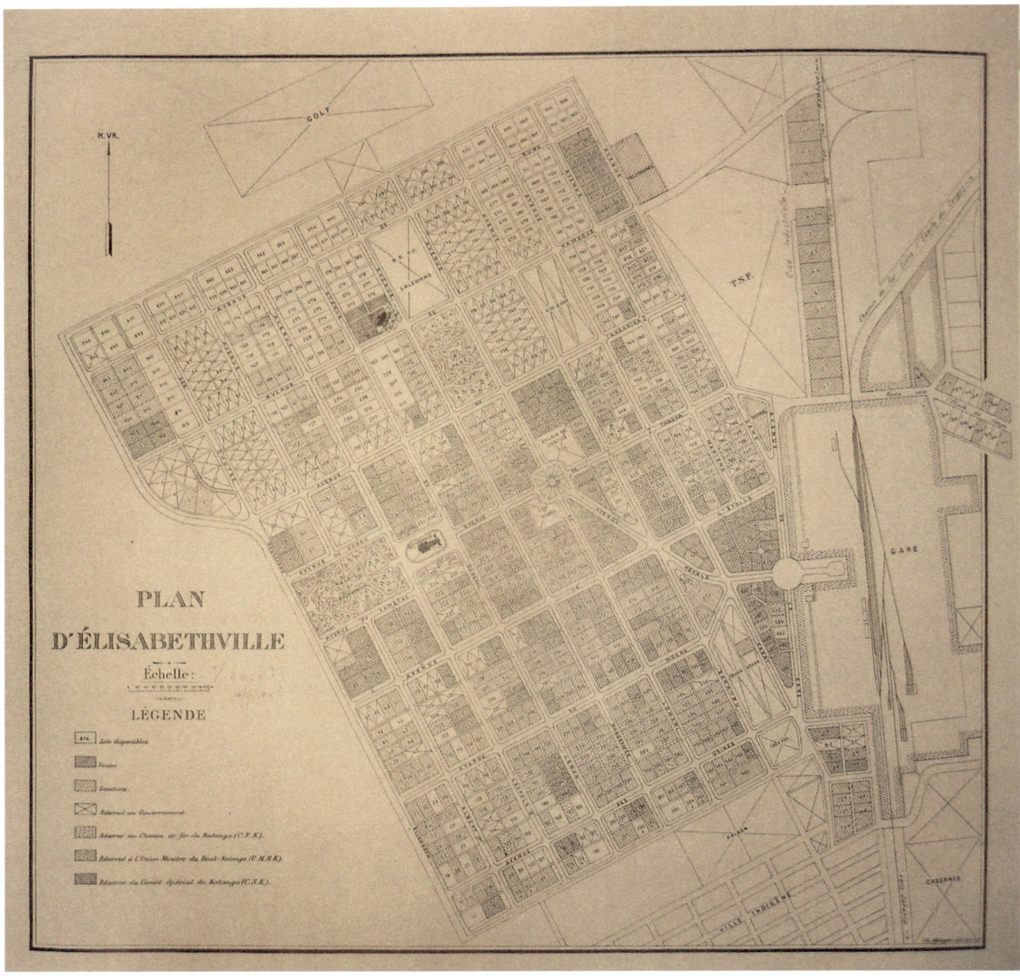

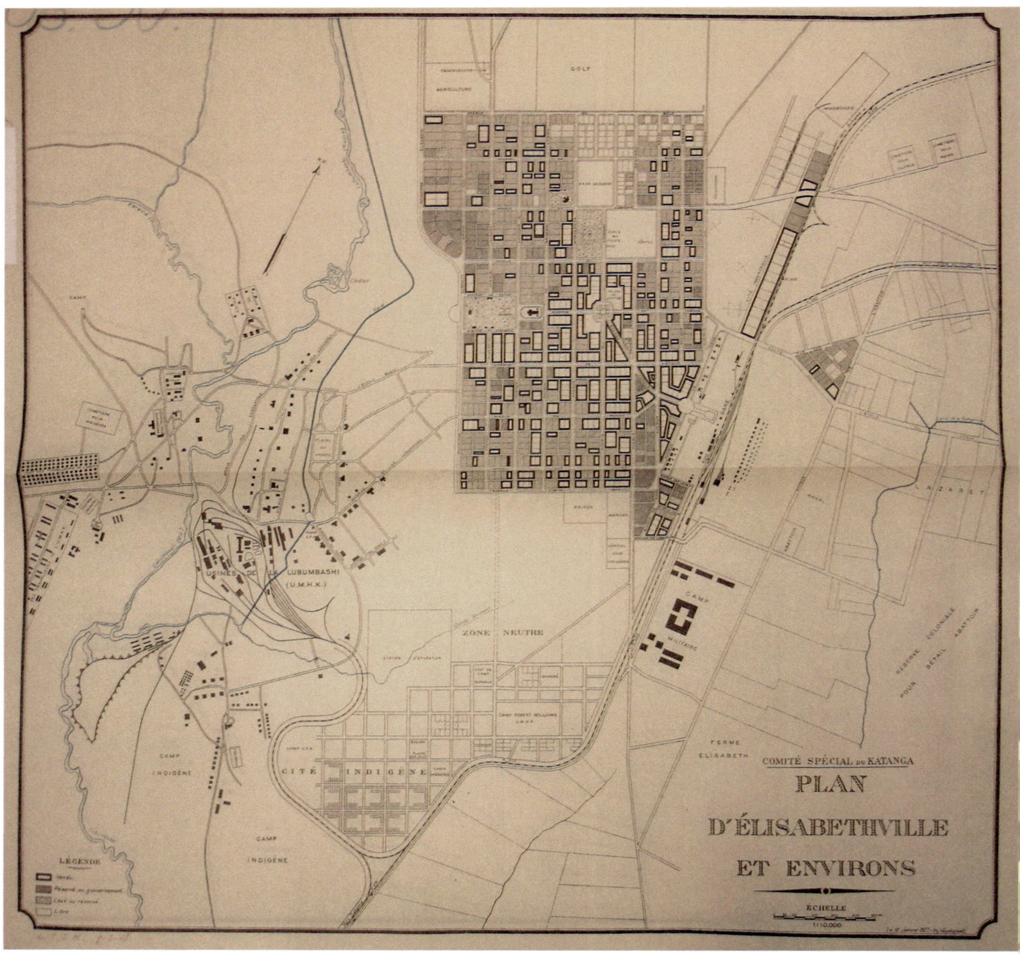

↑ Between 1921 and 1929, Elisabethville's first *cité indigène* was partly demolished and relocated to create a wide buffer zone, the so-called *cordon sanitaire* that anticipated the later institutionalized scheme for an ideal colonial city proposed by Schoentjes. Plan d'Élisabethville, undated map (ca. 1921), and Plan d'Élisabethville, 1927.

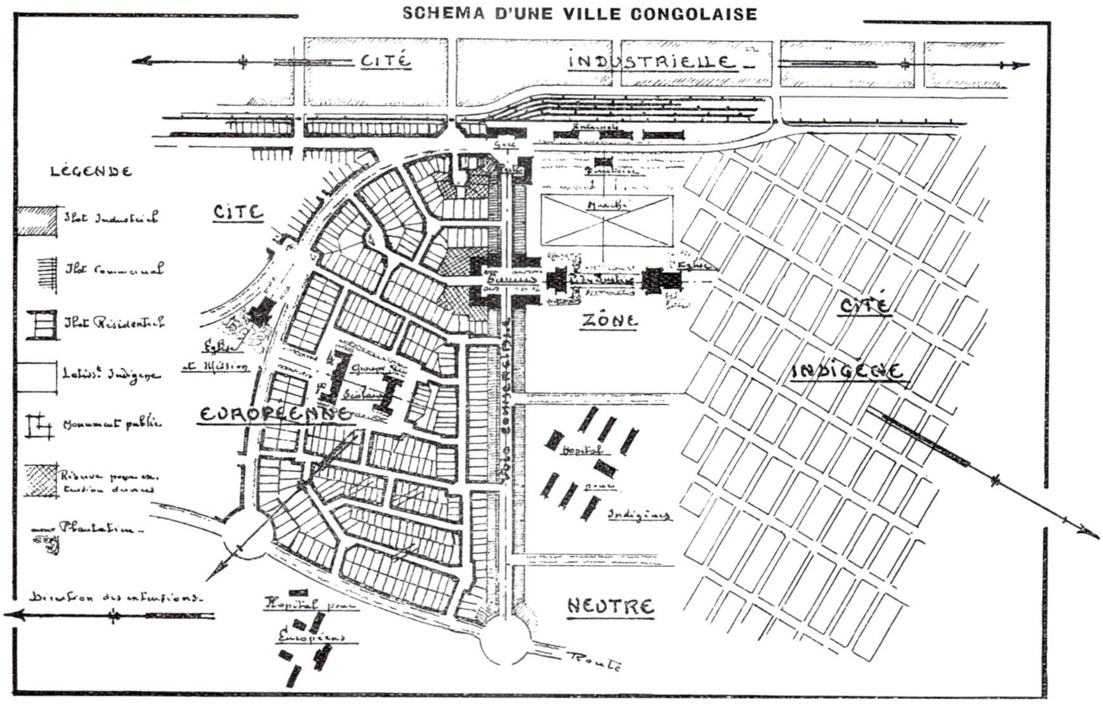

→ "Schéma d'une ville congolaise," published in 1933 by Brussels-based engineer-architect René Schoentjes in his text "Considérations générales sur l'urbanisme au Congo belge," which is based on a talk he gave the previous year to members of the Royal Belgian Colonial Institute.

Belgian engineer-architect employed at the Ministry of Colonies, presented a template to the Royal Belgian Colonial Institute for the design of more orderly, efficient, and sanitized Congolese towns.[7] The plan outlined four constitutive elements: an industrial zone linked to a transport network (railway or river), a European part with a picturesque spatial layout, a *cité indigène* or native town based on a grid structure, and, in between, a *zone neutre* or buffer zone that included some public facilities, such as a hospital for Africans, a market, and a church. The width of this "neutral zone"—500 meters—was defined by the alleged distance a mosquito carrying malaria could fly. Moreover, to further avoid contagion, the European parts of town were to be positioned upwind from the *cité indigène*.[8]

While a segregationist logic had already informed the development of urban centers such as Elisabethville and Matadi in the previous decade, Schoentjes's template quickly started to circulate widely within the colonial administration.[9] Its actual implementation, however, often proved difficult. Throughout the history of urban planning in Belgian Congo, Schoentjes's template, with its clear-cut binary structure between a European and a "native" part separated by a "neutral zone," often remained an idealized scheme rather than a reality on the ground.

Elisabethville: A Model *Cordon Sanitaire*?

Situated in the copper-rich Katanga province, the mining city of Elisabethville (today Lubumbashi) was founded in 1910 and built *ex nihilo* on a plateau.[10] The first urban plans speak to the colonial logic of *mise en valeur* (economic exploitation) and display a grid organization for the *ville européenne*, with wide avenues delineating rows of plots up for sale. An African quarter soon sprang up next to this center, separated by a narrow *non aedificandi* (nonbuilding) zone 170 meters wide. In 1912, the colonial state issued new legislation that required all Africans previously living in the ville européenne to move to this new *cité indigène*.[11] Official sources and early maps suggest that this native town also had spacious lots and wide avenues. Yet locally based doctors would quickly lament its deplorable sanitary conditions and lack of basic urban infrastructure. When in 1921 the Governor General Maurice Lippens visited the area, he was reportedly shocked by the native town's "saleté repoussante"—its "disgusting filth."[12]

Lippens consequently ordered the relocation and reconstruction of the native town further from the European city center, following practices in use at the time in southern Africa.[13] By 1929, the urban form of Elisabethville prefigured Schoentjes's binary scheme with a wide *zone neutre*, which in 1931 was described by the head of the provincial Public Works Service as a *cordon sanitaire:*

> The neutral zone prohibits promiscuity between the white and black population. It separates the two cities by an almost completely open space of at least 500 meters, a distance that corresponds with the regular range of the flight of a mosquito that transmits malaria. The neutral zone thus separates the life of blacks from those of whites, thereby sheltering the latter from the breeding grounds of malaria.[14]

Reality on the ground was different, however. As a pole of economic opportunities, connected to southern Africa via a new railway that ran all the way down to Cape Town and the port city of Beira in Portuguese-ruled Mozambique, Elisabethville immediately attracted *des gens d'ailleurs* (people from elsewhere) and quickly turned into a globalized melting pot. The resulting cosmopolitan nature of Elisabethville's urban society cannot be grasped by the binary framework of colonial discourse. Telling, in this respect, is a 1921 map that indicates a section of the existing native town to be demolished for the new *zone neutre* advocated by Lippens. It lists the names of those who would need to be expropriated, including not only African names but also Belgian and several Italian and Portuguese names. Such non-African presence continued after the implementation of new African quarters in 1921, as so-called "Hindous"—an ambiguous state category that lumped together both Muslim Africans and Indian-Pakistani migrants—occupied parcels in the European city, as well as the new *cité indigène*.[15]

Similarly, Italian and Portuguese residents, together with Greek and Jewish traders, were often described as *blancs de second rang* (second-rate whites).[16] Throughout the colonial period, they often occupied lots on the southern edge of the European part of the city. As "middle figures" in colonial society, they created a commercial contact zone serving primarily African clientele. Further complicating

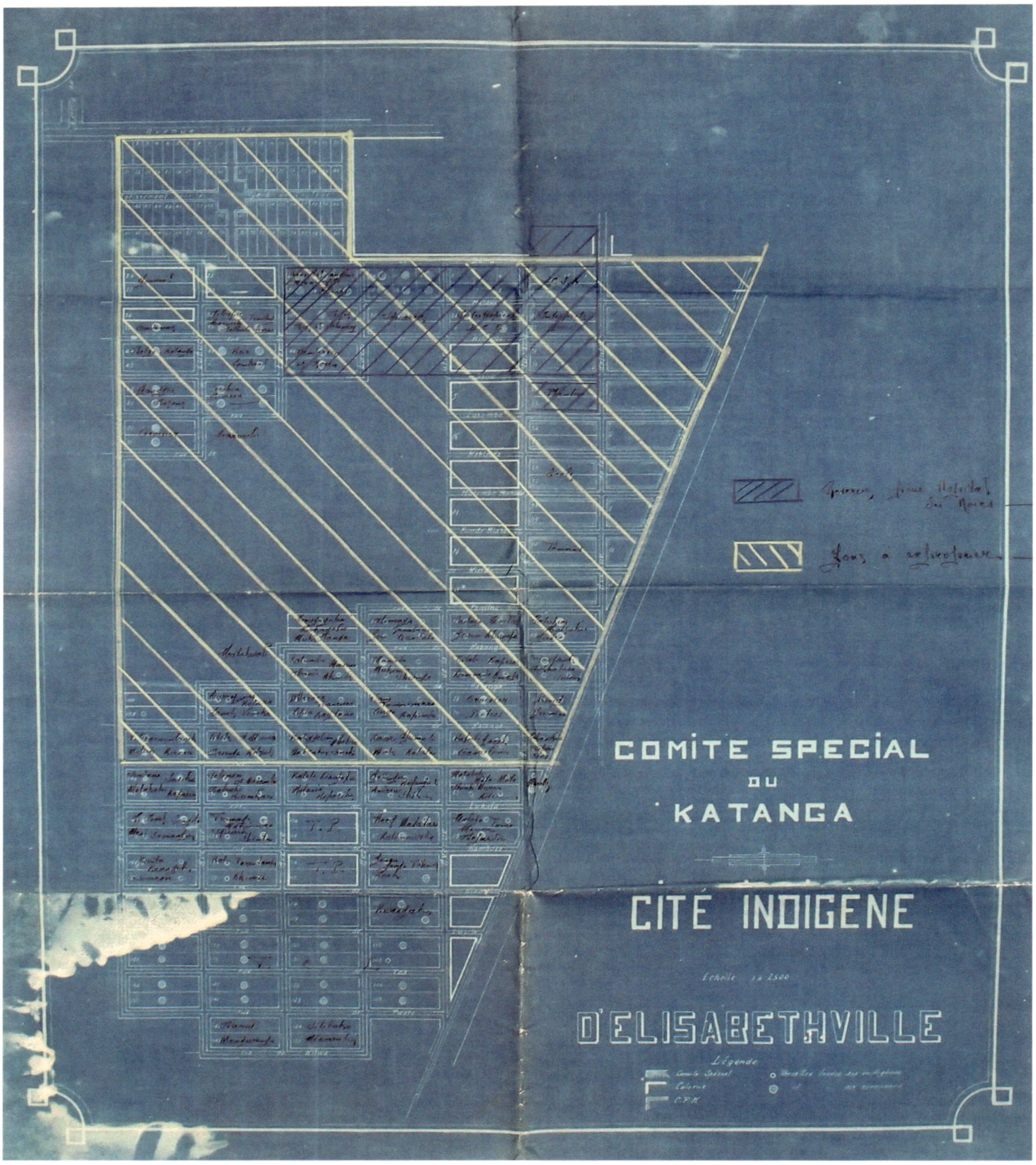

← Comité Spécial du Katanga, Cité indigène d'Elisabethville (Special Committee of Katanga, Native Town of Elisabethville), scale 1/2500, 1921.

→ Sketch included in the minutes of a meeting in Matadi on the issue of the "final location of the native towns and the Construcol workers' camp," September 20, 1928.

this strict division were African domestic servants, who lived in the European city but who would often cross the neutral zone. If the clear-cut *zone neutre* in Elisabethville's maps seems to align neatly with the ideal Congolese city proposed by Schoentjes, it masks a more complex reality, with "middle figures," African domestic servants, and Muslim Africans and Asian migrants living on both sides and blurring the boundaries of the segregated city.

Matadi: A Fictitious *Cordon Sanitaire*

Just as in Elisabethville, the introduction of a *zone neutre* in the port city of Matadi preceded the 1931 Paris conference and the publication of Schoentjes's scheme. An outbreak of yellow fever in late December 1927 impelled local authorities to segregate Europeans and Africans living in the area close to the harbor and the railway yard. This situation had long existed in the area, as Matadi was for centuries the endpoint of important (slave) trade routes linking the Congo River to the Central African hinterland. By the mid-1920s, Matadi had become a modern harbor and a crucial transfer node in the infrastructural network that girded the *mise en valeur* of the colony. Although the epidemic was almost completely contained by the end of January 1928, it had caused major collateral damage by bringing harbor activities to a standstill for two entire months.

The outbreak would also have a major impact on the future of Matadi's urban form.[17] Spatial segregation along racial lines was instigated by doctors who lamented the deplorable sanitary conditions in large parts of the port city, and in its workers' camps in particular. A sketch drawn by an engineer during a meeting in Matadi on September 20, 1928, prefigures Schoentjes's template and adds emphasis on controlling mobility in the segregated city. The drawing suggests that laborers accommodated in the *ville noire* (African city) were to have direct access to the harbor and railway yard via a road that bypassed the *ville européenne*. Similar to the situation of the military camp in Elisabethville, key to this proposal was the strategic location of a police station at the intersection of this road with the *zone neutre*.

Because of the extreme topography of the site—a hilly area with steep, rocky slopes—and the hot and humid climate, urban planning in Matadi proved a complicated affair. The 1928 scheme illustrates how the existing natural environment was instrumentalized for segregating the city along racial lines. The so-called Ravin Léopold, a natural ravine almost perpendicular to the Congo River's edge, with a small stream running through it, was to delimit the *ville européenne*, with a number of bridges connecting to the *ville noire* on the other side. This ran counter the idea of the *zone neutre* acting as a *cordon sanitaire:* not only was the ravine much narrower than the width of 500 meters, but during long periods of the year, it was full of pools of stagnant water—an ideal breeding ground for mosquitos. The colonial authorities seemed well aware of the risks of contagion near the ravine and developed ambitious schemes to canalize the stream that ran through it.

As was often the case in planning matters in interwar Congo, this major reengineering project was deemed financially unfeasible. In the end, pragmatics prevailed. On occasion, squads of African auxiliaries were sent into the ravine with buckets full of petrol to destroy the mosquito larvae, a practice known as *pétrolage* (oiling), in use since the 1910s in several tropical colonies.[18]

The implementation of the 1928 scheme also had another shortcoming. The topography of the site forced the planners to access the new, extensive *ville noire* mainly via a single, centrally located bridge, today known as the Pont Kiamfu, from which a radial network of roads and pathways connected the various *cités* and workers' camps situated uphill. As a consequence of its centrality, the majority of inhabitants of the *ville noire* thus needed to pass through the heart of the *ville européenne* on their way to work. To get to the harbor or railway yard, they would need to walk directly across the central square where the governor's house, the church, the city's main hotel, and various other important buildings serving Matadi's white population were situated.

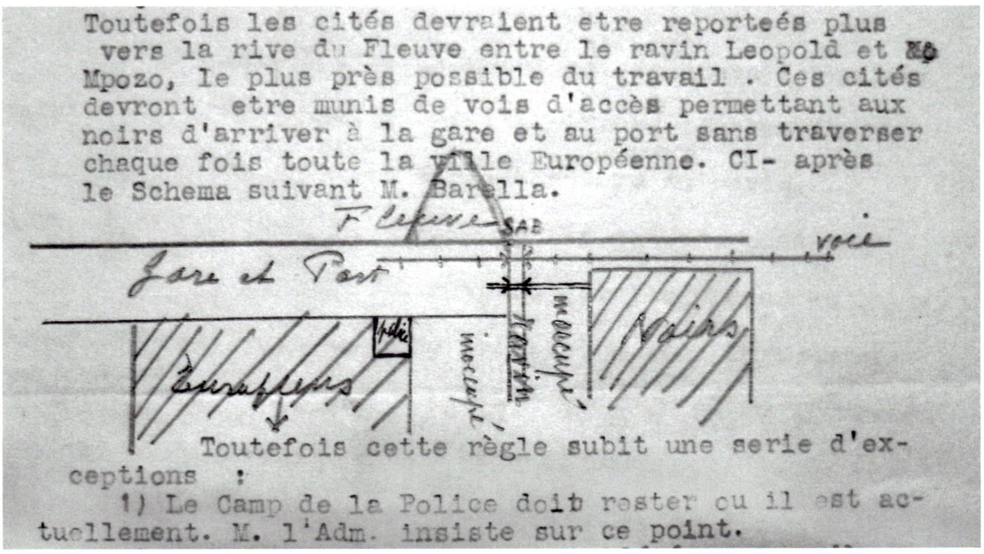
Toutefois les cités devraient etre reporteés plus vers la rive du Fleuve entre le ravin Leopold et la Mpozo, le plus près possible du travail . Ces cités devront etre munis de vois d'accès permettant aux noirs d'arriver à la gare et au port sans traverser chaque fois toute la ville Européenne. CI- après le Schema suivant M. Barella.

Toutefois cette règle subit une serie d'exceptions :

1) Le Camp de la Police doit rester ou il est actuellement. M. l'Adm. insiste sur ce point.

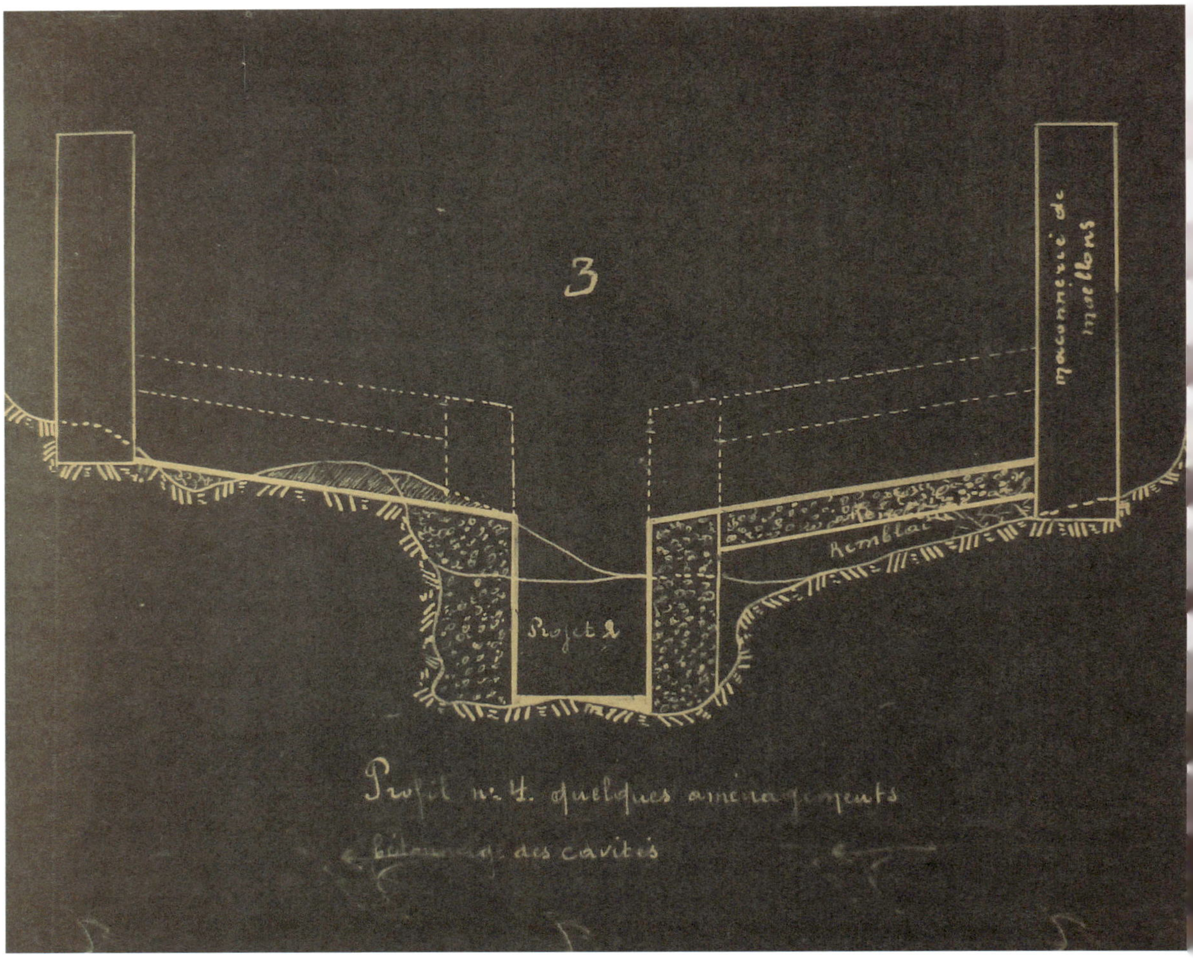

→ Proposal to canalize the stream running through Ravin Léopold, designed by the technical services of the Ministry of Colonies in Brussels, ca. 1932. Source file "Assainissement des ravins à Matadi."

Even with the police station and a large army camp located close to the bridge, in the end this bridge would prove to be the city's Achilles' heel. When on November 26, 1945, the dockworkers went on strike, they immediately blocked the bridge, forcing the port city into a complete standstill for three full days. The Police Urbain, a particular faction within Matadi's police squad, together with the colonial army, or Force Publique, crushed the strike with force, killing several people.[19] Rather than displaying the power of the colonial state, the event starkly reveals the fragility of the colonial spatial strategy. Colonial urban planners were unable to anticipate, let alone cope with, resistance, as lines drawn by colonial powers on urban maps imagined as neat borders quickly proved fictitious on the ground.

Leopoldville: The Porous *Cordon Sanitaire*

The complexity of successfully implementing a *cordon sanitaire* became particularly evident in Leopoldville in the 1930s. During a mission to the city in 1928 and 1929, René Schoentjes was shocked by what he described as an inexcusable "interpenetrating" of the *ville européenne* and the *cité indigène*. His 1933 "Schéma d'une ville congolaise" was, in fact, in large part intended as a way to solve this "deplorable" situation of spatial mixing that, he stressed, was "not allowed in any colony."[20] Several local policymakers had already lamented the "promiscuity" caused by such "coexistence of two races" and had initiated a buffer zone to separate white and black neighborhoods by the end of the 1920s. Schoentjes's project sought to segregate Leopoldville's commercial center based on the template he had presented to the members of the Royal Belgian Colonial Institute in 1932.

As it made an abstraction of an already existing, dense urban fabric that accommodated the trade activities of the city's "middle figures," the implementation of the planned *zone neutre* in Léopoldville proved more cumbersome than Schoentjes anticipated. Expropriating the group was too expensive, and so the *zone neutre*, initially conceived as an 800-meter-wide no-man's land, was implemented as an incomplete, narrow, and fragmented belt of buffer zones. Moreover, the existing hospital for Africans was situated on the "wrong," European side of the *cordon sanitaire*, while according to Schoentjes's project, it should have been situated within the *cité indigène*. As was argued in a local popular newspaper, this "out-of-place" hospital went against any sound policy of urban sanitization. This was endorsed by several high-ranking officials, who declared it was impossible to ensure public hygiene "with the maintenance of the hospital of Blacks at its current location."[21]

Despite extensive protest, the hospital was never relocated, as again no budget was available for the operation. In the end, colonial authorities erected a wall to seal off the hospital as an enclave and mask the life inside the facility, despite the fact that its very location defied the city's new segregated order. Already questionable as an effective sanitary strategy, neither the wall nor the *cordon sanitaire* were able to stop the flows of sick African patients "penetrating" the *ville européenne* on their way to the hospital. This phenomenon would continue to frustrate European residents over the next decades. Due to the fragmented nature of the *cordon sanitaire* in Leopoldville, the porosity of the colonial city became an intrinsic part of urban life, even more so than in Elisabethville or Matadi.

Colonial Residues of the "Nervous State"

The "segregation mania" that pervaded colonial Africa during the interwar years went hand in hand with colonial authorities' obsessive desire to sanitize colonial cities across the continent.[22] This resulted in a widely agreed practice of dividing cities through the introduction of a *zone neutre* that was to act as a *cordon sanitaire* between the *ville européenne* and the *ville noire*. Yet, as the histories of Elisabethville, Matadi, and Leopoldville demonstrate, such spatial policies were cumbersome and most often proved ineffective. Despite medical circles increasingly starting to question the "politics of skin" in the postwar years, local urban authorities continued to stubbornly pursue racial segregation—often by shrouding it in a functionalist discourse of urban zoning.[23] Caught between plan and reality, the histories of segregation in Congolese cities, then, speak of what historian Nancy Hunt has evocatively called the "nervous" colonial state, a term that highlights how these states, rather than being omnipotent, well-oiled machines, were "unsettled, combining vigor, force, and determination with excitation, weakness, timidity."[24]

If repressive excess and impotence had embodied the "two faces" of the "nervous state," "juxtaposing the clinical and the carceral" in the interwar planning and policing of the *cordon sanitaire*, the postwar insecticide campaigns marked its crude apogee.[25] In Leopoldville and beyond, the neutral zone proved more porous than planned, and colonial authorities quickly resorted to chemicals to maintain their medical ambitions. Although decontaminating the European parts of town had been the first priority, which authorities widely disseminated as colonial propaganda, the capital's medical service redirected its 1952 DDT campaign toward Congolese *cités indigènes*, which were still feared as the hotbed of tropical disease. Here, the colonial administration went much further than sending helicopters to decontaminate water pools and public spaces from afar. Mobile squads were dispatched on the ground, checking over fifty thousand African parcels annually, and went door to door, lining up all of the area's African habitants outside their houses for chemical spraying before entering the privacy of the home to (de)contaminate the interior, often in the presence of the inhabitants. These campaigns proved not only extremely costly but also increasingly ineffective, as, by the late fifties, insects developing resistance against DDT had become a recurring problem.[26]

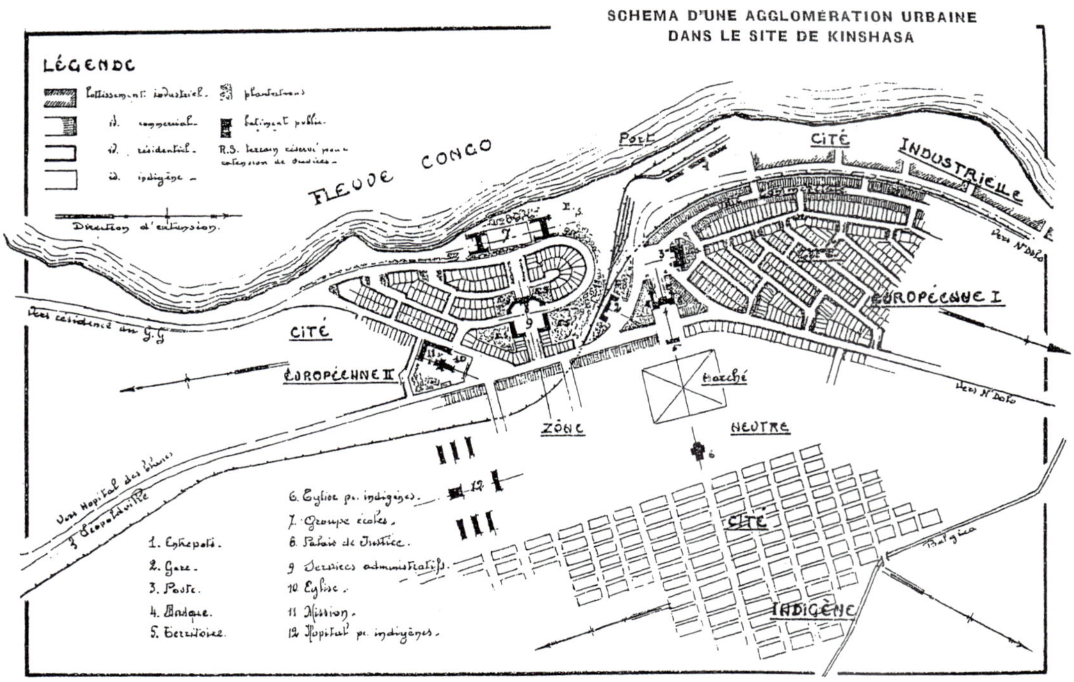

← Scheme of an urban agglomeration at the site of Léopoldville, including the introduction of a *zone neutre*. Reproduced from Réné Schoentjes, "Considérations générales sur l'urbanisme au Congo belge," *Institut Royal Colonial Belge, Bulletin des Séances* 2 (1933): 528–572.

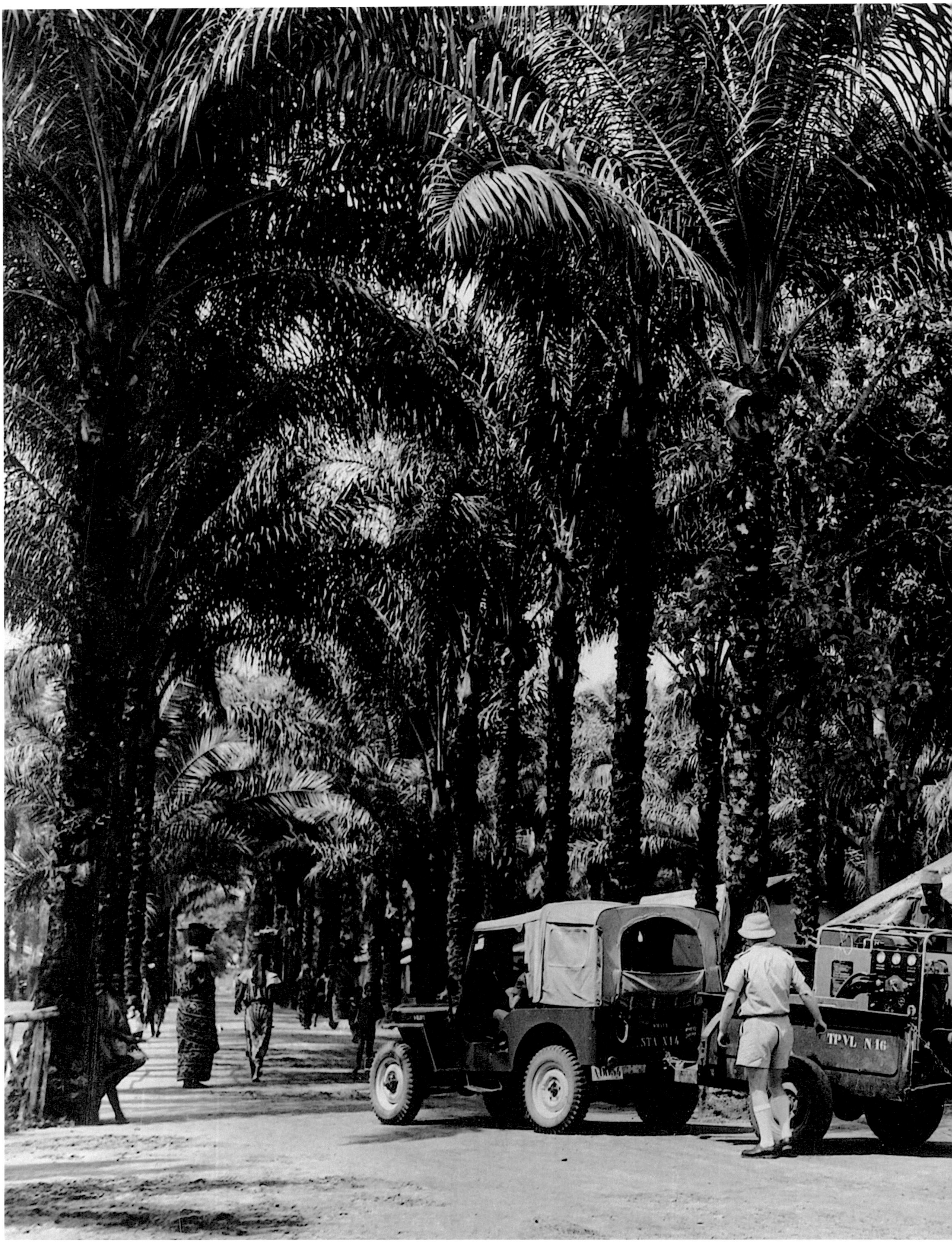

↑ Towed thermal fogger in the *cité indigène* of Léopoldville, 1950s. Photo: C. Lamote.

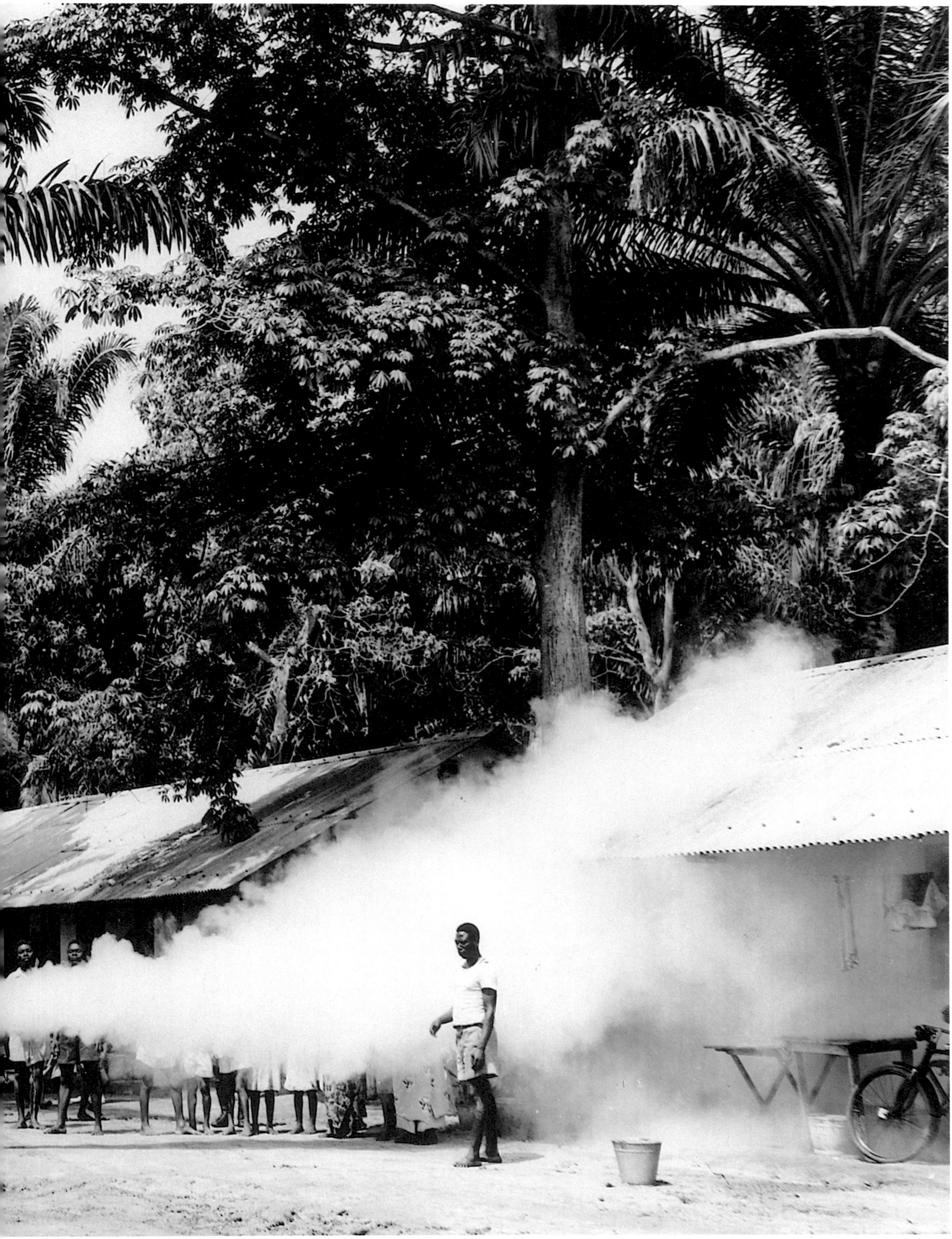

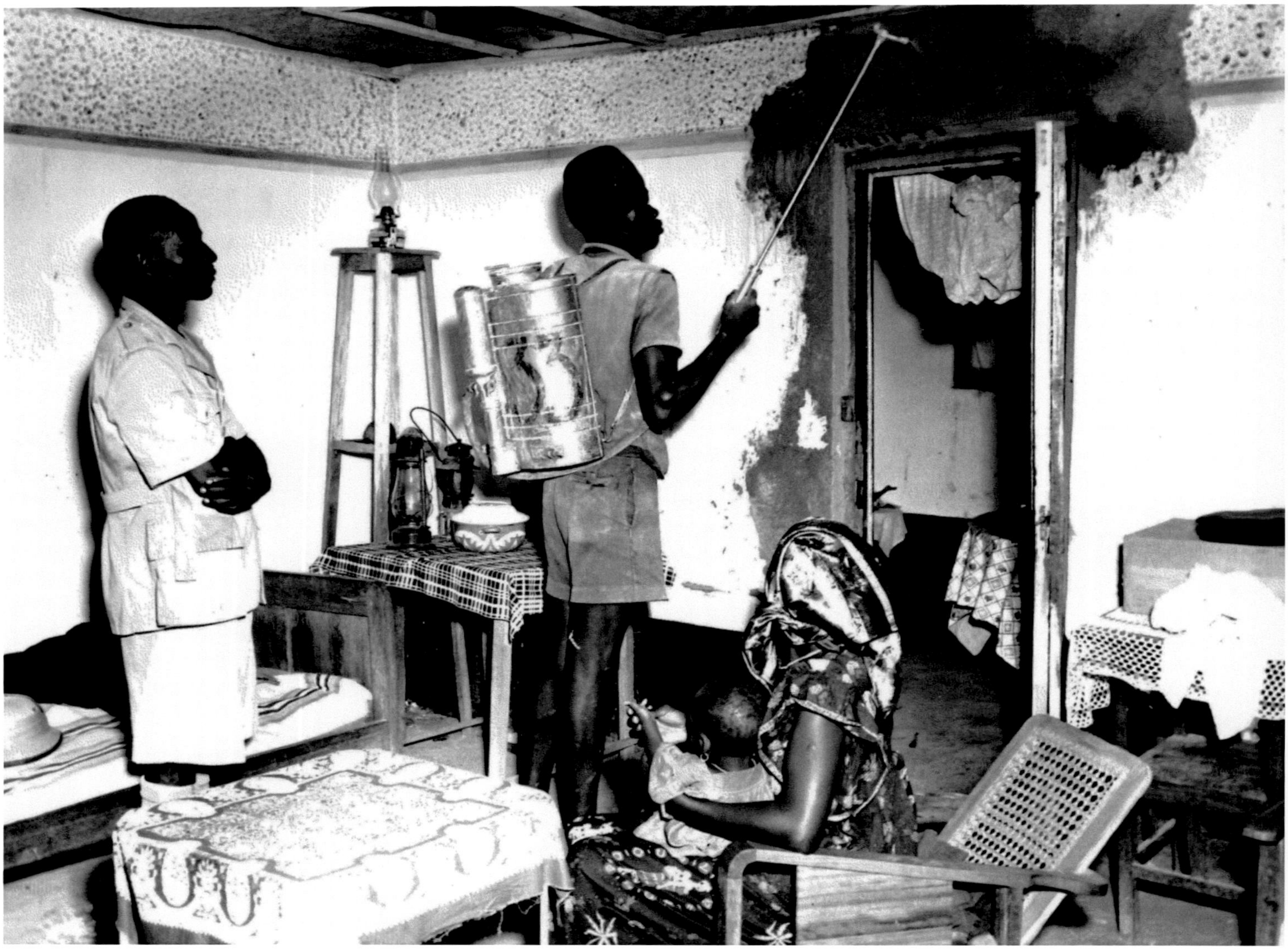

Investigating these practices of planning and pesticides not only allows us to properly understand the extent of the colonial "nervous state," but also forces us to think more explicitly about the residues of its "colonial toxicity."[27] Whereas the *cordon sanitaire* formerly separated black and white, and continues to spatially structure the city's social strata, the aftereffects of years of chemical campaigns likely go beyond urban form. Just as the carcinogenic fallout of these invasive programs must have been extensive, epidemiologists are still piecing together the extent to which such campaigns have increased mosquito resistance against chemicals and contributed to the prevalence of malaria in Congo's urban centers today.[28] Even if such residues are hard to trace, resurfacing these histories of toxic urbanism not only underlines how coercion and weakness crudely coincided in the colonial city as symptoms of the "nervous state." It also reveals that the fallout of such toxic urbanisms is not confined to the (colonial) past, but impacts lives and space in the present and future.

↑ Indoor spraying in a Congolese household, Bas-Congo, 1951. Photo: H. Goldstein.

1. We will refer to cities in today's DRC using their colonial place names as they also appear in the historical sources and maps on which this article is based. We will thus write Leopoldville instead of Kinshasa, and Elisabethville instead of Lubumbashi, while the name of the port city Matadi has remained the same.
2. By then, DDT had been in use in Congo for some years, particularly in Leopoldville, with its booming population. A mere decade after it was introduced, the use of DDT was banned due to the growing recognition of its toxicity. For a discussion of the use of DDT in colonial Congo, see Karel Proot, "Clouds of Health: Insecticide Use as a Lens for Writing an (Urban) History in Belgian Congo" (master's diss., Ghent University, 2023).
3. John Latouche and André Cauvin, *Congo* (New York: Willow, White & Co, 1945), 100, 110.
4. Nancy Rose Hunt, *A Nervous State: Violence, Remedies, and Reverie in Colonial Congo* (Durham: Duke University Press, 2016), 10. Hunt borrows the phrase "engineers of happy land" from Rudolf Mrázek, *Engineers of Happy Land: Technology and Nationalism in a Colony* (Princeton: Princeton University Press, 2002).
5. Philip D. Curtin, "'The White Man's Grave': Image and Reality, 1780–1850," *Journal of British Studies* 1, no. 1 (1961): 94–110; Daniel R. Headrick, *The Tools of Empire: Technology and European Imperialism in the Nineteenth Century* (New York: Oxford University Press, 1981), 59.
6. Maynard W. Swanson, "The Sanitation Syndrome: Bubonic Plague and Urban Native Policy in the Cape Colony, 1900–1909," *Journal of African History* 18, no. 3 (1977): 387–410.
7. For the broader context of this event, see Patricia A. Morton, *Hybrid Modernities: Architecture and Representation at the 1931 Colonial Exposition, Paris* (Cambridge, MA: MIT Press, 2000).
8. René Schoentjes, "Considérations générales sur l'urbanisme au Congo Belge," *Institut Royal Colonial Belge, Bulletin des Séances* 2 (1933): 542–543.
9. These measures indicate how from the early 1930s onward spatial segregation in Belgian Congo "evolved from an improvised practice into an institutionalized policy." See Luce Beeckmans and Johan Lagae, "Kinshasa's Syndrome-Planning in Historical Perspective: From Belgian Colonial Capital to Self-Constructed Megalopolis," in *Urban Planning in Sub-Saharan Africa: Colonial and Post-Colonial Planning Cultures*, ed. Carlos Nunes Silva (New York: Routledge, 2015), 205.
10. Even if it was previously uninhabited, this space was not a *terre vacante* as colonial law would define it, but a territory embedded with indigenous claims and uses. For a history of the city, see Maurice Amuri Mpala-Lutebele, ed., *Lubumbashi, cent ans d'histoire* (Paris: L'Harmattan, 2013).
11. Sofie Boonen, "Une ville construite par des 'gens d'ailleurs': Développement urbain et 'gouvernementalité' coloniale à Elisabethville (RDC)" (PhD diss., Ghent University, 2019), 136.
12. Lippens cited in F. Grévisse, *Le centre extra-coutumier d'Élisabethville: quelques aspects de la politique indigène du Haut-Katanga industriel* (Brussels: Institut Royal Colonial Belge, 1951), 5–6.
13. Carl Nightingale, *Segregation: A Global History of Divided Cities* (Chicago: University of Chicago Press, 2012).
14. R. Hins, "L'urbanisme au Katanga," *Essor du Congo*, special issue published on the occasion of the 1931 Elisabethville International Exhibition (1931).
15. Boonen, "Une ville construite par des 'gens d'ailleurs,'" 308–312.
16. Michel Lwamba Bilonda, *Histoire de l'onomastique d'avenues et de places publiques de la ville de Lubumbashi (de 1910 à nos jours)* (Lubumbashi: Presses Universitaires de Lubumbashi, 2001).
17. Johan Lagae, Jacob Sabakinu Kivulu, and Luce Beeckmans, "Pour Matadi la question [de la ségrégation] est encore plus grave qu'ailleurs: The Making and Shaping of a Congolese Port City during the Interwar Years," in *The Belgian Congo between the Two World Wars*, ed. J. Vanderlinden (Brussels: Koninklijke Academie voor Overzeese Wetenschappen, 2019), 129–158.
18. This practice of *pétrolage* was only one of the strategies of so-called *petit assainissement* (minor sanitation), others being *désherbage* (clearing of vegetation), *curage* (leveling ground to eliminate standing water), and the removal of refuse. See Proot, "Clouds of Health," 67.
19. Johan Lagae and Jacob Sabakinu Kivilu, "Policing the City: Colonial Urban Planning and the Politics of Order in the Port City of Matadi, DR Congo, 1928–1960" (International Conference African Urban Planning, Lisbon, 2017). On colonial policing, see Simon De Nys-Ketels, "Colonial Policing and Urban Space in the Notorious Commune Rouge of Lubumbashi, Democratic Republic of Congo," *Urban History* 49, no. 1 (2022): 129–148.
20. Schoentjes, "Considérations générales sur l'urbanisme au Congo Belge," 542–543.
21. Note from Head-Engineer Gustave Itten, File GG 14927, Belgian State Archives, Brussels. For a full analysis see Simon De Nys-Ketels et al., "Spatial Governmentality and Everyday Hospital Life in Colonial and Postcolonial DR Congo," in *Neocolonialism and Built Heritage: Echoes of Empire in Asia, Africa, the Middle East and Europe*, ed. Daniel Coslett (New York: Routledge, 2019), 147–167; Simon De Nys-Ketels, "Myths and Realities of the Belgian Medical Model Colony: A Genealogy" (PhD diss., Ghent University, 2021), 223–252.
22. Nightingale, *Segregation*.
23. Johan Lagae, Sofie Boonen, and Maarten Liefooghe, "Fissures dans le 'cordon sanitaire': architecture hospitalière et ségrégation urbaine à Lubumbashi, 1920–1960," in Mpala-Lutubele, *Lubumbashi, cent ans d'histoire*, 247–261; Benoît Henriet, *Policing in Colonial Empires: Cases, Connections, Boundaries (ca. 1850–1970)*, ed. Emmanuel Blanchard, Marieke Bloembergen, and Amandine Lauro (New York: Peter Lang, 2017).
24. Hunt, *A Nervous State*, 5.
25. Hunt, *A Nervous Sate*, 167–168.
26. Proot, "Clouds of Health," 135.
27. Samia Henni, *Colonial Toxicity : Rehearsing French Radioactive Architecture and Landscape in the Sahara* (Amsterdam: Framer Framed, 2024).
28. Proot, "Clouds of Health."

p49 *Belgique d'Outremer*, no. 277 (April 1958), collection Johan Lagae.
p50 Courtesy of Fund Cartothèque, National Archives 2 – Joseph Cuvelier repository.
p51, 57 Reproduced from René Schoentjes, "Considérations générales sur l'urbanisme au Congo belge," *Institut Royal Colonial Belge, Bulletin des Séances* 2 (1933): 528–572.
p52, 53, 54 Courtesy of Belgian State Archives, Brussels: File GG 15.840 (52), GG 16485 (53), GG 1477 (54), Courtesy of Fund Cartothèque, National Archives 2 – Joseph Cuvelier repository.
p56–57 Photo: C. Lamote. Collection of Royal Museum for Central Africa (RMCA), Tervuren. HP.1956.15.10218.
p58 Photo: H. Goldstein. Ghent University, BIB. FOT.001216/01. © 2024 Goldstein – SOFAM.

"THE FINEST IMMIGRATION STATION IN THE WORLD"

JEREMY LEE WOLIN

The Covid-19 pandemic provided a recent reminder that international borders pervade far beyond their physical sites in order to alienate from within. In the United States, one study found that people who read and answered personal questions about Covid-19 were roughly twice as likely to choose not to live with Hispanic and Asian roommates as those who did not.[1] Yet reminders of the long history of racial ostracism often lay in plain sight. On the very same day that former House Speaker Nancy Pelosi traveled to San Francisco's Chinatown to support its businesses hard-hit by the anti-Chinese hysteria of the early pandemic, one of the Bay Area's largest dailies ran a headline posing the question, "Where did our quarantine facilities go?" atop an image of nearby Angel Island.[2]

Angel Island first served as a Miwok fishing ground before the Union Army established a fort on its Western tip during the Civil War.[3] In 1888, a smallpox outbreak in Hong Kong prompted the US Public Health Service to establish a quarantine facility for ships arriving from the Pacific on Angel Island's Ayala Cove. The quarantine station's forty-five structures included a fumigation shed, a hospital, employee lodgings, and quarantine facilities accommodating up to 500 people.[4] From the start, however, race and class determined who was quarantined on Angel Island. First-class passengers often disembarked in San Francisco after cursory checks in the privacy of their own cabins, while passengers in steerage,

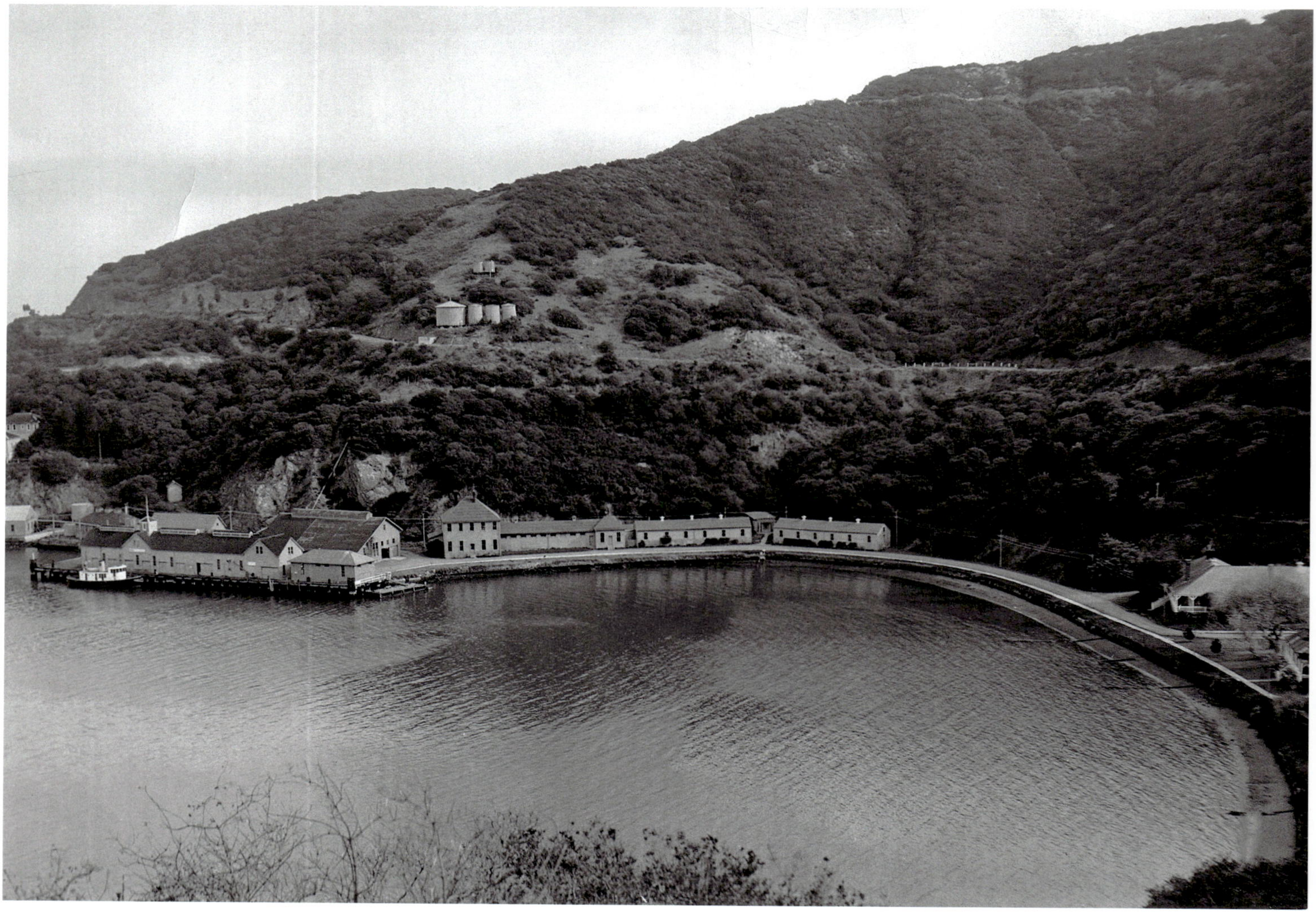

← The forty-five structures of the quarantine station, Ayala Cove, 1948.

→ Well before the station was completed, the *San Francisco Chronicle* printed a full page of praise for the station's architect.

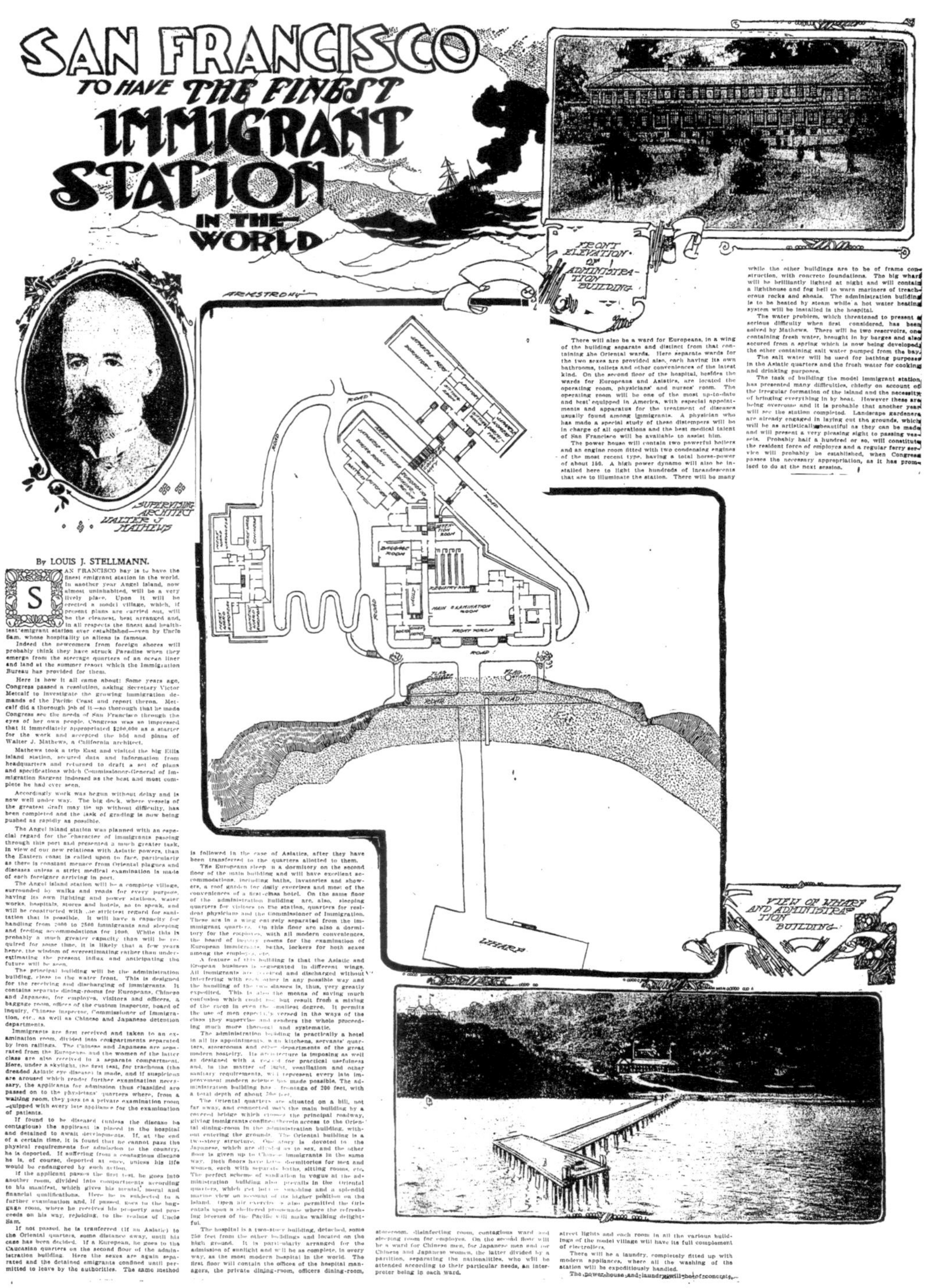
SAN FRANCISCO
TO HAVE THE FINEST
IMMIGRANT
STATION
IN THE
WORLD
SUPERVISING ARCHITECT WALTER J. MATHEWS
FRONT ELEVATION OF ADMINISTRATION BUILDING
VIEW OF WHARF AND ADMINISTRATION BUILDING
By LOUIS J. STELLMANN.

largely Asian laborers, spent two weeks on the island while officials bathed and inspected them.[5]

Segregated quarantine procedures reflected the anti-Chinese, medicalized political atmosphere of the time. In 1862, American surgeon Arthur B. Stout conflated Chinese labor with racial impurity and national decay.[6] Despite the critical role of Chinese labor in the construction of the transcontinental railroad in the 1860s, by 1882 the *Daily Alta California* surmised that "the State is diseased by the presence of the Chinese," and the federal Chinese Restriction Act from the same year made working-class Chinese men the first group to be barred from naturalization.[7] Six years later, President Grover Cleveland expanded the ban, describing the arrival of Chinese labor as "injurious to both nations."[8] One year after that, the San Francisco satirical weekly, *The Wasp*, published a political cartoon depicting Uncle Sam struggling to stop a flow of Chinese men depicted as the size of rodents, invoking a plague.

With Chinese labor seen as a disease to the country, Angel Island became an ideal laboratory for testing new modes of prevention. In 1910, the US Immigration Bureau replaced the Ayala Cove quarantine station with a larger immigration station complex to its northeast. Over the next three decades, the Angel Island Immigration Station processed about half a million people, deported about one in five, and

↑ The interior divisions of the administration building separated arrivals by race and gender for the duration of their stays. Daniel Quan, administration building, ground-floor plan, 2015.

↓ An original drawing of the immigration station complex showing the four main buildings before the construction of the staff cottages and fumigation shed. Walter J. Mathews, Angel Island Immigration Station, 1907.

→ Julia Morgan's spartan staff cottages allowed station workers to live on the island rather than take the ferry daily. Julia Morgan, four-room cottage, foundation, plan, and section, 1910.

detained several hundred at once.[9] For those allowed entry to the mainland, Angel Island disciplined new arrivals into a rigid racial hierarchy in which they would be marked as perpetually foreign. The station's brutality was imposed on a broad swath of Pacific passengers, giving it an outsized role as a tool of Chinese exclusion. Lengthy investigations used to enforce the Chinese Exclusion Acts created prolonged detention periods that required specific architectures of containment, and the complexity of the station was a point of pride within the city of San Francisco. Three years before the station opened in 1910, the *San Francisco Chronicle* lauded its anticipated methods of segregating and analyzing arrivals, calling it "The Finest Immigration Station in the World."[10]

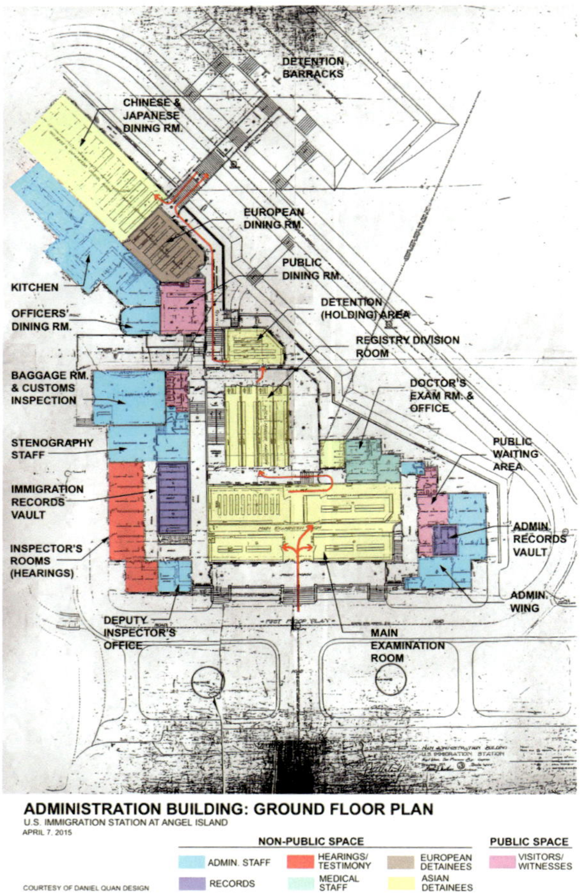

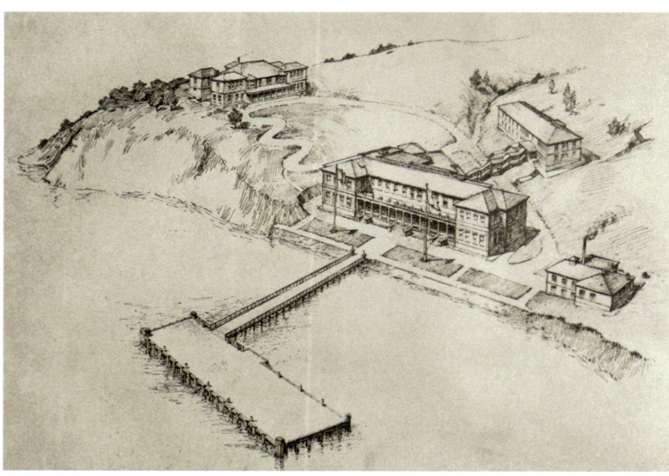

Designing Segregation

When Walter J. Mathews received the commission to design the station in 1904, his oeuvre was limited to Bay Area municipal buildings.[11] Mathews conducted considerable research for the project, visiting warehouses used as immigration detention barracks on the mainland and traveling to Ellis Island to observe the main station building completed there in 1900.[12] Ellis Island's new complex inspired Mathews, who modeled Angel Island on its East Coast predecessor by organizing the station in a similar "cottage system" of multiple buildings, each devoted to a single purpose: hospital, barracks, powerhouse, and administration. The result is Ellis Island's typology scaled down to suit a smaller port of entry and realized on a tighter budget ($250,000 for the entire complex versus $1.5 million for Ellis Island's main building alone).[13]

After its opening, Julia Morgan designed staff cottages that relieved workers from traveling to the island each day and a disinfection room that streamlined the hospital's operations. Morgan was already well known in California for her work with the Hearst family and Mills College. Angel Island's attraction of such a prominent architect might be explained by her personal connection to station commissioner Hart Hyatt North, her sister's husband.[14]

After depositing their luggage at the dock and stepping over the administration building's windswept threshold, passengers entered a carefully calibrated architecture of immigration. A main hall divided into four metal pens divided passengers by race and gender. Officers took the most visibly ill aside but only examined them after processing. The remainder continued down four metal corridors into a registry room so that station staff could individually observe each person. Based on new arrivals' race, class, and profession, officers decided their fate: detention or passage to the mainland.[15]

Those detained traveled further into the station, where spaces reinforced strict hierarchies. Station officials lodged Europeans on the administration building's second floor while relegating Asian

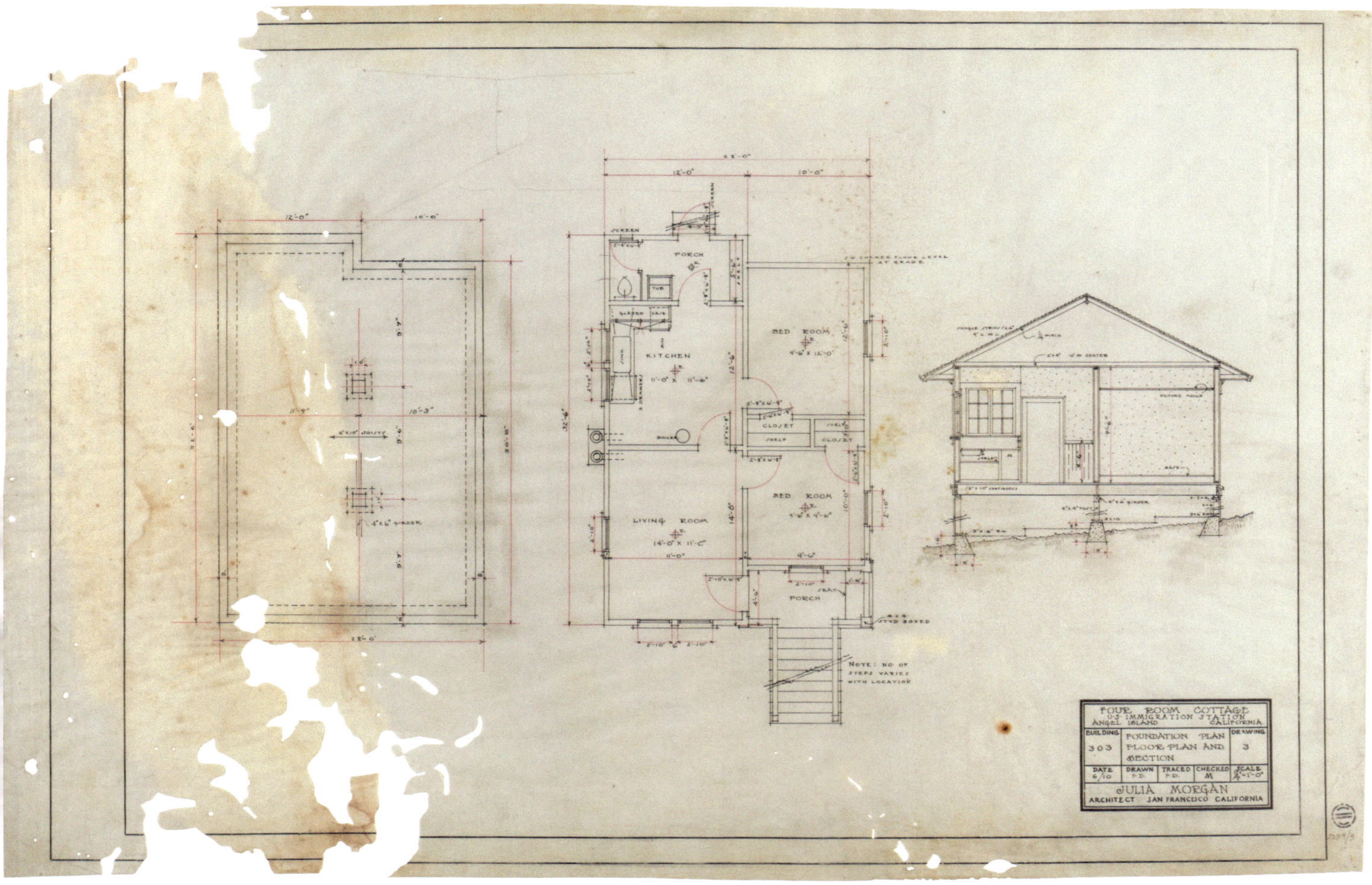

immigrants to separate barracks. These buildings held separate wards for Chinese men, Japanese and other Asian men, Asian women, and federal prisoners. Despite the *Chronicle*'s claim that the station could process two thousand arrivals and house one thousand at a time, in reality the barracks could safely sleep barely one-fifth of this estimate. According to the newspaper the European accommodations were on par with a first-class hotel, with fresh water supplied by barge, while showers in the simply "sanitary" Asian barracks pumped in saltwater from the bay.[16] In practice, any attempt at sanitation would have been difficult in the Asian barracks, which were designed to sleep 192 detainees at a time in bunks stacked three beds high but which often hosted between three and four hundred men.

At the time, California did not legally enforce segregated dining in the same way as the Jim Crow South, but historians have noted that many Chinese knew of and avoided establishments where staff would not serve them.[17] They perhaps learned this self-segregation through the experience at Angel Island, whose four dining rooms segregated Europeans, Asians, staff, and visitors. Contracted firms could spend fifteen cents per European meal compared to fourteen cents per Asian while providing the latter fewer options. Distinctions continued into the décor: tables in the European dining room had tablecloths while those in the Asian dining room did not.[18]

Hugging the slope behind the administration building, the station's hospital provided examination rooms where doctors let white men and women remain clothed but undressed Chinese men to examine their bodies for physical abnormalities. A chief cause of deportation was a diagnosis of trachoma, a degenerative eye disease, which despite a higher prevalence in European arrivals was diagnosed more in Asians.[19] The station's medical staff also made noncontagious hookworm, threadworm, and liver fluke, all parasites common in China, into deportable diagnoses.[20]

The segregated nature of medical examination reveals its intent to limit Chinese immigration rather than strictly keep disease out of the United States. In fact, the hospital did little to limit disease. Its facilities even encouraged transmission. In 1914, for instance, twenty-nine detainees caught cerebrospinal meningitis from a single case. A Public Health Service report published on the outbreak in 1921 revealed that though the first cases originated in the hospital, much of the spread occurred in overcrowded barracks.[21]

Inside the administration building, a wing of investigation rooms held officers whom the

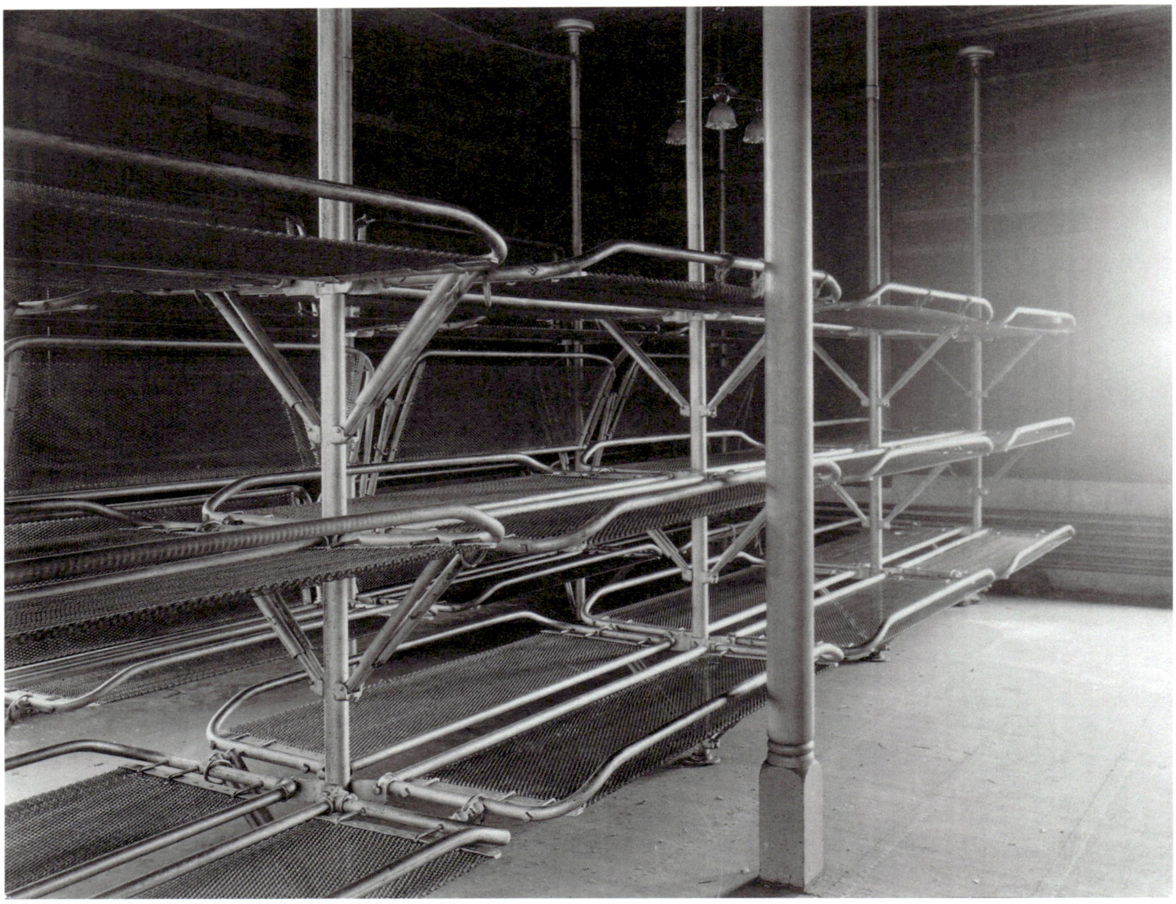

← Immigrants slept in bunks stacked three high, directly adjacent to another stack of bunks on one side and a narrow walkway on the other. Angel Island Immigration Station, 1910.

↓ An officer performs an eye examination on a child, 1923.

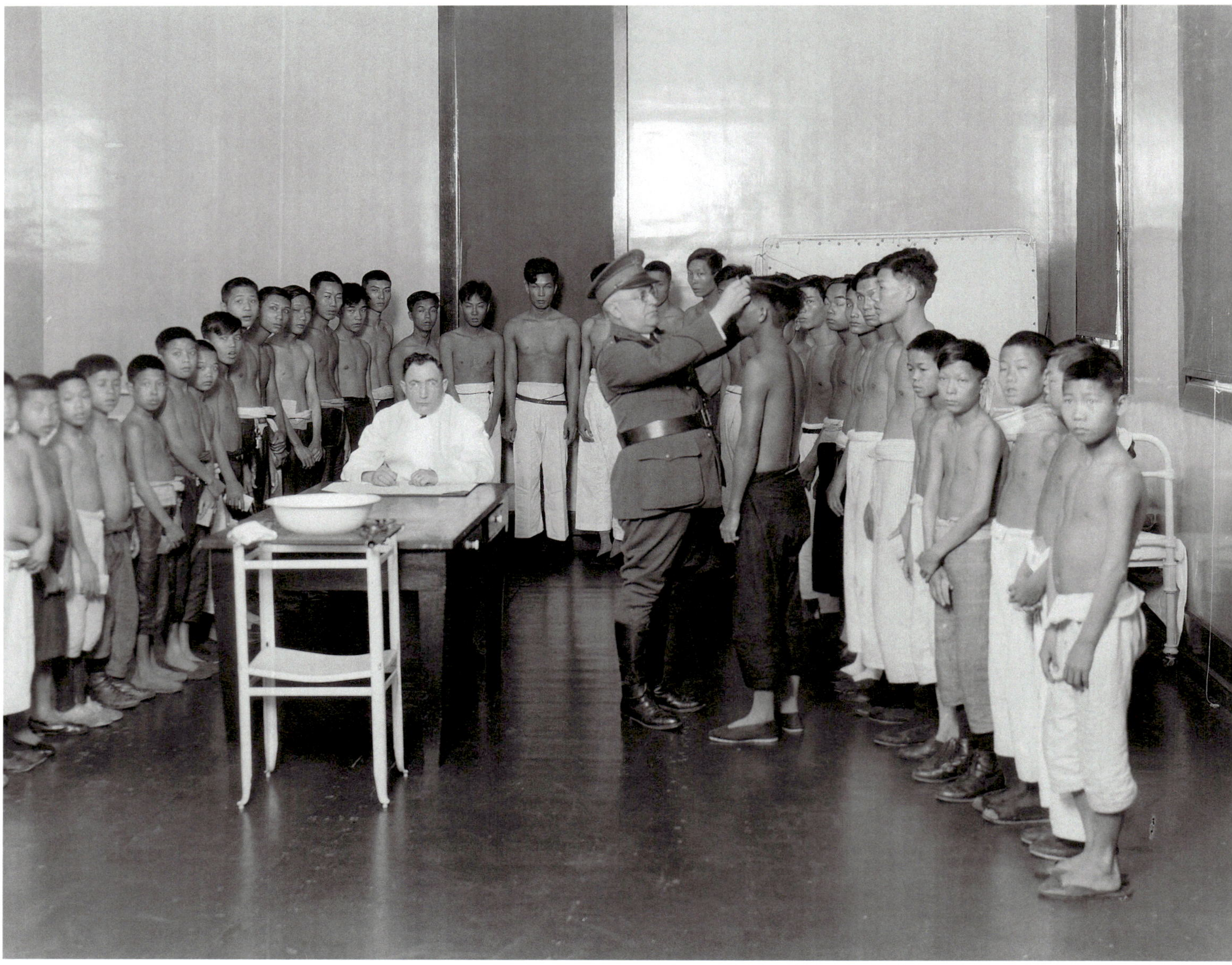

Immigration Bureau tasked with disproving arrivals' claims of profession and familial relation to existing US residents. Many claims were fabricated; a lack of records at arrivals' points of origin and the burning of birth records during the San Francisco Earthquake of 1906 enabled Chinese immigrants to deceive administration officials. However, even true relatives languished in an investigation process that involved extensive minutiae designed to trick anyone, regardless of status. Viewed together, the investigation wing and the hospital constructed twin systems of examination, both personal and physical, to impede or exclude as many as possible.

Though Angel Island housed vastly more men, the experience of women gives insight into the station's reinforcement of gendered concepts of labor and family. Marriage was one of few avenues for Asian women to enter the country, so interrogations of women attempted to reveal sexual immorality or prostitution in order to discredit matrimonial claims.[22] Limited means of immigration also meant that fewer women stayed at Angel Island in general. In a 1915 report Michi Kawai, General Secretary of the YWCA of Japan, noted that due to their small numbers, Asian and European women dined together on the island. Yet this proximity made blunt the station's racial distinctions: "Europeans have meat, beans, and even better silverware."[23]

In addition to testimony like Kawai's, detainees criticized their treatment by writing vivid poems on the barracks' wooden walls, some scrawled in ink or pencil and others inscribed in an elegant classical Cantonese technique. One detainee recounted:

> I have been imprisoned on Island for seven weeks.
> In addition, I do not know when I can land.
> It is only because the road of life has many twists and turns
> That one experiences such bitterness and sorrow.

Attempts at resistance also included the formation of the Zizhihui, or Self-Governing Association, in 1922 to advocate for better living arrangements. Older members of the Zizhuihui educated new arrivals on how to survive the station, collected money, purchased books, held meetings, and coached detainees through their immigration investigations.[24]

Not every Chinese immigrant passing through Angel Island underwent the same brutal system; the Chinese Exclusion Acts allowed the wealthy to enter relatively unscathed. I. M. Pei, for instance, left the station the day he entered. His Notice of Admission declared that his father, a manager of the Bank of China, could support him, that he held a telegram proving his acceptance to the University of Pennsylvania, and that he had an American reference to support him in traveling from San Francisco to the East Coast.[25]

↑ Railings divided the main examination room into pens according to race and gender. Angel Island Immigration Station entry and main examination room, 1910.

↓ Unlike its European counterpart, the Chinese and Japanese dining room had no tablecloths, lower-quality silverware, and cheaply cooked meals, 1933.

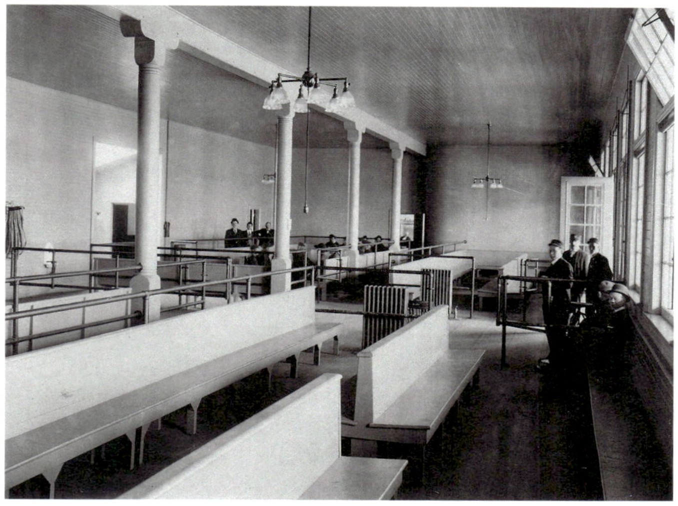

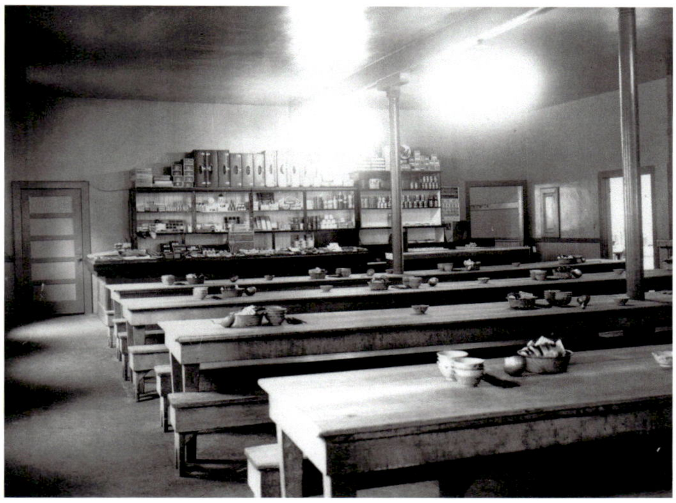

Afterlives of an Immigration Station

Despite the high-profile design commissions and press interest, the station at Angel Island quickly fell into disrepair. A US Immigration Bureau representative called it a "veritable firetrap" in 1922, just twelve years after its opening.[26] Morgan's worker cottages and hospital renovations made it moderately more functional, but the Immigration Bureau evaluation proved accurate when the administration building burned down in 1940. Coinciding with the beginning of World War II and a need for healthier diplomatic relations between the United States and China, station officials transferred the last detainees to the mainland and shut down the operation.

Following the station's decommissioning, local conservationists formed the Angel Island Foundation and, in partnership with private boaters represented by the California State Marine Parks and Harbors

Association, advocated for the island's recreational reuse. However, the island's preservation as a site of memory was never guaranteed, as the first proposals for reuse did not see the station structures as significant. When the California legislature hired Frederick Law Olmsted Jr. to evaluate the island in 1947, one of its proposals sought to level the island into an airport. Olmsted flatly rejected the proposal but suggested that the island's structures be repurposed for lodging tourists. He further warned that reusing the buildings as prisons or asylums would "seriously impair the recreational values of the adjacent lands." Like Mathews, Olmsted also looked to New York for architectural inspiration, suggesting that Angel Island could offer a recreational opportunity for San Francisco on par with what the "States of New York and New Jersey jointly have long been providing ... at the Palisades Interstate Park."[27] Two decades later, a 1966 report by Marshall McDonald and Associates finally acknowledged the complex's difficult past but suggested demolishing all structures save for the barracks and hospital, which would be renovated into contemporary museum spaces.[28]

The existing condition of the immigration station's abandoned buildings complicated renovations. This became clear in 1970, when park ranger and San Francisco State College student Alexander Weiss visited the barracks ahead of their proposed demolition and discovered the hundreds of poems carved by former detainees into the wooden walls.[29] These poems—unmatched evidence of the trauma experienced—came to light during a time of emerging Asian American political consciousness. Weiss brought the poems to the attention of his professors, who in turn shared them with ethnic studies faculty members at San Francisco State College, who were only recently hired in the aftermath of the Third World Liberation Front's 1968 march and the foundation of the first School of Ethnic Studies in the nation.[30]

Even still, the site's preservation was not guaranteed. In 1973, Norman Gilroy, architect and founder of the Institute for the Human Environment, suggested hosting a summer design workshop for California College of Arts and Crafts environmental design students on Angel Island to construct outdoor recreation structures on the immigration station site. Unaware of the site's history, the students planned areas for barbecuing, picnicking, and lawn games, and with the assistance of the US Army, demolished the station's pier to make way for a planned private marina.[31]

Advocacy by local preservationists and activists, including many descendants of former detainees themselves, prevented further destruction, stabilized the remaining barracks building, and drew attention to its poems. In 1978, a $250,000 grant from the State of California allowed architect Philip Choy to make fire and accessibility code improvements on the barracks and to reinforce the poem-laden walls with seismic bracing. Choy was resolute that the preserved barracks not be reappropriated into a rosy narrative of opportunity, telling historians Erika Lee and Judy Yung that he wanted "none of this tourist stuff."[32] Instead, the preservation effort would expose the brutal conditions of the barracks: walls, floors, and ceilings were left rough, and a few remaining bunks were outfitted with personal items.

This first wave of preservation work attempted to relay the psychological trauma of the barracks to visitors and allow those who had experienced this trauma to reenter. Former detainees who returned had a visceral experience. Richard Lee told the

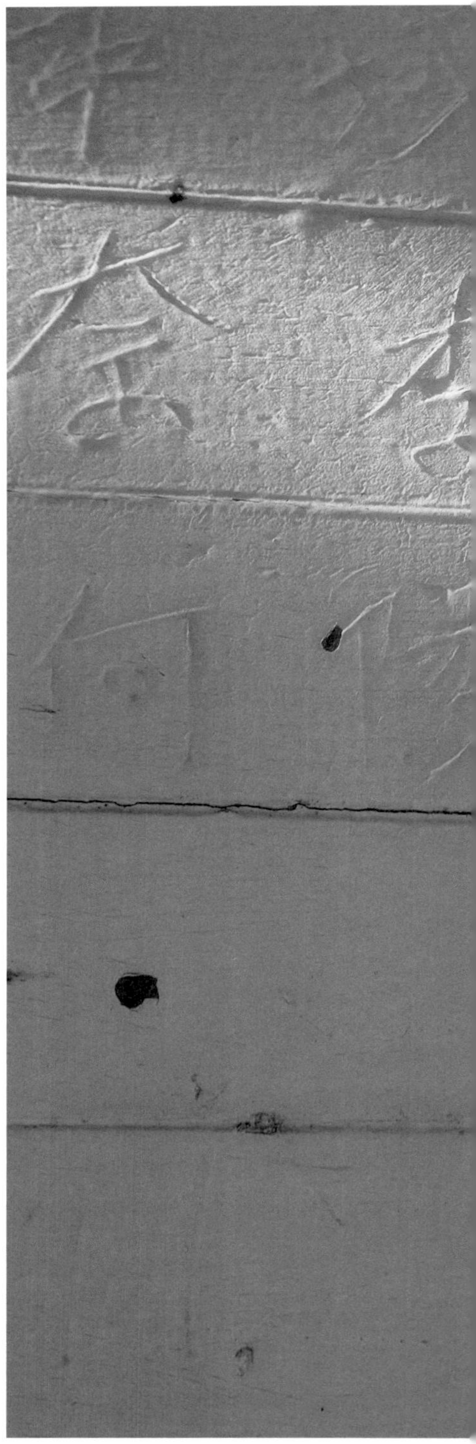

Chronicle that the sounds of guards rapping the bunk posts still rung in his ears; Paul Chow told the *New York Times* that he saw his father, Wan Gai Chow, cry for the first time upon their visit.[33] Others found catharsis in returning of their own accord. Li Kei Wong's writing teacher encouraged her to face the station, and in doing so, she found the confidence to write her 2006 memoir *Good Fortune: My Journey to Gold Mountain.*[34] The opening of the barracks also introduced the island to a second generation of preservationists and activists, some of whom did not even know of their own families' connection to the island prior to its reopening.[35]

Remembering Angel Island

A common shorthand for the Angel Island Immigration Station is "the Ellis Island of the West," but this false equivalence downplays Angel Island's brutality. Ellis Island detained twenty percent and deported two percent of its largely European population. Angel Island detained over half and deported one in five of its largely Asian population. An Ellis Island of the West did in fact exist on Angel Island, it was just found on the other side of a wall, upstairs or downstairs, or on the opposite side of a dining room; manifested in differences at the level of a tablecloth, silverware, shower water, or the interrogation table.

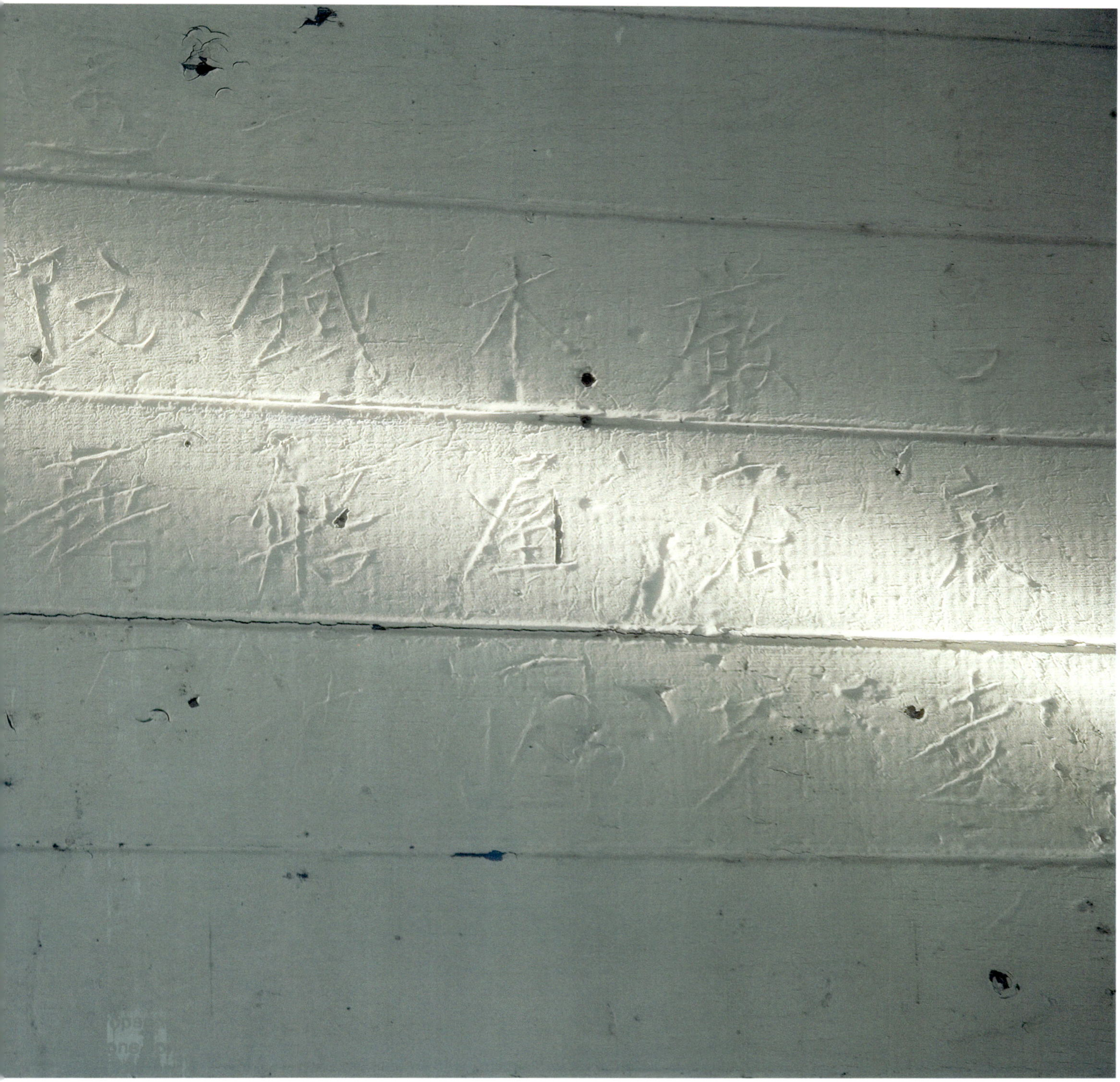

↑ A patch of light reveals Chinese carving on the barracks wall at Angel Island internment camp, 2006.

The imbalance between the two sites continues into the present. Though Angel Island prominently displays a plaque noting the "Sister Park" status of Ellis Island, the plaque's language makes clear that Ellis Island is a national park while Angel Island is only a state park. A dedicated ferry takes tourists to Ellis Island and the Statue of Liberty; visitors to Angel Island board a ferry mostly used by passengers seeking recreation. The state did not even guarantee public access until the private company operating the route for years abruptly ended its service in 2021 and advocates lobbied the Golden Gate Bridge Highway and Transportation District to take over the route.[36]

Nonetheless, the preservation and dissemination of Angel Island's legacy provides an opportunity for what Viet Thanh Nguyen has termed "just memory" when he writes that "any project of the humanities ... should also be a project of the inhumanities, how civilizations are built on forgotten barbarism toward others."[37] Demonstrating this potential, in 2003 Angel Island's traveling exhibition "Gateway to Gold Mountain" opened at the Ellis Island Immigration Museum with a lion dance performed by students from the Chinese Community Center of New Jersey. In doing so, it argued for inclusion of those historically excluded from the wider narrative of American immigration. Local papers described Asian American visitors seeing their own stories in the museum for the first time.[38] Speaking to the press, Ellis Island's curator of exhibits and media maintained that the exhibition "enables us to tell the larger story."[39] As an antidote to the mythologies of Ellis Island and American immigration, the preservation and dissemination of Angel Island demonstrates that architectures of exclusion existed on both shores and were unequally applied along lines of race and class, with disease labeled as the culprit.

Until I boarded a ferry to Angel Island in the summer of 2021, I had not fully understood the geographic isolation of the immigration station. The trip from San Francisco to the island today takes about thirty minutes, though the journey would have been longer one century earlier. High waves and strong winds coming off the Pacific buffeted the boat as the San Francisco skyline faded behind fog. I went to Angel Island assuming I would find little personal connection to it. My father and grandmother had flown from Seoul to San Francisco long after the immigration station shut down, and I had always assumed that the one great-grandfather who had left Korea to pursue a graduate degree in New York had passed through Ellis Island unscathed, just as my Ashkenazi Jewish great-grandparents had done around the same time. Reading about I. M. Pei's itinerary prompted me to double-check my great-grandfather's immigration records. To my surprise, Chough Pyung-Ok had not only been detained at Angel Island but had been treated for hookworm in the station's hospital at the expense of all of the money he had brought with him.

I struggled to reconstruct what his experience would have been. The immigration station sits on the island's far north shore, completely out of sight of the cities that line the Bay. New arrivals were truly alone, with vast stretches of wind and water separating them from where they had left, where they hoped to go, and anyone who would have aided them on either shore. Chough was among the more privileged; his records also noted that a white missionary, M. C. Harris, accompanied him from Yokohama, undoubtedly helping his case.[40] Coming from Korea via Japan, he was subject to a different set of immigration standards set by the Gentleman's Agreement of 1907 between the United States and Japan that relied more on exclusion at his port of departure. Finding him personalized the distinction between Angel Island and Ellis Island for me. While my Eastern European family could arrive in New York via steerage with little network in the United States, Chough could only enter the country via wealth and connections to whiteness. And even in his privileged position, he still entered the country marked as diseased.

Covid-19 revealed what many Asian Americans already understood: that a country could simultaneously refer to itself as a nation of immigrants and still mark some immigrants as perpetually dangerous. If an Ellis Island of the West existed, it comprised just one part of a larger immigration apparatus that gave out vastly different treatment based on race and class, setting a precedent for an immigration system that continues to separate and detain migrant families from nonwhite countries. Thus, the political potential of the preservation of Angel Island and similar sites is reparative. Preserving its legacy does not merely bring more groups into a popular understanding of the United States as a "nation of immigrants," but rather redefines the country as a nation produced by exclusion.

An earlier version of this essay was originally published by e-flux Architecture in 2022.

1. Yao Lu et al., "Priming COVID-19 Salience Increases Prejudice and Discriminatory Intent against Asians and Hispanics," *Proceedings of the National Academy of Sciences* 118, no. 36 (September 7, 2021), https://doi.org/10.1073/pnas.2105125118.
2. "Pelosi Remarks at Media Availability Following Visit to San Francisco's Chinatown and Meetings with Local Business Owners: Press Release" (Office of the Speaker of the House, February 24, 2020), https://www.speaker.gov/newsroom/22420; Lisa M. Krieger, "Coronavirus: Where Did Our Quarantine Facilities Go?," *Mercury News*, February 24, 2020, https://www.mercurynews.com/2020/02/24/coronavirus-where-did-all-our-old-quarantine-facilities-go/.
3. Luigi F. Lucaccini, "The Public Health Service on Angel Island," *Public Health Reports (1974-)* 111, no. 1 (1996): 92.
4. Lucaccini, "The Public Health Service on Angel Island," 92.
5. Michael C. LeMay, *Doctors at the Borders: Immigration and the Rise of Public Health* (Santa Barbara, CA: ABC-Clio, 2015), 101.
6. Arthur B. Stout, *Chinese Immigration and the Physiological Causes of the Decay of a Nation* (San Francisco: Agnew & Deffebach, 1862).
7. Untitled article ["The Anti-Chinese Convention Has Adjourned"], *Daily Alta California*, March 14, 1886, California Daily Newspaper Collection, UCR Center for Bibliographical Studies and Research.
8. Grover Cleveland, "October 1, 1888: Message Regarding Chinese Exclusion Act," Presidential Speeches | Miller Center, University of Virginia, October 20, 2016, https://millercenter.org/the-presidency/presidential-speeches/october-1-1888-message-regarding-chinese-exclusion-act.
9. Though Chinese immigrants were the most targeted, arrivals from other Asian countries and some Europeans were subject to similar, though not as stringent, systems of segregation, detention, and deportation as the station aged. Future uses of "Asian" in place of "Chinese" refer to instances in which all Asian immigrants, not just Chinese, were subject to specific conditions. See Erika Lee and Judy Yung, *Angel Island: Immigrant Gateway to America* (Oxford: Oxford University Press, 2012), 4.
10. Louis Stellmann, "San Francisco to Have the Finest Immigrant Station in the World," *San Francisco Chronicle*, August 18, 1907, 4.
11. Stellmann, "San Francisco to Have the Finest Immigrant Station in the World."
12. Ellis Island's original building opened in 1892 but burned down in 1897; Metcalf visited the rebuilt structure. "Metcalf to Make Inspection Tour," *San Francisco Examiner*, September 28, 1904; Stellmann, "San Francisco to Have the Finest Immigrant Station in the World," 4.
13. Interior Department, National Park Service, "Statue of Liberty National Monument (N.M.) and Ellis Island, Ellis Island Development Concept Plan: Environmental Impact Statement, " Executive Agency Publications, 2005, 5.
14. National Historic Landmarks Survey, National Park Service, "US Immigration Station, Angel Island, USDI/NPS NRHP Registration Form," October 15, 1995, 4, National Register of Historic Places.
15. While detention and deportation were overwhelmingly applied to Chinese immigrants under the Chinese Exclusion Acts, the apparatus was applied in increasing cases to other Asians and Europeans in later decades of the station's operation. In particular, the 1924 Immigration Act established quotas on immigrants from many countries aside from China, who were also detained or deported if the number of arrivals already processed from their country of origin had already reached their countries' quotas. See Lee and Yung, *Angel Island.*
16. Stellmann, "San Francisco to Have the Finest Immigrant Station in the World," 4.
17. Beth Lew-Williams, *The Chinese Must Go: Violence, Exclusion, and the Making of the Alien in America* (Cambridge, MA: Harvard University Press, 2018), 110, 230–231.
18. Lee and Yung, *Angel Island*, 61.
19. Lee and Yung, *Angel Island*, 39; Stellmann, "San Francisco to Have the Finest Immigrant Station in the World."
20. H. M. Lai, "Island of Immortals: Chinese Immigrants and the Angel Island Immigration Station," *California History* 57, no. 1 (1978): 94, https://doi.org/10.2307/25157818.
21. Joseph Bolten, "Cerebrospinal Meningitis at Angel Island Immigration Station, Calif," Public Health Reports, 1921, 593–594, http://archive.org/details/jstor-4575931.
22. Lee and Yung, *Angel Island*, 22.
23. Michi Kawai, "A Day on Angel Island," *Joshi Seinen-Kai* 12, no. 8–9 (September 1915): 49–53.
24. Lai, "Island of Immortals," 97.
25. "Pei, Ieoh Ming—Case Number: 35527/015-16," Department of Justice. Immigration and Naturalization Service. San Francisco District Office, August 28, 1935, 35527/015-16, National Archives at San Francisco (RW-SB).
26. "Immigration Station Needs Pointed Out: Elimination of Disease and Greater Efficiency Will Follow," *San Francisco Chronicle*, December 20, 1922.
27. Frederick Law Olmsted Jr., "Report on the Recreational Possibilities and Values of Angel Island, San Francisco Bay," 1947, 3, Angel Island Foundation Committee Records, 1950–1966 vol. 1, Bancroft Library, University of California, Berkeley.
28. Marshall McDonald, "Recommendations for the Historical Recreational Development of Angel Island," 1966, Him Mark Lai Papers, Box 2, Folder 4, Ethnic Studies Library, Asian American Studies Archives, University of California, Berkeley.
29. Him Mark Lai, Genny Lim, and Judy Yung, eds., *Island: Poetry and History of Chinese Immigrants on Angel Island, 1910–1940* (Seattle: University of Washington Press, 2014), 19.
30. Karen Umemoto, "'On Strike!' San Francisco State College Strike, 1968–69: The Role of Asian American Students," *Amerasia Journal* 15, no. 1 (January 1, 1989): 25, https://doi.org/10.17953/amer.15.1.7213030j5644rx25.
31. Institute for the Human Environment, "Proposal," ca. 1973, California Marine Parks and Harbors Association records, BANC MSS 86/155, Bancroft Library, University of California Berkeley; Harter G. Hudson, "Letter to Commodore George C. Berticevich," ca. 1973, California Marine Parks and Harbors Association records, BANC MSS 86/155, Bancroft Library, University of California, Berkeley.
32. Lee and Yung, *Angel Island*, 307.
33. Katherine Bishop, "Angel Island Journal: Saving Voices of the Other Ellis Island," *New York Times*, November 11, 1990.
34. Patricia Leigh Brown, "Poetic Justice for a Feared Immigrant Stop," *New York Times*, December 7, 2005.
35. Notably, the descendants of detainees were affected by the site's preservation, though in different ways than their parents and relatives. This perhaps demonstrates what Marianne Hirsch has termed "postmemory," or a remembering of trauma of generations before, passed down both directly and indirectly, as well as the "reading of silence" Gabriele Schwab identifies in such a "post-generation." Marianne Hirsch, *The Generation of Postmemory* (New York: Columbia University Press, 2012), 6.
36. Carly Graf, "Some San Francisco Ferries Could Stop Running to Angel Island and Tiburon," *San Francisco Examiner*, December 20, 2020; "Push to Retain Ferry Service to Historic Angel Island a Reminder of Its Dark History," KTVU News, FOX 2, April 8, 2021, https://www.ktvu.com/news/push-to-retain-ferry-service-to-historic-angel-island-a-reminder-of-its-dark-history; Ron Downing, James P. Swindler, and Denis J. Mulligan, "Authorize Actions for Implementation of a Demonstration Project to Provide Golden Gate Ferry Service Between the San Francisco Ferry Terminal and Angel Island," Golden Gate Bridge Highway & Transportation District, October 21, 2021, https://www.goldengate.org/assets/1/25/2021-1021-transcomm-no5-estabdemoprojangelislandferryrev.pdf?7401.
37. Viet Thanh Nguyen, *Nothing Ever Dies: Vietnam and the Memory of War* (Cambridge, MA: Harvard University Press, 2016), 19.
38. Merry Firschein, "Angel Island, the Other Ellis Island: Exhibition Tells the Story of Chinese Entry in California," *The Record* (Hackensack, NJ), March 9, 2003.
39. Corey Takahashi, "West Coast Legacy of the 'Paper People,'" *Newsday*, March 30, 2003.
40. Cho, Pyeng Ok, Case Number: 13203/012-02, *China* Passenger, January 26, 1914; Immigration Arrival Investigation Case Files, 1884–1944, Record Group 85: Records of the Immigration and Naturalization Service, 1787–2004.

p60, p65 (bottom) San Francisco History Center, San Francisco Public Library.
p61 Reproduced from "San Francisco to Have the Finest Immigrant Station in the World," *San Francisco Chronicle*, August 18, 1907.
p62 (bottom) California History Room, California State Library.
p63 Julia Morgan/Forney Collection, University of California, Berkeley, Environmental Design Archives.
p64 (top), 65 (top) National Archives and Records Administration.
p64 (bottom) Photo: Western Photo Company. National Library of Medicine.
p66–67 Photo: Carol Highsmith. Library of Congress.

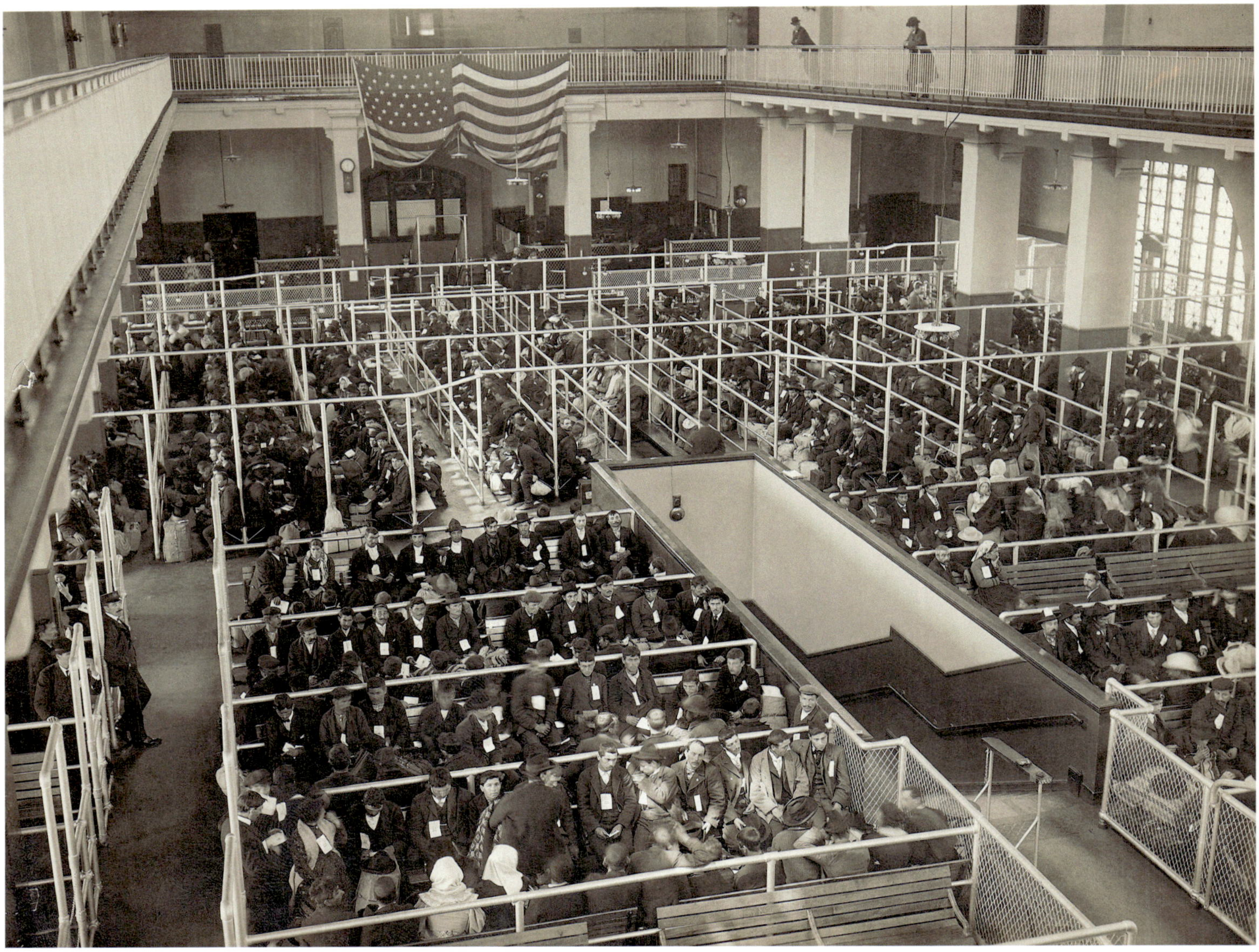

ANATOMY OF A BORDER

GUILLERMO S. ARSUAGA

The development of immigration stations, quarantine facilities, and hospitals at the main ports of entry to the United States in the early twentieth century medicalized the architecture of its border.[1] From the mid-nineteenth to the mid-twentieth century, New York was the primary destination for European and Middle Eastern working-class immigrants entering the United States, with over twelve million people inspected at the Ellis Island Immigration Station alone.[2] Although Ellis Island is a single location in the vastly distributed border apparatus, it embodies the complexity of the entire immigration system as a site of entanglement between ideas of modernity, health, race, and class, and played a crucial role in the enactment and perpetuation of these biopolitical narratives and norms.

Through a mediatized spectacle, Ellis Island shaped the way the US public came to view immigration, inherently linking it to concepts of health and social desirability. The press carried significant coverage of the opening of a new immigration station in 1900, with the *New York Times* even calling it an "amphitheatre."[3] The island and its process of medical screening were also open to visitors, attracting individuals awaiting their family members' arrivals as well as those curious about the immigration process and seeking a glimpse into the lives of new arrivals. The popularity of Ellis Island as a visitor destination underscored its emblematic role in the American immigration narrative at the turn of the century. It also drew prominent personalities and immigration officials, who at times were encouraged to experience the medical inspections firsthand.[4] Concurrently, medical processes at Ellis Island were particularly well publicized and communicated prejudices that some immigrants were more likely to import contagious disease or have weaker physical and mental conditions than others.[5]

Medical processes also dictated Ellis Island's architecture. The island's screening routines identified and segregated unhealthy and undesirable working-class immigrant bodies from healthy and desirable ones.[6] Within its first two decades, the immigration inspection center at Ellis Island became an assembly line of medical assessments. By establishing the process of medical screening as the defining experience of becoming an American citizen, the architecture of Ellis Island normalized the social construct of a healthy, productive, and morally pure body.

The Creation of the Ellis Island Immigration Station

For many years, the only manmade intervention on Ellis Island was a small naval powder magazine constructed during the Civil War. In 1892, an immigration station was built, only to be destroyed by a fire in 1897.[7] Following this, the federal government released funds to enlarge the island's land mass and to build a new immigration station, hospital, kitchen, and dining hall.[8] The New York-based architectural office Boring & Tilton won the federal competition with a design that integrated modern industrial materials into a Beaux-Arts historicist style. Ellis Island grew exponentially over the following decades, together with new immigration laws, procedures, and buildings.

The process of design and construction of the new Ellis Island Immigration Station took two years. US Public Health Service officials were concerned with the spread of contagious diseases during the process of immigration, which often brought many bodies from different places into close proximity with one another.[9] Architecture was therefore used to guarantee proper airflow, social distance, and other hygienic measures. For instance, the Great Hall—the central space where new arrivals were inspected and sometimes held for hours—could use a combination of mechanical air extraction and gear-operated windows

← The pens at Ellis Island, Registry Room (or Great Hall). The people seen in the photograph have passed the first mental inspection, ca. 1902–1913.

→ Historical development of Ellis Island as an immigration station.

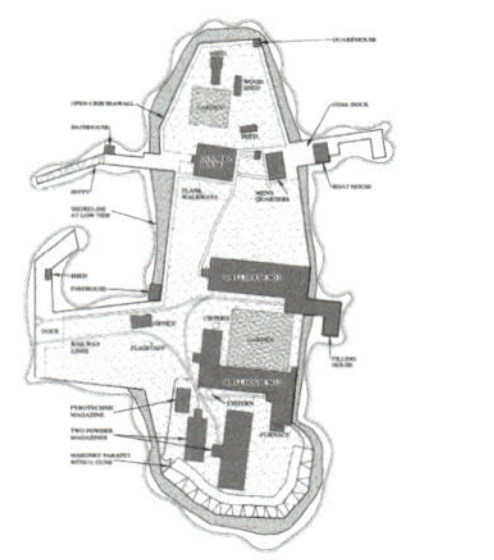

1890

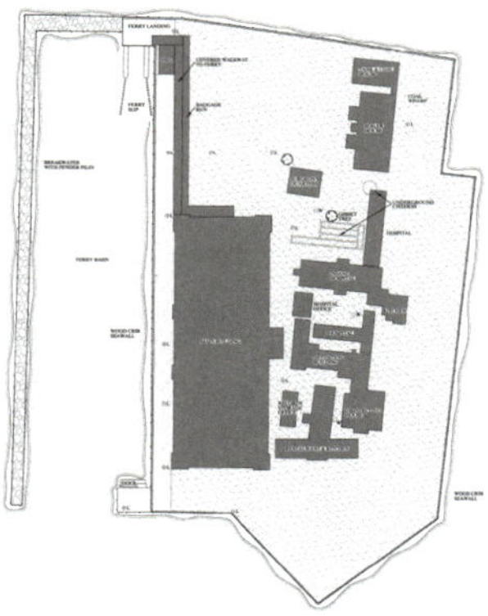

1897

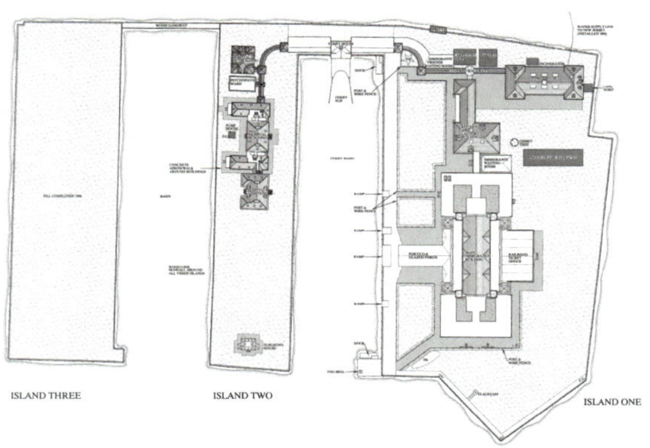

1907

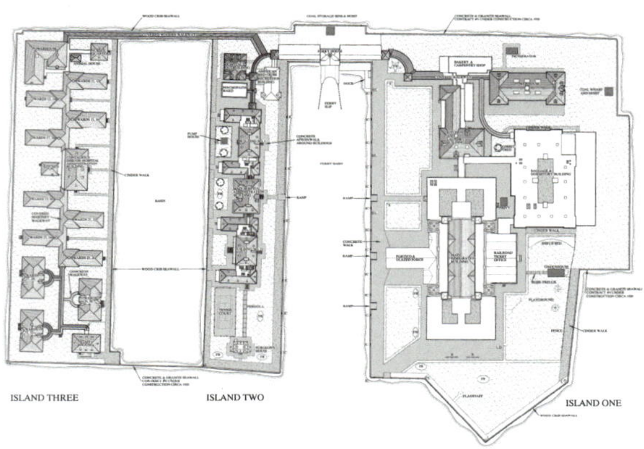

1920

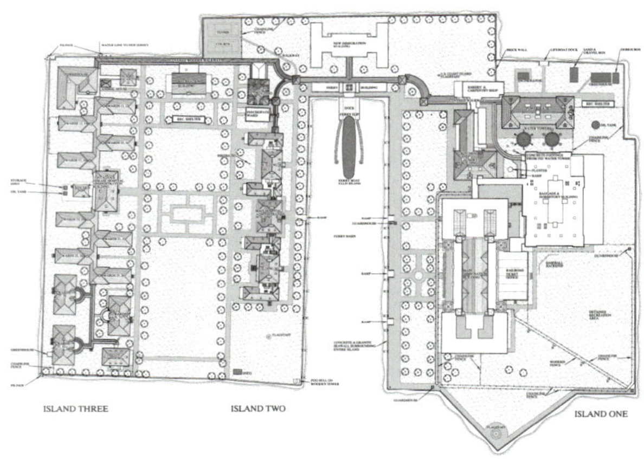

1954

to have its air fully renovated in fifteen minutes. Railings throughout the station created a "network of [aisles], in which the immigrants are placed in alphabetical order, according to nationality."[10]

Hygiene was not only incorporated into the architectural design, but also mandated for the immigrants' bodies. A bathing house was built, "where 200 immigrants can be bathed at a time, 8,000 being about the number that can be thus refreshed during an ordinary day."[11] According to an Assistant Commissioner of Ellis Island: "We expect to wash them once a day, and they will land on American soil clean, if nothing more."[12]

Arrival at Ellis Island

For the majority of its new arrivals, the immigration process began many weeks before and many miles away from Ellis Island. Private steamship companies often performed their own medical checks on travelers at ports of origin, both to avoid carrying sick individuals and to prevent being held liable for the cost of passengers' return journeys if they were deported for medical reasons. The steamboats had first- and second-class cabin passages reserved for US citizens and other travelers already admitted to the US, while new arrivals would stay in third-class cabins. Before arriving at Ellis Island, boats would first anchor in the New York Lower Bay, where Public Health Service (PHS) physicians would examine first- and second-class passengers for cholera, plague, smallpox, typhoid fever, yellow fever, scarlet fever, measles, and diphtheria.[13]

Steamships then moved to Ellis Island, where upon arrival medically checked first- and second-class passengers could head to the ferry station and purchase a ticket to New York. Meanwhile, third-class passengers were taken for medical examinations at the Immigration Station. After stepping ashore, immigrants passed through an "imposing private entrance, made as nearly as possible free from the observation of the curious," and poured into a waiting area under a pergola connected to the Station. Here, a first medical examination was carried out in which doctors used a metal hook to lift the eyelid and check for traces of trachoma, a highly contagious eye disease.[14] If any evidence of this disease was found, the doctor used a piece of chalk to mark the immigrant with a "T" on the front of their right shoulder.[15]

After the trachoma check, the flow of immigrants was bifurcated as they moved into the Station: those with trachoma would take the right-hand lane, and those without would take the left. Those suspected of having the disease would then be led to a different part of the Station for further medical checks and would ultimately either be sent to the Contagious Disease Hospital (if they could afford it) or deported.[16] Immigrants considered free of trachoma took a route toward the Great Hall (also known as the Examination Room), which involved climbing from the dark ground floor up a steep stairway into the voluminous bright Hall. Although they did not realize it, as they climbed up the stairs a second medical test was being performed, with a doctor standing at the top watching for signs of lameness or heavy breathing that might indicate a heart condition.[17]

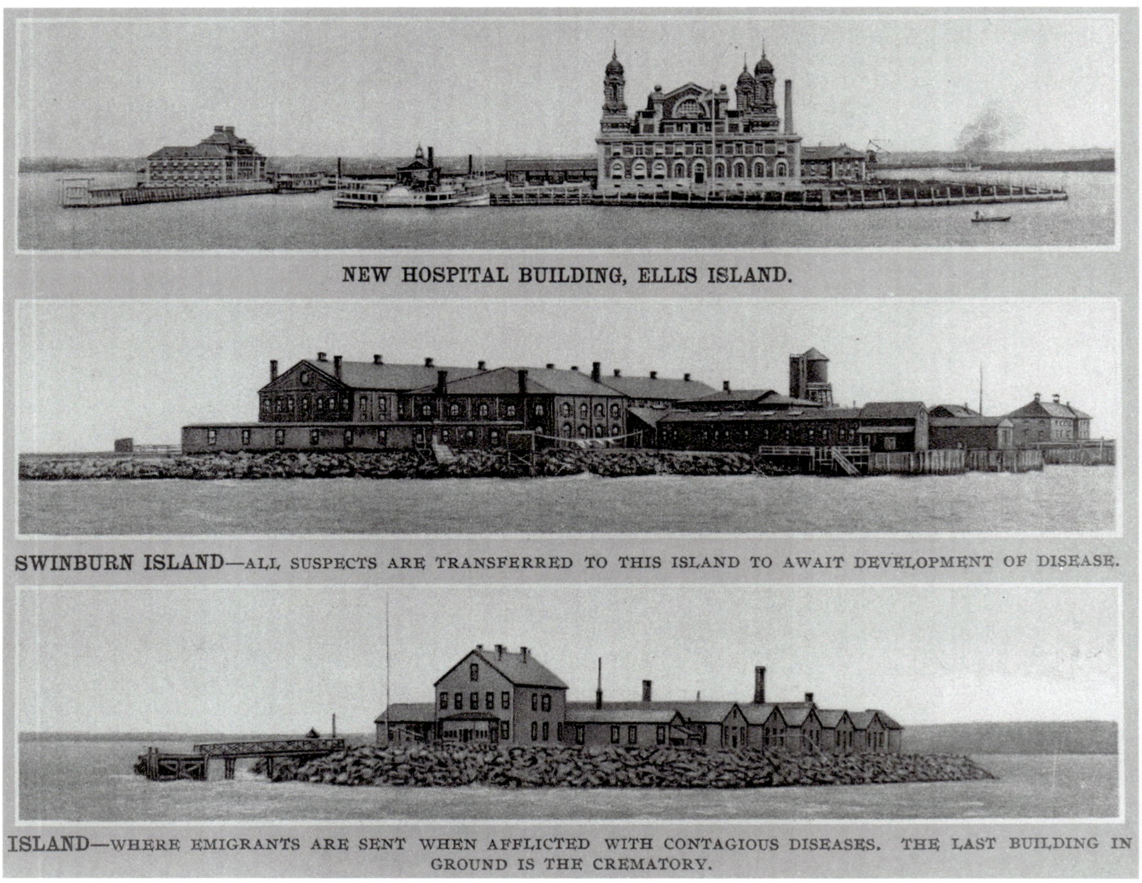

→ New hospital building, Ellis Island; quarantine buildings on Swinburne Island, where all suspects were transferred to await development of disease; and Hoffman Island, where emigrants were sent when afflicted with contagious diseases.

Entering the Great Hall

The Great Hall was the most important space in the immigration screening process, large and centrally located. It was also the most modern room in the whole complex; industrial metal trusses and pillars, similar to the ones that were used in railway stations at the time, liberated the brick facade from any load and allowed enormous windows, thirty-six feet in height, to be placed on all four sides of the room. This structural operation also freed the floor to serve as an open multifunctional space where paths of circulation could be recombined and reshaped depending on medical and immigration requirements and the number of people to be examined.

As they entered the Great Hall, immigrants were segregated by nationality into different aisles. In contrast with the heavy-looking Beaux-Arts exterior, the aisles in the Great Hall were built with lightweight metal pipes and chicken wire.[18] Here immigrants waited seated in cagelike conditions, sometimes for many hours, for further medical examinations. The protocol to segregate the new arrivals by nationality emphasized the PHS's belief that disease was linked to specific origins.[19] Certain populations—such as those from the Mediterranean or Eastern Europe, who were not considered to be white at the time—were profiled as more likely contagious or feeble-minded, and thus subjected to more exhaustive inspections.[20]

As immigrants were called to be examined, they walked through aisles that zigzagged across the Hall in a way that facilitated the physicians' work. The aisles made two right-hand turns to enable the PHS officers to check both sides of an immigrant's face and body and facilitate the detection of deformities or disease.[21] As weary immigrants marched forward, a doctor examined their face, hair, neck, and hands.[22] Following the same protocol as the trachoma check, should an immigrant be suspected of mental defects, the doctors marked an "X" on their shoulder with chalk. An "X" within a circle meant some definite mental symptom had been detected. A "B" indicated possible back problems, while "Pg" stood for pregnancy, and "Sc" a scalp infection. If an immigrant received any mark, they were directed to rooms set aside in the Great Hall for further examination.

Serving as a crucible for the multifaceted processes of immigrant inspection and categorization, Ellis Island systematically interwove medical, social, and moral scrutiny within its architecture. Approximately twenty percent of the immigrants passing through inspection at the Great Hall were held for further examination, and here they encountered a bifurcated fate.[23] Some, after additional inspection, found release, while others were relegated to Ellis Island Hospital, where their "curability" was probed—not merely through a medical lens but also considering their financial capacity to bear treatment costs.[24] Immigrants who were free of disease could

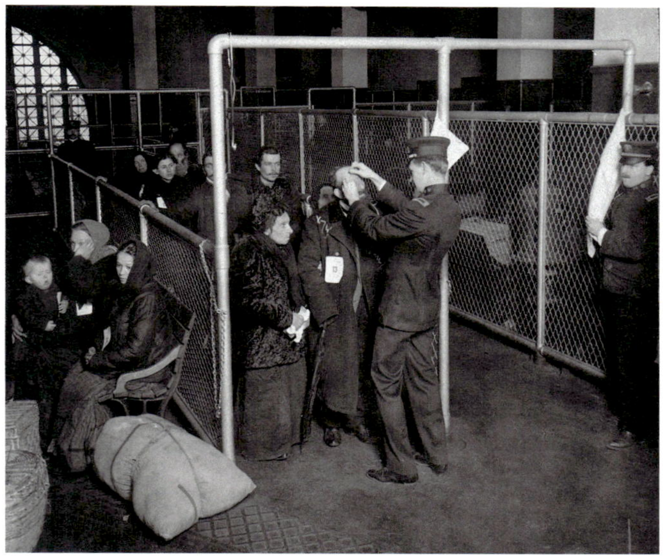

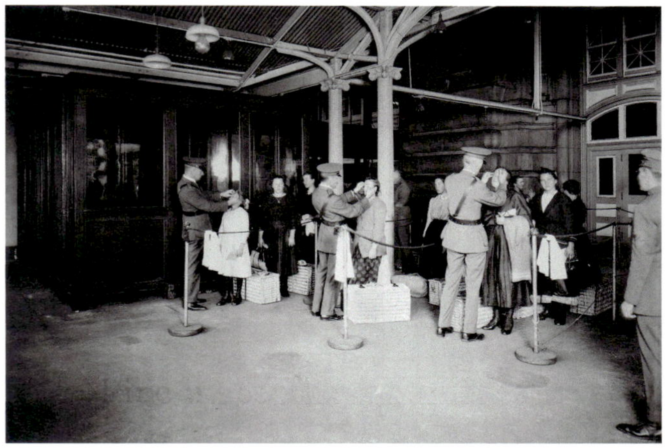

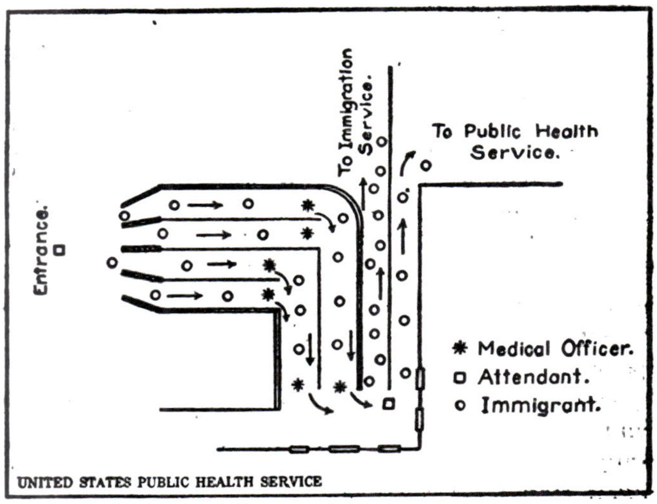

↑ US inspectors examining eyes of immigrants, Ellis Island, New York Harbor, ca. 1913.

– Line inspection of arriving immigrants, including trachoma examinations, ca. 1923.

↓ Spatial diagram of the medical inspection at Ellis Island by E. H. Mullan, Surgeon, United States Public Health Service.

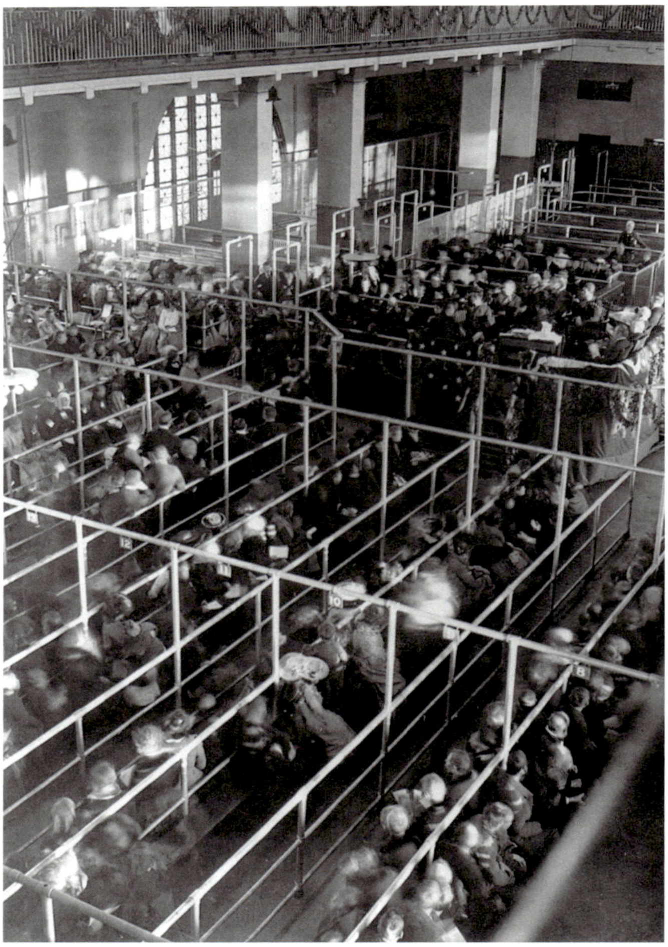

still be given the label of "likely to become a public charge" if they were determined to be unable to work and make a living during medical screening. They could, for example, be categorized as having a "poor physique" or "deformities," judgments often rooted in racialized and eugenicist ideas, which were reason enough for them to be deported.[25]

The architecture of Ellis Island crystallized and instrumentally participated in the exclusionary processes of immigration. The meticulously articulated spaces—from the segregating inspection areas of the Great Hall to the strategically organized hospital wards—were pivotal in facilitating a rigorous examination and categorization of immigrants. In this architectural and administrative matrix, terms like "poor physique" and "deformities" transcended rudimentary medical evaluation, subjecting immigrants within a network of classist and racist predispositions, actively selecting a demographic landscape and safeguarding a government-defined societal profile. The architecture, in its ability to mediate, segregate, and publicize this process, emerged as a potent tool, enacting regulatory and exclusionary practices. And not only through coverage in the media but also by opening its doors to the public, this very architecture helped broadcast social norms and draw correlations between immigrants, health, and disease well beyond the limits of the island.

Shaping Immigration Narratives

In 1907, the US Department of the Treasury published the *Book of Instructions for the Medical Inspection of Immigrants*, which aimed to categorize immigrants denied entry to the United States on the basis of medical reasons into two groups. "Group A" was described as "Aliens excluded from admission in the country because of disease or abnormal condition," and was subdivided into "(1) Persons suffering from dangerous contagious disease, (2) Persons suffering from loathsome disease, (3) Insane persons, (4) Idiots." "Group B" was described as "Aliens, who present some disease or defect, physical or mental, that be regarded as conclusive as an alien 'likely to become a public charge.'" These diseases or defects were subdivided into "(1) Hernia, (2) Valvular heart disease, (3) Pregnancy, (4) Poor physique, (5) Chronic Rheumatism, (6) Nervous diseases, (7) Malignant disease, (8) Deformities, (9) Senility and debility, (10) Varicose veins."[26]

The book also provided design instruction, largely informed by the design of Ellis Island, on the spatial qualities of inspection rooms, along with guidelines on how to medically perform the examinations. It highlighted the importance of "natural light" and advocated for examinations to be conducted on "even level surfaces" to ensure consistent footing for immigrants, enabling them to keep their gaze directed straight ahead during the examination process.[27] The book furthermore outlined organizational and spacing protocols for managing immigrant queues, recommending a single-file, evenly spaced line with individuals at ten-foot intervals to facilitate an orderly inspection process.[28] This was optimized through the use of the "right angle," in which the queue would make a ninety-degree turn immediately in front of the examiner. This setup, the book argued, allowed both sides and the back of the individual to be observed, expediting the inspection while aiding in the identification of lameness or defective eyesight as immigrants adjusted their vision and position during the turn.[29]

The architectural and organizational design of Ellis Island orchestrated the flow, waiting, and passage of bodies. Its layout serves as a tangible manifestation of the era's laws and social constructs concerning immigration and health. Situated within a wider socioeconomic and epistemic framework of border control and exclusion, Ellis Island Immigration Station materialized a complex mechanism of inspection. The spaciousness of the Great Hall normalized the medical assessments that filtered out undesirable bodies and crafted the idea of a proper citizen. By exposing the process of medical examination, Ellis Island's architecture crystallized and broadcast a particular social ideology of immigration. The island not only mirrored but actively shaped and perpetuated biopolitical norms, crystallizing them into the

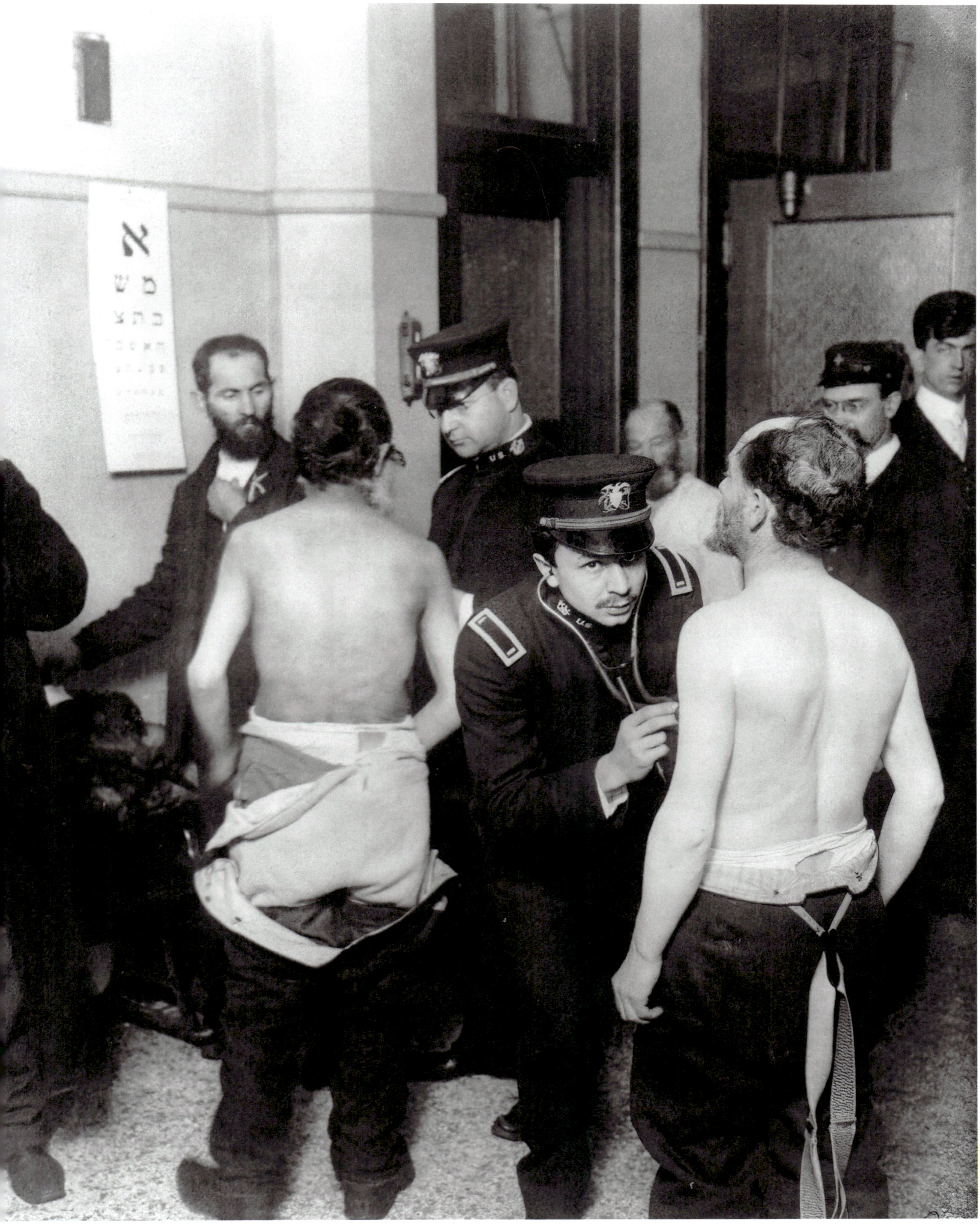

← Emigrants in "pens" at Ellis Island (probably on or near Christmas, given the decorations), ca. 1906.

↑ Physicians examining a group of Jewish immigrants; an eye chart using Hebrew characters hangs on the wall, ca. 1907.

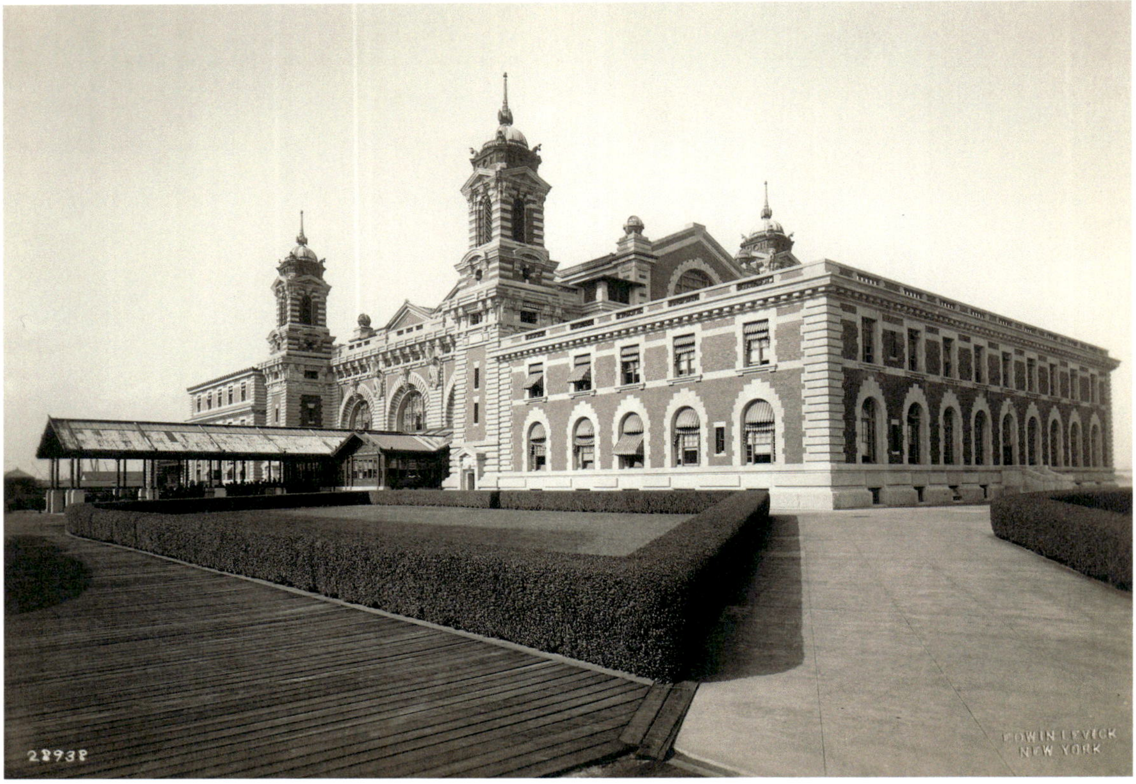

tangible daily realities of society and consequently facilitating the broad acceptance and internalization of these medically and racially charged perceptions of immigrants.

Ellis Island still has a pivotal role in the history and narrative around immigration in the United States, today as the Museum of Immigration. The mediatized spectacle of immigration once observed live by visitors now unfolds within a curated setting. Through a collection of personal objects, the recreation of historical spaces, and the didactic explanation of the immigration and medical process, the museum upholds romanticized narratives of hope and triumphant arrivals while often forgetting histories of exclusion. The once hectic traffic of immigration arrivals and procedures now unfolds as static and historicized. Meanwhile, the border has moved elsewhere and largely remains an architecture of exclusion.

An earlier version of this essay was originally published by e-flux Architecture in 2020.

1. In the context of the early twentieth century, Michel Foucault's concept of "biopower" and Achille Mbembe's "necropower" provide a crucial theoretical lens to understand the policy and spatial tactics employed to control populations—determining who lives and who dies, with intersections in public health, medicine, and surveillance. While existing scholarship has addressed these themes, this essay explores the specific historical and architectural elements that positioned Ellis Island as a focal point for such policies. For further reading, see Michel Foucault, François Ewald, and Alessandro Fontana, *Security, Territory, Population: Lectures at the Collège de France, 1977–1978*, ed. Michel Senellart, trans. Graham Burchell (New York: Picador, 2009); Michel Foucault, *The History of Sexuality* (New York: Pantheon Books, 1978); Achille Mbembe, "Necropolitics," trans. Libby Meintjes, *Public Culture* 15, no. 1 (2003): 11–40; Sandro Mezzadra and Brett Neilson, *Border as Method, or, the Multiplication of Labor* (Durham: Duke University Press, 2013).
2. Harlan D. Unrau, *Ellis Island, Statue of Liberty National Monument, New York-New Jersey* (Denver: US Dept. of the Interior, National Park Service, 1984), xix. Additional inspection stations were established at the main ports of entry, such as the one on Angel Island (operating from 1910 to 1940) dedicated to the inspection of Asian migrants. The island is examined by Jeremy Wolin in this volume.
3. "New Immigrant Station," *New York Times*, December 3, 1900.
4. On known individuals visiting and the firsthand experience in Ellis Island, see for example a 1905 *New York Times* article that describes how the delegates of an immigration conference in New York City were taken to Ellis Island: "At Ellis Island the delegates obtained an admirable idea of the workings of the immigration law. They saw the steerage passengers of the *Kaiser Wilhelm II*, passed through the doors, and inspected the buildings from top to bottom. The visitors watched the process of passing the immigrants from the gallery of the main inspection hall. A few of them submitted themselves to the examination, being cheered by their comrades as they were marshaled into the pens. Archbishop Ireland was one of the most interested of all the visitors. He was recognized by the immigrants as a dignitary of the Church, and many knelt and kissed his ring. After his return to the city, he said: 'I was much impressed with what I saw. The immigrants are well fed, clean quarters are provided for them.'" "Immigration Conference Musters 500 Delegates," *New York Times*, December 7, 1905.
5. For instance, in 1912, *Popular Science Monthly* published an article titled "The Medical Side of Immigration." The article, written on pseudo-medical evidence, describes how some immigrant races are more desirable than others from a medical point of view, taking as example some of the immigrants arriving to Ellis Island: "According to the law, the feeble-minded, as well as idiots and imbeciles, are absolutely excluded. It is of vast import that the feeble-minded be detected, not least because they are predisposed to become public charges,

↑ Front facade of the Ellis Island Immigration Station after completion in 1900, 1902–1913.

ut because they and their offspring contribute so largely to the criminal element." It continues: "In general, it may be said that the best class is drawn from northern and Western Europe and the poorest from the Mediterranean countries and Western Asia. Among the worst are the Greeks, South Italians, and the Syrians, who emigrate in large numbers. The Greeks offer a sad contrast to their ancient progenitors, as poor physical development is the rule among those who reach Ellis Island, and they have above their share of other defects." On European immigration into the US and whiteness, see David R. Roediger, "New Immigrants, Race, and 'Ethnicity' in the Long Early Twentieth Century," in *Working toward Whiteness: How America's Immigrants Became White: The Strange Journey from Ellis Island to the Suburbs* (New York: Basic Books, 2018).

6. On Ellis Island and the industrialized inspection process, see Jay Dolmage, "Ellis Island and the Inventions of Race and Disability," in *Disabled upon Arrival: Eugenics, Immigration, and the Construction of Race and Disability* (Columbus: Ohio State University Press, 2018), 14.

7. Unrau, *Ellis Island*, 3.

8. Unrau, *Ellis Island*, 35.

9. On the American peak of immigration see Alan M. Kraut, *Silent Travelers: Germs, Genes, and the "Immigrant Menace"* (Baltimore: Johns Hopkins University Press, 1995), 4.

10. "New Immigrant Station."

11. "New Immigrant Station." "The plans and specifications for the new structure were selected from the designs submitted by the architectural firm of Boring & Tilton of this city. ... The style is a conglomeration of several styles of architecture, the predominating style being that of the French Renaissance. The material used in the construction is brick, with light stone trimmings, harmonized so as to make the general effect as attractive in appearance as possible. ... But the interior arrangements are what, after all, make the station a model of completeness. Every detail of the exacting and confusing service to which its uses are to be dedicated were considered in perfecting the interior plans. The transportation, examining, medical, inquiry, and various other departments of the service being assigned quarters that, while they are practically separate in every detail, yet are so arranged as to follow one after the other, according to its proper place in the department. ... Every inch of space on this floor is utilized. The railings forming the network of the aisles, in which the immigrants are placed in alphabetical order, according to nationality, gives the great amphitheatre the appearance of an immense spider web. ... Surrounding this room, from the third floor, is the observation gallery, where visitors can watch the inspectors at work. ... One of the greatest of the improvements will be the. bathing house, where 200 immigrants can be bathed at a time, 8,000 being about the number that can be thus refreshed during an ordinary day. 'We expect to wash them once a day, and they will land on American soil clean, if nothing more,' said Assistant Commissioner McSweeney a few days ago. ... The floors are of concrete and slate, the railings of iron, while the beds are combinations of iron and wire netting. ... The spending of the million and a half dollars by the US Government on Ellis Island will be, according to those best fitted to judge, the beginning of a new era in the complicated system of the immigration service."

12. "New Immigrant Station."

13. US citizens were excluded from these checks, and very few passengers from the first and second classes were sent to further inspection when they arrived on Ellis Island. On first-class tickets and immigrant regulation, see Unrau, *Ellis Island*, 226. Specifically: "Notice Concerning Sale of First Class Transportation to Immigrants at Ellis Island," November 24, 1911, William Williams, Commissioner, Taft Papers, Library of Congress.

14. Already, the architecture of the island facilitated the medical examinations (indeed, in 1911, the Unites States Health Service published a diagram for the trachoma checks that translated them into a floor plan). The trachoma protocol outside the Immigration Building at Ellis Island was introduced in 1911, after some structural reforms in the building. Previously this check was performed indoors at the Great Hall.

15. Howard Markel, *When Germs Travel: Six Major Epidemics That Have Invaded America and the Fears They Have Unleashed* (New York: Vintage Books, 2005), 83.

16. Interestingly, there is a clear connection in plan between the holding medical examination rooms, the detection center, and the exit to the quarantine and infectious disease hospital on the other side of the island.

17. Kraut, *Silent Travelers*.

18. On the origin-related differences in inspection procedures at Ellis Island, see Alison Bateman-House, "Medical Examination of Immigrants at Ellis Island," *AMA Journal of Ethics* 10, no. 4 (April 1, 2008): 235–241.

19. Markel, *When Germs Travel*, 83.

20. David Roediger has written how these populations were perceived as separate ethnic groups not belonging to the "white America" and were later considered white in the United States. See Roediger, "New Immigrants, Race, and 'Ethnicity' in the Long Early Twentieth Century."

21. Lorie Conway, *Forgotten Ellis Island: The Extraordinary Story of America's Immigrant Hospital* (New York: Harper Collins, 2007). The United States Public Health Service, *Book of Instructions for the Medical Inspection of Immigrants* (Washington, DC: GPO, 1903).

22. Based on what can be deduced from the photographs, this preliminary inspection was performed at the same time and in the same space for both men and women who were segregated in groups by nationality. However, those with chalk marks were detained in holding areas and separated by gender and suspected medical affliction.

23. Conway, *Forgotten Ellis Island*, 34.

24. As Alan M. Kraut describes, in many cases, the payment for the hospitalization was covered by immigrants' own networks. Kraut, *Silent Travelers*, 56.

25. During the first half of the twentieth century, there are several examples of deportation at Ellis Island of immigrants qualified by the medical inspectors at Ellis Island as "likely to become a public charge." See for example "Report of a Special Inquiry Held at Ellis Island Regarding the Deportation of Italian Immigrants, 6/5/1915." The archive document reports on the interview and findings for the status of Giuseppe Giorni, a twenty-seven-year-old male immigrant from Italy. The inquiry determined Giorni was to be deported because of his varicose veins which would lead to him likely becoming a public charge. The topics of the eugenic nation and the design implications exceed the scope of this paper but open a rich research possibility, already developed by authors such as Alexandra Minna Stern, *Eugenic Nation : Faults and Frontiers of Better Breeding in Modern America* (Berkeley: University of California Press, 2005), and Howard Markel and Alexandra Minna Stern, "Which Face? Whose Nation? Immigration, Public Health, and the Construction of Disease at America's Ports and Borders, 1891–1928," *American Behavioral Scientist* 42, no. 9 (June 1, 1999): 1314–1331. "Report of a Special Inquiry Held at Ellis Island Regarding the Deportation of Italian Immigrants, 6/5/1915, European War—German Refugees—Deportation of Italians—Alien Deportations, Subject and Policy Files 1906–1957," Records of the Immigration and Naturalization Service 1787–2004, National Archives at Washington, DC, https://catalog.archives.gov/id/12013855. Within the eugenic rhetoric, the categories of race, physical and mental disabilities were created for racist purposes. See "Disability" and "New Racism" in Jay Dolmage, "Ellis Island and the Inventions of Race and Disability," 23.

26. United States Public Health Service, *Book of Instructions for the Medical Inspection of Immigrants*.

27. According to the instructions, "The medical examination should be made by daylight and never, except in an emergency, attempted in poorly lighted rooms or by artificial light. The preliminary line inspection should be conducted on an even, level surface, so that the passengers may not be tempted to look where they are stepping." United States Public Health Service, *Book of Instructions for the Medical Inspection of Immigrants*, 6.

28. "Care should be taken to prevent crowding, to maintain a single file evenly spaced, with the individuals well separated (10 feet)." See United States Public Health Service, *Book of Instructions for the Medical Inspection of Immigrants*, 6.

29. "The file should make a right angle turn immediately in from of the examiner's position. This enables the examiner to observe both sides and the back of the passenger in the shortest possible time, beside bringing out lameness, defective eyesight (through the efforts to adjust his vision to a new course), artificial eyes, corneal opacities or roughened cornea (through striking eye at changing angles of incidence and passenger turns)." United States Public Health Service, *Book of Instructions for the Medical Inspection of Immigrants*, 6.

p70, 76 Photo: Edwin Levick. Courtesy of the New York Public Library.
p71 Courtesy of the Library of Congress.
p72 Illustrated in *Quarantine Sketches* (Brooklyn, NY: Maltine Company, 1902). Courtesy of the Library of Congress.
p73 (top), 74, 75 Photo: Underwood & Underwood. Courtesy of the Library of Congress.
p73 (middle) Photo: Department of the Treasury, Public Health Service. Courtesy of the National Archives, Washington, DC.
p73 (bottom) Reproduced from E. H. Mullan, "Mental Examination of Immigrants: Administration and Line Inspection at Ellis Island," *Public Health Reports* 32, no. 20 (1917): 734.

GOLD FEVER: NORMALIZING PREJUDICE THROUGH HEALTHCARE

REBECCA KELLAWAN

→ United States Marine Hospital, author unknown, 1853. The first publicly funded building in the state of California and designed by architect Robert Mills, the hospital was severely damaged following two earthquakes and was abandoned by the Marine Hospital Service in the 1870s.

California and its northern population center, San Francisco, owe much of their character and development to disease. "Gold fever," as it was called, was undoubtedly the most powerful sickness to transform the small colonial village, Yerba Buena, into an international metropolis in less than a decade. The California Gold Rush (1848–1857) facilitated the largest recorded mass migration to a United States territory, with roughly 300,000 people descending upon northern California on their way to the goldfields, most passing through San Francisco.

Although gold fever provided the human capital to transform former satellite settlements of the Spanish and then Mexican empires, the human cargo also carried a vicious cocktail of Old and New World diseases. While these pathogens found fertile breeding grounds in the filth emblematic of Gold Rush-era San Francisco, disease would ultimately drive federal and local government institutions and immigrant communities to design semiautonomous healthcare systems to primarily serve and support their constituents. In this sense, San Francisco's first hospitals were not only early monuments of health, but the materialization of co-dependent social practices.

If a chaotic collection of dispersed, mobile, and ephemeral architecture was one of San Francisco's first material expressions of gold fever, the establishment of modern hospitals can be imagined as the beginnings of an architectural cure. These hospitals, their origins, and visual representations on city maps, postcards, and advertisements reflected and reified a particular social order that normalized the bodies and architectures of certain groups while stigmatizing those of others. In other words, in an effort to control the spread of microscopic organisms yet to be called bacteria, an epidemic of racial prejudice and discrimination was transmitted and reproduced. This gave way to a system of healthcare that was dominated by Western European immigrants, despite the city's founding diversity.

From Gold Fever to Modern Hospitals

While non-native migration to California was minimal under Spanish (1769–1821) and Mexican rule (1821–1848), the gold rush functioned as a catalyst to realize the westward ambitions of a rapidly expanding US population. As the popular story goes, in January 1848, an American carpenter from New Jersey, John Marshall, discovered a piece of gold on the American River just days before the signing of the Treaty of Guadalupe Hidalgo, officially ending the Mexican-American War and transferring over half of Mexico's land holdings that would eventually become parts of Arizona, California, New Mexico, Texas, Colorado, Nevada, and Utah. However, Congressmen in Washington long knew of the mineral wealth of California, as did many of San Francisco's first merchants, some of whom had previously mined for gold and silver in Mexico, Chile, and Peru.[1] Gold fever was thus initiated by President James Knox Polk when he publicly confirmed the mineral wealth of California in his 1848 State of the Union address and declared he was "deeply interested in the speedy development of the country's wealth and resources."[2]

When the land now known as California formally came into the possession of the United States that same year, the territory was characteristic of a North American borderland. It was represented by the intermixing and cohabitation of descendants of one of the largest and most diverse precontact Indigenous populations in the Western hemisphere, Spanish missionaries, Mexican colonial authorities, Californios, and Russian fur traders, among others.[3] In its rapid population gains and transformation from a territory to a state, settlers brought racist ideologies with them from other parts of the country.[4] While, after much debate, California was not admitted to the nation as a slave state, its first elected governor, Peter Hardeman Burnett, was a slaveholder from the south who openly championed the idea of an exclusively white American West.[5] As such, the

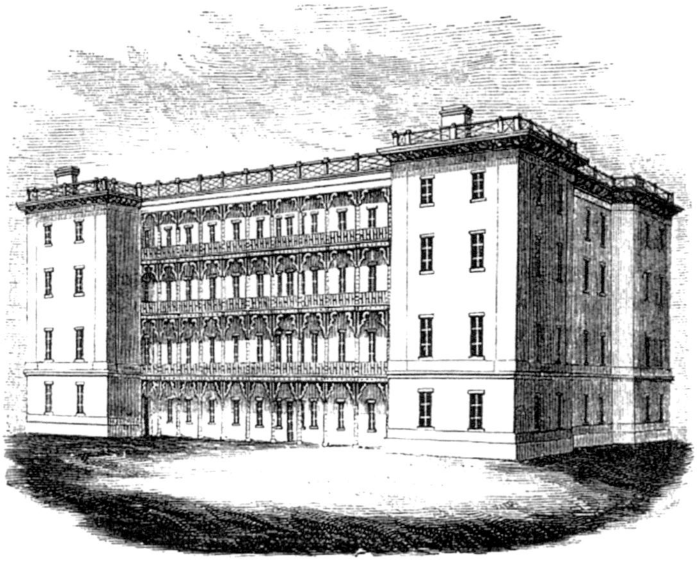

state's earliest legislation was dependent on a suite of labor, vagrancy, voting, citizenship, and tax laws that prevented Indigenous peoples, Blacks, Mexicans (or Californios), and Asians from equality or justice, and regulated their participation in the development of the state.[6] In the impromptu urban quarters of San Francisco, for instance, an overseas Chinese community grew alongside other immigrant enclaves, but was instantly subject to processes of racialization and ultimately equated with vice and disease.[7]

Just over a year into the gold rush, in 1849, a cholera epidemic raged in New York and New Orleans, and the mass migration westward gave the *Vibrio cholerae* microbe the opportunity to penetrate the Pacific coast. San Francisco was the epicenter of the first outbreak.[8] With nearly 40,000 emigrants passing through the city on their way to the goldfields in 1849, lack of proper housing and shelter, limited freshwater supplies, and inadequate or nonexistent sewer systems fostered a deluge of disease. As one observer reported, many houses stand on "made land, composed of offal, manure, rotten and decayed vegetables and animal matter."[9]

While the 1850 federal census indicates that California contained more physicians per capita than any other state at the time, hospitals and a formalized system of healthcare were nonexistent.[10] In addition to cholera, San Francisco was also struck with outbreaks of malaria, yellow fever, typhoid, ophthalmia, smallpox, and scurvy. As the city's population expanded, its healthcare needs increased exponentially, which led to the construction of San Francisco's first formalized network of hospitals. These institutions not only managed the sick and dying, but also solidified group membership and citizenry. Co-ethnic, co-national, and co-religious healthcare promoted assimilation by normalizing a predominately Western European population.

Given that city migrants came from all corners of the globe and diversity defined the population and character of San Francisco from its beginnings, migrants often sought refuge within urban communities that offered some form of familiarity such as language, religion, nationality, or race. Nineteenth-century city directories confirm that benevolent societies were prevalent in San Francisco, numbering over eighty by 1871. Several were organized around nationality or nativity specifically and were represented by British, Jewish, Greek, Russian, Slovenian, Italian, Irish, Mexican, Portuguese, West Indian, and Chinese citizens, among others.[11] While a main feature of most benevolent societies was to take care of sick and indigent and to bury the dead, only a small minority of these organizations were able to transform early health wards into city institutions that would come to define healthcare and modern hospital architecture in San Francisco at the turn of the twentieth century.

Between 1850 and 1890, several private hospitals and wards were established within the city to manage the sick and dying. In the following period, however, modern hospital complexes sponsored by just a few benevolent societies and government institutions emerged as permanent fixtures: the French Hospital (1895), the Public Service Hospital (1931), St. Mary's Hospital (Catholic, 1911), the Franklin Hospital (German, 1908), St. Luke's Hospital (Episcopal, 1914), the City and County Hospital (1915), and Mt. Zion Hospital (Jewish, 1917). Many of these hospitals' original facilities were damaged by earthquakes or fire, and most were unable to accommodate the city's growing population. Furthermore, since advances in medicine were unfolding concurrently with hospital design, many were not adaptable to modernization. Therefore, successful institutions were able to fund new healthcare facilities that solidified the influence these organizations accumulated during the state's tumultuous early history.

Through an act of Congress, the US Marine Hospital was the first publicly funded building in the state of California. It was designed by Robert Mills, who is often described as the first American-born architect.[12] Built in 1853 on Rincon Point, along the eastern (bay) side of the city, it was described at the time as "large, strongly built, and luxurious."[13] However, following two earthquakes, it was abandoned and by 1875 was rebuilt in the new French-derived "pavilion system" as a healthcare compound at a rural location within the city's adjoining US military installation, the Presidio. The new timber-framed complex with brick foundations overlooked a natural lake and included three long rectangular wards that radiated from a central reception building. Several additional ancillary support structures were placed on either side of the wards.[14] Within fifty years, however, the hospital was functionally obsolete and considered a severe fire hazard. In 1928, federal legislation appropriated funds to the newly named

→ Postcard of the French Hospital, San Francisco. This is the fourth and final iteration of the French Hospital, designed by Franco-American architect M. G. Morin-Goustiaux, in collaboration with M. Mooser. The cornerstone was laid in 1894, and on completion the building was celebrated as the most modern hospital on the Pacific Coast. Considered a model for hospital planning, it featured courts, gardens, and state-of-the-art equipment, and it hosted one of the first nursing schools in the city.

↘ Postcard of Franklin Hospital, San Francisco. Renamed the Franklin Hospital due to Germany's involvement in World War I, the new hospital was designed by architect Hermann Barth, who was born in Germany and immigrated to San Francisco in 1881. Barth was a practitioner of numerous types of architecture, designed several hospitals for the city, and was a member of the San Francisco Chapter of the American Institute of Architects.

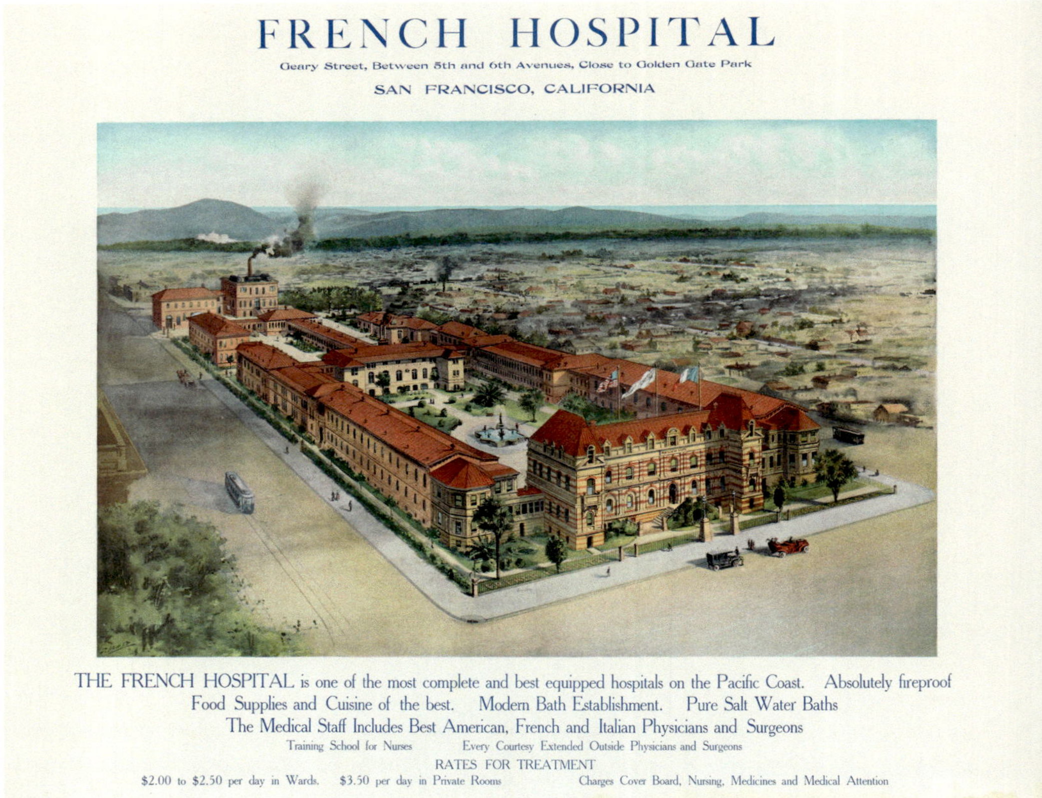

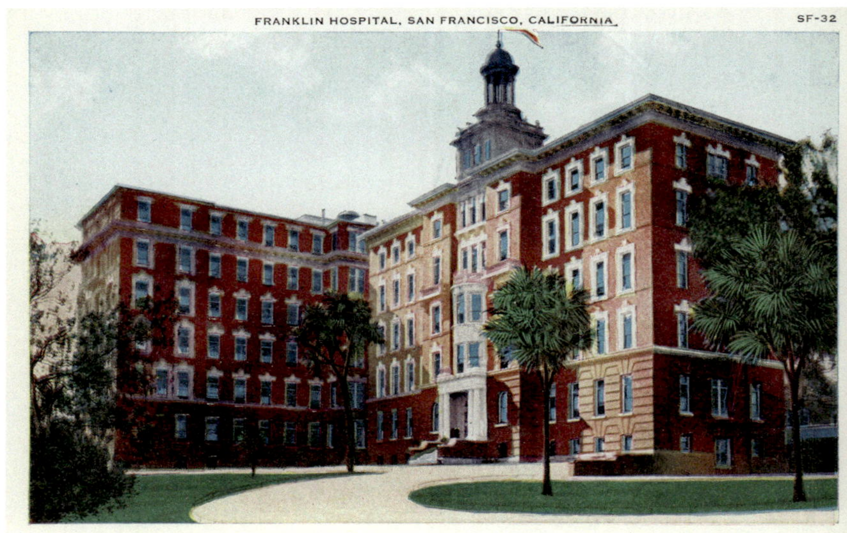

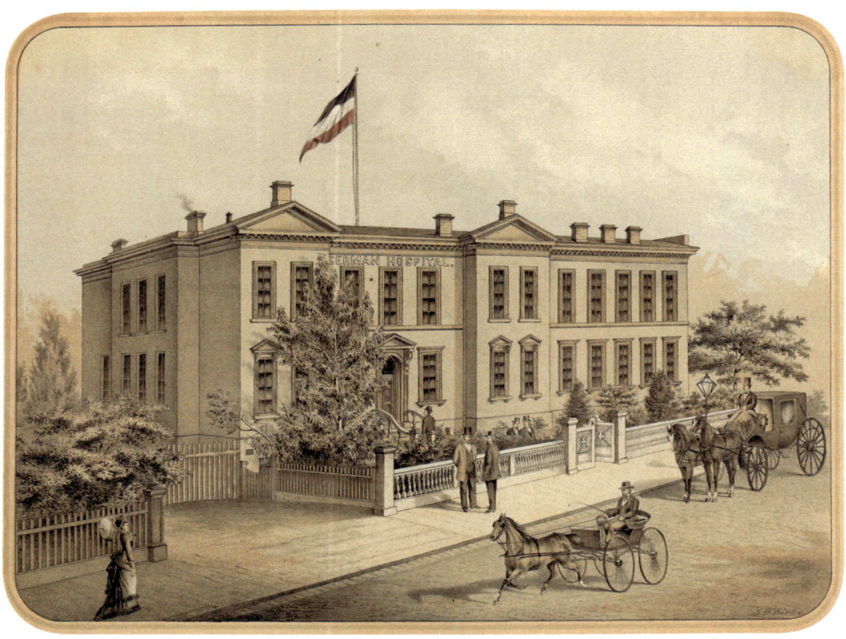

← Postcard of the Hospital of the German Benevolent Society, San Francisco. The society's founder, Joseph N. Rausch, also created one of the first known prepaid health plans whereby German-speaking immigrants could pay one dollar a month to secure a private hospital bed at a rate of one dollar per day. Completed in 1858, this first iteration of the hospital was destroyed by fire in 1876.

Public Health Service for another (third) Marine Hospital, which was considered to be one of the agency's most ambitious building projects at the time. The main hospital was now a six-story reinforced concrete structure that accommodated growing advances in medicine.[15] It was also representative of a "crucial period" of hospital design, when American hospitals shifted from pavilions to high-rises.[16]

Similarly, the French Hospital, first built in 1851, was reimagined and rebuilt for the fourth time in 1895. When it was completed, the complex of fourteen buildings was said to have utilized five miles of electric wire, one of the most extensive electrical projects completed in the city.[17] A little over a decade later, a third iteration of the German Hospital was erected and touted as "the most complete and perfect, as well as the largest hospital in the Western half of this continent." Its modern Renaissance-style complex also represented the "new departure in modern hospital construction" that favored two compact high-rise buildings to facilitate "the administration and economy" of the hospital.[18] Collectively, the evolution of the city's first hospitals and the ideals they represented transformed a city of crude architecture and disease into a symbol of modern medicine and design. Indeed, by the close of the nineteenth century, San Francisco contained the largest number of hospital beds in relation to its population of any city in the nation.[19]

Normalizing Stigma through Public Health

Since pestilence was inherent to most nineteenth-century urban spaces, cities all over the world established public health organizations with broad authority to survey, monitor, and in effect "police" the health offenses of their inhabitants.[20] In San Francisco this was manifested through the authority of state and local "health experts" who organized health boards to prioritize issues and enact remediation. This system of oversight incorporated architects and architecture as essential participants in constructing modern and acceptable notions of health and sanitation.

Following the first two decades of statehood, in 1871 California's State Board of Health defined a range of statewide health problems that were common to the nineteenth century. Miasma theory—the notion that noxious air transmitted pestilence—was still accepted as the main cause of disease at the time. Sanitary architecture and municipal practices that incorporated proper design, building materials, and legislation tested and vetted by English, French, and German "authorities" were discussed in relation to hospitals and other public buildings, practices for managing the dead and burial grounds, sewerage, land reclamation, and water supply.[21]

In San Francisco, health concerns specific to Chinese immigrants—such as personal hygiene, living conditions, and their complicity in prostitution—were

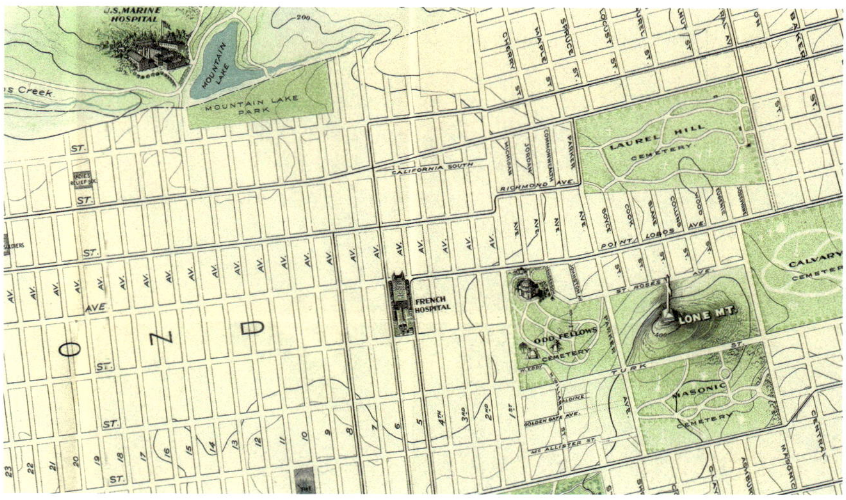

↗ The French Hospital, detail from "The Commercial, Pictorial, and Tourist Map of San Francisco, in colors and illustrated with litho-engraved pictures of all public buildings, parks, monuments, and recommended business houses, etc.," 1904.

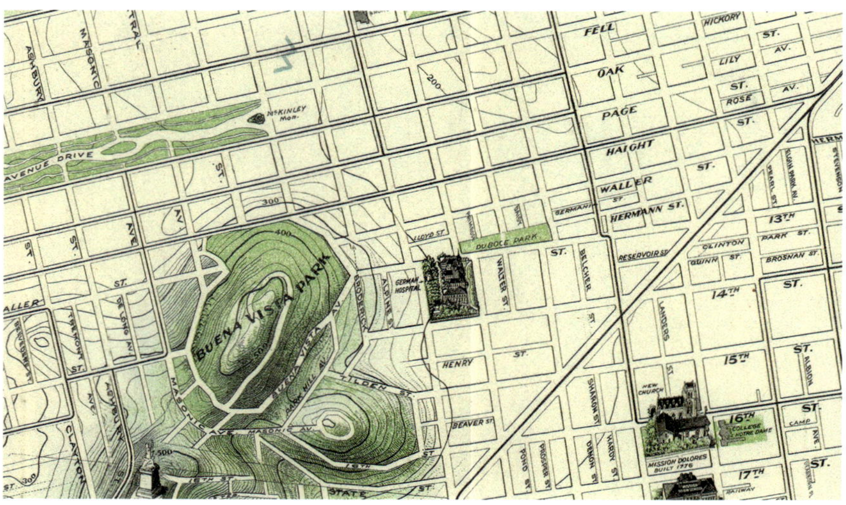

→ The German Hospital, detail from "The Commercial, Pictorial, and Tourist Map of San Francisco, in colors and illustrated with litho-engraved pictures of all public buildings, parks, monuments, and recommended business houses, etc.," 1904.

considered "special questions" of the Board.[22] From the Board's perspective, the Chinese represented not only a public health concern but a nefarious presence that needed swift remediation. The report stated that the "Mongolian portion" of the population were not only "totally regardless of all sanitary laws ... but none who have ever witnessed the midnight orgies of this hebetated people in San Francisco, can imagine the depths of depravity into which they are sunk."[23] An account of a midnight survey of the "Chinese quarter" by doctors, a medical heath officer, and a city police officer details a visit to "the lowest dens of degraded bestiality." The account describes "foul labyrinthine passages" that connect dark rooms housing "dusky human beings, lying on tiers of broad shelves, like the berths of a ship." Rooms were described as "pens" absent of proper ventilation.

In the slowing California economy of the 1860s–1870s, white workers formed racist associations throughout the state such as the "Anti-Coolie Association," which largely blamed male Chinese laborers—who had primarily come to California in response to labor demands—for their inability to find work.[24] They also successfully pressured public health officials to enact sanitary laws to encourage Chinese immigrants to return to China.

If modern hospitals constructed by French, German, Christian, Jewish, and government organizations represented normality, citizenship, and the cure, San Francisco's Chinatown and its working class were abnormal, alien, the disease. As one scholar puts it, "Chinatown was not simply associated with smallpox, plague, and syphilis: it was made metonymous with these diseases. That is, its labyrinthine alleyways, mysterious josshouses, and grimy brothels were construed not just as spawning these diseases or containing them, but as actually becoming a part of them."[25] While San Francisco's modern hospitals were monumentalized in city maps, Chinatown became a monument to both disease and vice, reinforcing both an architectural and "spatial pathologization."[26] The backlash the Chinese experienced as a result of their alienation in San Francisco and beyond supported the passage of federal legislation such as the Chinese Exclusion Act of 1882, the Geary Act in 1892, as well as a host of other localized legislation to limit Chinese immigration to the United States as a whole, but particularly California.[27] Moreover, laws specific to architecture like the Cubic Air Ordinance of 1870, which required at least 500 cubic feet of air per tenant, were unevenly enforced in Chinese neighborhoods.[28]

Given the special attention and pathological blame the Chinese population experienced for the degeneration of city health, they were almost completely forbidden access to most of the city's healthcare facilities.[29] As a result, Chinese residents relied on their own traditional health practices and transnational networks to fund benevolent health institutions in San Francisco. Subterranean "chambers of tranquility" to aid recovery or death and herbal shops scattered throughout Chinatown constituted an alternative healthcare support system but were subject to constant scrutiny.[30] In 1899, the community established the Tung Wah Dispensary, which is considered to be the first iteration of a Chinese hospital in San Francisco that incorporated medical practices from China and the West. The new dispensary offered free care to the poorest Chinese residents and was networked with herbal drug stores in Chinatown to fill prescriptions.[31]

The dispensary was undermined shortly after its opening by the arrival of the bubonic plague, which was leveraged to enact new city health regulations that continued to police and control Chinatown and its residents. Chinatown was quarantined, and the dispensary became a locus of conflict between federal and city health regulators and the community. Western medical practitioners working out of the dispensary were also targeted by authorities and were subject to regulations that purposely challenged and disrupted their authority and autonomy under the leadership of the dispensary until anti-plague operations officially came to an end in 1905.[32]

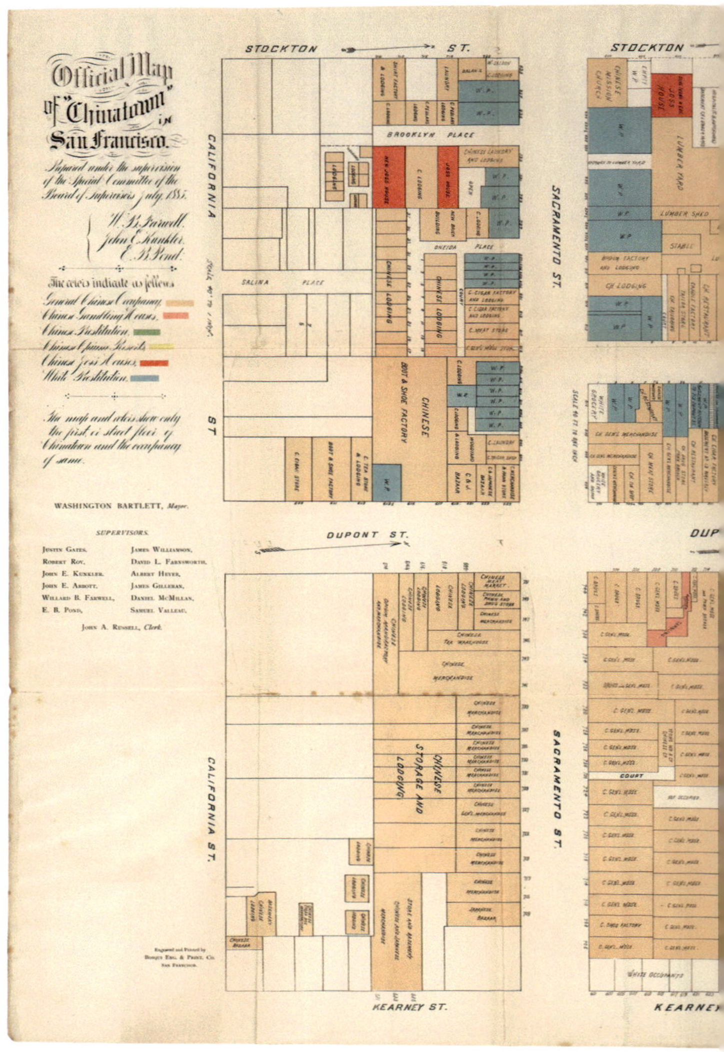

→ Chinese Hospital. Published in "San Francisco's First Chinese Hospital" by T. J. Gintjee and Howard H. Johnson, M.D., in *Modern Hospital* 25, no. 4 (October 1925): 283–285.

↓ Official Map of "Chinatown," San Francisco, July 1885. Engraved and printed by Bosqui Eng. & Print. C°., San Francisco. Color-coding distinguishes between Chinese and white prostitution as well as different types of Chinese businesses.

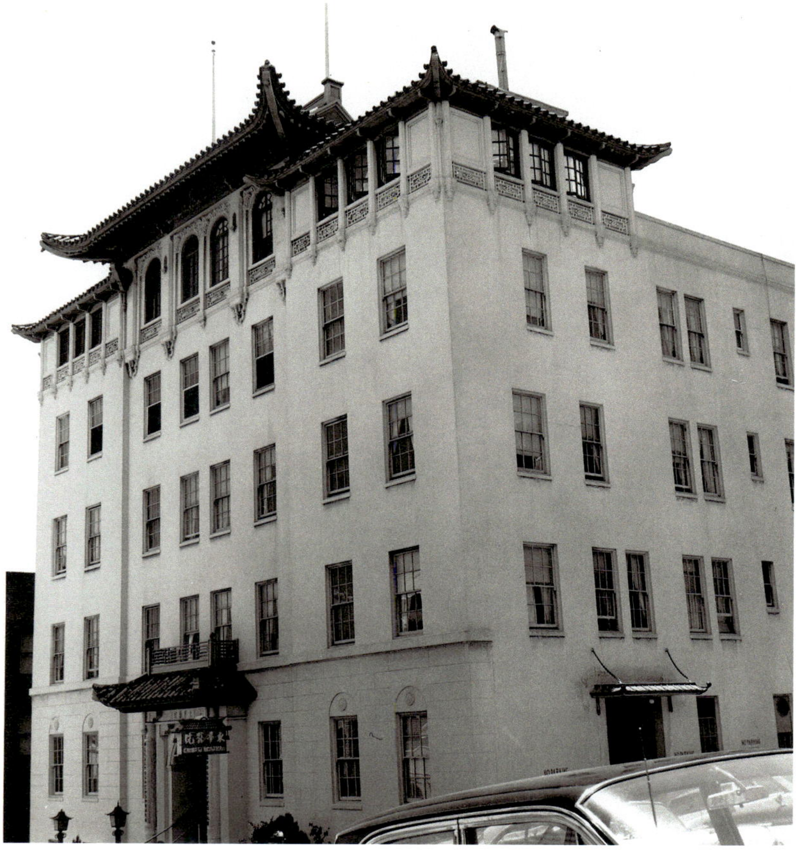

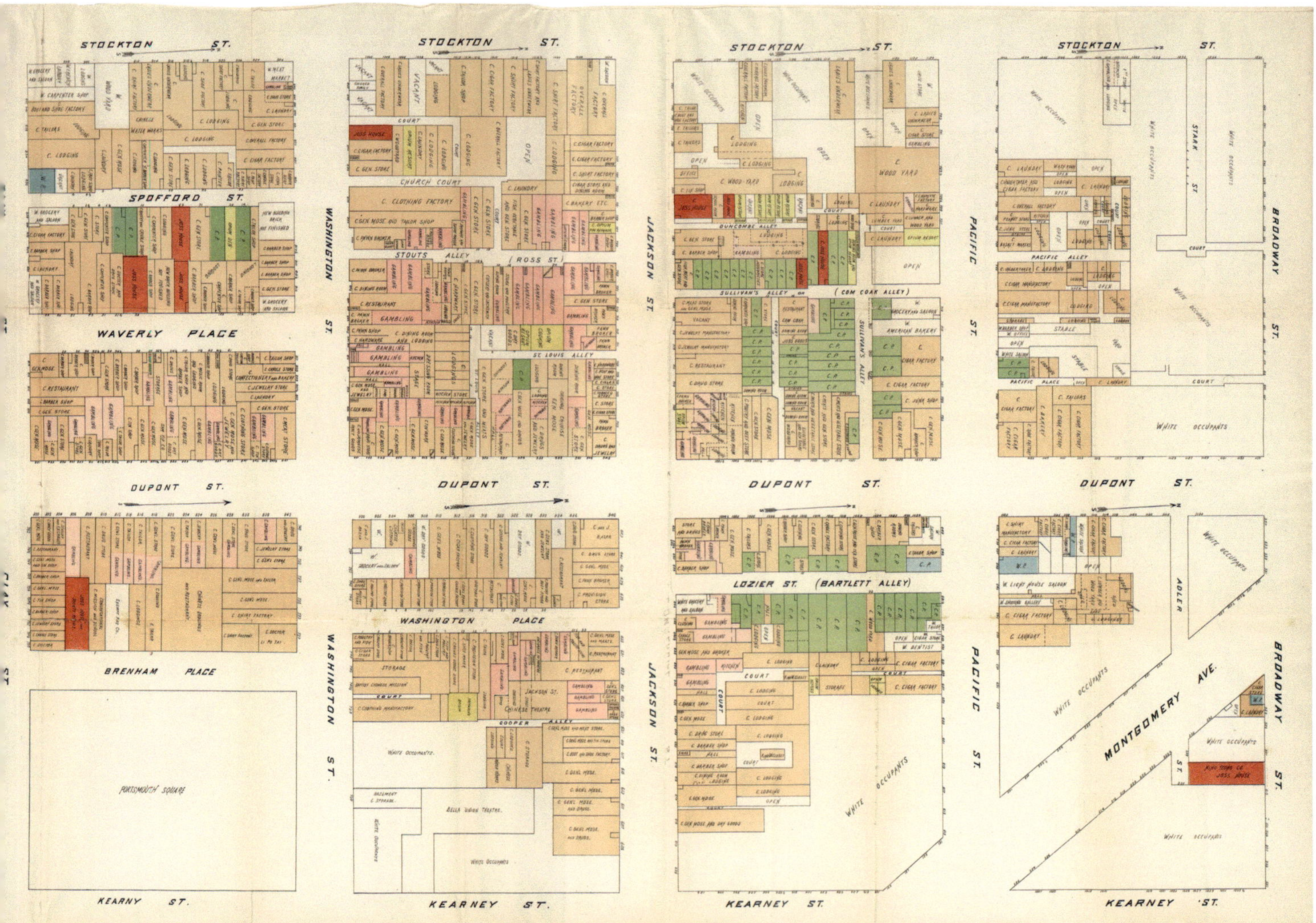

The 1906 earthquake was a seminal moment in the city's architectural history, as the shaking and subsequent fires destroyed some 28,000 buildings—including all of Chinatown. Its complete destruction was touted as a purification for the city, and its rebuilding was predicated on a "sanitary plan" that catered to tourism and police surveillance. New buildings were carefully designed by white architects from firms such as Ross & Burgren to promote a new "Oriental City," donned in an "imitation oriental" style that crudely translated ancient Chinese forms into a new Sino-architecture using Western construction methods and local materials, and in compliance with local building codes.[33] Despite the fact that this new Oriental City was believed to encourage its Chinese residents to adopt more sanitary practices, San Francisco's Chinese and Chinatown continued to be associated with disease.[34]

Meanwhile, many of San Francisco's nineteenth-century hospitals either continued to operate or were remodeled or rebuilt following the earthquake. Images of these hospitals were used in early twentieth-century postcards and advertisements not only to communicate an image of modern health and normality, but also to effectuate practices of citizenship and civic pride.[35] Trade journals such as *Modern Hospital* (established in 1913) also served to publicize the interiors and floor plans of some of San Francisco's hospitals, normalizing a new relationship between private spaces, public consumption, and mass media.[36]

It took almost twenty years after the earthquake and the architectural reform of Chinatown for San Francisco's civic leaders to commit to actually improving, and not simply regulating and criminalizing, the living and social conditions of the Chinese community. The emergence of a new population of educated second-generation Chinese Americans "helped bridge the chasm between the Chinese American Community and dominant white society" in this task.[37] After the earthquake, charitable Chinese, American, and Christian organizations pledged money and sought ways to integrate traditional Chinese medical knowledge and Western medicine. Given the decades of pathologizing Chinese bodies, practices, space, and architecture, a compromise was reached by both communities by looking again to Hong Kong for inspiration on how to successfully, or acceptably, comingle Western medical science with traditional Chinese practices.[38]

Finally, in 1925 the Chinese Hospital (東華醫院) was constructed in Chinatown. To this day, it is the only Chinese hospital in the United States, and was described at the time of its opening as "marking the most modern advance of Orientals in this country."[39] The four-story reinforced-concrete building originally accommodated fifty-five beds, a surgical department with two operating rooms, a maternity department with a delivery room, a pharmacy, a lab, and an outpatient department. The hospital reflected the general trend of Chinatown's rebuilding to embrace an overtly stylized version of Sino-architecture.[40] Its form was said to have been copied from the hospital of the Rockefeller Foundation in Peking, China. Of the forty-four doctors originally employed, only five were Chinese, along with twelve Chinese "girls" trained in nursing.[41]

Following the hospital's opening, the 1930s and 1940s marked an "extraordinary switch from demonizing San Francisco's Chinese residents to assisting them as deserving citizens."[42] Concurrently, no longer associated with disease and vice, Chinatown was rebranded to create a family-friendly tourist destination for white, middle-class Americans. This transformation was dependent on public health reform, but also necessitated the retention of an alien otherness.[43] The Chinese Hospital, therefore, along with other charitable support institutions, not only reshaped the physical geography of Chinatown but its social geography as well.[44]

Whereas the city's first Euro-American hospitals and associated medical practices mediated normalcy, citizenship, and a racialized social order, the Chinese Hospital mediated a prescribed assimilation process that necessitated a desire from Chinese residents to acculturate to Western norms, values, and standards of living, while never attaining the full benefits of citizenship. For instance, Chinese Americans struggled to find housing outside of Chinatown because of racially restrictive housing covenants. While these covenants lost their legal authority in 1948, Chinese Americans continued to be victims of lawsuits and overt acts of violence.[45] Prejudice had so effectively centered difference in the body, social habits, and architectures of Chinese Americans (amongst other minority groups in the United States) that they could never quite escape a racialized group identity. While the Chinese hospital was, in theory, a material and symbolic victory for the Chinese community, its racial ordering of immigrant groups and construction of normality ultimately evolved alongside public health reform and advances in hospital design.[46] The conditional acceptance of a Chinese community residing within the city, then, was predicated on an architectural cleansing, a prescribed cultural assimilation, and a commodification of San Francisco's largest nonwhite immigrant enclave.[47]

An earlier version of this essay was originally published by e-flux Architecture in 2020.

1. Gray A. Brechin, *Imperial San Francisco: Urban Power, Earthly Ruin* (Berkeley, 1999), 29.

2. Brechin, *Imperial San Francisco*, 30. Quote cited from Emil Theodore Hieronymus Bunje and James C. Kean, *Pre-Marshall Gold in California* (Berkeley: University of California Press, 1938), 44.

3. Pekka Hämäläinen and Samuel Truett, “On Borderlands,” *Journal of American History* 98, no. 2 (2011): 338–361. Californios can be described an ethnically mixed group of settlers that lived for several generations in California and descended from Spanish colonizers, African slaves, and Native Americans. For more information see Ryan Reft, “From Alta California to American Statehood: Race, Change, and the Californio Pico Family,” in *East of East: The Making of Greater El Monte*, ed. Romeo Guzman, Carribean Fragoza, and Alex Sayf Cummings, and Ryan Reft (New Brunswick, NJ: Rutgers University Press, 2020), 37–48.

4. For a thorough accounting of how racist ideas evolved in the United States, see Ibram X Kendi, *Stamped from the Beginning: The Definitive History of Racist Ideas in America* (New York: Nation Books, 2016).

5. Peter H. Burnett, “State of the State Address,” speech delivered January 6, 1851.

6. The state’s 1852 census, conducted to supplement the federal 1850 census, used “color” as a category and assigned individuals to white, negro, mulatto, or domesticated Indians (most Native Americans in California and the United States were not included in census reports prior to 1900). For a discussion of how race functioned in the first state and local laws of California, see Shirley Ann Wilson Moore, “‘We Feel the Want of Protection’: The Politics of Law and Race in California, 1848–1878,” in *Taming the Elephant: Politics, Government, and Law in Pioneer California*, ed. John F. Burns, Richard J. Orsi, and Marlene Smith-Baranzini (Berkeley: University of California Press, 2003), 96–125.

7. For a full account of the Chinese in San Francisco and the blame and stigma they experienced with regard to disease, see Susan Craddock, *City of Plagues: Disease, Poverty, and Deviance in San Francisco* (Minneapolis: University of Minnesota Press, 2000), 10; Guenter B. Risse, *Plague, Fear, and Politics in San Francisco’s Chinatown* (Baltimore: Johns Hopkins University Press, 2012); and Nyan Shah, *Contagious Divides: Epidemics and Race in San Francisco’s Chinatown* (Berkeley: University of California Press, 2001).

8. Mitchel Roth, “Cholera, Community, and Public Health in Gold Rush Sacramento and San Francisco,” *Pacific Historical Review* 66, no. 4 (November 1997): 527–551.

9. E. O. Kemble and J. E. Durivage, “Filth and the Cholera,” *Daily Alta California*, November 12, 1850.

10. Roth, “Cholera, Community, and Public Health,” 532.

11. Henry G. Langley, *The Pacific Coast Business Directory for 1871–73, Containing the Names, Business and Address of over Forty Thousand Merchants* (1873).

12. John Morrill Bryan, *Robert Mills: America’s First Architect* (New York: Princeton Architectural Press, 2001). Mills is best known for his designs in Washington, DC, including the Washington Monument, the Department of Treasury Headquarters, and the Post Office Headquarters to name a few. He was the first official architect and engineer to the federal government.

13. See John Woodworth, *1st Annual Report of the Supervising Surgeon of the Marine-Hospital Service of the United States for the Year 1872, Containing a Brief Historical Sketch of the Service from the Date of Its Organization in 1798*, cited in Norman E. Tutorow, “A Tale of Two Hospitals: U.S. Marine Hospital No. 19 and the U.S. Public Health Service Hospital on the Presidio of San Francisco,” *California History* 75, no. 2 (Summer 1996): 154–169.

14. “The Marine Hospital: Description of the New Buildings: The Pavilion Plan to Be Carried Out,” *San Francisco Chronicle*, May 10, 1874.

15. Tutorow, “A Tale of Two Hospitals,” 165.

16. Jeanne Kisacky, *Rise of the Modern Hospital: An Architectural History of Health and Healing, 1870–1940* (Pittsburgh: University of Pittsburgh Press, 2017), 4.

17. “Five Miles of Wire: For the French Hospital One of the Most Extensive Jobs of the Kind Ever Undertaken Here,” *San Francisco Chronicle*, July 11, 1894.

18. “New German Hospital Viewed from Noe Street: It Will Cost Four Hundred Thousand Dollars and Be the Finest Institution of Its Kind in the West,” *San Francisco Chronicle*, May 1, 1904.

19. John B. C. Saunders, “Geography and Geopolitics in California Medicine,” *Bulletin of the History of Medicine* 41 (1967): 293–324, cited in Guenter B. Risse, “Translating Western Modernity: The First Chinese Hospital in America,” *Bulletin of the History of Medicine* 85, no. 3 (2011): 413–447.

20. Shah, *Contagious Divides*, 3–4.

21. California State Board of Health, *First Biennial Report of the State Board of Health of California for the Years 1870 and 1871* (Sacramento: D. W. Gelwicks State Printer, 1871).

22. California State Board of Health, *First Biennial Report*, 9.

23. California State Board of Health, *First Biennial Report*, 44–46

24. California State Board of Health, *First Biennial Report*, 47. Coolie was a term that was originally assigned to unskilled indentured workers from South Asia and China that Britain exported to its colonies—largely following the abolition of slavery in the British Empire.

25. Craddock, *City of Plagues*, 10.

26. Craddock, *City of Plagues*, 11. This term is used to describe how geographic spaces, like Chinatown, can be pathologized with disease and deviance.

27. Several books and articles have been written on the exclusionary laws that targeted Asian migration to the United States. The Chinese Exclusion Act of 1882 was the first US law that excluded an entire ethnic group from immigrating to the US.

28. See Joshua S. Yang, “The Anti-Chinese Cubic Air Ordinance,” *American Journal of Public Health* 99, no. 3 (2009): 440.

29. Risse, “Translating Western Modernity.”

30. Risse, “Translating Western Modernity,” 413–419.

31. Risse, “Translating Western Modernity,” 420–433.

32. Risse, “Translating Western Modernity,” 437–440.

33. Philip P. Choy, *San Francisco Chinatown: A Guide to Its History and Architecture* (San Francisco: City Lights Books, 2012), 44–45.

34. Shah, *Contagious Divides*, 152–153.

35. Sara Anne Hook, “You’ve Got Mail: Hospital Postcards as a Reflection of Health Care in the Early Twentieth Century,” *Journal of the Medical Library Association* 93, no. 3 (2005): 386–393.

36. Beatriz Colomina, *Privacy and Publicity: Modern Architecture as Mass Media* (Cambridge, MA: MIT Press, 1994).

37. Shah, *Contagious Divides*, 226.

38. Yi-Ren Chen, “Chinese Hospital: A Study of San Francisco’s Chinatown Attitudes towards Western Medical Practices at the Turn of the Century,” *Herodotus* 16 (Spring 2006): 69–83.

39. “First Chinese Hospital Ready to Open: Chinatown to Celebrate Big Forward Step,” *San Francisco Chronicle,* March 19, 1925.

40. City and County of San Francisco Planning Department, “Draft Environmental Impact Report: 835–845 Jackson Street Chinese Hospital Replacement Project,” IV.B.2., 2012.

41. “First Chinese Hospital Ready to Open.”

42. Shah, *Contagious Divides*, 2.

43. Ivan Light, “From Vice District to Tourist Attraction: The Moral Career of American Chinatowns, 1880–1940,” *Pacific Historical Review* 43, no. 3 (1974): 367–394.

44. Shah, *Contagious Divides*, 208.

45. Shah, *Contagious Divides*, 246–247. Racially restrictive covenants date back to the nineteenth century in the United States but were especially used in the early to mid-twentieth century. They were deemed unconstitutional in 1948 in the Supreme Court ruling *Shelly v. Kraemer*. See Eli Moore, Nicole Montojo, and Nicole Mauri, “Roots, Race, and Place: A History of Racially Exclusionary Housing in the San Francisco Bay Area,” Haas Institute for a Fair and Inclusive Society, University of California, Berkeley (October 2019), haasinstitute.berkeley.edu/rootsraceplace. And Richard Rothstein, *The Color of Law: A Forgotten History of How Our Government Segregated America* (New York: Liveright, 2017).

46. Rothstein, *The Color of Law*, 252–253.

47. Ching Lin Pang and Jan Rath, “The Force of Regulation in the Land of the Free: The Persistence of Chinatown, Washington, DC, as a Symbolic Ethnic Enclave,” *The Sociology of Entrepreneurship: Research in the Sociology of Organizations*, ed. M. Ruef and M. Lounsbury (Leeds: Emerald Group Publishing, 2007), 191–216.

p79 University of California San Francisco Archives and Special Collections.
p80 (top) California State Library, Digital Collections.
p80 (middle) East Carolina University’s Digital Collections.
p80 (bottom) Image courtesy of California State Library, California History Section Picture Catalog.
p81, 83 (bottom) David Rumsey Map Collection.

THE BIRTH OF A MODERN CHINESE SANATORIUM

CHENCHEN YAN

In May 1919, the literary magazine *Xin qingnian / La Jeunesse* published a short story by Chinese writer Lu Xun called "Medicine," in which Old Chuan and his wife save every penny to buy a folk medicine cure—a roll of steamed bread soaked with blood—for their son, who is dying of tuberculosis.[1] As the reader soon learns, the blood is from a young radical who was executed for revolutionary activities. The image of the bread dripping with blood not only represents the superstition of traditional Chinese medicine, but is also a metaphor for the political ignorance of the public. As a medical student turned writer who studied in Japan, Lu Xun saw a profound interconnection between the physical and social illnesses of his time. Looming large was the Xinhai Revolution of 1911 that overthrew the Qing dynasty and in 1928 resulted in the establishment of the Nationalist Party (Kuomintang, KMT) and the Republic of China, which quickly fell into political chaos and internecine warfare. In this regard, Lu's story "Medicine" asks if the revolution was really a cure for the ailing nation when it still conformed to traditional values.

The publication of "Medicine" coincided with the onset of the May Fourth Movement, which arose from massive student protests in Beijing against the government's inaction in response to the Treaty of Versailles, which allowed Japan to take over territories in eastern China that had previously been colonized by Germany. The outbreak of student protests marked the culmination of years of intense cultural debates known as the New Culture Movement. Disillusioned with Confucianism and the failures of the Nationalist government, intellectuals called for the reformation of the Chinese language and the emancipation of women, and promoted Western ideals like democracy and science. In many Chinese political and literary texts, social problems were medicalized in order to decry China's failure to catch up with a modernizing and globalizing world.[2] For Chinese reformers at the time, diseases like tuberculosis became the perfect arena for questioning Chinese medicine in particular, and traditional Chinese culture in general.

While tuberculosis helped to modernize architecture in Europe, it also prompted a group of Chinese doctors and architects to build one of the earliest examples of International Style architecture in China: the Hongqiao Sanatorium, completed in 1934 in Shanghai.[3] Unlike most contemporary architectural production at the time, which was built in Chinese,

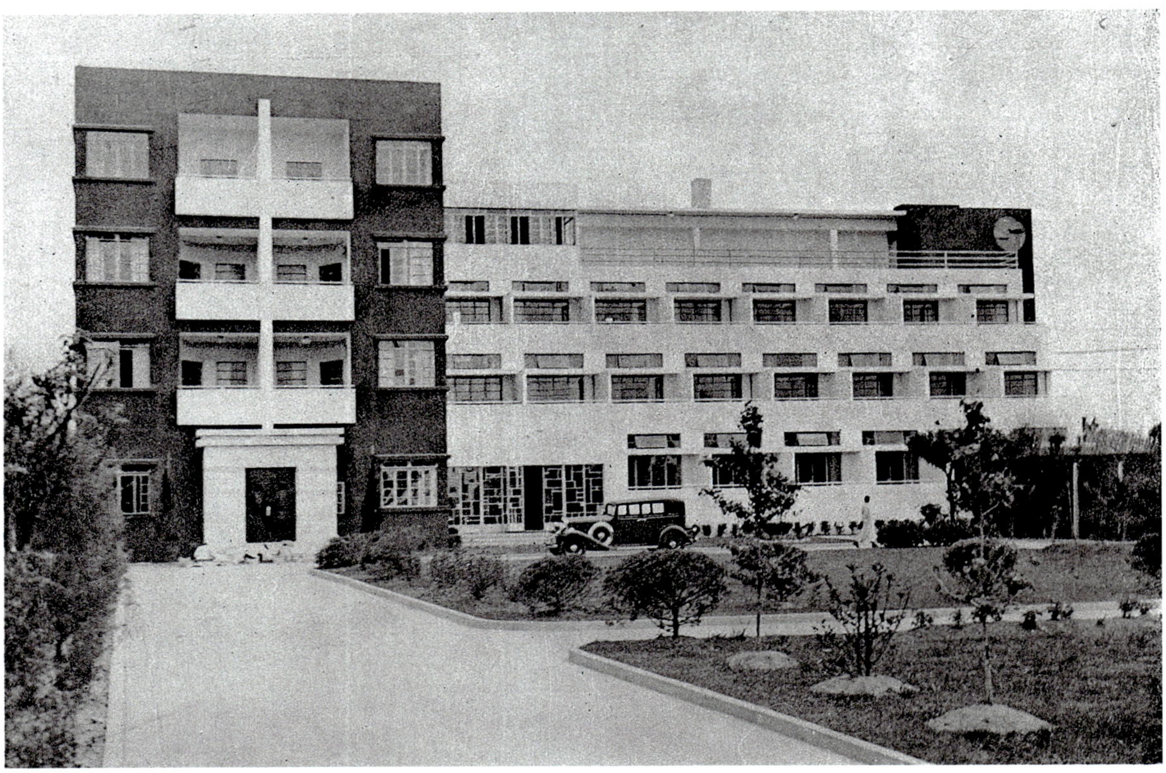

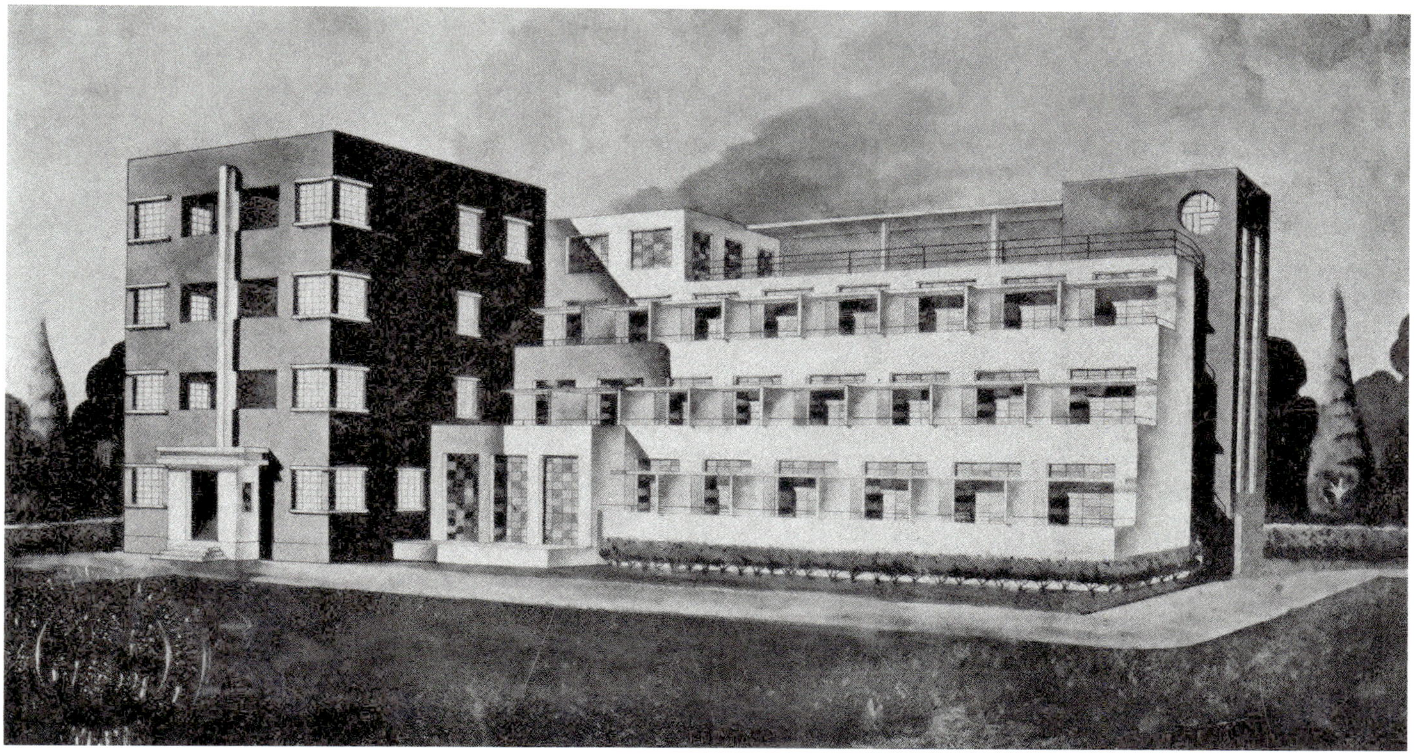

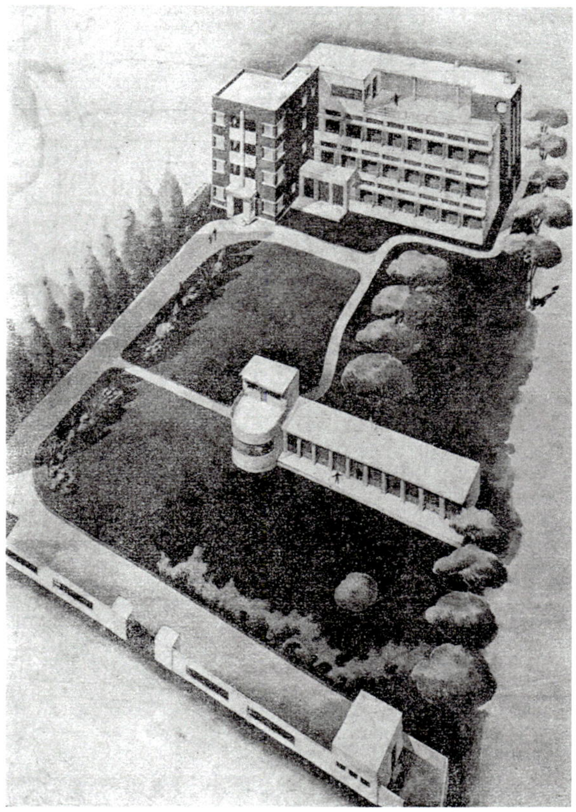

neoclassical, art deco, or other revival styles, the Hongqiao Sanatorium is regarded as "the most representative work of modernist architecture" in Republican China.[4] For many architectural historians, the sanatorium marked a brief period of "serious modernism" in Chinese architectural history, characterized by the emergence of the idea of "functionalism" in tandem with the first translations and studies of Western architects such as Le Corbusier and Bruno Taut.[5]

This historiographical desire for a "pure" modernism can be read as a response to the predominant nationalism of early twentieth-century China that confined the discourse of architecture to the nation's cultural identity. When China's first generation of modern architects returned home after studying in the US, Europe, or Japan in the 1920s and 1930s, most collaborated closely with the government, which was struggling to centralize power through nation-building projects.[6] To further create a sense of national sovereignty and belonging, in 1929 the Nationalist government officially mandated an "inherently national style" for all public buildings, which led Western architectural styles to become associated with foreign settlements, imperialism, and the loss of economic and cultural autonomy.[7] At the same time, state architects fashioned this traditional Chinese style with a language drawn from their Beaux-Arts training and other Western architectural theories.[8]

A similar nationalist sentiment can also be discerned in medicinal discourse. In 1928, following the lobbying of John B. Grant at the Rockefeller Foundation and a group of practitioners of Western medicine, a proposal was unanimously passed to

↑ With its flat roofs and stepped terraces, the sanatorium is considered as "the most representative work of modernist architecture" in Republican China.

↓ A bird's-eye view of the Hongqiao Sanatorium.

← The facade of the main building in the Hongqiao Sanatorium complex.

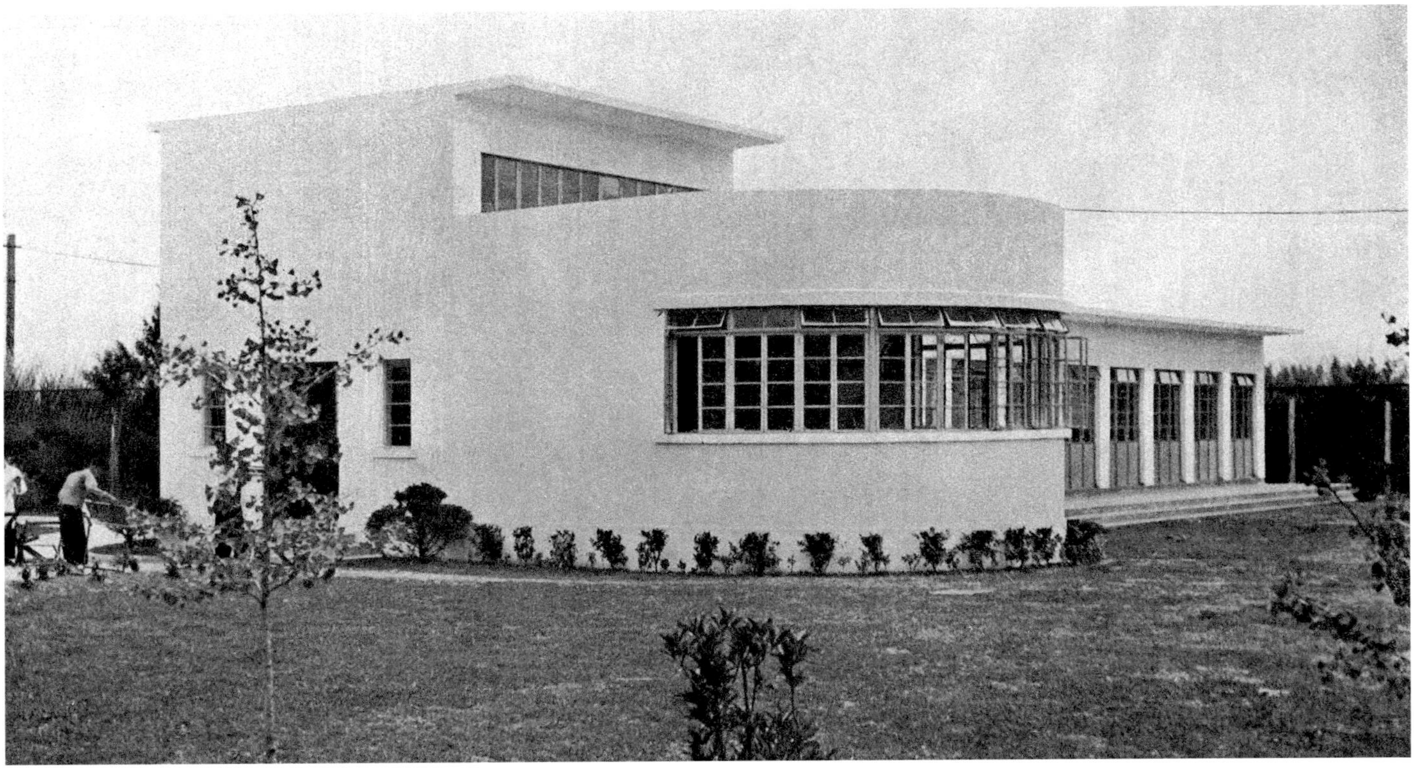

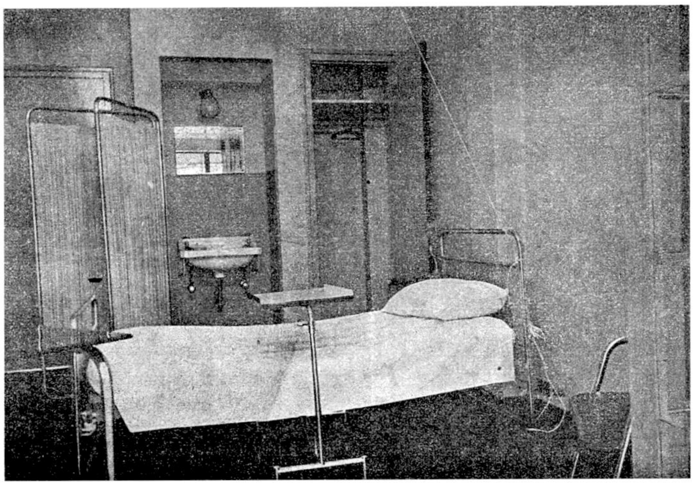

abolish the practice of Chinese medicine at the first National Conference on Public Health. However, the resolution quickly backfired and mobilized the previously unorganized practitioners of Chinese medicine into a National Medicine Movement (*guoyi yundong*). Motivated by the need for a uniquely Chinese identity in the midst of social and cultural convulsions, the National Medicine Movement actively competed with Western medicine and successfully forged a closer alliance with the Nationalist government.[9]

Seen in this light, the flat roofs and stepped terraces of the Hongqiao Sanatorium represent a remarkable break from the predominant nationalist discourse in the name of public health and modernization. The sanatorium was conceived by the father and son Ding Fubao and Ding Huikang, both of whom were members of the newly founded National Anti-Tuberculosis Association of China (Zhongguo Fanglao Xiehui, NATAC). Ding Fubao was a doctor, translator, and one of the earliest reformers of Chinese medicine.[10] After a study trip to Japan in 1909, he became a proponent of Western medicine in China and established the Sino-Western Medical Research Society. From 1912, he devoted himself to commercially publishing a popular series of medical guides called *Mr. Ding's Medical Compendium*, which comprised translations from Japanese texts on Western medicine. Deeply influenced by his father, Ding Huikang received his doctorate of medicine from the University of Hamburg in 1924, specializing in tuberculosis and pneumonic diseases.

Despite the establishment of China's first Ministry of Health in 1928, the country had no public-health-centered policy throughout the 1920s and 1930s.[11]

↑ A separate building at the sanatorium, designed for cheaper wards.

↓ Inside the "first class" ward.

Tuberculosis in particular was not considered a public health crisis until campaigns by NATAC.[12] Established in Shanghai in October 1933 and independent of the government, NATAC was the only organization active in the 1930s and 1940s dedicated to the elimination of the tuberculosis.[13] Its efforts included weeklong educational campaigns, radio talks, and public lectures, as well as founding clinical facilities and increasing beds across hospitals in Shanghai for tuberculosis patients.[14]

NATAC produced and publicized often exaggerated statistics in popular newspapers and magazines to make the tuberculosis crisis "visible." As medical historian Sean Hsiang-lin Lei has argued, the pathology of the emergence of the tuberculosis crisis in Republican China is not *Mycobacterium tuberculosis*, but the internalization of the colonial gaze that objectified the Chinese as the unhygienic, uncivilized, and unhealthy other.[15] Tuberculosis became associated with traditional lifestyles within an extended family. In her article "The Chinese and Tuberculosis," Ge Chenghui, one of first woman doctors in China and a graduate of Yale Medical School, identified three "unhygienic" habits within the family as causes of contagion: sharing meals, sharing the bed, and sleeping with closed windows.[16] In this sense, Western medical thinking represented not only scientific and epistemological difference to Chinese tradition, but also cultural and behavioral difference. By appropriating the tuberculosis crisis as a cultural critique of tradition, NATAC appointed itself as the "doctors of enlightenment" and thereby worked to create a modern, hygienic subject.

Inaugurated on June 17, 1934, the Hongqiao Sanatorium became a media sensation. Photos of the general and mayor of Shanghai Wu Tiecheng with a crowd of celebrities, politicians, and doctors were reproduced in newspapers and magazines across the country.[17] The sanatorium, advertised as "the latest and most up-to-date" medical facility in Shanghai and the best of its kind in East Asia, instantly became a source of national pride and a tourist attraction, drawing national politicians like Cai Yuanpei and Sun Ke (son of Sun Yat-sen) for visits.[18] Located in the suburbs to the west of Shanghai and surrounded by small farms and gardens, the sanatorium claimed to offer peace and tranquility to the sick. Constructed in reinforced concrete and oriented to the south, the complex consisted of one four-story building and another single-story structure that together provided thirty-nine wards, all of which were directly connected to balconies, allowing patients access to sunlight throughout the day. Costs to stay at Hongqiao were low compared with other contemporary medical facilities in Shanghai, but the sanatorium was still unaffordable for most of the population. The hierarchically organized complex boasted "first-class wards" with en-suite bathrooms

↑ The Hongqiao Sanatorium differs from the European models in its partitioning of terraces.

↓ Titled "an analysis of sunlight," this drawing also shows the architect's careful consideration of patient privacy. The terraces are set back in such a way that a patient upstairs would not be able to look out and easily see a patient downstairs, and vice versa.

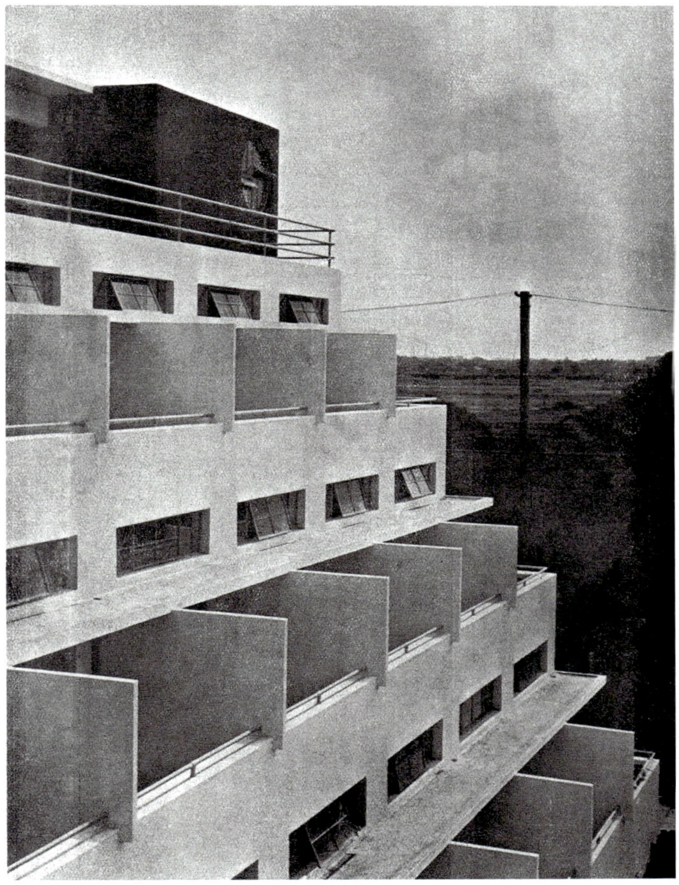

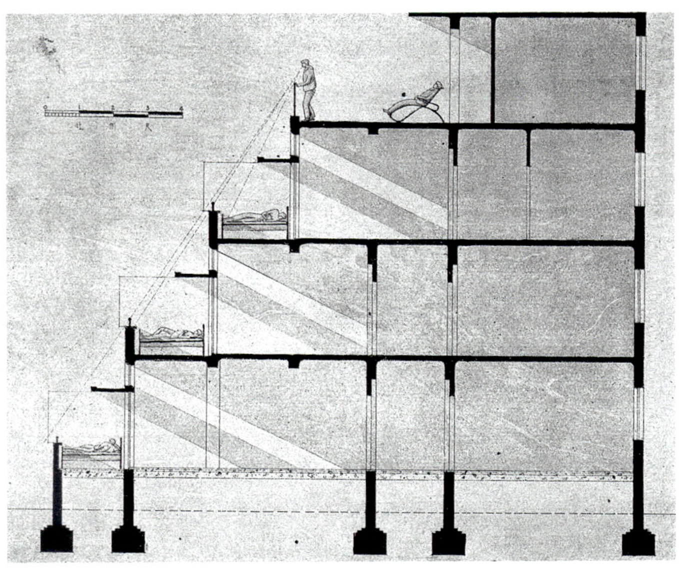

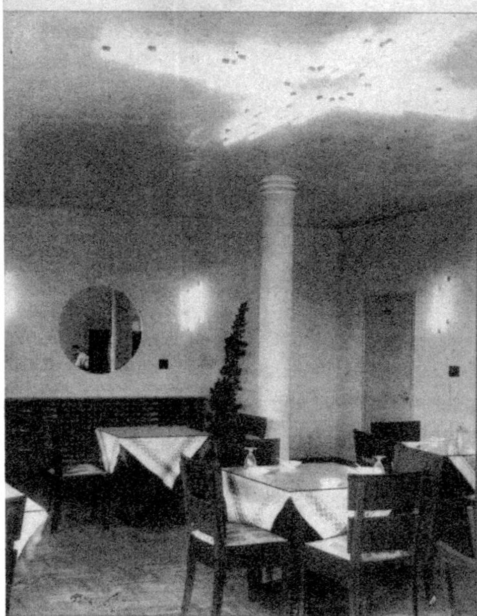

院中餐廳，亦出於美術專家之設計。

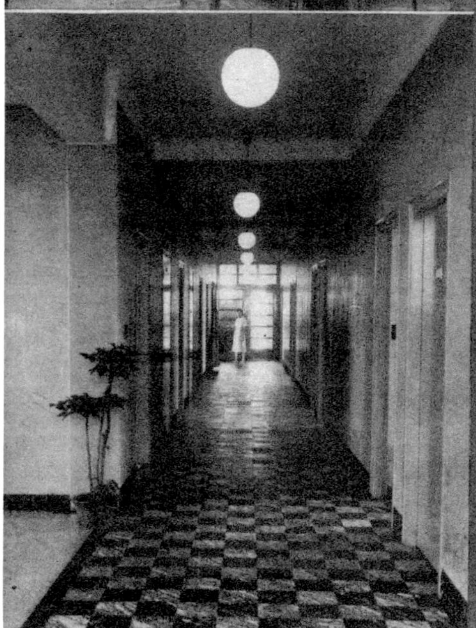

走廊爲橡皮地板，美觀清潔，避去步行聲浪，使病人得充分靜養。

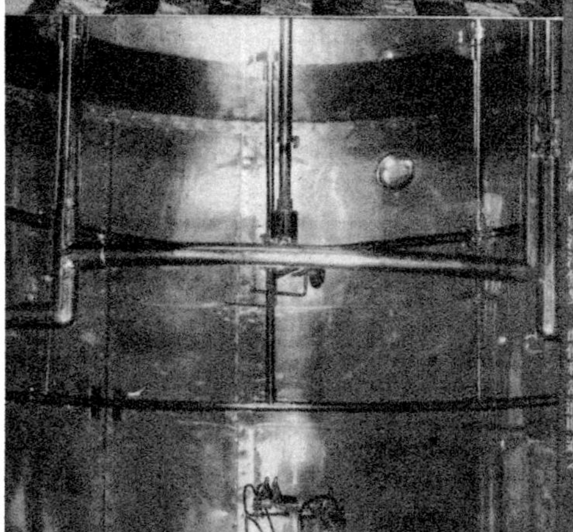

太陽燈浴室，同時容十六人，且有反射光線，與海浴無異，而便利舒適則過之。

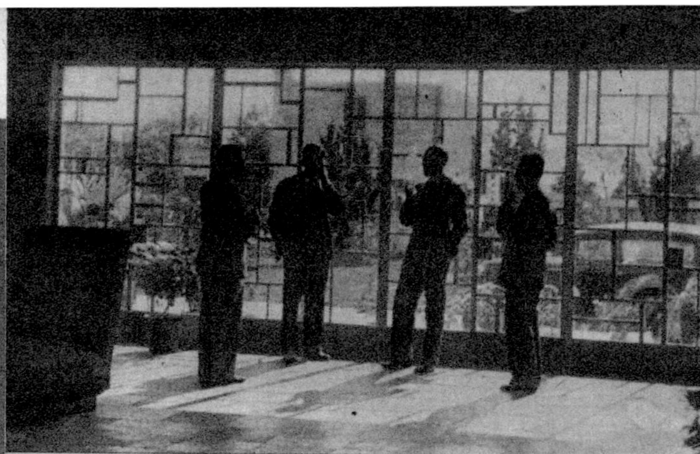

院中會客室，於病人施手術前召集專家討論病情。

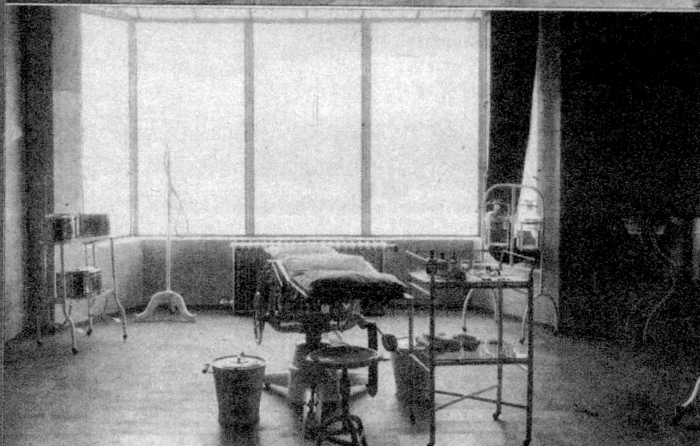

手術室用橡皮地板及最新式無影燈光，並有調節氣溫之冷熱機裝置。

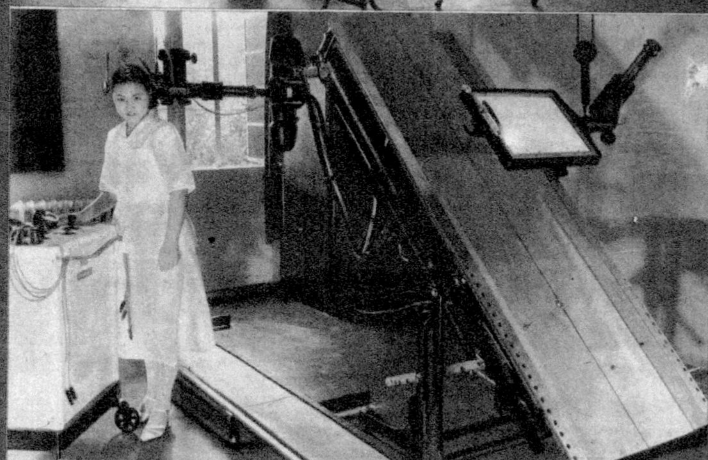

愛克司光機，有透視之設備，爲世界最近發明者，旁爲短波治療機，國內醫院，尚少此項設備。

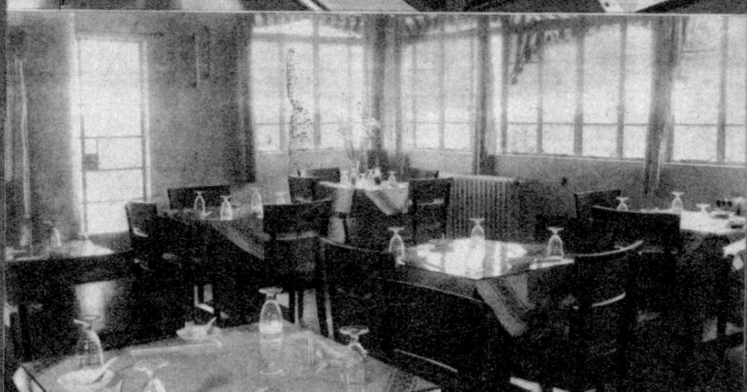

（→）病院樓之小廚房，有冷藏及水爐等，極爲清潔。
（←）會食室一隅，位於全院最高層。

室。該院之特點，爲所有臥室，悉數南向，每室均有互相隔離陽台，以備橫臥休憩之用。每高一層，卽向內縮進六七尺，故每層臥室之光線空氣，異常充足，爲國內最新式之醫院建築。而環境幽靜，接近村鄉，尤適合於療養。並新闢日光療養所，上供長期曝養及戒患之用，可免醫藥等費。創辦人爲無錫丁福保氏及其哲嗣惠康醫師，經營設計，歷二年有餘，全屋於今夏落成，由吳市長行開幕禮。

　　歐美各國致富強之由，要非一端，而國勢之隆，實與醫藥衛生之進行爲正比例。上海爲吾國第一大埠，其間不乏規模宏大之醫院，但皆由外人所設，國人自辦而足與比美者，當推虹橋療養院。編者參觀，歎其設備之完美，乃攝圖刊於本報，使國人知吾國療治界有現代最高標準之設施，亦國家進步之一端也。（梁得所誌）

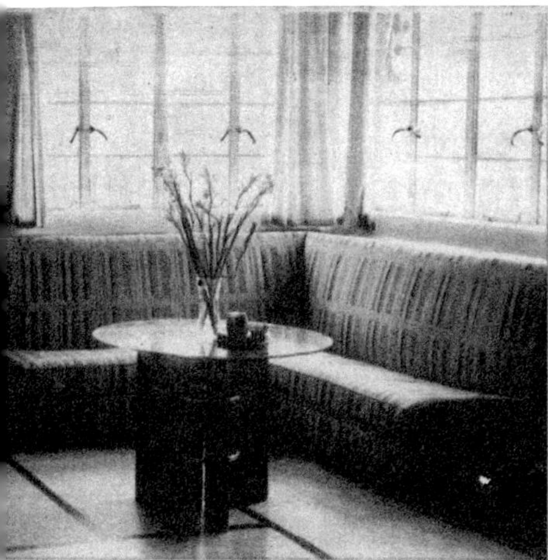

會客室之一隅，佈置簡潔而幽雅。

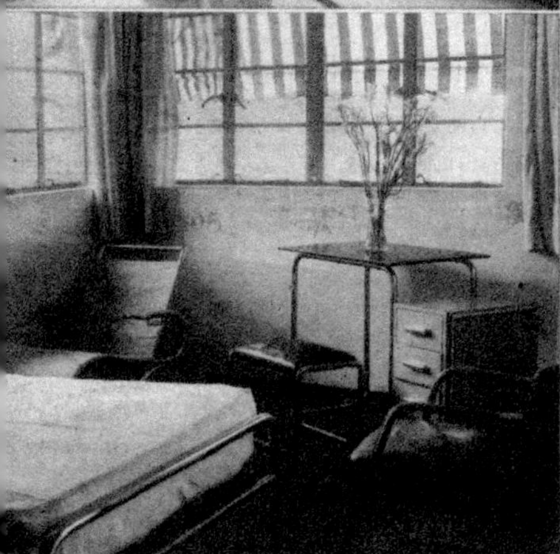

臥房三面闢窗，空氣光線充足，另有個人平台以供休憩之用。

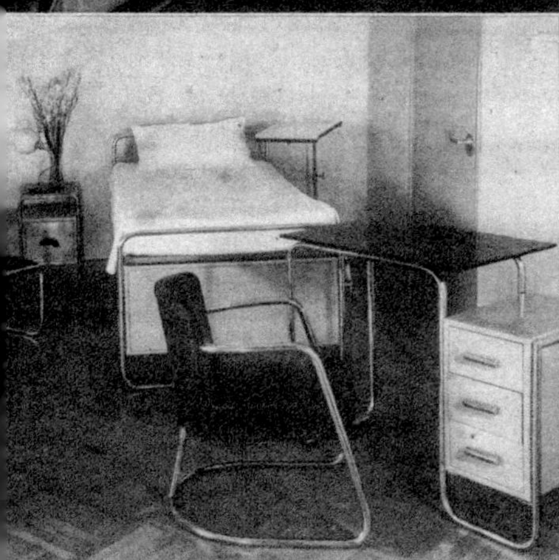

特制臥室內部，均爲最新式之陳設。

療病者之一個福地

THE HUNGJAO SANATORIUM

Founded by the well-known Dr. F. P. Ting, and inaugurated last summer, the Hungjao Sanatorium, on Hungjao Road, Shanghai, is the newest of its kind in China. With its construction and equipment based entirely on modern medical science, it spells real comfort and assured convalescence to the patient. The sanatorium is under the able management of Dr. W. K. Ting (Inset), son of its founder.

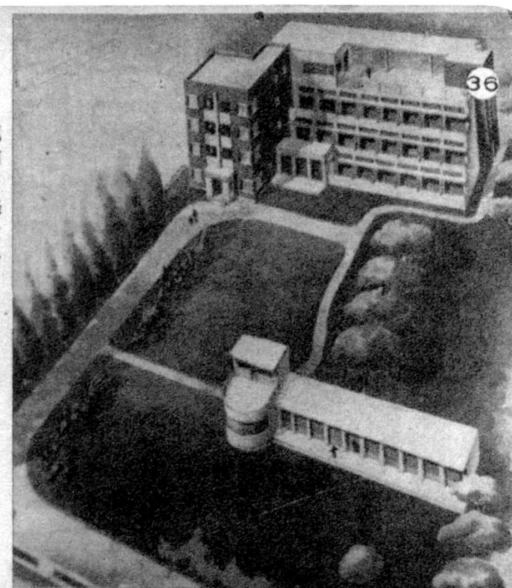

滬西新築虹橋療養院鳥瞰

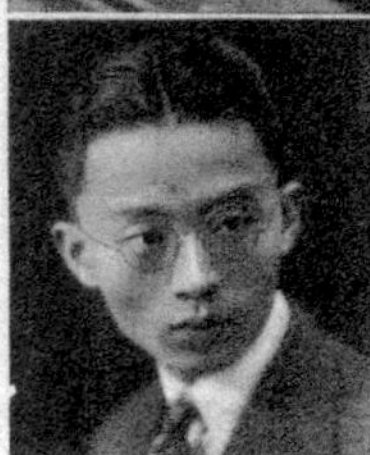

院主任丁惠康醫師

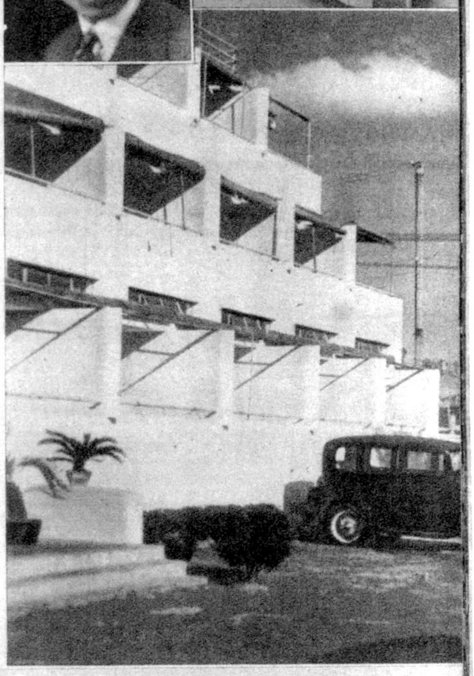

該院堆疊式建築爲科學化之最新設計

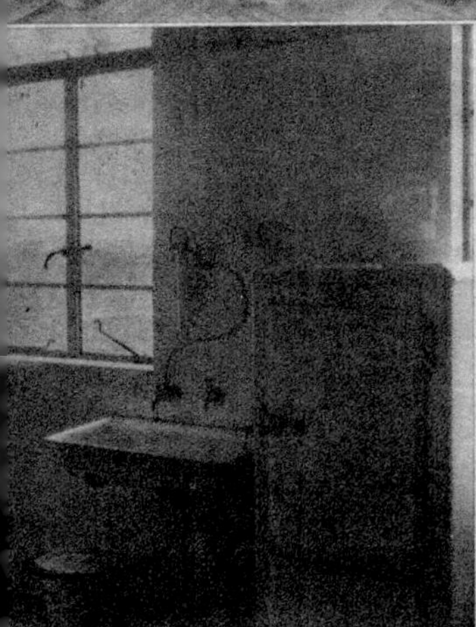

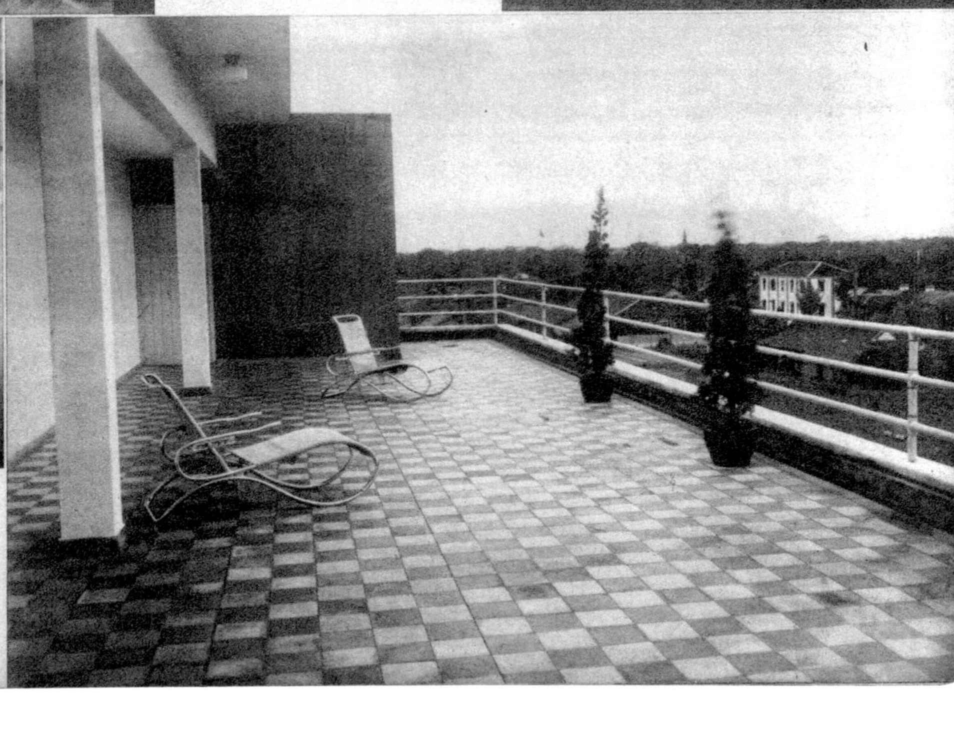

上：頂層遼闊陽台，平整雅潔，憑欄遠眺，郊野風景瞭然入目

虹橋療養院，位僻於滬西虹橋路，完全爲最新立方體，作堆疊階梯式，疊立郊外，倍覺雄壯。全廈外部，用紅白二色，莊嚴美麗。入門後，左爲覺生室，右爲交誼廳，鵝壁淡綠，古雅宜人。第一關有看護室，愛克司光室，太陽燈室，存生臥登；第二

while standard, cheaper accommodation was located in the separate one-story structure across the lawn from the main building.[19]

The facility's "splendid equipment," as Mayor Wu remarked, included hot and cold running water, electricity, air conditioning, UV light-permitting windows, and modern furniture. In addition to sunbathing rooms, operation rooms, sanitation rooms, observation rooms, and labs, the sanatorium provided recreation spaces, a dining hall, lounge, library, music room, and a kitchen. Hallways and corridors were covered with rubber flooring imported from the Netherlands intended to reduce the noise of foot traffic. The most advanced light therapy and ultrasound (or short-wave diathermy) therapy machines had been imported from Germany, as well as X-ray machines and shadowless surgical operating lights.[20]

Designed by Xi Fuquan, who had studied in Germany from 1922 to 1929, the architecture was described in the *China Times* as "great" and "cubist."[21] Visitors expressed amazement at the building's terraces and reinforced concrete structure, as well as the rounded edges and corners in the interior designed to prevent the accumulation of dust.[22] While bearing many similarities to its European counterparts, the Hongqiao Sanatorium differs in its partitioning of terraces. In European sanatoria such as the County Hospital in Waiblingen by Richard Döcker or Alvar and Aino Aalto's Paimio Sanatorium, the terraces usually ran continuously along the building. At Hongqiao, however, partitions separated the outdoor space into individual terraces. As Mayor Wu perceptively commented: "the planning of the institution made it possible for every patient to enjoy privacy."[23] Indeed, individual privacy is meticulously represented throughout the building. In addition to partitions, the terraces are set back in such a way that patients above were not able to look out and easily see a patient below, and vice versa.

After its inauguration, the Hongqiao Sanatorium continued to be publicized. Its representation in professional journals mainly covered how the sanatorium contributed to contemporary discourses of

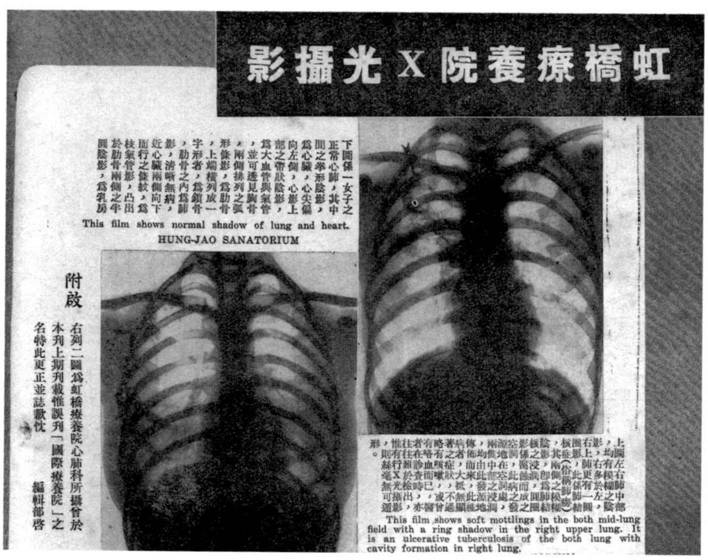

medicine and architecture. Its media presence in popular magazines and newspapers consisted primarily of promotions placed by the sanatorium itself. One photo showcased X-ray equipment with a female nurse, thereby associating modern technology with the trope of the modern woman.[24] An array of photographs in another double-page feature titled "Patients' Paradise" presented the sanatorium as a resort rather than a hospital. It would also appear in the news whenever a celebrity or politician was admitted.

The tuberculosis crisis in Republican China ultimately elevated questions of health from the level of the personal to the national and tied "hygiene" to China's place in the global order. The Hongqiao Sanatorium represents an exceptional case in which the private sector replaced the state-controlled public health system as a leading force in the politicization of a disease. Emerging out of the constant struggles and confrontations between Chinese and Western medicine and architecture, the sanatorium adds a colonial twist to the often-cited alliance between modern architects and doctors: Western medicine helped architects overcome the limits of the predominant nationalistic discourse of "the Chinese style," while Western architecture functioned as a visual rhetorical device that promoted the professional image of Western medicine. As an unambiguous rejection of Chinese tradition (both architectural and medical), the sanatorium could not have been realized without this alliance as well as the power vacuum left by the lack of state-controlled public health measures. Its adaptation and appropriation of Western forms and ideologies allowed NATAC doctors and architects to claim authority over China's modernization processes at a time when the state power was still weak, confounding the binary narrative of imperialist domination and anti-imperialist resistance.

This transient independence from nationalism and "serious modernism" ended with the onset of the Sino-Japanese War in 1937. This forced the sanatorium's medical team to abandon the buildings, which faded into oblivion as the Communist Party took over in 1949 and nationalized the healthcare system. While the complex no longer stands, the tension between Chinese and Western medicine continues to exist in a new yet equally politicized fashion. Although Chinese medicine has largely been integrated into the country's technoscientific healthcare system, it remains a nationalistic symbol, which came to the fore as treatment against Covid-19 was exported as part of relief missions intended to boost China's soft power.[25]

← An advertisement for the sanatorium, described as a "paradise for patients."

↙ X-ray images from a popular magazine showing healthy and infected lungs.

1. Lu Xun, "Yao [Medicine]", *Xin Qingnian / La Jeunesse* (*Xin Qingnian*) 6, no. 5 (1919).
2. Carlos Rojas, *Homesickness: Culture, Contagion and National Transformation in Modern China* (Cambridge, MA: Harvard University Press, 2015); Yang Nianqun, *Remaking Patients: Space Politics under the Conflict between Chinese and Western Medicine (1832–1985)* (New York: Peter Lang, 2020).
3. Beatriz Colomina, *X-Ray Architecture* (Zurich: Lars Müller, 2019).
4. Yongyi Lu and Yan Chen, "The Idea and Form of Functionalism in Early Chinese Modern Architecture: A Case Study on Hongqiao Sanatorium in Shanghai," *Jianzhu shi* (October 2017): 49–58.
5. Jianfei Zhu, *Architecture of Modern China* (London: Routledge, 2009), 71.
6. Although the Qing dynasty was toppled in 1911, China was not unified until 1928, when the KMT was finally able to consolidate its control over most of the country and relocated the capital from Beijing to Nanjing, ushering in an era of relative stability before the outbreak of the Sino-Japanese war in 1937. The notion of the architect as an individual artist did not exist in China before the twentieth century. The emergence of the architectural profession is also manifested in an epistemological shift of the concept of architecture. The traditional term for architecture, *yingzao*, was replaced by a new term, *jianzhu*, to emphasize the new notions of architecture as an art, a discipline, and a profession (as opposed to a craft).
7. Lai Delin, *Zhongguo Jindai Jianzhu Shi Yanjiu* [Studies in Modern Chinese Architectural History] (Beijing: Qinghua Daxue Chubanshe, 2007).
8. To be clear, this reinvented "Chinese architectural tradition" is a modern construction underpinned by the Beaux-Arts tradition and various Western architectural theories such as structural rationalism and organicism, and its development involved a history of orientalist scholarship and a legitimizing process in which Western architecture was taken as the universal point of reference. However, it has been deemed to be "traditional" by reformers and historians in pursuit of a Western-centric notion of modernity. Jeffrey W. Cody, Nancy S. Steinhardt, and Tony Atkin, eds., *Chinese Architecture and the Beaux-Arts* (Honolulu: University of Hawaii Press, 2011).
9. Sean Hsiang-lin Lei, *Neither Donkey nor Horse: Medicine in the Struggle over China's Modernity* (Chicago: University of Chicago Press, 2014), 116.
10. Bridie Andrews, *The Making of Modern Chinese Medicine, 1850–1960* (Vancouver: UBC Press, 2014), 122–133.
11. Sean Hsiang-lin Lei, "Habituating Individuality: The Framing of Tuberculosis and Its Material Solutions in Republican China," *Bulletin of the History of Medicine* 84, no. 2 (2010): 255.
12. In his 1923 proposal for a department of hygiene at the Peking Union Medical College (PUMC), John B. Grant, a professor at PUMC and the representative of the International Health Board of the Rockefeller Foundation, argued against implementing tuberculosis control at the early stage of managing public health in China. While Grant estimated that China had an extremely high death rate of fifteen per thousand, he maintained: "In China, where funds and personnel are limited, it would be unwise to concentrate inadequate resources on tuberculosis until the attack on the more easily controllable gastrointestinal diseases had been well organized." This proposal was readily accepted by the government. John B. Grant, "A Proposal for a Department of Hygiene" (1923), 17, Rockefeller Foundation Archives, Rockefeller Archive Center, Sleepy Hollow, New York (hereafter RAC), box 75, folder 531. Quoted in Lei, "Habituating Individuality," 253.
13. Lei, "Habituating Individuality," 256.
14. Despite being called "national," the range of their impact was relatively local and concentrated in the Shanghai region.
15. Lei, "Habituating Individuality."
16. Ge Chenghui, "Zhongguoren yu jiehebing [The Chinese and Tuberculosis]," *Kexue* [Science] 10, no. 5 (1935): 587–596. Quoted in Lei, "Habituating Individuality."
17. "New Sanatorium Opened, Hungjao Institution Presents Many Modern Features," *North-China Herald and Supreme Court & Consular Gazette*, June 20, 1934, 430.
18. *China Times*, June 16, 1934, 2.
19. *Shi shi xin bao*, June 26, 1934.
20. *China Times,* June 10, 1934, 9.
21. Fuquan studied under the name Fohzien Godfrey Ede, he received his diploma in engineering from Technische Hochschule zu Darmstadt in 1926, and his doctorate in engineering under the direction of architectural historian and Sinologist Ernst Boerschmann from Technische Hochschule zu Charlottenburg in 1929. Eduard Kögel, "Early German Research in Ancient Chinese Architecture (1900–1930)," *Berliner Chinahefte/ Chinese History and Society*, no. 39 (2011), 81–91.
22. *Shi shi xin bao*, December 21, 1934.
23. "New Sanatorium Opened," 430.
24. *The Modern Girl Around the World: Consumption, Modernity, and Globalization* (Durham: Duke University Press, 2008.)
25. Syed Raza Hassan, "Pakistan Says Trial of Chinese Traditional Medicine for COVID-19 Successful," *Reuters*, January 17, 2022; Zhuang Pinghui, "World Health Organization Chief Given Report on Use of Traditional Chinese Medicine in Fighting Covid-19," *South China Morning Post*, January 21, 2022; Victoria Amunga, "China Exports Its Traditional Medicine to Africa," *VOA News*, January 21, 2022; Ian Johnson, "Chinese Medicine in the Covid Wards," *New York Review of Books*, November 4, 2021.

p86, 87, 88, 89 Reproduced from *Zhongguo jianzhu/ Chinese Architect* 2, no. 5 (1934): 11 (86), 9 (87 top), 3 (87 bottom), 12 (88 top)), 33 (88 bottom), 16 (89 top), 9 (89 bottom)
p90–91 Reproduced from *Dazhong huabao/The Cosmopolitan* 14 (1934): 23.
p92 Reproduced from *Zhanwang/The Outlook* 19 (1940): 23.

An earlier version of this essay was originally published by e-flux Architecture in 2022.

LIVE FREE OR DIE? PSYCHO-POLITICAL INFRASTRUCTURES OF DENIALISM

EMILY APTER

"Spirit of molestation, spirit of abuse, get out right now!" Locke commanded.

"Every spirit of homosexuality, lesbianism, come out, come," his wife ordered.

"Transgenderism, gender dysphoria, come out."

"We rebuke it, we rebuke it!" Locke yelled. The tent slowly took on a spirit of its own. Worshipers began writhing as if in pain. Others waved their hands in the air in benediction. "Amens" began to mix with the guttural sound of growling, moaning and praying in tongues.

"If you've had the Covid-19 shot, I'm telling you you've got poison in your veins," Locke thundered. "We call out the Covid-19 vaccine out right now. Keep that demonic spirit out of you right now in the name of Jesus!"

Some fell to the ground, pawing at cedar chips, or retched into silver vomit buckets that had been set at the end of each row of white folding chairs.[1]

This scene, described in an article about the way "patriot" celebrations of the January 6, 2020, insurrection in the US Capitol have become imbricated with white evangelical Christianity, focuses on pastor Greg Locke addressing his congregation at the Global Vision Bible Church in Mt. Juliet, Tennessee. The article is accompanied by video clips of book burnings—Harry Potter and the Twilight series, both alleged to communicate Satanic instructions—and chanting, mesmerized crowds of believers. Images such as these trigger disturbing flashbacks to Nazi Germany, southern lynch mobs, and secretive cults of the kind masterminded by Charles Manson, Jim Jones, David Koresh, and more recently, David Raniere, leader of sex cult Nxivm. More disturbing, perhaps, is something without any single historical precedent: the gathering specter of a pandemia-driven political form (or array of forms) that combines structures of psychosis, neurosis, phobia, paranoia, delusional narcissism (monomania), sadism, and the *Todestrieb* (death drive); this last considered to be more death wish (in Freud's sense of *Wunsch,* unconscious wish fulfillment) than blind *Trieb*, the Nirvana principle or sadistic side of Eros.

No one schema maps onto the political cartography of Covid denialism, or denialism *tout court* for that matter. Though one might want to confine Covid denialism to a conservative ideology that exploits the psychic reflex of flight from a threatening reality or inconvenient truth for political gain (overriding scientific evidence of contagious disease to bolster unregulated capitalism and libertarian ways of life), denialism as such is impossible to pin down as a single phenomenon or right-wing political mindset. As a psychopolitical form it manifests as something viral, continually mutating and adding on.[2] Slavoj Žižek describes this phenomenon aptly when he characterizes viruses as "zombie agents":

> neither alive nor dead in the usual sense of these terms, they are a kind of living dead. A virus is alive in its drive to replicate, but it is a kind of zero-level life, a biological caricature not so much of a death-drive as of life at its most stupid level of repetition and multiplication. ... [T]hey are a case of what Schelling called "*der nie aufhebbare Rest*": a remainder of the lowest form of life that emerges as a product of the malfunctioning of higher mechanisms of multiplication.[3]

Like the "poison," the "vax" toxin has been mysteriously subbed in for the virus itself that requires expulsion from the bio-organism and the spiritual body alike by means of an exorcism ritual of collective vomiting. Denialism mimes (and thereby sustains) the virus metaphor. One could even say, following Žižek's indications, that denialism as such, in the era of social media reproducibility, has become viral: translating viral microbiology from one medium to another, morphing and metastasizing in the guise of political memes and "alternative facts" that "go viral," in conspiracy-mongering that becomes contagious, in crossovers of science denialism into the "pandemic is a hoax" credo, and in political crossovers of the kind seen at anti-vax rallies that blur the lines between political left and right (as when Greens joined forces with constituents of the far-right Alternative for Germany party, or as when Trump-convert Robert F. Kennedy Jr. yokes vaccine skepticism and anti-fluoride conspiracy theory to progressive stances against ultraprocessed food and Big Pharma).

Covid denialism denotes a state of "being" (of being in *le déni*, as denialism is rendered in French) that activates a "tauto-teleological," suicidal way of thinking.[4] This is encapsulated in the oft-heard phrase "I'd rather die than take the vaccine," with its strange ultimatum of dying for the sake of death. What imprints itself in this statement is a kind of "loving dying" paradigm that carries over to the Eros-infused "attraction" to morbid conspiracy theories and Malthusian prophecies.

The suicidal subtext of Covid denialism is found in climate change denialism too. As Elissa Marder has observed, with respect to the term "ecocide" (which to her ears is a reminder that "the murder of the primal other is also a form of suicide"), "ecocide is always also egocide."[5] The same could be said for Covid denialism: it is always also egocide to the extent that in fixing the vaccine in its sightlines, it targets an "existential threat" that is ultimately inextricable from its own egoic extinction. What Marder says about denialism as a self-defeating expression of reality negation also applies:

> The unbearable reality of climate change exposes the psyche to a primordial tear in reality itself. The inexorably real threat of climate change threatens the psyche's ability to establish a rational relation to reality. There is no merely sane relation to climate change. It has made us crazy, and it will make us crazy. Denial is our only defense, but it is also our undoing. There is no outside to denial. There are only different forms of denial that will have different side-effects and unintended consequences. Some of the most "well-meaning" forms of denial may turn out to be the most insidious as they attempt to rationalize, humanize, and normalize actions and events that ought to force us to reckon with what we cannot bear to know.[6]

"Denial is our only defense": a giant defense mechanism, as it were, shielding us, if unsuccessfully, from the crazy, from the prospect of psychosis, itself induced by the unbearable "reality" of epidemic and ecological catastrophe.

Marder has recourse to Freud, and specifically his propensity for civilizational diagnoses that take psychoanalytic complexes tailored to the individual psyche and scale them up to collective phenomena: war, mass psychology, mass extinction events, and climate change; the last, in her view, a threat to the psyche that defies processing to the point of elevating denialism to new heights. Marder's focus on "psychoanalysis and ecocide," and on denialism's role in the simultaneous staving off and bringing on of collective psychosis in the face of a climate catastrophe being experienced now—and not in some future temporality—prompts a more careful parsing of Freud's actual vocabulary of denial: particularly its foregrounding of negation, and the interplay between *Verneinung* (negation, denial), and *Verleugnung* (the refusal or disavowal of a fact imposed by the external world). According to Jean Laplanche, the strange and troubling concept of negation—crucial to Freud's concept of the death drive—springs from the peculiar phrasing in the text of *Beyond the Pleasure Principle:*

> [W]e find in this text a new, entirely original, and even unheard-of conjunction of the different modes of what might be designated, in all its generality, as the "negative": aggression, destruction, sadomasochism, hatred, etc.
>
> Profoundly baffling, Freud's discourse is only sporadically and superficially subordinated to logical imperatives: it constitutes a mode of thought that is free (in the sense of free associations) ... and implies a series of *"about-faces," acts of virtual repentance, and denials*. ... [T]he holes in the reasoning constitute so many traps; the sliding of concepts results in blurring terminological points of reference; the most far-reaching discussions are suddenly resolved in the most arbitrary manner. ...
>
> At stake then is an effort to grasp what is most "driven" in the drive—ataraxy, Nirvana as the abolition of every drive—and what is most vital in the biological—death, explicitly designated as the "final aim" of life.[7]

In underscoring the unsettling effect on the reader of Freud's negation/denial concept as a misfit joint between thought and biology that wants to capture "what is most driven in the drive"—even at the risk of canceling itself out—Laplanche identifies what is so discomfiting about Covid denialism: its defiance of medical risk is nothing short of a courtship of the death drive. Thus, if it cannot divine the cause of the drive—always ungraspable—it will tarry with the form of its negation.

What form denial takes is itself, as I have already suggested, an unsettled matter. Though Didier Fassin draws a distinction between "denial," defined as "the empirical observation that reality and truth are being denied," and ":denialism," defined as "an ideological position whereby one systematically reacts by refusing reality and truth," my sense is that denial and denialism, like negation and negationism (on the order of slavery negationism, Holocaust negationism, AIDS negationism), are impossible to neatly disintricate.[8] Both entangle "empirical observation" in questions about the coincidence of external and psychical reality, credulity and belief. Both also share the deep structure of *Verneinung* whereby repressed content makes its way backhandedly into consciousness without being fully acknowledged.[9]

Symptomatic in this regard are statements of credulous incredulity—statements of belied belief often expressed through double-negative affirmation, as in: "I would not deny it ..." (which leaves the door open that you might still sort of deny it). Octave Mannoni took such statements as the classic prototype of psychoanalytic fetishistic disavowal: "Je le sais bien, mais quand même" ("I know well, but all the same").[10] As Alenka Zupančič has observed, "all the same" in this construction plays the role of the fetish: a displaced, disavowed form (the foot, the woman's panties or glove) of the "fact of castration." The fetish, she says, "believes in my place, belief is thus outsourced to the fetish."[11] This "believing in my place" creates a kind of closed self-circuitry, allowing the fetish to confirm a delusion that the subject already "knows" or wants to believe in. Lacan's variant term for *Verneinung*, *Bejahung* (affirmation), places this foreclosing, autoaffirmative psychic infrastructure of fetishism in even starker relief. It is characterized as a "three-card trick or juggler's game between the symbolic, the imaginary, and the real." In identifying the voice of the other within the ego as an address from without, *Bejahung* paves the way to an order of delusion in which "the allocution is the response" and the Big Other of the symbolic is entirely excluded.[12]

In his analysis of Robert Faurisson's Holocaust negationism, Jean-François Lyotard would give the name "differend" to this hedged way of thinking, typically found in instances where a plaintiff becomes a victim because "the author of the damages turns out directly or indirectly to be one's judge."[13] The differend is a good example of how denial and denialism, or negation and negationism, are bound together in expressions of "both-and" that suspend the execution of a critical judgment.[14]

Daniel Hoffman-Schwartz further complicates and enriches our understanding of *Verneinung* as a both-and structure of denial/denialism by insisting on a third term: "deniability." Deniability may be a more apt term than "negationism" to describe the politics of Covid denialism, since it homes in on the doubt-seeding hypothetical as a viral factor or hypnotic suggestion that hobbles the faculty of judgment.[15] The equivocal logic of the differend remains operative, but here a small element of undecidability is mobilized to discount a mountain of evidentiary proof.[16] In the contemporary Covid denialist version, this argument goes something like this: "vaccines kill you because you can't prove they never do." Deniability (and its close cousin, plausible deniability) functions as a kill mechanism; a preemptive refusal on the order of a *Verwerfung* (*forclusion* or foreclosure) in Lacan's theory of psychosis, whereby the subject rejects an element outside the symbolic order by treating it as if it had never existed.

When approached from the angle of political theory, the *Todestrieb* of Covid denialism aligns with the logic of "live free or die" libertarianism. New Hampshire's official motto was adopted in 1945 and borrowed from a toast ("Live free or die: Death is not the Worst of Evils") made by Revolutionary War hero General John Stark, who himself was borrowing it from the French Revolutionary slogan "Vivre libre ou mourir." Under conditions of pandemia, this libertarian rallying cry is weaponized in a paroxysm of individual choicism that gains energy and positive reinforcement from in-group identification and the community support structures of fellow denialists. One could say, then, that pandemia denialism produces a singular community: a company of Lockean self-property owners, possessive individualists whose ego ideal is based on the kind of self-sufficing "ownness" (*Eigenheit*) that Max Stirner outlined in his controversial 1844 book *The Ego and Its Own* (*Der Einzige und sein Eigentum*).[17] Stirner's theory of the ego was castigated by Marx as little more than a smokescreen for petty bourgeois individualism and self-interest, but Marx was shortsighted in dismissing its potential for the kind of anarchist individualism that we see animating entrepreneurial philosophy in the tech industry. Nor could he foresee its importance for Freud's theory of *das Ich*, of the ego as a subjective agency that, in misrecognizing itself, and engaging in a dreamlike distortion of reality to justify its own ends, enables grandiose fantasies of self-possession. Psychosis, as Freud would note in this instance, becomes a way of making good on the loss of reality.[18]

"Ownness" in the context of Covid denialism fulfills the wish *to own one's own death*, arrogating to oneself God-like powers to control one's destiny. In *Beyond the Pleasure Principle*, Freud singles out this attitude in describing a key aspect of the death drive: "What we are left with is the fact that the organism wishes to die only in its own fashion."[19] Here we could say the either-or logic built into the credo of "live free or die" gives way to the both-and fetish logic of "die and be free" (with the belief in death outsourced to a fetish of libertarian "freedom" that guarantees a saving oblivion). Covid denialist self-ownership also affords the privative satisfaction of denying self-safety to others, especially the immuno-compromised. It represents supreme social indifferentism.[20] It implies contempt for any public interest served by marshaling healthcare resources, protecting others from sickness, and lowering economic and social costs through mask mandates and the adoption of vaccines. In their willful ignorance of the social and racial subsidy of health (assured by a social contract that assumes the willingness of low-paid healthcare workers to die for the cause of supporting the lives of others), together with their cognitively dissonant resistance to personal taxation for socialized medicine, anti-vaxxers have evolved a radically self-centric political brand that peddles magical financial thinking: a right to health resources without having to pay for it. It is along these lines as well that Covid denialism has evolved into a veritable plank of alt-right ideology.

In a protracted period of lockdown and political impasse, a period that witnessed the channeling of anti-vax sentiment into a host of alt-right causes encompassing January 6 insurrectionism, education censorship, anti-abortion, voter suppression, anti-gun control laws, stymied environmental protection measures, and opposition to "plandemia" (David Mamet's repugnant term for public health strategies designed to reduce the risk of epidemic infection), Covid denialism stakes a special claim to the word "freedom," particularly that form of negative liberty identified as "freedom from" something—government interference, state control, federal regulation, and so on.[21] It was just this populist negative liberty that resounded in Florida governor Ron DeSantis's appeal to "freedom from the judgmentalism of pro-mandate libs"—a no-fault antimoralism credo. (And who doesn't identify with that?) Denialism's political weaponization by the far right caters to the negative liberty of libertarianism (*freedom from* government interference) even as it promotes the positive liberty of neoliberal entitlement, the *freedom to* enjoy absolute safety on one's own terms and at others' expense. Both freedoms envisage a fully privatized world of the self in which the right not to be vaccinated vies with the demand for a space entirely controlled by oneself ("my home is my castle") and socially inoculated against the dangers of others.

We get a glimpse of what that world looks like in Todd Haynes's prescient 1995 film *Safe*, in which Julianne Moore embraces her autoimmunity and makes her living environment—an antiseptic igloo reinforced by a mobile oxygen tank—into a reflection of self-love that doubles as a death of the social. "Safe" is the form the death drive assumes as a social capsule of one: an apotheosis of the bourgeois concept of the private and endpoint of social distancing. Materially literalizing the psychopolitical infrastructure of "safetyism" in the architecture of an isolation chamber, *Safe* identifies "safe" as a condition of surviving "life as a disease": a condition that affords narcissistic fulfillment through existential subsistence at the minimal edge of bare life.[22]

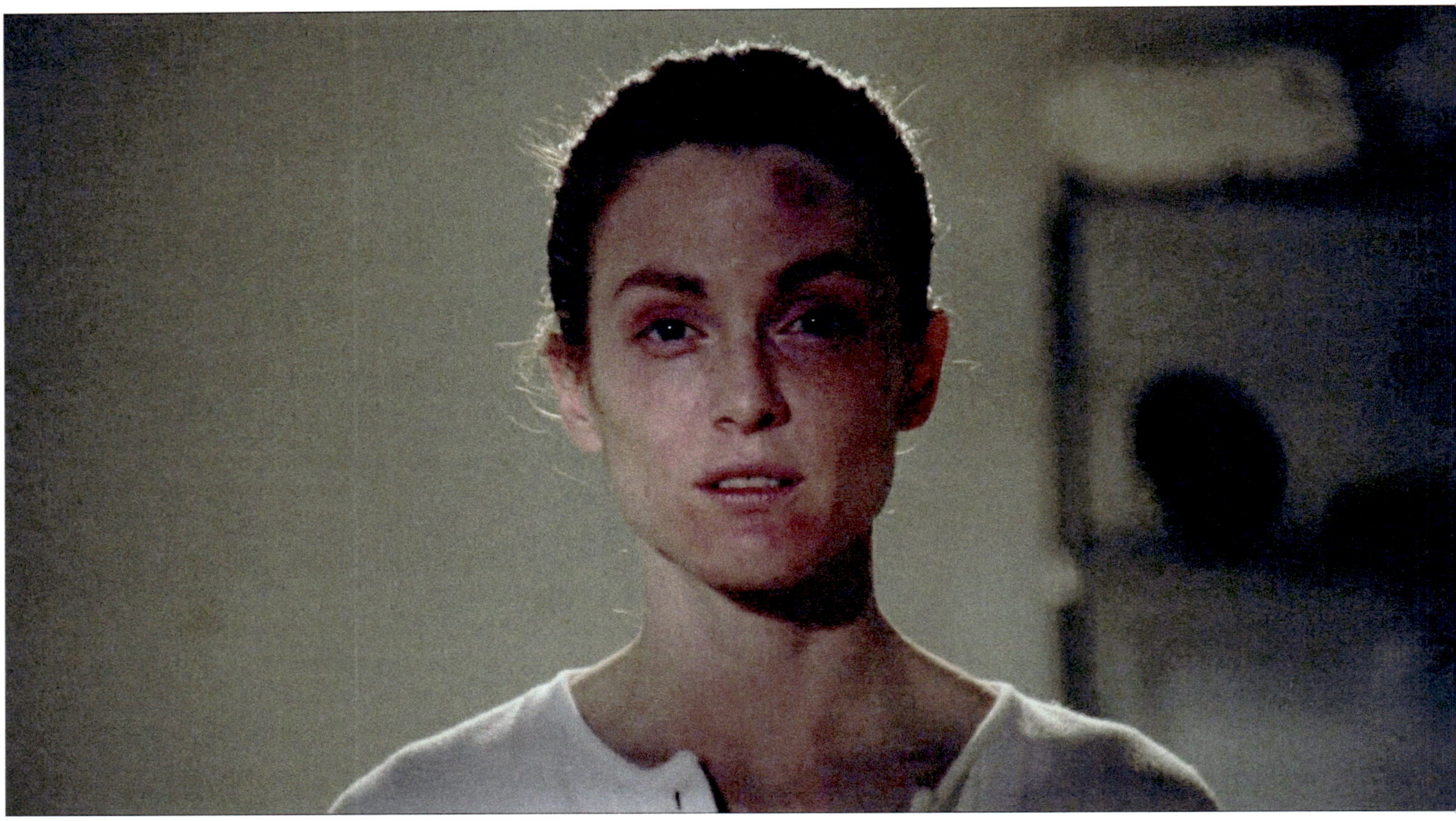

Extending the political infrastructure of narcissistic safetyism, the late Jean-Luc Nancy coined the expression "neo-viralism" for specific offshoots of neoliberalism that flourish under conditions of pandemia. Neo-viralism is characterized by the virality of discourses that corrode civic bonds, by the mutations of a world-organism sickened by the predations of technocapitalism, by neo-Malthusianism ("let the over-seventy die to strengthen the species"), by a resentment that breeds more resentment, by a nihilist penchant for "autodestruction," and, last but not least, by a denunciation of the *communovirus*—"le virus qui vient du communisme, le virus qui nous communise" ("the virus that comes from communism, the virus that communizes us")—that Nancy ironically invokes to describe "the dethroning (if not decapitation) of the *corona* of the old imperial monarchies to make way for an anti-Chinese specter of the 'communo.'"[23]

Nancy conjures communoviralism as the phobic specter of communism and as a manifold symptom of neoliberal autoimmunity.[24] But with Covid denialism, the politics are all over the map. Think here of anti-vaxxers who fall into neither the neoliberal nor the alt-right camp: those committed to minimizing toxins in the body; those who believe that an immunity induced by jiggering RNA genetic sequences is transgressive of a natural or divinely sanctified concept of the bodily human; those with a rational skepticism toward big pharma; vaccine-hesitant people of color traumatized by a bad history of protocol-testing; those who reject the superstitious logic that says if we make a strong enough gesture of sacrifice that brings our entire social life to a standstill, then maybe we can expect mercy; as well as critical thinkers averse to the medical biopolitics and control apparatuses of a hyperstate.[25] The point here is not to reduce Covid denialism to an "ism" or politics of party, but rather to see it as a complex political groundswell whose signs are everywhere on the populist right, in neoliberal discourses of self-securitization and anti-regulation, as well as in the work of thinkers who hail from a left-anarchist repudiation of state power and institutional structures of domination like Giorgio Agamben, Mehdi Belhaj Kacem, and the anonymous authors of the *Manifeste conspirationniste* (*The Conspiracy Manifesto*).[26]

What is fundamentally at stake in Covid denialism is a fight for power, a desire to master mastery. It is this power struggle at the heart of the death drive (characterized by Aaron Schuster as Freud's "metaphysical biology" as well as the "gap or rupture that is [psychoanalysis's] proper object") that most clearly defines the psychic life of Covid denialism as political form.[27] It is also why we can identify left denialism in its relation to anarchism, and more generally to forms of philosophical politics engaged with the deconstruction of power.

In a chapter on Derrida's "responsible anarchism" Catherine Malabou tries to imagine anarchism as a pure political force (*puissance*) untethered to structures of domination (*pouvoir*). Malabou wants to make anarchism's pulsive energy available to *an other* mode of political organization; one that is *inédit*

↑ Film still from *Safe*, directed by Todd Haynes, 1995.

(yet to be invented or road-tested) and revolutionary. When she poses the question "Is deconstruction an anarchism?" or the related question "Is the death drive anarchic or anarchist?" or when she ponders whether the drive to mastery is deconstructible (subject to being undone), or indestructible as it assimilates deconstructive *différance* to the mechanism of *Zwang* (compulsion, constraint, force), the answer in each instance is an equivocal "yes and no." This "yes and no"—the classic formulation of *Verneinung* that Freud assigned to the death drive and that Derrida references through the ambivalent figures of aporia, autoimmunity, and virus—limns a porous border between deconstruction and anarchism. "Yes and no" *is a kind of anarchy*, Malabou affirms, even as she calls it out as a *flagrant délit*—a scandal or trick that distracts us from the harder task of imagining an anarchist denegation unsusceptible to deconstruction.[28] What kind of denial would this be?

Malabou calls it "another difference," one that is *hors différance* (outside the difference machine), which is to say, an example of "pure power" untethered from law, government, and the principle of *Herrschaft*, the Hegelian concept of lordship or mastery that binds identity to its fate of endless self-reappropriation. Blocking the automaticity of the compulsive *Zwang* of life toward death with a power derived from the nonlife that precedes it (what Freud referred to in somewhat mysterious terms as an inorganic order of the living, or original state of matter that gives cells their quality of living), Malabou locates in Derrida's speculations on Freud "a death drive independent of its relation to power."[29] This nonprincipial non-life-form takes political shape as the "nongovernable" that must never be confused "with the ungovernability of difference."[30] Its undeniable existence is affirmed in its denegation. In other words, denial (*Verneinung*) is the sign that anarchism exists.[31] And yet, having guided us to an anarchism sited in the "beyond" of the pleasure principle (and the beyond of deconstruction), Malabou leaves us to mull questions posed along the way: What happens when "the principle" is transgressed, the state suspended, and the government overturned?[32] How does anarchism manage base instincts for power along with the urge to destroy, harm, or commit acts of cruelty?[33] How does the power of anarchism resist being assimilated into what Malabou calls the "dynamic of dynasty," referring to the recognition that "power can never be overcome by something that wouldn't itself be power"?[34] And finally, how does anarchism—affirmed as denial—resist being denied by the undeconstructible force of its own negation?

Malabou's quandary of a structure of denial that throws into question the possibility of unbinding power from the deathly telos of the death drive, or of realizing an anarchist politics of "the ungovernable," helps explain how figures like Agamben and Kacem, both renowned for their militant opposition to all forms of biopolitical sovereignty and repressive governmentality, could get caught in the trap of a denialism of means without ends and culminating in both cases in Covid denialism. In her chapter on Agamben, Malabou skirts this issue, focusing instead on the power of his "profanation" of theopolitical sovereignty. By disrobing the incapacity of command beneath the trappings of glory and the exercise of sovereign exception, Agamben makes manifest the *energeia* of an essential force of being that disciplines itself, yet remains ungovernable.[35] The problem, however, is that once this energy is dispatched to a zone of indistinction that is everywhere and nowhere, the zone itself is resacralized.[36] This "theological anarchism" is another denialist trick. Like Derridian *différance* telegraphed in the ambivalent logic of "yes and no," it too, by Malabou's reckoning, is a case of theory *en flagrant délit*: caught in the act of committing a scandal. In Derrida's case, the *délit* impedes the way to nongovernable power. But in Agamben's case, it traps him in the void of destituent power, fated to endlessly critique the ontology of anarchy at the expense of a politics of anarchism.

This denialist trap, this place abstracted from reality, is where, according to Malabou's interpretation, "the death drive turns in on itself."[37] And it is here that denialism becomes especially vulnerable to the attacks of someone like Benjamin Bratton, who not only dresses down Agamben for comparing government vaccine and mask mandates to Nazis' requirements that Jews wear the yellow star, but takes him as a symbol of all left theory post-1968 that indulges in "the horizontal multiplication of conditional viewpoints as both means and ends, via the imaginary dismantling of public reason, decision, and structuration." This, he claims, is "how they can at once fetishize 'the Political' while refusing 'governmentality.'" Philosophy and the humanities, he goes on, have failed the pandemic because they refuse "the epidemiological reality of mutual contagion" and subscribe to an ethics beholden to "subjective moral intentionality and a self-regarding *protagonism* for which 'I' am the piloting moral agent of outcomes."[38]

In tracing a through line between Agamben's Covid denialism (cast as a salve to unreason and the refusal of veridiction) and the "self-regarding protagonism" of left theory, Bratton indiscriminately tosses all post-1968 thought into the den of libertarianism and possessive individualism. What gets lost in the mudslinging are more serious questions: how does left opposition to the biomedical security state keep itself from shoring up its libertarian counterpart on the alt right? How do we prevent denial from being taken over by a structure of belief that overrides scientific reason and becomes vulnerable to falsehoods and disinformation?[39] How do we keep denialism—especially coming from the left—from being coopted by conspiracy theory, such as Kacem's embrace of *complotisme* ("conspiracy") on the grounds that it honestly names how the "nightmare of culture," and its handmaiden, academic philosophy, have been used to cover up the truly persecutory, tortuous side of humanity?[40]

Drawing back from the conspiracy hornet's nest, I continue to wonder whether the desire to recover an anarchic power of the nongovernable that, as it were, *masters mastery* can ultimately resist supersession by a structure of negation that is all-consuming and politically indifferent? How can we overcome this indifference, which either settles all too easily into the groove of political impasse, or condones the kind of "both-sides-ism" that credentials delusion, conspiratorialism, lies, and weaponized deniability? I also wonder about the ways in which Covid denialism channels a psychic political form engorged with hate (itself a literalization, in Kleinian terms, of the death drive) and in love with the force of the negative—the spectacle of the instinct unchained—that culminates in collective rituals of exorcism, conspiracy-mongering, and targeted expulsory violence?

Denialism at its most delusional, the death drive at its most politically lethal: these unnerving aspects of Covid denialism lead me to ask how, going forward, it will be possible to resist falling in love with the death-driven spectacle of morphing viralities, including neoliberalism's morph into neo-viralism. These issues underwrite the theoretical stakes of Covid denialism as a singular phenomenon of the times, one that links "viral-think" to problems of belief, veridiction, anarchy, power, nihilist libertarianism, and denegation—the last tantamount to a death wish, insofar as death itself is desired over a vaccine that protects against it.[41]

An earlier version of this essay was originally published by e-flux Architecture in 2022.

1. Annie Gowen, "A Jan. 6 Pastor Divides His Tennessee Community with Increasingly Extremist Views," *Washington Post*, March 31, 2022. See also Jaclyn Preiser's earlier "Evangelical Pastor Demands Churchgoers Ditch Their Masks," *Washington Post*, July 27, 2021. See, too, a segment on Locke where he goes from "There is no pandemic" to false allegations about the "aborted fetal tissue in all these vaccines," https://www.youtube.com/watch?v=kAfgkWgLF70.
2. In a similar vein, Patrice Maniglier theorizes the "ontology of the virus" through a Latourian lens as "multiversal," its internal multiplicities (the multiplicity of viruses, produced by the constant mutation of genes, viral variants, and entangled endosymbioses) to be conceived as horizontally distributed across heterogenous assemblages encompassing every type of entity and agency: animate and inanimate, inert and active. See Patrice Maniglier, *Le philosophe, la Terre et le virus: Bruno Latour expliqué par l'actualité* (Paris: Les Liens Qui Libèrent, 2021), 51–62.
3. Slavoj Žižek, *Pandemic! COVID-19 Shakes the World* (London: Polity, 2020), 79. Žižek's take on the "zombie" virus is in line with his very particular interpretation of the death drive, which, in a departure from Freud, he attaches to the concept of undeadness: "The Freudian death drive has nothing whatsoever to do with the desire for self-annihilation, for a return to the inorganic absence of all tension of life; rather, it is the very opposite of dying—a name for the 'undead,' eternal life itself, for the horrible fate of being caught in the endless iteration of wandering in guilt and pain. The paradox of Freud's 'death drive,' then, is that Freud is using it to denote its very opposite, namely the way immortality appears within psychoanalysis, an uncanny excess of life, an 'undead' urge that transcends the (biological) cycle of Life and death, persisting from arising and passing away. The real lesson of psychoanalysis is that human life is never just 'just life.'" See Slavoj Žižek: *Parallax* (Frankfurt: Suhrkamp, 2006), 61.
4. I borrow the expression "tauto-teleological" from Catherine Malabou who uses it in her book *Au voleur! Anarchisme et philosophie* (Paris: Presses Universitaires de France, 2022), 188.
5. Elissa Marder, "The Shadow of the Eco: Denial and Climate Change," unpublished paper, February 20, 2021; my emphasis. My thanks to Elissa for sharing this work, which was originally delivered as a talk at a Das Unbehagen conference on "Psychoanalysis and Ecocide," February 23, 2021, http://dasunbehagen.org/ecocide-psychoanalysis-thoughts-times-elissa-marder/. A different version of the talk, "The Shadow of the Eco. Climate Change and Psychoanalysis," was delivered at Columbia University on March 11, 2022, https://www.youtube.com/watch?v=FdsDUDZyqvQ.
6. Marder, "The Shadow of the Eco."
7. Jean Laplanche, *Life and Death in Psychoanalysis*, trans. Jeffrey Mehlman (Baltimore: Johns Hopkins University Press, 1976), 106–107; my emphasis.
8. Didier Fassin, *When Bodies Remember: Experiences and Politics of AIDS in South Africa* (Berkeley: University of California Press, 2007), 115. See too Michael Specter's influential 2009 study *Denialism: How Irrational Thinking Harms the Planet and Threatens Our Lives* (New York: Penguin Press, 2009).
9. Sigmund Freud, "Negation" (1925), in *The Standard Edition of the Complete Psychological Works of Sigmund Freud*, vol. 19, *The Ego and the Id and Other Works (1923–1925)* (London: Hogarth Press, 1953–1974), 235. In this volume, see too Freud's essay "The Loss of Reality in Neurosis and Psychosis" (1924), 183–190.
10. Octave Mannoni, *Clefs pour l'Imaginaire ou l'Autre scène* (Paris: Éditions du Seuil, 1969).
11. Alenka Zupančič, "In the Wake of the Plague: Eros and Mourning," conference paper, Dartmouth College, April 21, 2022. Zupančič further glosses Mannoni's canonical formula (and its implications for Covid denialism) in *Disavowal* (Cambridge, UK: Polity, 2024), 22–44.

12. Jacques Lacan, "I've Just Been to the Butcher's," in *The Seminar of Jacques Lacan*, vol. 3, *The Psychoses* (1955–1956), trans. Russell Grigg, ed. Jacques-Alain Miller (New York: W. W. Norton, 1993), 46–47, 52. Lacan's most fundamental text of reference is "Introduction and Reply to Jean Hyppolite's presentation of Freud's *Verneinung*," in *The Seminar of Jacques Lacan*, vol. 1, *Freud's Papers on Technique (1952–1954)*, trans. John Forrester, ed. Jacques-Alain Miller (New York: W. W. Norton, 1988), 52–61.

13. Jean-François Lyotard, *Le Différend* (Paris: Minuit, 1983), 22–23. See my discussion of the differend in "Armed Response: Translation as Judicial Hearing," *e-flux Journal* 84 (September 2017), https://www.e-flux.com/journal/84/149339/armed-response-translation-as-judicial-hearing/.

14. In more strictly psychoanalytic terms this "both-and" dissolves Freudian dualisms according to which neurotic negation (expressed in symptoms of failed repression, egoic self-preservation and defense, a negation of the unconscious to the end of preserving a connection to reality) is opposed to psychotic denial (expressed as dominance of the id to the point of total denial of external reality).

15. Daniel Hoffman-Schwartz, "Lyotard and the Trolls: *The Differend,* Sophistry, and the Right," *Philosophy Today* (February 2022). In the case of doubt-seeding, we can say with Lacan that the subject is not psychotic, just subject to a hallucination. Lacan, "Introduction and Reply to Jean Hyppolite's presentation of Freud's *Verneinung*," 59.

16. This strategy will be especially familiar to readers of Naomi Oreskes and Erik M. Conway's *Merchants of Doubt*: *How a Handful of Scientists Obscured the Truth on Issues from Tobacco Smoke to Global Warming* (London: Bloomsbury, 2012), which tracked the honing of deniability as a political technology in the 1960s and 1970s.

17. Max Stirner outlined this in his controversial book *Der Einzige und sein Eigentum* [The ego and its own] (Leipzig: Otto Wigand, 1845).

18. Freud, "The Loss of Reality in Neurosis and Psychosis," 184.

19. Sigmund Freud, *Beyond the Pleasure Principle* (London; Vienna: International Psycho-Analytic Press, 1922), 33.

20. This is relevant to the larger "ethics of the (infected) neighbor," as diagnosed by Kenneth Reinhard in *The Neighbor: Three Inquiries in Political Theology* (Chicago: University of Chicago Press, 2005).

21. See Marc Tracy, "As Mamet Returns to Broadway, His Claims on Pedophilia Get the Spotlight," *New York Times*, April 13, 2022.

22. The term "safetyism" crops up in the faceoff between Greg Lukianoff and Jonathan Haidt, coauthors of *The Coddling of the American Mind: How Good Intentions and Bad Ideas Are Setting Up a Generation for Failure* (New York: Penguin Press, 2018), and Michael Roth, author of *Safe Enough Spaces: A Pragmatist's Approach to Inclusion, Free Speech, and Political Correctness on College Campuses* (New Haven: Yale University Press, 2019). Lukianoff and Haidt denounce campus "coddling" and "vindictive protectionism," while Wesleyan college president Roth proposes "safe enough spaces" (after Winnicott's "good enough parent") centered on inclusion and respect. Roth traces the origin of safe space back to postwar industrial psychology when émigré social psychologist Kurt Lewin was asked to help workers and supervisors adapt to a feminized workplace at the Harwood Manufacturing textile plant. Lewin associated safe space with an environment that allows for participatory decision-making on productivity and absenteeism without fear of retaliation or retribution. The safe space concept migrated from the factory to the therapist's office and, with the help of social movements in the 1960s and 1970s, became a rallying point of feminism (the Bluestocking feminist bookstore as safe space), black empowerment, and LGBTQI emancipation. Aaron Schuster, *The Trouble with Pleasure: Deleuze and Psychoanalysis* (Cambridge, MA: MIT Press, 2016), 30.

23. Jean-Luc Nancy, *Un trop humain virus* (Montrouge: Bayard, 2020), 8.

24. Another, more positive way of theorizing "communovirus," or neo-viralism for that matter, might emphasize a model of community-in-virus. This is arguably found in the community of barebackers. It came together around the rejection of the repressive moral apparatus of safe sex and has been known to willingly share HIV as an affirmative gesture of investment in a future dying-together. See Tim Dean, *Unlimited Intimacy: Reflections on the Subculture of Barebacking* (Chicago: University of Chicago Press, 2009).

25. Žižek, *Pandemic!*, 10.

26. The title plays on Gracchus Babeuf and Sylvain Maréchal's "Manifesto of the Equals" (*Le Manifeste des égaux*, 1796), which referenced an insurrection against the Directorate known as "The Conspiracy of the Equals."

27. Schuster, *The Trouble with Pleasure*, 32, 33 respectively. Schuster ponders whether Freud's theory of the death drive refers "to a demonic compulsion to repeat? Or to an aggressive force of self-sabotage and self-destruction? Or to a metaphysical biology that makes of life a painful detour of inorganic matter?" (32). He also provides a reading of Thomas Mann's *Magic Mountain* that vividly illustrates this notion of "life as a disease," or life not as "Vibrant Matter" (Jane Bennett) or "Bodies that Matter" (Judith Butler) but as "Sick Matter" (35). Schuster writes: "During his unexpectedly long stay in the Swiss mountain retreat, the novel's main character, Hans Castorp, is exposed to different views on the relationship between sickness and health, body and mind, suffering and spirituality, but remains undecided. In the section of chapter five titled 'Research,' Castorp undertakes his own scientific inquiry, reading numerous volumes on anatomy, physiology, and biology: What is life? What is its origin? By what mysterious leap did the first living protoplasm come into being? This investigation into the earliest stirrings of life eventually leads him from biology to physics, the gulf between the organic and the inorganic harking back to the perhaps even more mysterious and unfathomable breach between the material and the immaterial. At the end of this episode, Castorp comes to a thought that perfectly captures Freud's patho-biological speculations, while daringly pushing them one step further. 'Disease was a perverse, a dissolute form of life. And life? Life itself? Was it perhaps only an infection, a sickening of matter?'"

28. Malabou, *Au voleur!*, 162: "une dénégation cette fois non déconstruite de l'anarchisme."

29. Malabou, *Au voleur!*, 191.

30. Malabou, *Au voleur!*, 193.

31. Malabou, *Au voleur!*, 200–201.

32. Malabou, *Au voleur!*, 163.

33. Malabou, *Au voleur!*, 190.

34. Malabou, *Au voleur!*, 188.

35. Malabou, *Au voleur!*, 316.

36. Malabou, *Au voleur!*, 323.

37. Malabou, *Au voleur!*, 394.

38. Benjamin Bratton, "Agamben WTF, or How Philosophy Failed the Pandemic," Verso, July 28, 2021, https://www.versobooks.com/blogs/5125-agamben-wtf-or-how-philosophy-failed-the-pandemic.

39. This question solicits a rereading of Umberto Eco's essay "Faith in Fakes," and other writings on the semiotics of lying as a mechanism of fiction, falsification, error, secrecy, and conspiracy.

40. From an interview relating to his talk on "Artaud et la théorie du complot" at an event organized in 2014 by Pierre Michon. "'Des phrases qui sauvent la peau': Entretien with Mehdi Belhaj Kacem," *Inferno*, September 29, 2014, https://inferno-magazine.com/2014/09/29/des-phrases-qui-sauvent-la-peau-entretien-avec-mehdi-belhaj-kacem/. During the pandemic Kacem launched a full-blown conspiracy theory that the pandemic is a genocidal plot hatched by the totalitarian biopolitical state. In addition to his broadside *Colaricovirus: D'un genocide non conventionnel* (Exuvie, 2022), and an incendiary open letter to the mayor of Turenne (https://anthropo-logiques.org/il-ny-a-pas-eu-de-pandemie-mais-un-genocide-est-en-cours-lettre-ouverte-au-maire-de-turenne-par-mehdi-belhaj-kacem/), Kacem released a torrent of Covid-denialist videos at the height of the pandemic that were banned from internet diffusion but continued to circulate on alternative media. A more muted version of his Covid denialism appears in the anonymously published *Manifeste conspirationniste* allegedly coauthored by members of the now defunct Invisible Committee. Joseph Confavreux, reviewing the book in *Mediapart* (January 27, 2022), denounced it as a mass of meta-conspiratorial delusions in the name of collective revolt that promotes the hypothesis of a preplanned pandemic orchestrated to give cover to mass surveillance by the global order (https://www.mediapart.fr/journalculture-idees/270122/conspirationnisme-un-manifeste-qui-allume-la-mauvaise-meche).

41. Žižek writes: "We in the West less and less accept death as part of life, we see it as an intrusion of something foreign that can be indefinitely postponed" (*Pandemic!*, 11).

BOD

ES

→ Otto Wagner, section of Kirche St. Leopold am Steinhof, competition project, 1902–1903.

↘ Otto Wagner, plan of Steinhofkirche, Steinhof am Main, 1903–1904.

AUTISTIC SPATIALITY

PATRICK JAOJOCO

Resolution WHA67.8 was published as part of the World Health Organization's 67th World Health Assembly in 2014, which offered a point of action for the "comprehensive and coordinated efforts for the management of autism spectrum disorders."[1] While this call for the "management" of autism spectrum disorders (ASD) is a recent phenomenon, autistic activists and disability rights groups have long called into question the present-day psychiatric context of autism pathologization. Autism advocacy is divided in two camps: the despairing parents of autistic children on the one hand, and autistic individuals and disability justice advocates on the other. We see the former in the continued dominance of the nonprofit organization Autism Speaks, which prioritizes parental support over societal change, and the continued use of applied behavioral analysis (ABA) in institutions for neurodivergent children. Developed in the 1980s by psychiatrist and child abuser Ivar Lovaas, ABA is a form of curative education that pushes autistic people to "mask" autistic traits in order to complete tasks in society as a neurotypical person would. This particular form of "therapy" has received vocal and widespread critique from the autistic community as well as the queer community, due to its direct associations with gay conversion therapy. In both, "acceptable" thoughts and behaviors in social settings are rewarded, while unacceptable ones are punished with verbal abuse, confinement, and until recently, physical abuse.

"Masking" has protected a significant number of autistic people from harm by rendering them largely invisible to written history. But with the professionalization of and revolutionary responses to psychiatry as a diagnostic practice in the early twentieth century, a language has been developed for autistic people to reclaim agency and define themselves in opposition to regimes of behavioral control. The autist-run blog Neuroclastic, for instance, describes how "members of the autism civil rights movement adopt a position of neurodiversity that encompasses a kaleidoscope of identities that intersects with the LGBTQIA+ kaleidoscope by recognizing autistic traits as natural variations of cognition, motivations, and patterns of behavior within the human species."[2] Centering autistic experience expands the bounds of communicable subjectivity in the context of modern society as such.

Autistic modes of being are so internal to one's relationship to their own body that only full agency over one's bodily, psychological, and social activity is required for full autistic liberation. Conditions of living are of immediate concern to autistic folks, whose currents of thought run along a number of different pathways and are fundamentally resistant to generalization and typologization.[3] The urgency of understanding the spatial experiences of autistic people, then, stems from the root of sociopolitical anxieties imposed by urban modernity. The trajectory of autistic spatiality in an increasingly urbanized, territorialized Europe throughout the twentieth century has had fundamental implications for the conceptualization of liberatory autistic spaces as communities located at—and, therefore, challenging—societal limits of care.

Modernity, Psychiatry, and Otto Wagner's Steinhof am Main

Georg Simmel accounted for the large-scale, sociopsychological shifts that come with modern urbanization. As a totalizing and ordering force, urban forms emerging at the turn of the twentieth century challenged and restructured interactions between the individual and society at large. Technologies of order and rationality in the city—divisions of labor, maintenance of a standard time, spatial arrangements of dwelling space, etc.—had alienated individuals from both themselves and society. Simmel notes that "the deepest problems of modern life flow from the attempt of the individual to maintain the independence and individuality of his existence against the sovereign powers of society, against the weight of the historical heritage and the external culture and technique of life."[4] The psychological effects of such a society affect the internal life of the mind. Increasingly, "metropolitan individuality is erected" with the attendant "intensification of emotional life due to the swift and continuous shift of external and internal stimuli."[5] The metropolis as a whole is a totalizing sensory experience, imposing conditions in which one's "emotional life" is at risk. And at the core of urban metropolitan life are its institutions, where "such a tremendous richness [is to be found] of crystallizing, depersonalized cultural accomplishments that the personality can, so to speak, scarcely maintain itself in the face of it."[6] The silencing of one's internal life is endemic to Simmel's metropolis.

As a distinctly European project, the modern metropolis is a historical construct determined by a central governing state, elite interests in industrial expansion, and a social order that is both legible and controllable. It is within this context that "modern" psychiatric institutions were first used to pathologize autistic spatiality. Steinhof am Main, a psychiatric facility designed by Otto Wagner outside Vienna in 1907, is key to the history of autism diagnosis. The commission for the institutional complex arose out of a broader Austrian political shift toward the conservative Christian Social Party in 1896, which vowed to reform psychiatric housing and care in order to "elevate Lower Austria's status among civilized nations."[7] Steinhof am Main consisted of sixty buildings, a central church, agricultural land, an enormous kitchen that distributed meals, and an electric train running throughout the complex. Wagner's "white city," as art critic Ludwig Hevesi described it, was an "omen of modernity," and a microcosmic site for the enforcement of "correct" social behavior as a cure to psychological affliction of various kinds.[8]

With plenty of open space and opportunities for agricultural work and religious life, Wagner's design was based on an ideal model of the metropolis. As historian Leslie Topp remarks about its opening, "the

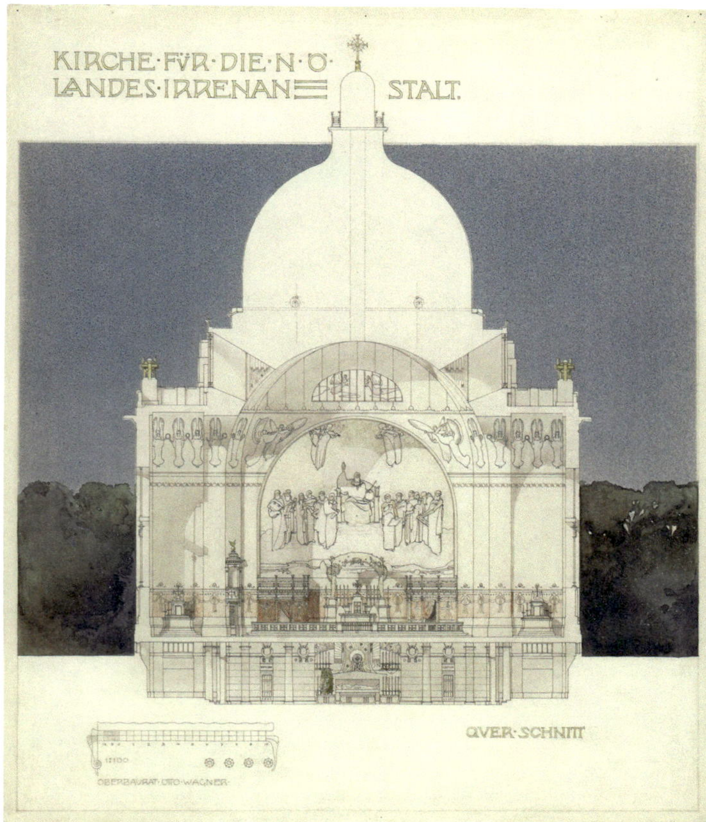

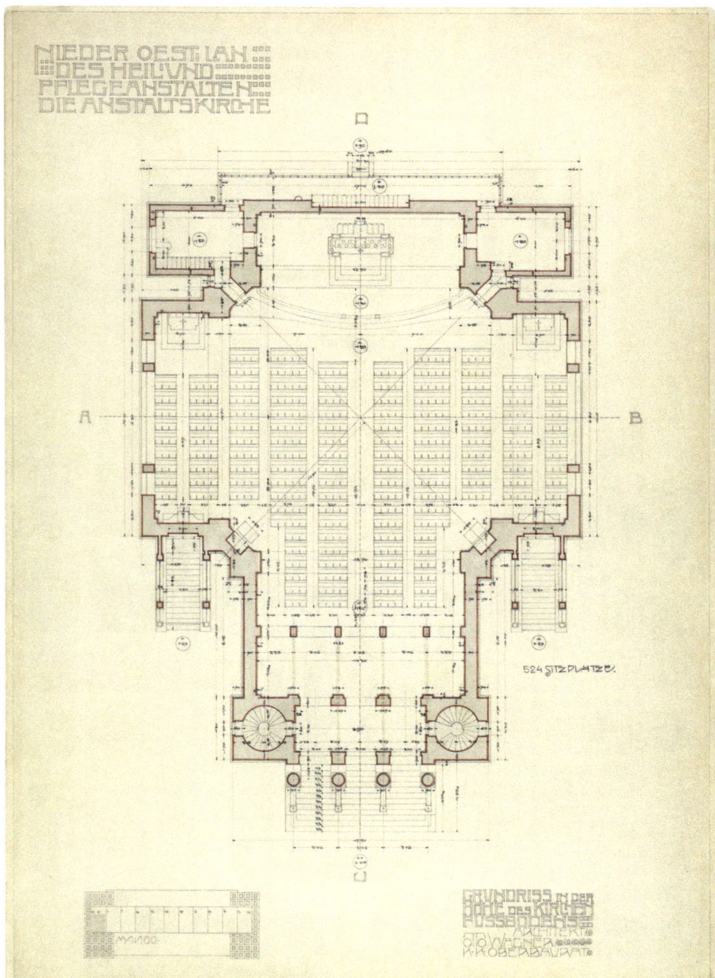

doctors and civil servants who planned Steinhof embraced an overblown psychiatric optimism, with a strong emphasis on publicity, and they sought to expand the influence of the mental hospital into the lives of the wider public." Functioning as an ideal city also requires an ideal society, which in turn requires compliance on the part of its residents. To this point, the pews of the church were specifically designed at such a height that should an individual deviate from expected behavior, Steinhof staff could forcibly lift the patient over the pew and remove them from service altogether. From there, the patient could be transported to a number of locations depending on the severity of the reaction. Clinics, holding rooms, and isolation cells were all included in Wagner's original designs, as were high walls, enclosing gardens, iron-caged verandas, and other methods of spatial control that gave the illusion of freedom but were in fact modes of confinement.

With the rise of Nazi rule in Vienna, Steinhof became the site of the Nazi pediatric clinic Spiegelgrund, which from 1940 to 1945 served as the location for the holding and euthanasia of "uneducable" children who could or would not conform to Nazi Youth education. In 1940, more than 3,200 neurodivergent or disabled adults living in Steinhof were executed in newly constructed gas chambers in order for nine of its thirty-four pavilions to be used for the reeducation, observation, or murder of hundreds of neurodivergent or disabled children. Scales of confinement at Steinhof under Nazi administration grew ever smaller, with "problematic" autistic

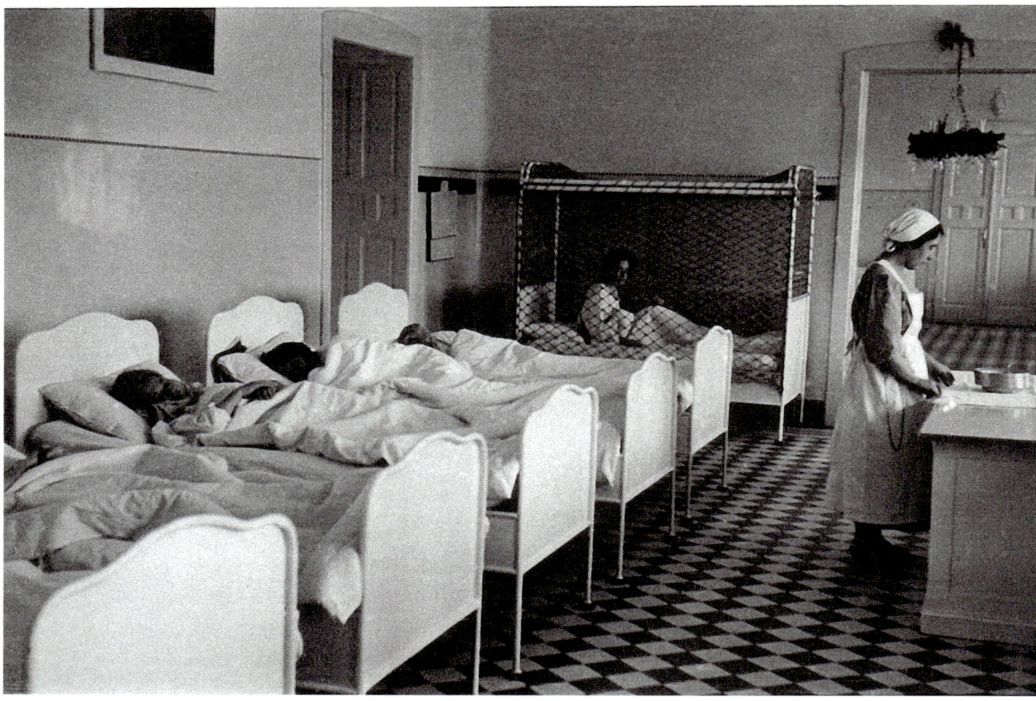

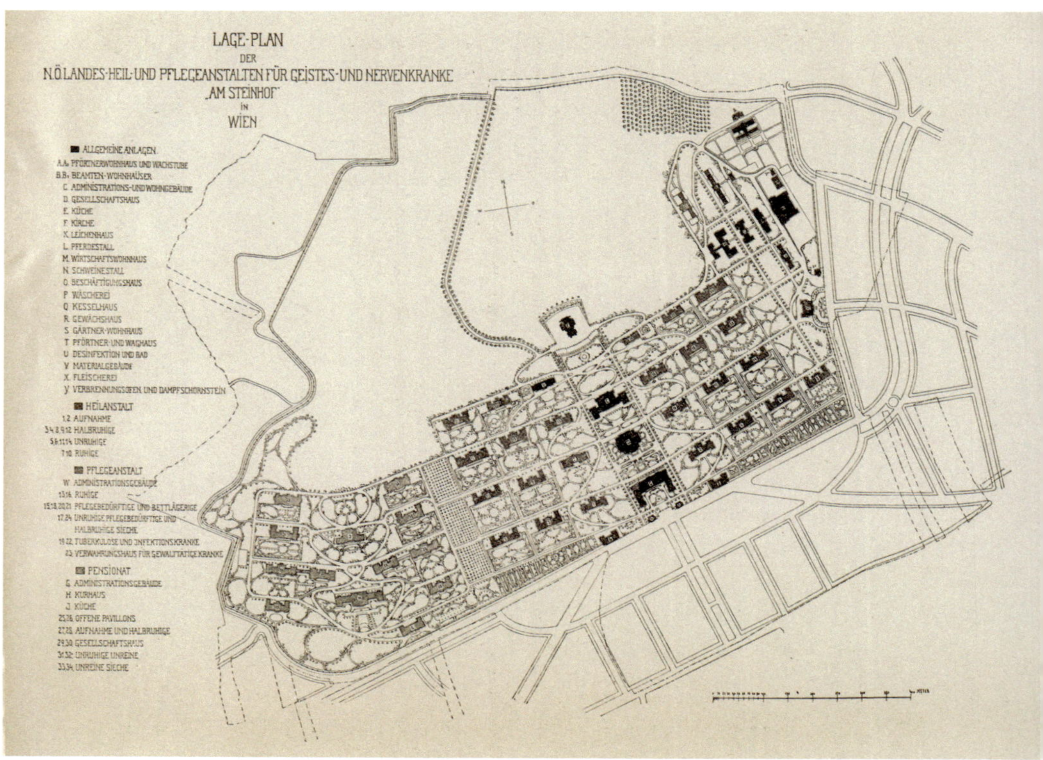

↗ Children at Am Spiegelgrund, 1938. Vienna.

→ Otto Wagner, site plan of Steinhof am Main.

children threatened with or placed in cages.[9] At the scale of the complex, the segregation of pavilions for "observation" and killing provided a horrific form of motivation for those in the curative education pavilions. The overarching goal of Nazi psychiatry, at Spiegelgrund and beyond, was not only to further genetic hygiene, but also to measure children's potential to be transformed into productive laborers for the ongoing reproduction of the Nazi state.

Hans Asperger, a pediatric psychologist who would become a central figure in autism research, developed his practice and his theories in this context. He earned his medical degree in 1931 at the University Children's Hospital in Vienna. During the rise of the Nazi state, Asperger was a participant in increasingly white-supremacist political activities, eventually joining the right-wing fascist Fatherland Front in 1934. In 1941, as an assistant director of the Vienna Children's Hospital overseeing organizational dynamics, Asperger consolidated Spiegelgrund and the Vienna Children's Hospital into a network known as the Vienna Society for Curative Education.[10] The administrators of the Society for Curative Education (*Heilpedagogik*) formed a network of state institutions that aimed to "educate" neurodivergent children to be able to contribute more broadly to Nazi society. The network facilitated the removal of uneducable individuals using existing psychiatric infrastructures compatible with the project of neurotypical supremacy. *Heilpedagogik* clinics were a crucial part of the Nazis' highly efficient network of concentration camps. On various scales, from Spiegelgrund's interiors to the infrastructures between *Heilpedagogik* psychiatric centers where initial diagnoses occurred, Asperger facilitated and maintained a network of spatial control that both activated and built upon Nazi principles.

Building on his experience at the Society for Curative Education, Asperger published his doctoral thesis in 1944, entitled "The 'Autistic Psychopaths' in Childhood," which considered individuals with milder social and executive functioning challenges—and put the "spectrum" in "autism spectrum." Despite Asperger's ties to the Nazi project, he continued his psychiatric scholarship after World War II and consulted at the Vienna Children's Hospital until his retirement in 1977. In 1981, British psychiatrist Lorna Wing rediscovered Asperger's thesis and publicized the diagnosis as "Asperger's Syndrome."[11] This diagnosis rapidly gained recognition in the global psychiatric community, and in 1994 Asperger's syndrome was adopted by the *Diagnostic and Statistical Manual of Mental Disorders* (DSM). In 2013, the DSM changed its criteria to combine Kanner-type (nonverbal) autism and Asperger's syndrome into a single diagnosis, autism spectrum disorder (ASD).

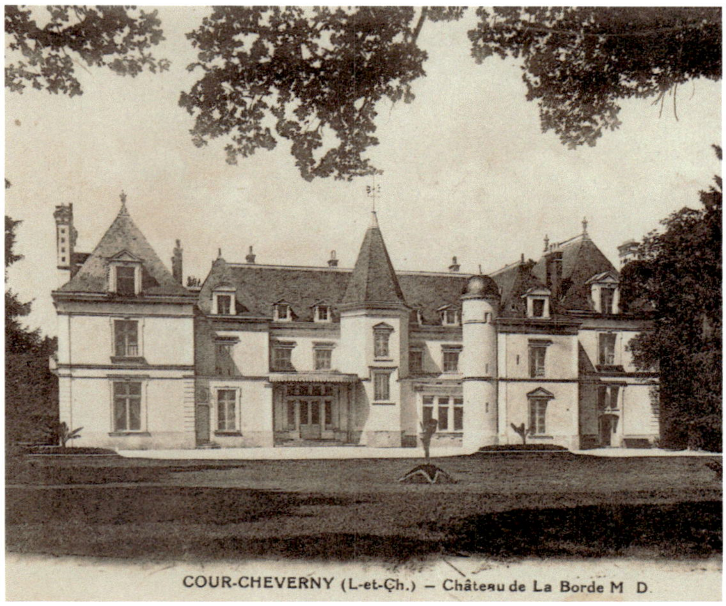

↑ Postcard of Clinic La Borde, Cour-Cheverny. 1922.

Institutional Psychotherapy and Radical Politics

The term "autism" was first coined in 1911 by Eugen Bleuler, a Swiss psychiatrist who described patients "who have no more contact with the outside world, live in a world of their own, they have encased themselves with their desires and wishes (which they consider fulfilled) or occupy themselves with the trials and tribulations of their persecutory ideas ... this detachment from reality, together with the relative and absolute predominance of the inner life, we term autism."[12] In 1925, Jewish Ukrainian psychiatrist Grunya Sukhareva studied and described autistic children, going on to lead the department of psychiatry in Kharkiv University in 1935.[13] The closest to Asperger was the Austrian-born psychiatrist Leo Kanner, who fled Weimar Germany to the United States in 1924 and published a study on "autistic" children at Johns Hopkins University in 1943. Kanner worked closely with Georg Frankl, who had been Asperger's diagnostician until he fled Vienna in 1937.[14] Kanner's diagnosis is slightly different from Asperger's and is commonly referred to as "classic" or "Kanner-type" autism, characterized by social and emotional withdrawal, little to no speech, and severe cognitive impairment. Kanner, Asperger, and Sukhareva would continue to define the field of autism research globally over the following decades.

In postwar France, critical responses to psychiatric institutionality formed a spatial language for radical psychological care.[15] At Saint-Alban, a clinic in the mountainous Lozère region, a group of leftist psychiatrists built a community with mentally ill patients that confronted existing forms of diagnosis, pathology, and treatment. Their challenges were less psychiatric than social, communal, and spatial. Saint-Alban was originally founded by Spanish socialist psychiatrist Fernand Tosquelles and saw the participation of other institutional psychotherapy (IP)

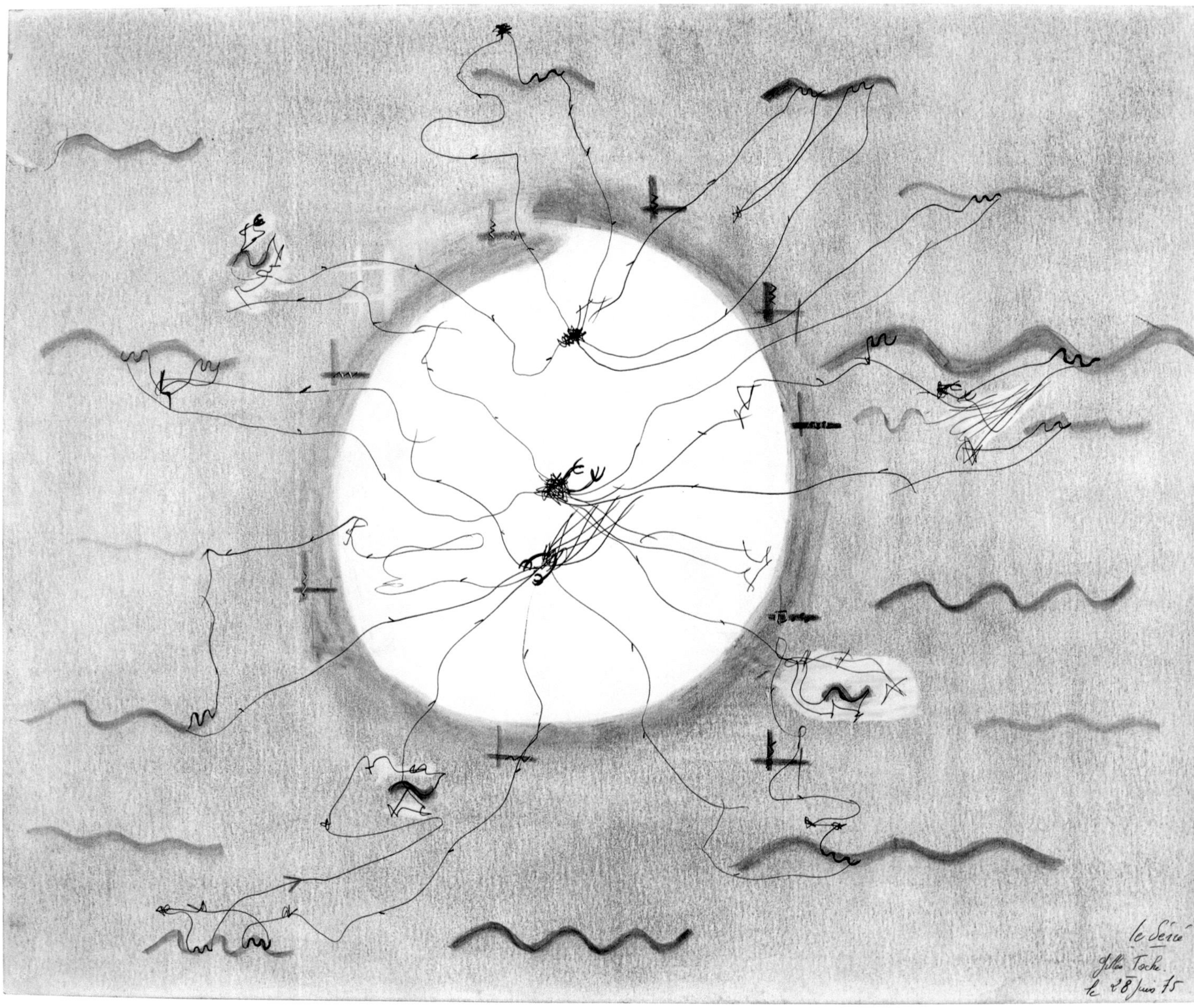

↑ Wander lines of Christophe B., Le Serret, June 28, 1975. Map drawn by Jean Lin.

practitioners and thinkers such as Frantz Fanon, Félix Guattari, and Michel Foucault.[16] Marxist thought was foundational to the psychopolitical spatial formations at Saint-Alban. Social divisions between doctor, patient, and nurse were blurred, contributing to the sense of an integrated community of people living together rather than a place of hierarchical treatment. The IP movement was not just about societal politics, but also about metropolitan/peripheral relationships.[17] The success of Saint-Alban can therefore be credited to the lack of architectural development around Lozère, which enabled nonstate and counterhegemonic institutions to take root.

Taking lessons from Saint-Alban, in 1952 Guattari joined fellow psychiatrist Jean Oury to help establish the clinic La Borde in an unused château in the middle of a park in Cour-Cheverny, a small commune in France's Loire Valley. At both Saint-Alban and La Borde, hierarchies established in industrial society were done away with as much as possible. Nurses and doctors wore the same kinds of clothing as the "patients." They shared tasks such as cooking and cleaning, as well as facilitating care and communication between residents of all types. Patients even took part in directing their own care, and the free communication of ideas and collective need was encouraged.

The château architecture of La Borde became a site of community and "transversality." As Guattari defines it, transversality is "the unconscious source of action in the group, going beyond the objective law on which it is based, carrying the group's desire."[18] Desire—and the psychoanalytic determination of it by some facilitator—was thus crucial to the group's functioning as an alternative psychiatric community. This meant prioritizing the shared experience of space in opposition to psychiatry's traditional ordering of diagnosis, movement, and segregation. As a refuge for difference, La Borde operated on three principles: democratic centralism, a rotating basis for the division of labor, and anti-bureaucracy. Patients were free to roam the grounds and actively participated in—or at least, had a standing invitation to—a central governing committee. By 1966, La Borde was well established among radical psychiatrists, philosophers, and political organizers.

That same year, Guattari invited the educator Fernand Deligny to La Borde. Deligny had known Guattari and others from Saint-Alban and from organizing with the French Resistance. After the war, Deligny started collective projects with other pediatric psychiatrists to form alternatives to harsh state-run psychiatric clinics and juvenile delinquent centers.[19] At Guattari's invitation, Deligny, whose treatment of autistic children reflected similarly radical modes of communal existence, saw an opportunity for continuing and expanding his work with mainly nonspeaking autistic children. However, he found the psychoanalytic approach at La Borde to be insufficient for his work. While most "patients" with mental differences at La Borde already had methods to communicate their desires, Deligny's children simply enacted their desires, disregarding social structure in favor of a total freedom of activity. Seeing this necessity for total spatial freedom, Deligny initiated an alternative psychotherapeutic project in a nearby unused house owned by Guattari.

In the desolate Cévennes mountains, Deligny and volunteers acted as monitors and occasional interactees with the nonspeaking children, who for the most part went about their business, wandering around and playing with sticks and other natural materials they could find. As the children wandered, Deligny and one of his volunteer staff, Gisèle Durand-Ruiz, instituted a daily practice of tracing each child's movements on a site plan. The resulting archive of over 300 "maps and wander lines," traced from 1969 to 1980, points to a counterinfrastructural practice of autistic agency removed from both legible social structure and any semblance of spatial prescription.

Deligny wrote extensively on the revolutionary and communal potential of what he called the "Arachnean Network."[20] Influenced by Karl von Frisch's *Animal Architecture* (1974), Deligny saw the autistic "Arachnean" as creating a relational web in refusal of the "thought-out project," a term he used to encompasses any planned activity from cooking to architectural production.[21] Deligny's dense, poetic theorization views the resulting lines as connections in which modernity—that is to say, urban plans, architectural programming, and attendant modes of conduct—is profoundly avoided. To quote Deligny: "can we say that the spider's project is to weave its web? I don't think so. We might as well say that the web's project is to be woven."[22] This network, based entirely in autistic creation, manifests as immediate sociospatial agency that otherwise defies easy accommodation in architectural theory and practice.

The abandoned spaces that Deligny and his community occupied were deliberately underdeveloped, offering only basic necessities and depending on the broader institutional psychotherapy community for material resources and connections. Deligny's focus on living in community with nonspeaking autistic subjects required immense creativity, both in spatial arrangements and interpersonal interpretation. The maps and wander lines offer a point of contact between the autistic child and the concept of the "thought-out project," drawing a dialectical tension between inhabitation and plan that undergirds the arachnean network. As Sabel Gavaldon writes:

> the maps drawn by Gisèle Durand-Ruiz combined the overlapping experiences of this territory as perceived and navigated by each of the children, revealing not just a rich universe of subjectivity,

> but in fact a plurality of inhabited worlds. … Each of those charts and drawings contained dozens of intersecting lines but no arrows, and thus no direction, no teleology … just network.[23]

This collective mode of psychosocial spatiality resists easy architectural classification and analysis. Instead, the network itself becomes the dominant form of spatial arrangement, and Deligny explicitly highlights its incompatibility with architecture: “If the observer had been present, his gaze alone would have disturbed the architecture of trajectories, and should his presence have lasted or recurred, the ‘vague’ space would have become vacant. This is where architecture disappears, and if the word seems excessive let us discuss the net of our trajectories.”[24]

The Limits of Care

Deligny’s network of simple dwellings, nonprescribed spaces, and objects “of no use” provided a free space for autistic life outside of the prescriptive, harmful binary of pathologization and cure so central to Asperger’s psychiatry. The arachnean network reflects an exit from the political hierarchy of the nation-state and the psychiatric hierarchy of doctor-nurse-janitor-patient. Deligny’s “primordial communist” network in the Cévennes required only the bare necessities and a handful of volunteer facilitators. However, the relations between the arachnean network, La Borde, Saint-Alban, the families of those housed within the facilities, and the broader French radical community were crucial to Deligny’s success. Deligny followed his arachneans’ trajectories, which were incommunicable except for the fact of their completion in space, with trust and acceptance. His network of arachneans crawled (and trotted, skipped, slept, and ran) relatively happily in the ridges of the Cévennes for almost thirty years. The arachnean network thus gestures toward what a more integrated psychotherapeutic urbanism might look like. From the periphery, architectural analysis and design are secondary to active creation, compelling us to rethink our very modes of living.

Deleuze, Guattari, other theorists, journalists, and psychiatrists would come to visit Deligny’s primordial community, offering support where and however needed. The self-organized, nonhierarchical political network of resources independent of the French state provided a foil to government-run institutions of the era. The creation of a network outside of the necropolitical psychiatric network of post-World War II society tells of an emergent need to confront the idealist conditions of Western political forms of organization. In responding to Nazi psychiatry, Guattari and Deligny were additionally responding to the material conditions of global

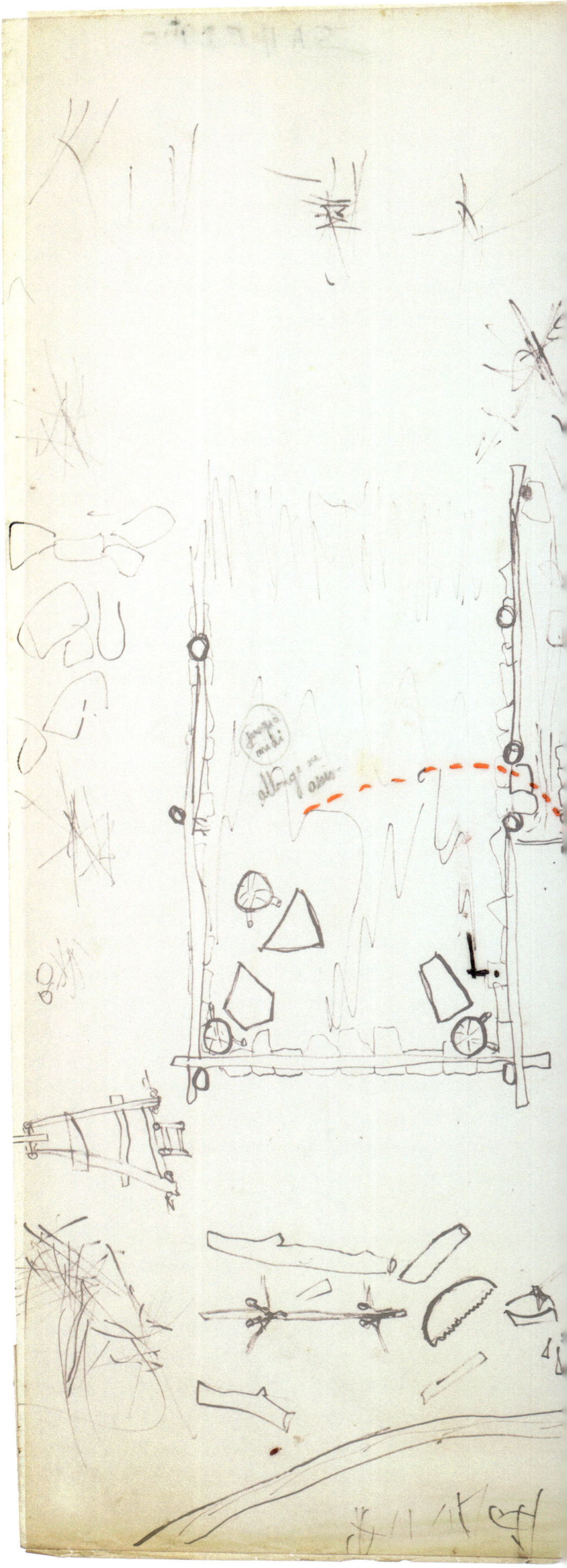

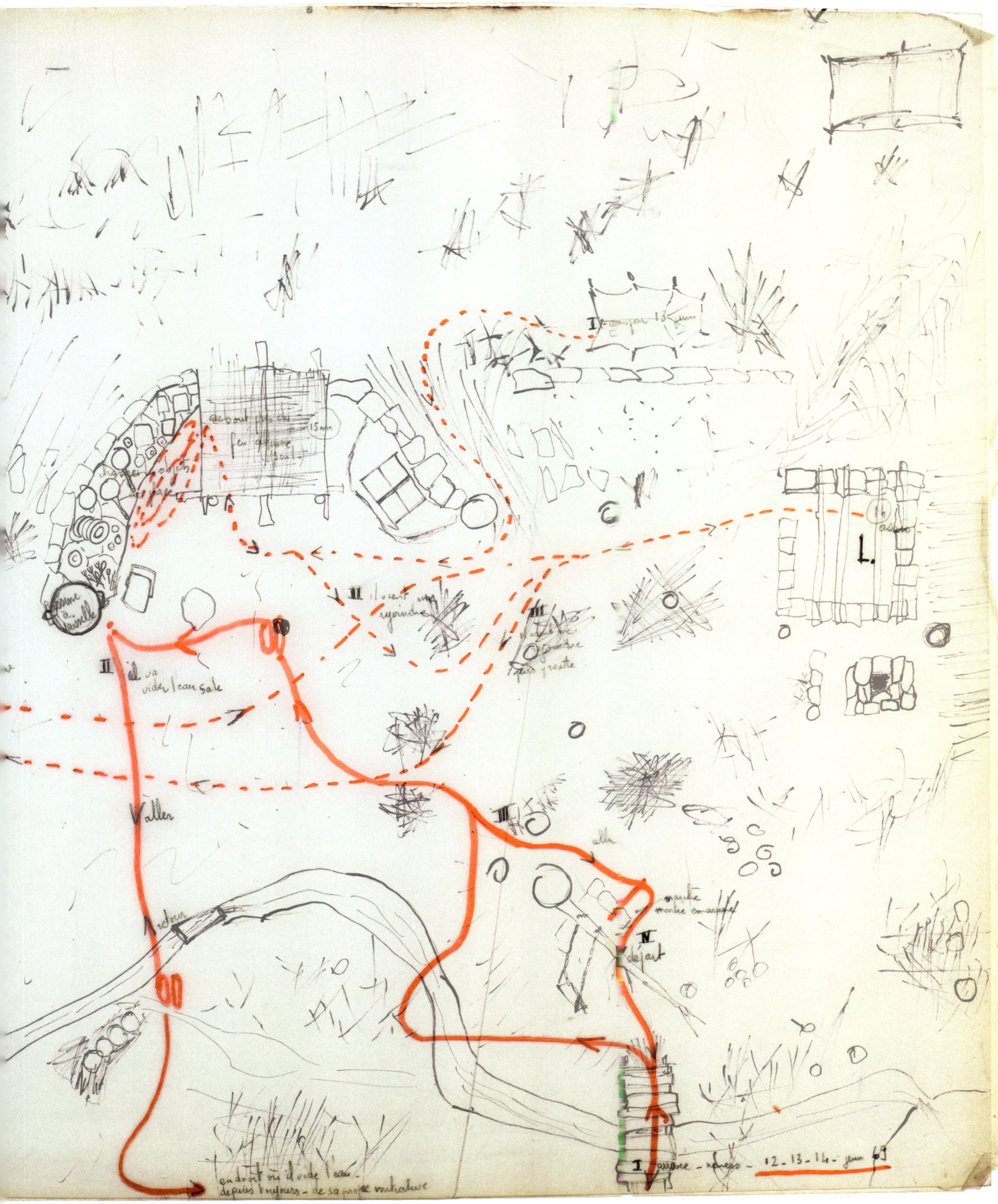

↑ Wander lines of Janmari et Gaspard, Ile d'en bas, June 12–13–14, 1969. Map drawn by Jacques Lin, India ink, 20 × 25 inches.

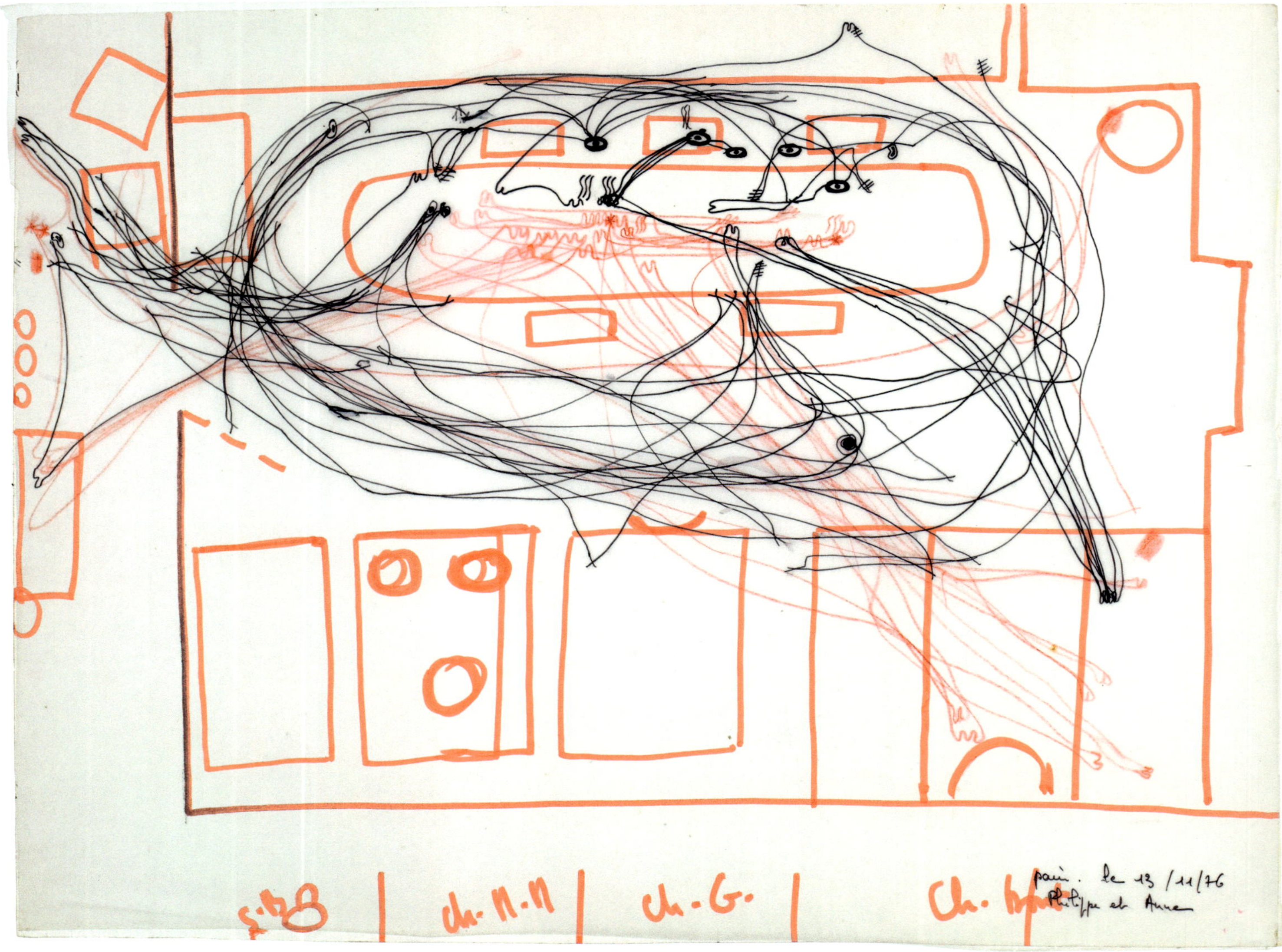

imperialist society, in which colonial frontiers and internal mental health paradigms can be described in extremely similar terms. Indeed, the presence of Frantz Fanon in Saint-Alban and the militant, revolutionary spirit of those involved in the institutional psychotherapy movement speaks not just to the evolution of anticapitalist philosophy, but also to the instituted praxis of independent communal mental health networks.

"If I wanted to indicate one of the constants of the network," Deligny writes, "I would note an 'outside' as one of the necessary components. That said, and when space becomes a concentration camp, the formation of a network creates a kind of outside that allows the human to survive."[25] This outside lies beyond communicable boundaries. It is the unknowable interiority of the autistic life of the mind, which must be protected and cultivated dearly. The evolution of psychiatric spatiality must center the internalities of the "patient" and enable the maintenance of healing, agentic, and self-organized communities.

↑ Wander lines of Philippe and Anne, Monoblet, Y house, November 13, 1976. Map drawn by Thierry Bazzana and Marie-Madeleine Godet, India ink, 15 × 20 inches.

An earlier version of this essay was originally published by e-flux Architecture in 2022.

1. The assembly urged member states "to give appropriate recognition to the specific needs of individuals affected by autism spectrum disorders and other developmental disorders in policies and programmes related to early childhood and adolescent development, as part of a comprehensive approach to address child and adolescent mental health and developmental disorders." Additional resolutions included dedicating resources to research, education, and "strengthen[ing] different levels of infrastructure for comprehensive management of autism spectrum disorders and other developmental disorders, as appropriate, including care, education, support, intervention, services and rehabilitation."
2. "What Is Autism?," Neuroclastic, https://neuroclastic.com/autism/what-is-autism/.
3. Charlotte M. Pretzsch, James L. Findon, and Declan G. Murphy, "Autism Spectrum Disorders in Adults," in *The Oxford Handbook of Adult Cognitive Disorders*, ed. Michael L. Alosco and Robert A. Stern (Oxford: Oxford University Press, 2019), 357–377.
4. Georg Simmel, "The Metropolis and Mental Life," in *The Sociology of Georg Simmel* (New York: Free Press, 1950), 324.
5. Simmel, "The Metropolis and Mental Life," 325.
6. Simmel, "The Metropolis and Mental Life," 338.
7. Leslie Topp, *Freedom and the Cage: Modern Architecture and Psychiatry in Central Europe, 1890–1914* (University Park: Pennsylvania State University Press, 2016).
8. Ludwig Hevesi, "Otto Wagners moderne Kirche (29. November 1899)," in *Acht Jahre Sezession (März 1897-Juni 1905). Kritik, Polemik, Chronik* (Vienna: Verlagsbuchhandlung Carl Konegan, 1906).
9. See the popular publication *Asperger's Children*, by Edith Sheffer (New York: W. W. Norton, 2018), for a comprehensive history of Asperger's methods of diagnosis and control, involvement in state-run psychiatric activities resulting in genocide, and other points of interest.
10. This work was done in collaboration with Max Gundel, head of Vienna's Public Health Office and municipal director of Spiegelgrund; Erwin Jekelius, medical director of Spiegelgrund; and Franz Hamburger, director of the University of Vienna Children's Hospital
11. See Lorna Wing, "Asperger's Syndrome: A Clinical Account," *Psychological Medicine* 11, no. 1 (February 1981): 115–129.
12. T. H. McGlashan, "Eugen Bleuler: Centennial Anniversary of His 1911 Publication of Dementia Praecox or the Group of Schizophrenias," *Schizophrenia Bulletin* 37, no. 6 (November 1, 2011): 1101–1103.
13. Dr. Grunya Sukhareva is an often-overlooked protagonist in the history of autism studies. Leo Kanner was aware of her work, citing her in 1949. Hans Asperger likely knew of her work but may have chosen not to cite or mention her because she was Jewish. See "Tribute to Grunya Efimovna Sukhareva, the Woman who First Described Infantile Autism," *Journal of Pediatric Neurosciences* 12, no. 3 (July-September 2017): 300–301.
14. Steve Silberman, *NeuroTribes* (London: Penguin, 2015). See also Herwig Czech, "Hans Asperger, National Socialism, and 'Race Hygiene' in Nazi-Era Vienna," *Molecular Autism* 9, no. 1 (December 2018): 1–43.
15. See Amit Pinchevski and John Durham Peters, "Autism and New Media: Disability between Technology and Society," *New Media and Society* 18 (2016). The authors describe how new media technologies have become critical tools for autistic communication and organization.
16. See Camille Robcis's recent publication *Disalienation: Politics, Philosophy, and Radical Psychiatry in Postwar France* (Chicago: University of Chicago Press, 2021).
17. As Susana Caló and Godofredo Pereira note, "the design of hospitals or clinical centers has always been a part of broader projects, concerning not only the types of health care provision, but also their relation with the wider territory." Susana Caló and Godofredo Pereira, "ICERFI: From the Hospital to the City," *London Journal of Critical Thought* 1, no. 2 (2017): 1.
18. Félix Guattari, *Psychoanalysis and Transversality: Texts and Interviews 1955–1971* (Cambridge, MA: MIT Press, 2015), 118.
19. For a brief biography of Deligny, see Leon Hilton, "Mapping the Wander Lines: The Quiet Revelations of Fernand Deligny," *Los Angeles Review of Books*, 2015, https://lareviewofbooks.org/article/mapping-the-wander-lines-the-quiet-revelations-of-fernand-deligny/.
20. Fernand Deligny, *The Arachnean and Other Texts*, trans. Drew S. Burk and Catherine Porter (Minneapolis: University of Minnesota Press, 2015).
21. Karl von Frisch, *Animal Architecture* (Boston: Harcourt, 1974).
22. Deligny, *The Arachnean and Other Texts*, 34.
23. Sabel Gavaldon, "Flowers That Matter," in *Lossy Ecology*, ed. Louisa Martin (self-pub., 2017), 68–69.
24. Deligny, *The Arachnean and Other Texts*, 37.
25. Deligny, *The Arachnean and Other Texts*, 35.

p104 Courtesy of Wien Museum, Vienna.
p106 (top) Courtesy of the Documentation Centre of Austrian Resistance, Vienna.
p106 (bottom) In Paul Gerin, *Auszug aus der Verwaltungstätigkeit der christlichsozialen Landtagsmehrheit in den Jahren 1902–1908* (Vienna, 1908). ÖNB/Vienna, 461.815-C.
p107 CC BY-NC-SA 2.0 Creative Commons.
p108, 110–111 © Archives Gisèle Durand-Ruiz. Photo: Anaïs Masson. Reproduced in *Cartes et lignes d'erre / Maps and Wander Lines—Traces du réseau de Fernand Deligny* (L'Arachnéen, 2013). www.editions-arachneen.fr.
p112 © Archives Marie-Dominique Guibal. Photo: Anaïs Masson. Reproduced in *Cartes et lignes d'erre / Maps and Wander Lines—Traces du réseau de Fernand Deligny* (L'Arachnéen, 2013). www.editions-arachneen.fr.

BODY CULTURE AND CONTROLOGY

IBIAYI BRIGGS

For all the scientific discovery and technological progress heralded by modernity, its lasting legacy is also one of disenchantment and alienation. This alienation was psychological and physical, and was manifested in the bodies of the growing rank of industrial workers. The monotony of factory work and the environmental effects of its production clouded the minds, lungs, and entire being of urban populations. Georg Simmel famously painted a picture of the mind of the modern, urban citizen that was so overwhelmed by external stimuli as to be rendered inert.[1] That static mind translated to a docile body. To a growing movement of doctors, scientists, gymnasts, and performers, this docility had to be corrected, through exercise.

Histories of health and exercise tell stories about human bodies and the ways they have been idealized, sculpted, and tortured into different forms. They capture evolving standards of strength, beauty, science, and medicine. As these relationships with bodies change, so do the spaces and apparatus used to hone them. A central theme within the historical development of exercise is its connection to martial and carceral histories. Military barracks and prison yards were often the first testing grounds for bodily improvement—or as it was understood there, for bodily correction and discipline. As exercise moved into the domestic realm, the corrections targeted by exercise were not explicitly tied to an innate criminality, but rather to a wider societal rot. Its discipline was not marshaled on the battlefield, but rather in the character of each citizen as a reflection of a larger national character.

The nineteenth and early twentieth centuries saw the rise of "body culture" (*Körperkultur*), an expanding movement that encompassed new trends in exercise and bodybuilding. It made celebrities of strongmen who performed great feats in front of adoring audiences that would go on to read their books and magazines, attend their gymnasiums, and adopt their lifestyles. These exercise spectacles provided a compelling counternarrative to the lassitude wrought by modernization. Bodies could be reclaimed from industrialization, and there was an expanding class of doctors, designers, and performers shaping the methods. To do so would take control, but also the very same mechanization that engendered both innovation and ennui.

Perfecting the Body through Gymnastics

Physical education had been an important component of classical education in Germany from as early as the fifteenth century, and the cultivation of a specific exercise practice was primarily the privilege of the aristocracy. Activities like horseback riding, fencing, and dancing were important components in shaping the image of the gentleman. These exercises were not only social signifiers, but also relied on aesthetic judgments like the purity of a jump, or the style and gracefulness of a dance. However, in the late eighteenth century, there was an increasing interest in maximizing the body's power rather than its artistry. In 1793, the book *Gymnastik*, written by Johann Christoph Friedrich GutsMuths, a teacher at a *Philanthropinum* (Enlightenment-inspired German educational institution) in central Germany, attempted to detach exercise from gentility.[2] Instead of foregrounding the aesthetic aspects of exercise, GutsMuths emphasized the body's performance—the ability for specific exercises to improve strength, endurance, or balance—which he saw as a morally ideal masculine practice.[3] In the exercise regime outlined in *Gymnastik*, the pommel horse was positioned as a training apparatus that could produce a new range of activities. Vaulting and jumping were no longer valued for purity, but instead for their measurability.

GutsMuths's teachings were centered around the university and other institutions of higher education. In 1809, Friedrich Ludwig Jahn built on GutsMuths's philosophies and moved the space of exercise outdoors. He established a sports field in Berlin that made gymnastics a spectator sport, where curious audiences could watch groups of gymnasts performing different exercises. This public performance of gymnastics helped Jahn's pupils establish gymnastic clubs and similar sports fields in other cities. These new clubs were rooted in the same culture of masculinity established by GutsMuths, but also included a more nationalist philosophy. In the aftermath of the Prussian army's defeat by Napoleon in 1806 and the expanding power of the French Empire, there was a growing desire to bolster German heritage. Jahn tied his gymnastics to the cultivation—or recultivation—of a virile primitive man from ancestral Germanic tribes and encouraged his students to join the military as an opportunity to seek revenge on the French.[4] In 1819, the princes that then ruled the various regions of Prussia banned Jahn's form of gymnastics as they feared its potential to foment subversive activities. While Jahn's influence lingered, by the 1830s other practitioners of German gymnastics attempted to deemphasize his politics, allowing the sport to expand through the establishment of independent gymnastics clubs. This form of gymnastics was aligned with dietetics, a philosophy that advocated for a holistic perspective of health that encompassed a person's nutrition, environment, and daily habits. Advocates for dietetic gymnastics saw exercise as a means to balance the body with the environment.

Daniel Gottlob Moritz Schreber was a particularly strong voice of nineteenth-century middle-class German health and exercise culture. After graduating from medical school 1833, he lectured on dietetics at the University of Leipzig and further channeled these interests into founding a local gymnastics club. In his work with youth, he emphasized the importance of exercise as a matter of ethics and hygiene. When his career in academia faltered, he fully committed to professional practice as an orthopedic physician and medical doctor in pediatrics. When an accident ended that line of work, however, he began to write extensively on the benefits and philosophy of gymnastics. In the opening lines of Ärztliche *Zimmergymnastik* (*Medical Indoor Gymnastics*), Schreber proclaims that modern science, in its overreliance on "so-called medicinal substances," has overlooked exercise as a way to reconnect with nature.

> [Home gymnastics] is the most natural method for bringing the constantly rising tide of culture in each rank of society into harmonious cooperation with the physical laws which govern our human organism. It completes and perfects the whole development of the body, preserves it from countless defects and disorders, while laying the necessary foundation for the development of the mind.[5]

Schreber brought together his practice in orthopedics with his promotion of dietetics' natural remedies to promote normal bodily development.[6] He is particularly noted for the creation of orthopedic devices that materialized corrective postures such as the *Geradehalter*, a device consisting of a back and neck brace secured to the wearer's forehead and chest to produce upright posture. Some of his devices, like those designed to prevent masturbation, made the moralizing dimension of his work clear. Even after his sudden death in 1861, Schreber's influence continued to shape German ideas of the importance of access to nature and exercise. For instance, in 1846 a group of educators in Leipzig who were inspired by Schreber's writing built his proposal for a playground which included a small garden plot. The popularity of this playground-garden hybrid grew, and allotment gardens specially leased in cities to give children space to exercise—called *Schrebergartens*—spread throughout Germany.[7]

Schreber's son, Daniel Paul, was raised according to dietetic principles and with orthopedic devices. Born in 1842, Daniel Paul Schreber would become a well-established judge in Leipzig until he suffered a nervous breakdown. The initial onset of his nervous breakdown was attributed to overworking. What began as a bout of insomnia quickly spiraled into severe anxiety, paranoia, depression, and suicidal thoughts. The younger Schreber describes hearing voices and witnessing "miracles" during his breakdown, and one such memory seems to evoke the chest-constricting posture of his father's *Geradehalter*.[8] The experience became an important case study for Sigmund Freud, who interpreted that the orthopedics experiments undertaken by the looming figure of Moritz were directly tied to Daniel Paul's anxieties.[9] This was instrumental in Freud's understanding of dementia praecox, contemporarily known as schizophrenia.

Eric Santner highlights the recurring theme of degeneration that appears in Daniel Paul's *Memoirs of My Nervous Illness* (1903), which documented his breakdown. Santner connects this to wider sentiments of exhaustion and disillusionment that were prevalent in nineteenth-century ideas about medical conditions like hysteria and their relationship to rapid technological advancement.[10] As Anson Rabinbach notes, the belief that a mass intellectual degeneration was caused by modernity was a common refrain in medical literature in the 1870s, and fatigue and exhaustion were cited as the symptoms of the body's resistance to industrial labor.[11] Fatigue was further pathologized into a range of disorders, but most notably neurasthenia, a nervous exhaustion that nineteenth-century physicians tied directly to modernity.[12] Yet in 1847 the second law of thermodynamics was discovered, allowing scientists and engineers to conceive of a new relationship between the body and technology as a matter of energy conservation. The human body was thus recast as a technical object, which could be optimized by replacing human energy with new technologies, or inanimate technical energies.[13] Technology could save, rather than destroy, human energy. Through a deeper medical and scientific understanding, the body could grow with—rather than against—modernity.

Pilates and the Birth of Contrology

Joseph Pilates was born in 1883 into this post-Schreber world in Mönchengladbach, Germany. Although his family was poor, his father was an avid gymnast and took Joseph and his younger brother to gymnasia as children. His father

↓ Eugen Sandow demonstrating an exercise on his leg machine from his book *Sandow on Physical Training: A Study in the Perfect Type of the Human Form* (1894).

→ Photographs reproduced from from Bess Mensendieck's book *Die Körperkultur des Weibes* (*The Body Culture of Women*), 1906.

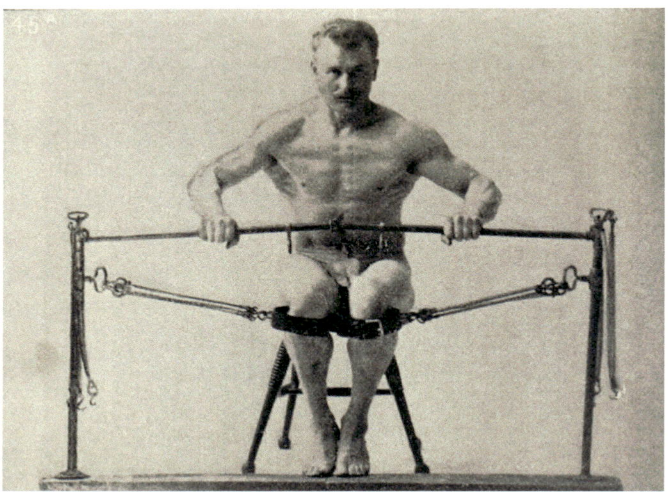

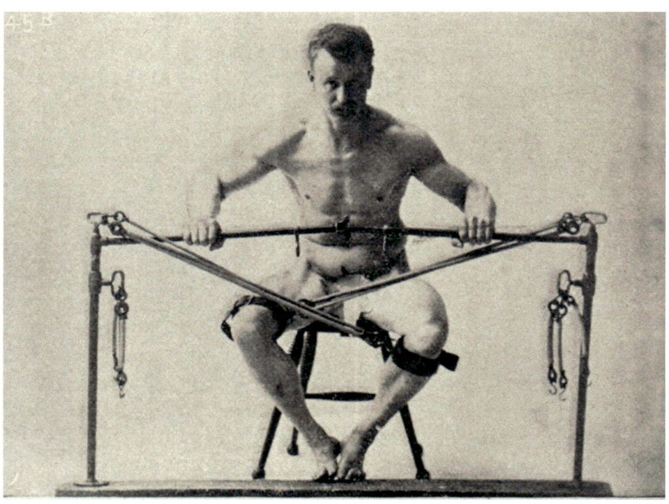

demonstrated how to use each apparatus and hoped that an interest in gymnastics would make Joseph, his frail son, strong. Joseph was also introduced to boxing, which not only led to a lifelong passion for techniques of boxing and gymnastics, but also a deep intellectual curiosity about the workings of muscles. As his interest in exercise grew, Pilates was particularly drawn to the work of two figures, Eugen Sandow and Bess Mensendieck.

Eugen Sandow was a world-renowned strongman and celebrity of late nineteenth-century *Körperkultur*. Although born and raised in Königsberg, Germany, Sandow initially made a name for himself in Britain where he performed feats of strength like breaking an iron chain around his arm simply by flexing his muscles, bending iron rods, and even fighting a lion. Sandow channeled this fame into business—opening his own gyms, publishing a magazine, and writing books. Sandow also created and sold his own exercise machines and apparatuses. Pilates was especially inspired by *Strength and How to Obtain It* (1897), in which Sandow laid out a definition of body culture that stressed training "to get rid of the defects that civilization and the changes it has brought about are responsible for making humans neglect their own body."[14] Sandow further emphasized the rehabilitating power of his exercise methods in a chapter titled "Why Body Culture Is the Best Cure for Some Diseases," which advocated for his methods as a cure for "rheumatism, hip pain, pulled muscles, inflamed joints, scoliosis, flat feet, [and] rickets."[15]

The work of the American Bess Mensendieck presented gymnastics in a way that emphasized grace and beauty. Her book *Die Körperkultur des Weibes* (*The Body Culture of Women*, 1906) built on a method of training that was popular with dancers, the Delsarte system, which emphasized breathing and relaxation along with strengthening. Mensendieck was also unique in her method of documenting her exercises. Like the subjects of the book's photogaphs, Mensendieck encouraged her students to do their exercises nude. She believed that nudity allowed the instructor and pupil to see, and therefore better understand, the muscles that were being exercised.[16]

By 1914 Joseph Pilates had been married, widowed, and was a single father. Compelled to follow in the footsteps of his hero Sandow, he decided to try to make a name for himself in Britain. Arriving in Blackpool that summer, he worked a series of odd jobs until the outbreak of World War I. That autumn he was arrested with other German citizens and interned as an "enemy alien."[17] Pilates used his time of internment as an opportunity to establish his training practice. He organized activities among his fellow internees and, using his knowledge of boxing, led self-defense courses and group exercises.[18]

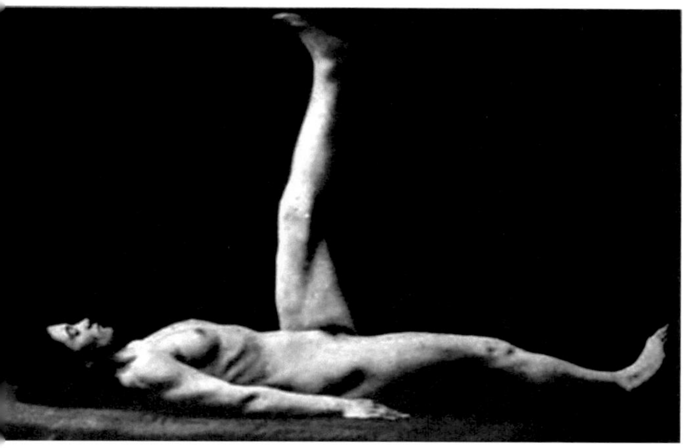

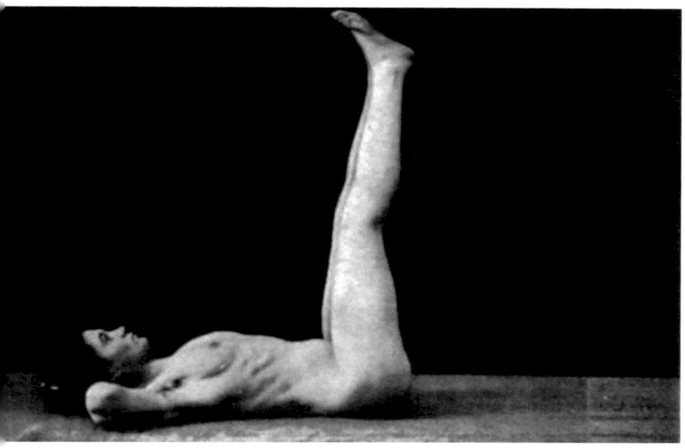

In 1915 Pilates was transferred to the largest internment camp for German civilians in Britain, Knockaloe on the Isle of Man.[19] There he continued to develop his exercise method and was inspired by his observations of local stray cats, developing more natural stretching techniques that mirrored the cats' lithe movements. At Knockaloe, Pilates had a captive audience of fellow internees. He often worked with sick or injured internees to test his methods as a form of rehabilitation. This, in particular, was crucial to what became his primary inspiration in the years to come: creating apparatuses that could stretch while also developing strength. His recent biography claims that "the springs from the camp beds that were provided in the hospital barracks—as opposed to the wooden bedsteads with straw bags the internees had to sleep on in their barracks—may have provided an inspiration for Pilates to design machines for rehabilitation using the resistance that springs offer."[20]

Although politically agnostic, Pilates related everything to the body. He thought that the economic and political failures of post-World War I Germany could be resolved by citizens who had a healthier and more thoughtful relationship to their bodies, and his life after internment was dedicated to spreading this idea. After the war ended in 1918, Pilates returned to Germany with proven success of his methods, friendships with German boxers, and a headful of new ideas on how to spread his technique. He remarried, had another child, and moved to Hamburg to open his own boxing gym. Although he never had a winning record, Pilates pursued a career as an amateur boxer, but he became better known locally as a respected trainer. As he worked with and competed against other boxers, he started building his first piece of exercise equipment. In 1922 he filed German patent number 375,001 for a "device for removal and improvement of foot and leg dysfunctions," which relied on elasticity to provide resistance.[21]

As he juggled his work as a boxing trainer and waited for the approval of his first patent (granted in 1923), Pilates set out to expand the scope of his apparatuses by designing something that could correct and strengthen the entire body. He also began training members of the Hamburg police in self-defense. At the time, police training was based on jiu-jitsu and boxing. Working with the police, then, allowed Pilates to buttress his expertise in boxing with a mastery of basic jiu-jitsu skills, which in turn introduced him to methods of resistance training with a partner. He was also reintroduced to ideas about nudism that he first saw in Bess Mensendieck's exercises when an officer introduced him to the *völkisch* movement. While it is unclear what Pilates's feelings were about that movement's latent antisemitism, racism, and fascism, he strongly supported its belief in the connection between

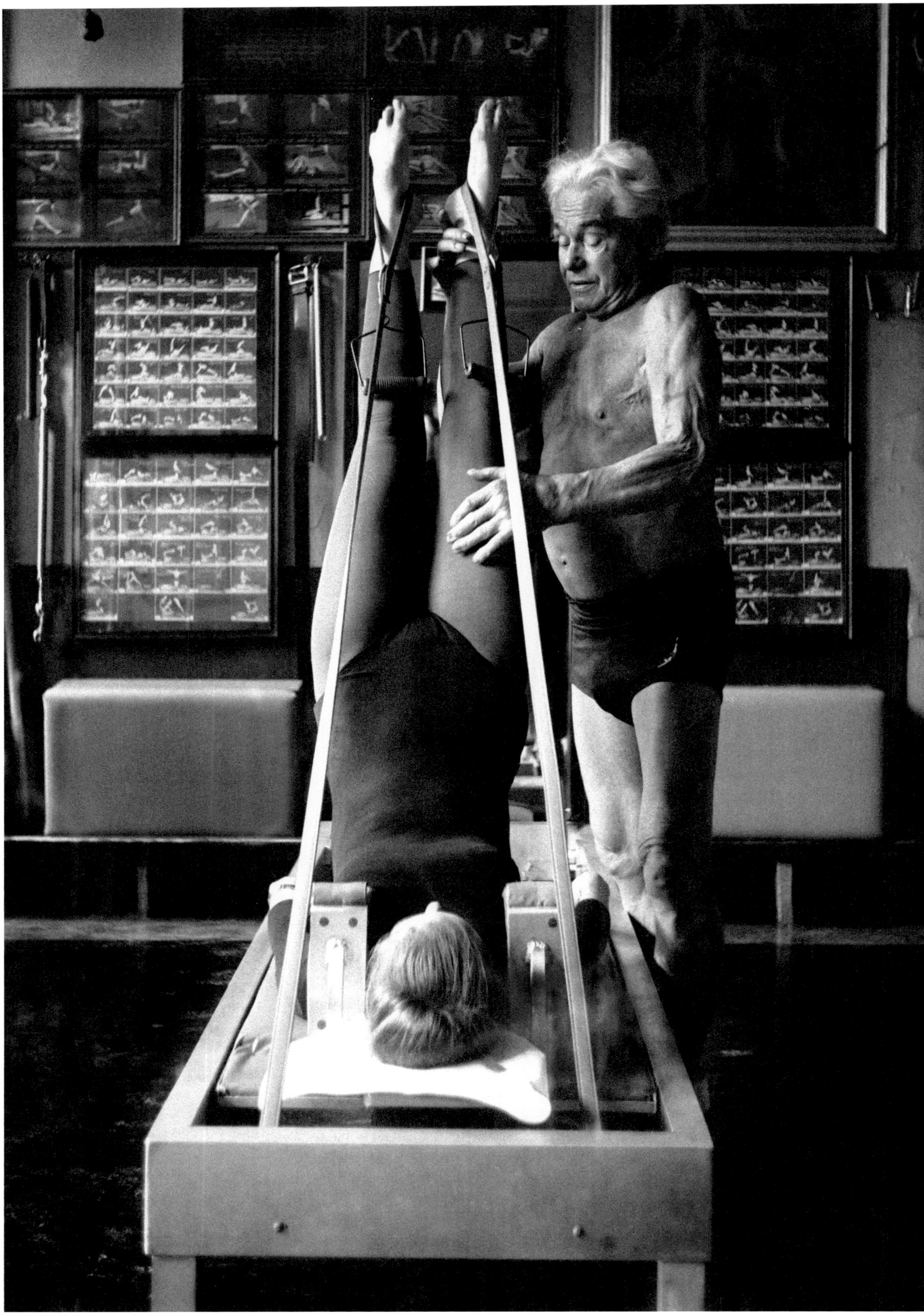

← Joseph Pilates instructing a client on the reformer. I. C. Rapoport, *Pilates Long Spine*, October 4, 1961.

→ The first Pilates studio in New York.

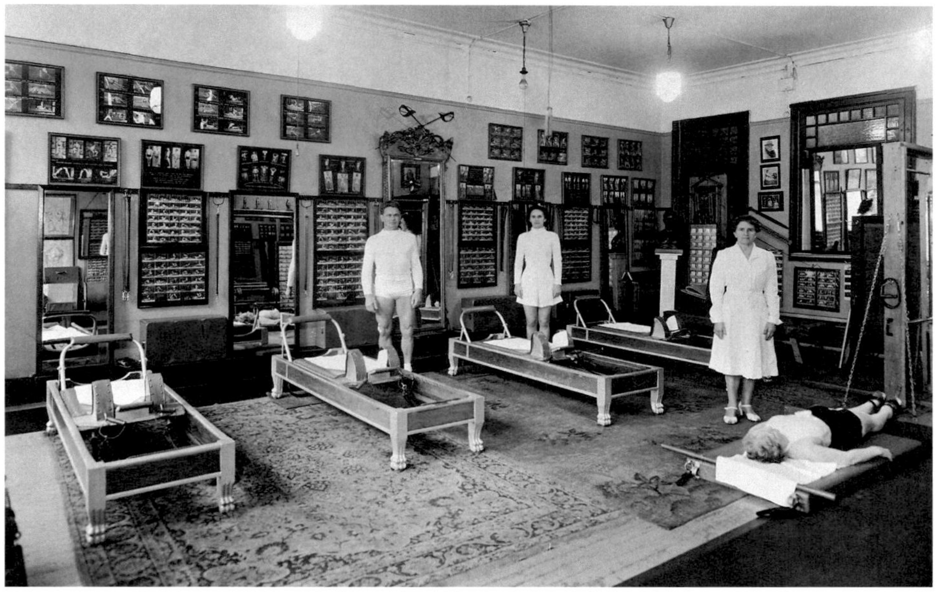

exercise and nature.[22] The free naked body in nature provided an idyllic counterimage to the hunched toiling of industrial work.

In 1924, Pilates filed German patent number 427,705 for the "Körperübungsgerät," a full-body "physical training device." Consisting of a small table with a wheeled platform on top that was moved via a system of ropes and pulleys, the apparatus could be "adjusted to different degrees of resistance to accommodate any type of person whether healthy or unwell, large or small." Similar to his "Foot Corrector," it relied on resistance to ensure the user was performing the exercise correctly.[23]

The large number of soldiers returning from war with missing limbs had resulted in an expansion of the medical field of orthopedics, and Pilates's new apparatus allowed him to partner with doctors in Hamburg for its use in rehabilitation. Pilates had first connected with Dr. Wilhelm Kotzenberg at the University Hospital in Hamburg Eppendorf over a mutual fascination with Sandow. Kotzenberg himself had developed a nonsurgical arm prosthesis inspired by the bodybuilder's ability to break a chain by flexing his upper-arm muscles. A shared obsession with strongmen and orthopedic inventions led Kotzenberg to open his roster of patients to Pilates, and the results of the full-body training apparatus received glowing recommendations:[24] Julius Philipp raved that he had "legs so crippled I could hardly take three steps with a cane. ... After three months of [Pilates's training method] ... I can walk 100 meters without assistance."[25]

Once Pilates had proved the efficacy of his training apparatus and methods, which he now called Contrology, he sought to expand his influence. He saw America as the perfect place to foster his entrepreneurship and immigrated to New York in 1926. That same year, he filed US patent 1,621,477 for the "Körperübungsgerät," which he called the "Reformer," and opened a studio at 939 Eighth Avenue in Manhattan with the help of his new wife and business partner Clara, whom he met on the journey from Germany. The location of this studio, between 55th and 56th Street, put him in proximity to the world of dance and performance. Pilates ended up drawing an important part of his clientele from Broadway. His influence in the world of dance was confirmed in 1929 when he successfully rehabilitated Ruth St. Denis, an icon of modern dance, from what she thought would be a career-ending knee injury.

Over the next several years he would invent more apparatuses for his growing clientele of dancers, performers, and society people. In 1930 Pilates designed two items—a chair, and a bed that also served as a couch—that adopted the generic language of domestic furniture and could double as such. He filed US patent 1,874,613A for the "Chair," which aimed to use his experience with springs to better support a relaxed seated posture. The chair employed a pivot as a tipping mechanism, so that when a person sat in the chair and leaned back, the back of the chair would adjust to the "body to assume a proper position necessary for complete relaxation and comfort."[26] A similar goal was implemented in his design of a V-shaped piece of furniture that served as either a bed or a couch, US patent 1,876,743, which he believed conformed better to the body and provided superior resting qualities.[27] In 1931, he reconfigured the chair and filed US patent 1,969,901A for the design of a more portable, apartment-friendly version that was dubbed the "Wunda Chair." Instead of functioning like traditional furniture, however, the Wunda Chair was also a device for exercise. It could be oriented on different sides to correspond with various exercises, and was light and portable enough to be carried outside for exercise *en plein air.*[28]

↓ US patent 1,621,477 for the Körperübungsgerät, now called the “Reformer,” filed by Joseph Pilates, 1926.

↓ US patent 1,874,613 for “Chair,” filed by Joseph Pilates, 1930.

↓ US patent 1,874,613 for “Chair,” filed by Joseph Pilates, 1930.

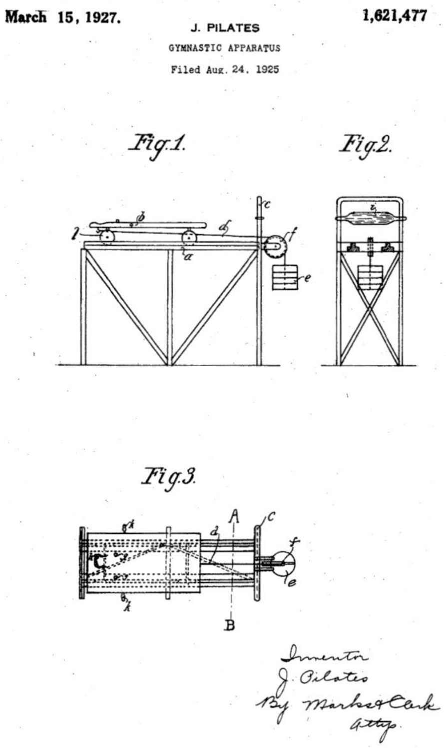

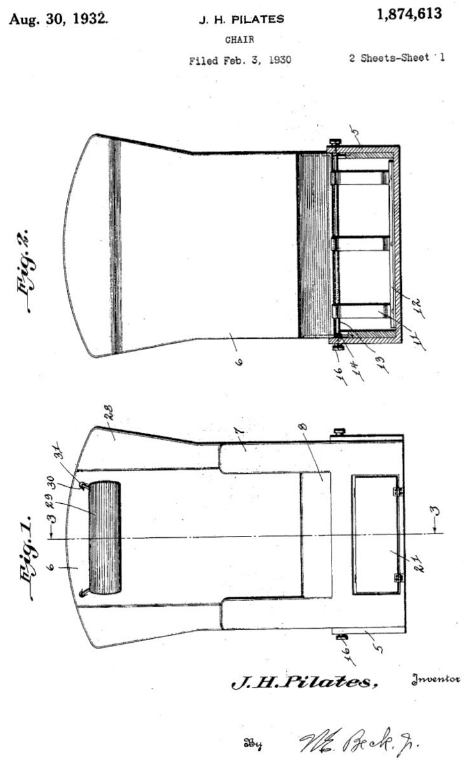

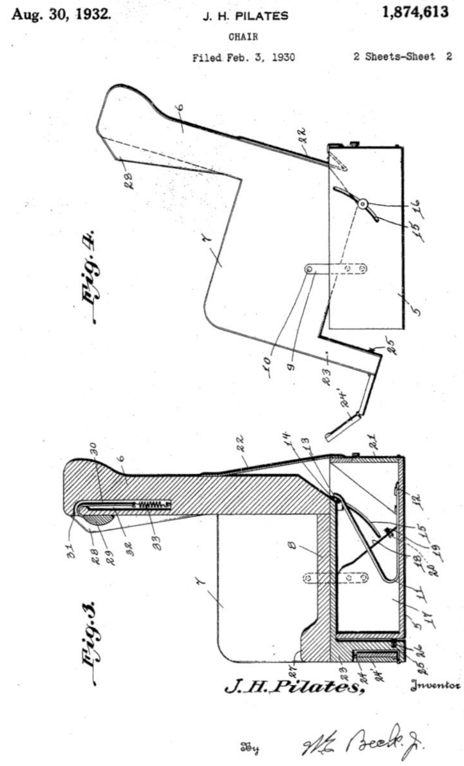

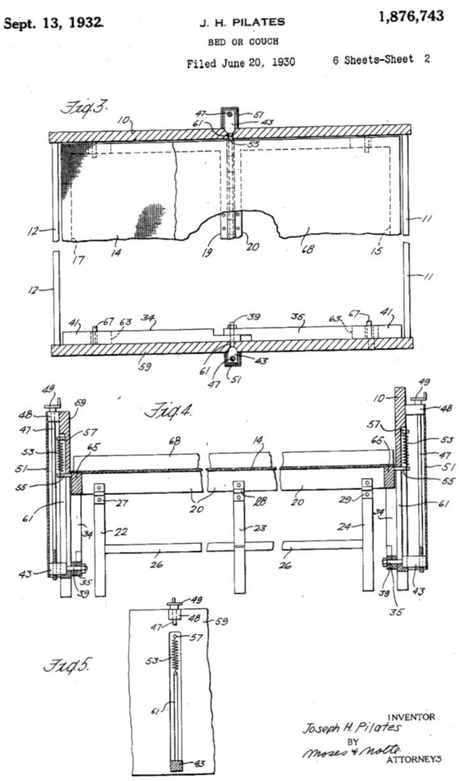

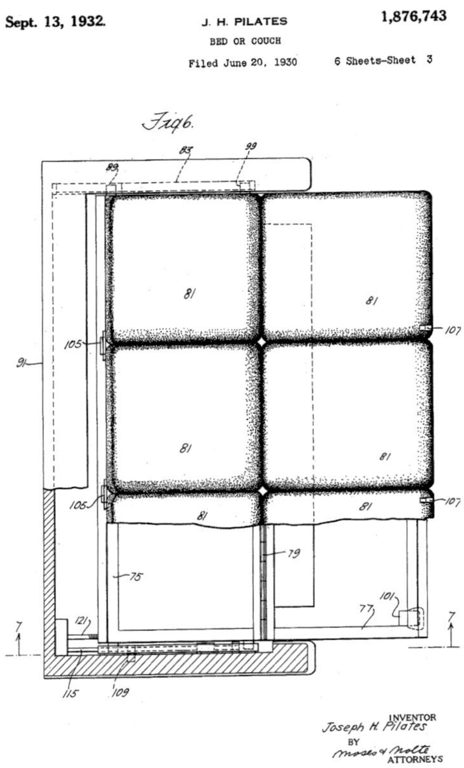

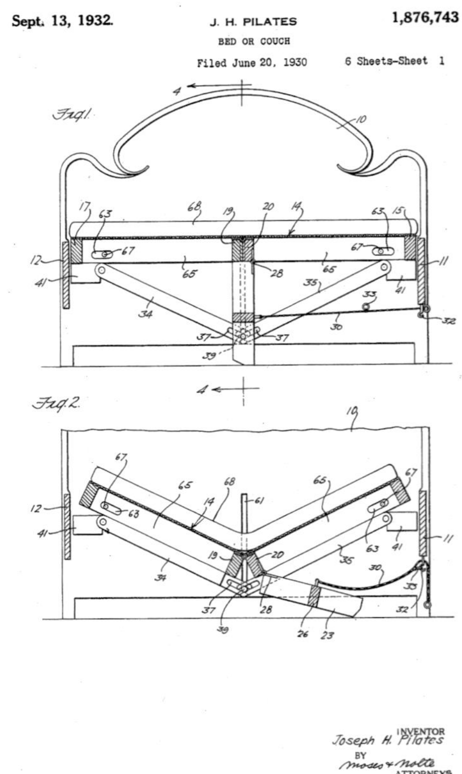

↗ US patent 1,876,743 for “Bed or Couch,” filed by Joseph Pilates, 1930.

↘ US patent 1,969,901 for "Chair," filed by Joseph Pilates, 1931.

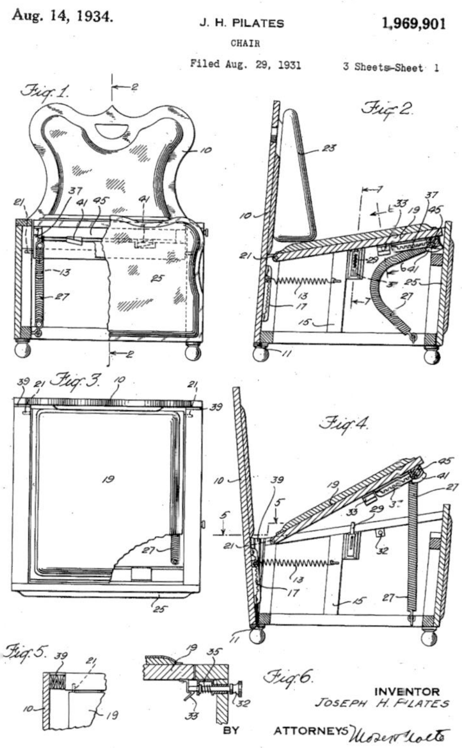

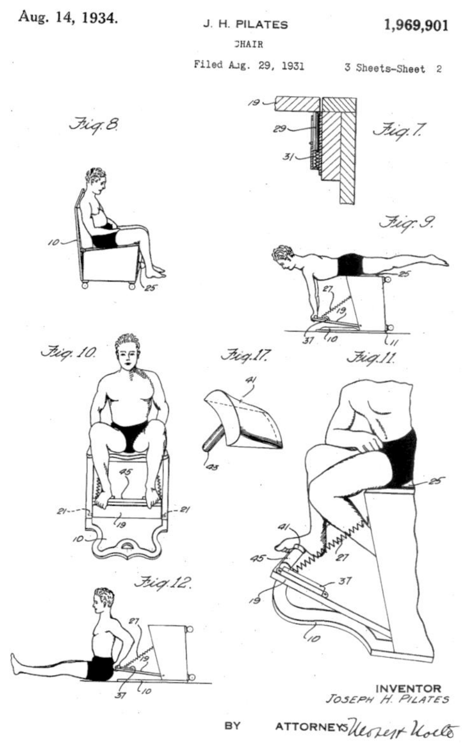

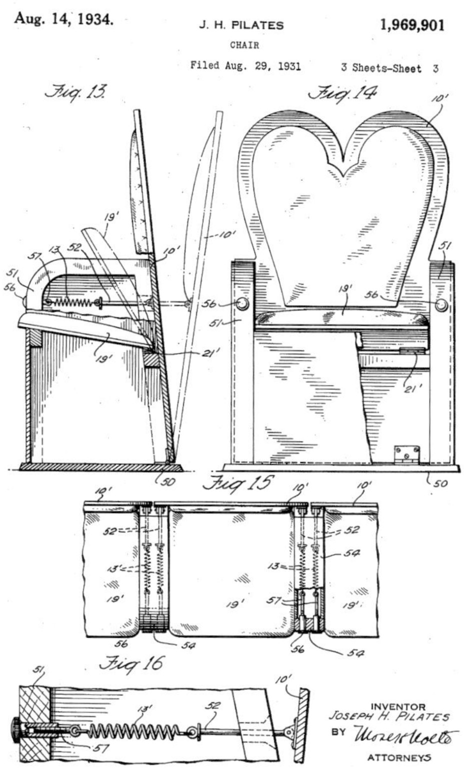

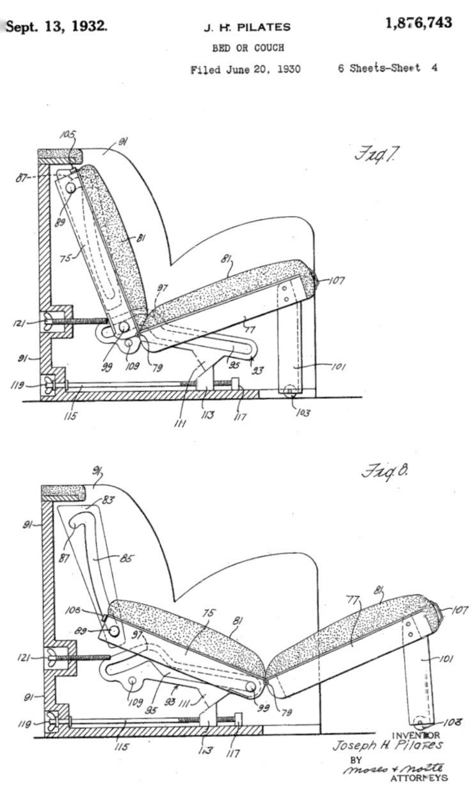

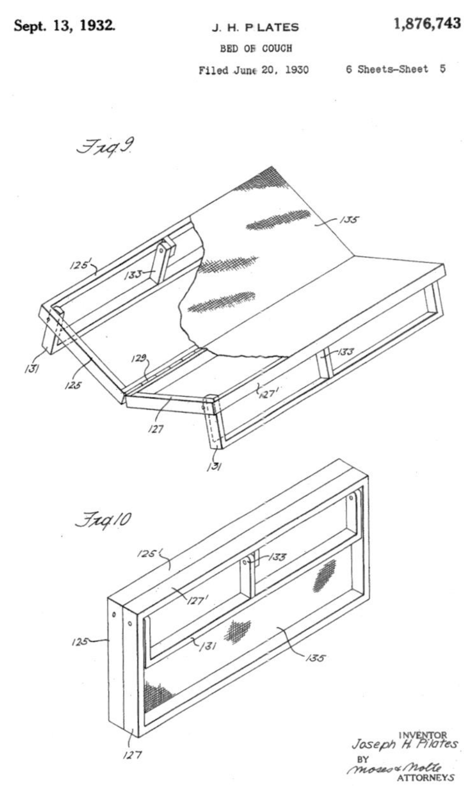

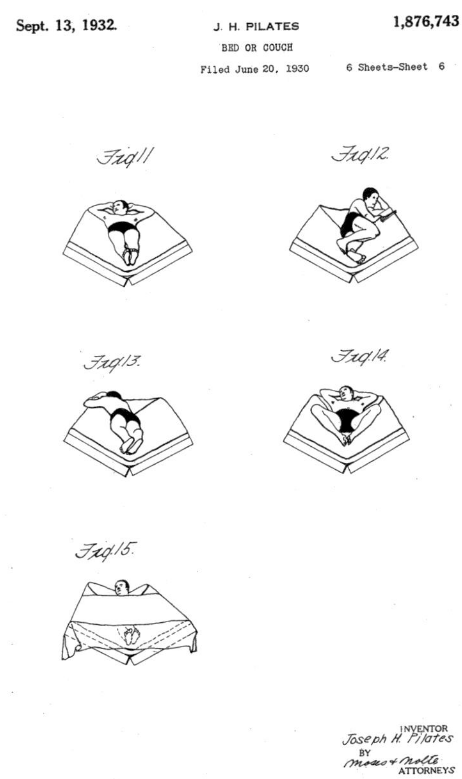

→ Exercises on the Pilates Reformer.

↑ Eve Gentry training with Joseph Pilates post-mastectomy, 1955.

↓ Joseph Pilates teaches Pedipole, 1955.

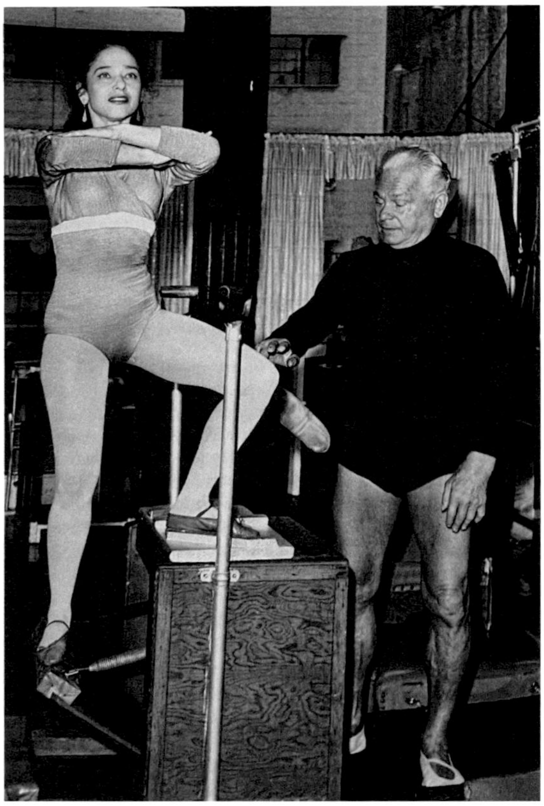

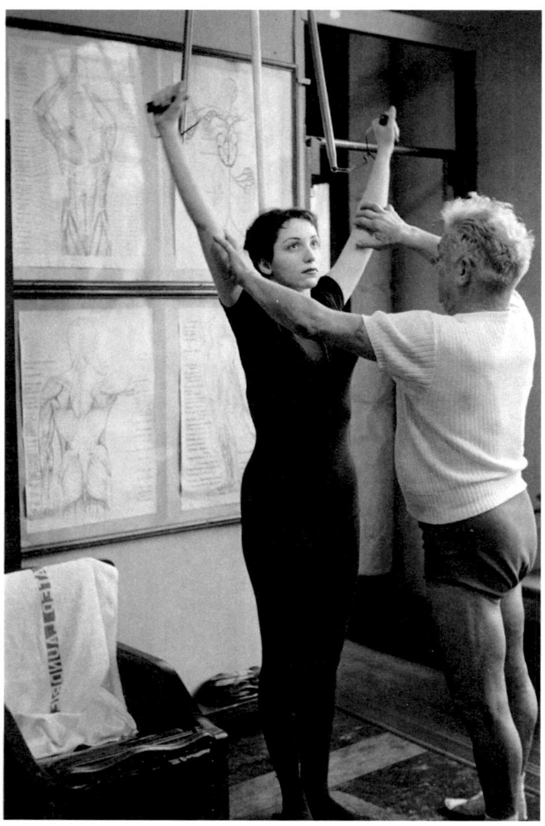

In 1955, Pilates had another breakthrough rehabilitation case with the invention of what he called the "Ped-a-Pull" apparatus. Although he did not file for a patent due to its similarity to other products, he was particularly proud of its results. The apparatus was made of "two long springs with leather loops at the end, which could either be mounted to a pole with a ground support or directly to the wall."[29] The device was inspired by an apparatus in Sandow's London gym for women and attained special significance after the dancer, and Pilates's longtime friend and client, Eve Gentry underwent a mastectomy to remove a lump in her breast. The surgery removed her entire breast as well as the pectoral muscles crucial for the mobility of her upper body. Gentry was "agitated, desperate, and almost hysterical" at the prospect of losing mobility, but Pilates created exercises with the Ped-a-Pull to strengthen the muscles around the excised pectorals, and after one year Gentry was able to move normally again.[30]

Inspired by her progress, Joseph and Clara Pilates with Eve and her husband Bruce Gentry eagerly filmed the training sessions and presented the footage to a group of physicians, hoping to get an endorsement and legitimization from doctors at Lenox Hill Hospital. Doctors were dubious of the results at first, so Pilates and team reshot the film, making Eve's mastectomy more obvious. Yet even after being convinced and impressed by Pilates's results, the physicians rejected an official partnership because his methods lacked scientific backing.

The unshakable core of Pilates' technique was his development of a system of corrective postures and apparatuses to support them. Although the postures generally stayed consistent, with room for adaptation to specific cases, the scope of "correction" was ever expanding. Rehabilitation was central to the development of Contrology, but its definition was malleable. As Pilates's clientele expanded, he expanded his explanation of the system's benefits. Rehabilitation was no longer just for a specific injury, illness, or disease; injury, or the deviation of the body from its natural movements, was now a condition of life. The need for rehabilitation was universal. In a 1934 profile in *Collier's* magazine, Pilates describes the value of his exercise methods over sports as follows:

> Sports are wonderful for the constitution generally, but they are of little value for correcting what's wrong with you—and there's something wrong with almost everyone. Corrective exercise is a nasty pill to most people, but it's the only way to build a beautiful, strong, youthful and one hundred percent healthy body.[31]

This diagnosis of a fundamental and universal sickness that required correcting was further elaborated in the 1945 book which summarized Pilates's life

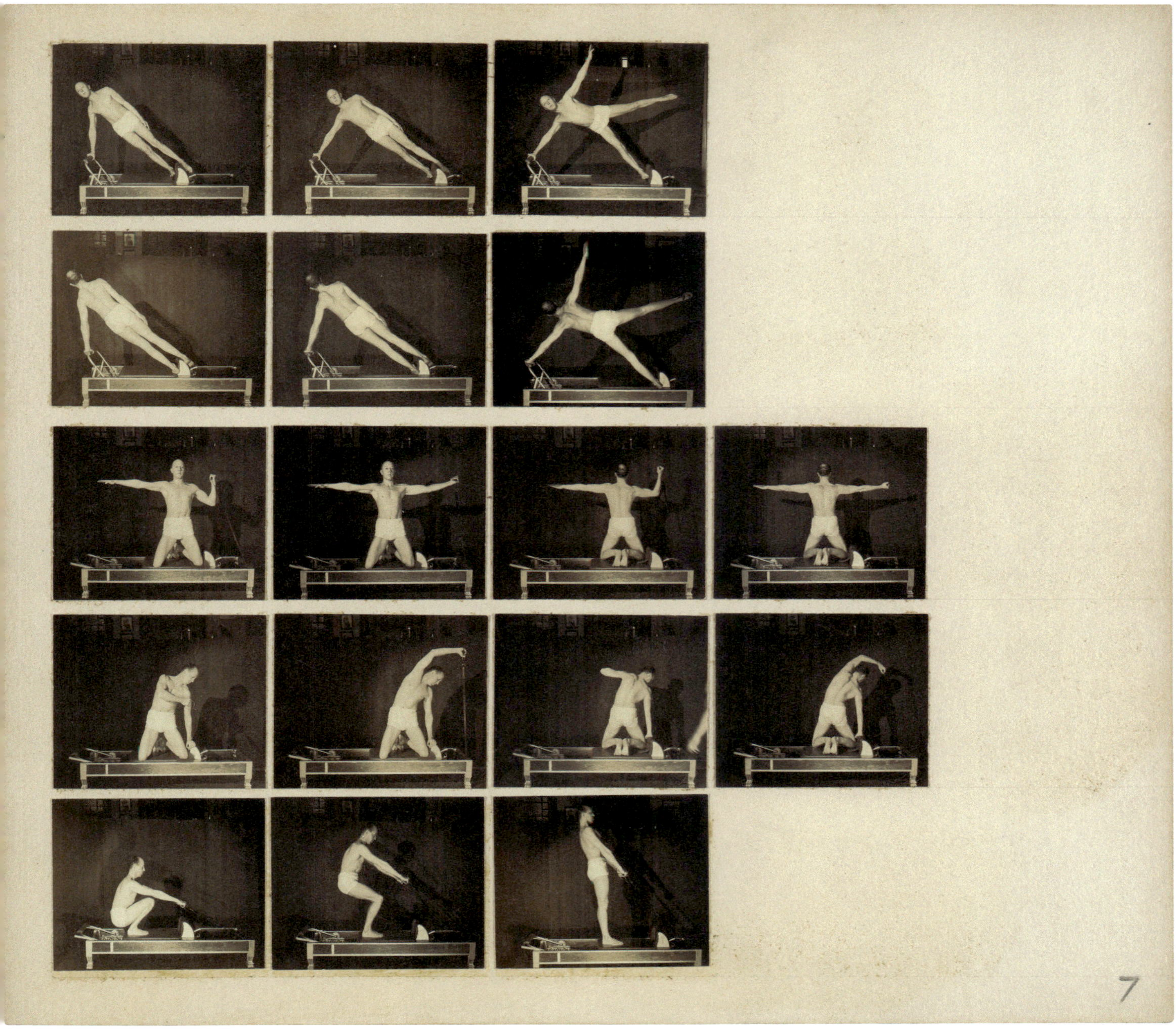

work, *Return to Your Life through Contrology*. Before demonstrating his postures in a series of photographs, Pilates and his coauthor (and client) William John Miller wrote extensively about Contrology as a cure for modernity:

> This very rapidly progressing world with its ever-increasing faster tempo of living demands that we be physically fit and alert in order that we may succeed in the unceasing race with keen competition which rewards the "go-getter" but by-passes the "no-getter." Physical fitness can neither be acquired by wishful thinking nor by outright purchase. However, it can be gained through performing the daily exercises conceived for this purpose by the founder of Contrology whose unique methods accomplish this desirable result by successfully counteracting the harmful inherent conditions associated with modern civilization. ... Even those of us who work in the city and are fortunate enough to live in the country must counteract the unnatural physical fatigue and mental strain experienced in our daily activities. Telephones, automobiles, and economic pressure all combine to create physical letdown and mental stress so great that today practically no home is entirely free from sufferers of some form of nervous tension.[32]

Return to Your Life through Contrology summarizes the appeal of Pilates as a project of both mental and physical health. Pilates's apparatuses were designed to make the exerciser think more deeply about what her body was doing and therefore emphasized the

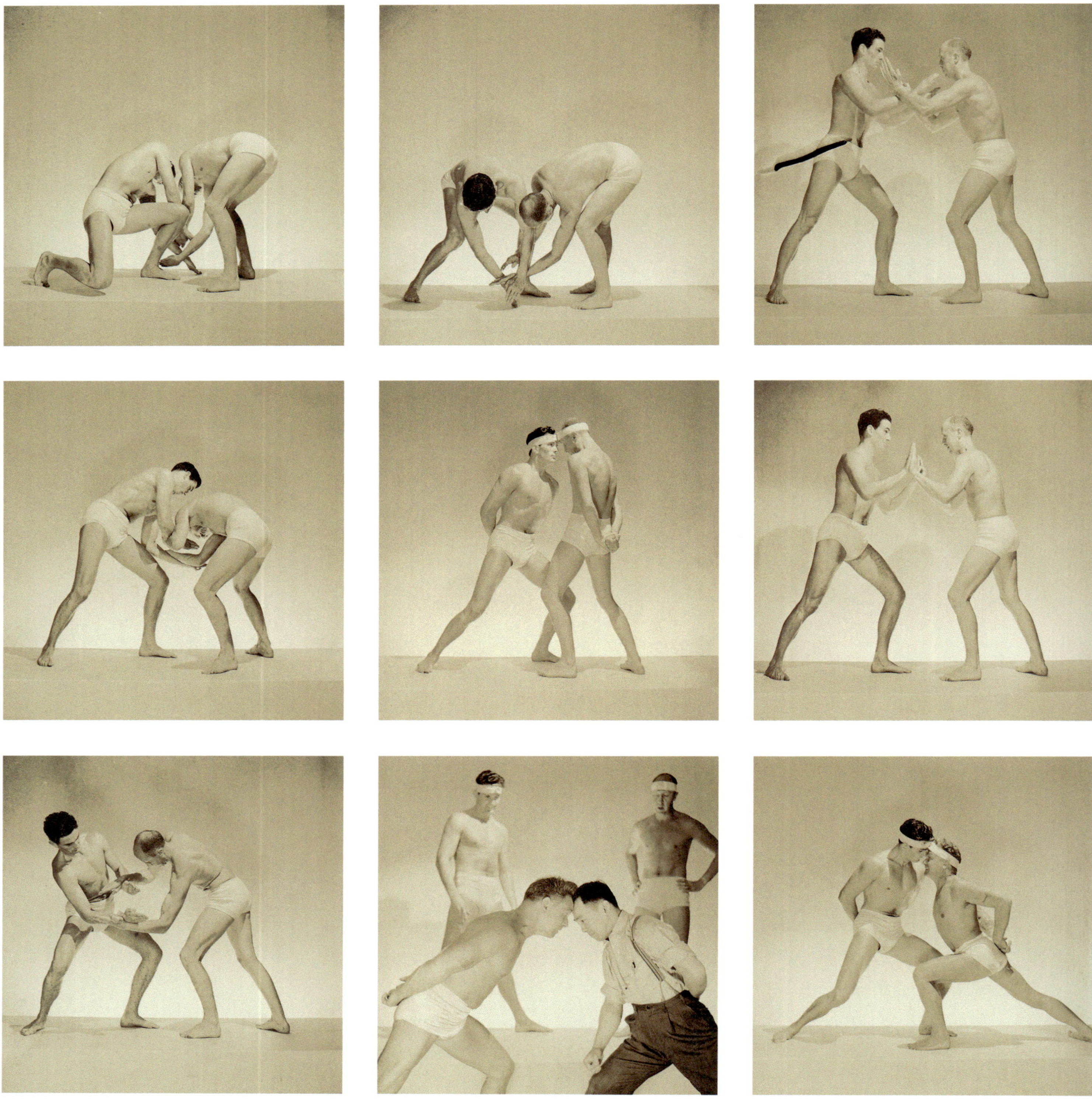

↑ Floor exercises.

use of mechanization as a bridge, rather than split, between human modes of thinking and feeling. Furthermore, Contrology exemplifies the ouroboros-like etiology of modern exercise: modernity—made evident by expanding industrialization and urbanization—was the illness, but it was also the cure. By harmonizing the body and mind through movement and breathing, Contrology could be a corrective for a world made dizzy by new technologies. At the same time, the body made technical through mechanized furniture that incorporated pulleys and cables into this corrective system of movement returned the body to its productive use and made it more capable of dealing with modern life.

An earlier version of this essay was originally published by e-flux Architecture in 2022.

1. Georg Simmel, "The Metropolis and Mental Life, 1903," in *On Individuality and Social Forms: Selected Writings* (Chicago: University of Chicago Press, 1971), 329.
2. Heikki Lempa, *Beyond the Gymnasium: Educating the Middle-Class Bodies in Classical Germany* (Lanham, MD: Lexington Books, 2007), 73.
3. Lempa, *Beyond the Gymnasium*, 76.
4. Lempa, *Beyond the Gymnasium*, 80.
5. Daniel Gottlieb Moritz Schreber, *Medical Indoor Gymnastics* (London: Williams & Northgate, 1899), vi, https://wellcomecollection.org/works/sydxrdff.
6. Schreber, *Medical Indoor Gymnastics*.
7. Lempa, *Beyond the Gymnasium*, 239.
8. He recounts the horrifying "so-called compression-of-the-chest-miracle, which I endured at least several dozen times; it consisted in the whole chest wall being compressed, so that the state of oppression caused by the lack of breath was transmitted to my whole body." Giorgina Samira Paiella, "Madness, Modernity, and Mechanization: Daniel Paul Schreber's Memoirs of My Nervous Illness, the Feminized Industrial Laborer, and the Rise of Automation," *Configurations* 28, no. 2 (2020): 264.
9. In this interpretation of Daniel Paul Schreber's condition, Moritz Schreber was "demonized as the sadistic paterfamilias whose pedagogic practices and orthopedic devices allegedly produced his son's psychotic predisposition." Eric Santner, *My Own Private Germany: Daniel Paul Schreber's Secret History of Modernity* (Princeton: Princeton University Press, 1996), 3.
10. Santner, *My Own Private Germany*.
11. Anson Rabinbach, *The Human Motor: Energy, Fatigue, and the Origins of Modernity* (New York: Basic Books, 1990), 38.
12. One doctor noted that neurasthenia was "even more a malady of civilization augmented in intensity as a result of the progress of the past century" and went on to explain how an increase in intellectual work resulted in an increase in intellectual exhaustion. Rabinbach, *The Human Motor*, 154.
13. Rabinbach, *The Human Motor*, 2–3.
14. Eva Rincke, *Joseph Pilates: A Biography*, ed. Nichole L'vov (Hightstown, NJ: Inner Strength Publishing, 2019), 33.
15. Rincke, *Joseph Pilates*, 33.
16. Rincke, *Joseph Pilates*, 37.
17. Rincke, *Joseph Pilates*, 44.
18. Rincke, *Joseph Pilates*, 46.
19. Rincke, *Joseph Pilates*, 47.
20. Rincke, *Joseph Pilates*, 54–55.
21. In German the device was called, "Vorrichtung zur Beseitigung oder Besserung von Bein- und Fussfehlern o.dgl." Pilates described the essence of the "Foot Corrector" as "the sliding pressure pad which is being moved by overcoming an elastic counter pressure. The shape of the pressure pad can be measured according to the kind of disease. It can be pressured down by guide rails or something of the kind and it is placed in the middle of a footrest plate." Rincke, *Joseph Pilates*, 65–66.
22. Rincke, *Joseph Pilates*, 71.
23. Rincke, *Joseph Pilates*, 72.
24. Kotzenberg wrote that Pilates's "methods are without a doubt excellent for the whole musculature ... particularly legs, back, stomach, lower extremities, hip accidents (hence) any sport. ... Especially advised instead of walking." Rincke, *Joseph Pilates*, 74.
25. Rincke, *Joseph Pilates*, 75.
26. Joseph H. Pilates, "Chair," United States US1874613A, filed February 3, 1930, and issued August 30, 1932, https://patents.google.com/patent/US1874613A/en?assignee=joseph+pilates&oq=joseph+pilates.
27. Joseph H. Pilates, "Bed or couch," United States US1876743A, filed June 20, 1930, and issued September 13, 1932, https://patents.google.com/patent/US1876743A/en?assignee=joseph+pilates&oq=joseph+pilates.
28. Joseph H. Pilates, "Chair," United States US1,969,901A, filed August 29, 1931, and issued August 14, 1934, https://patents.google.com/patent/US1969901A/en?assignee=joseph+pilates&oq=joseph+pilates. Rincke, *Joseph Pilates*, 101.
29. Rincke, *Joseph Pilates*, 151.
30. Rincke, *Joseph Pilates*, 151.
31. Quoted in Rincke, *Joseph Pilates*, 108.
32. Joseph H. Pilates and William John Miller, *Return to Life through Contrology* (New York: J. J. Augustin, 1945), 3–4.

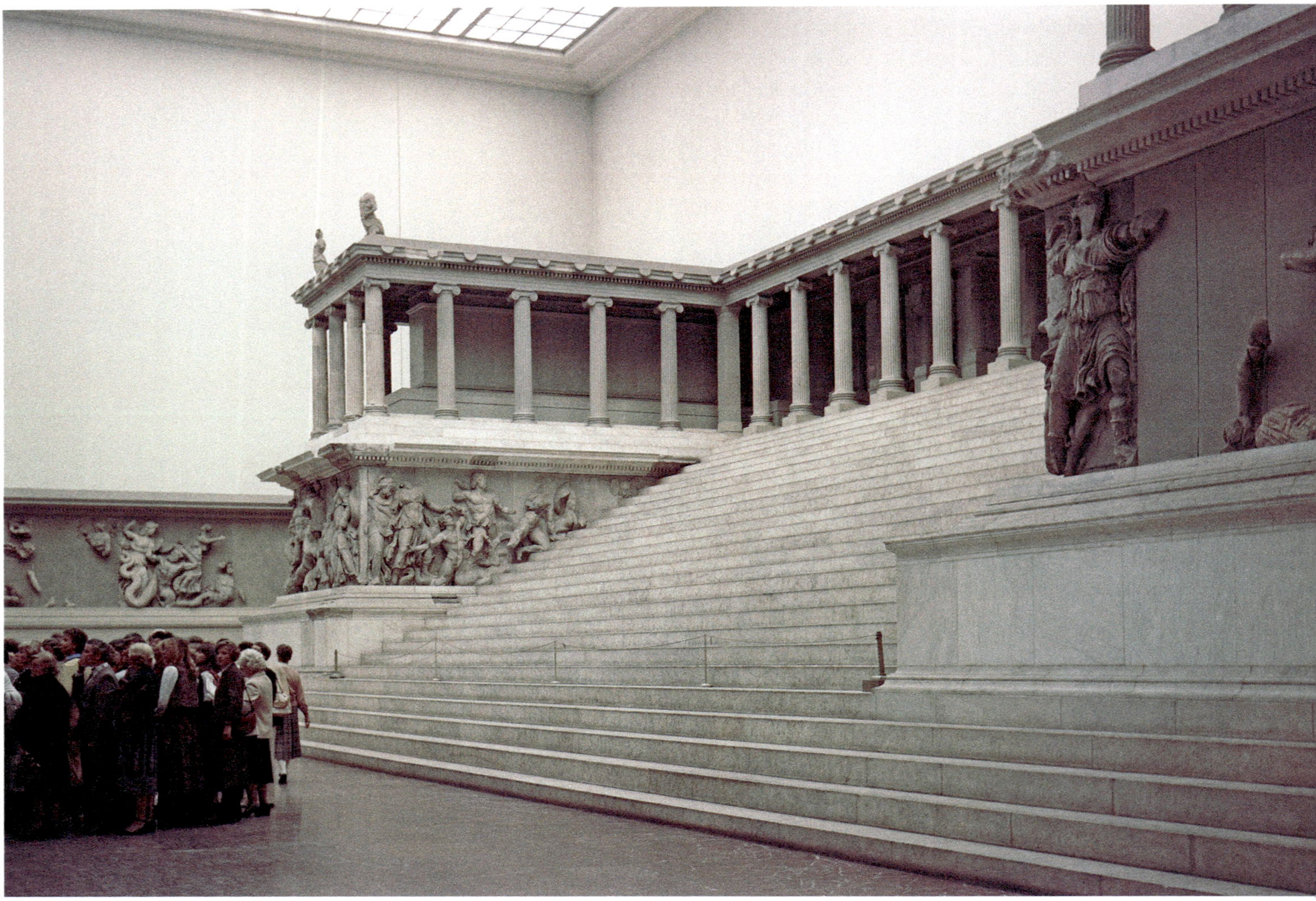

DISABLING FORM

DAVID GISSEN

↑ The Pergamon Altar, ca. 200–150 BCE. Pergamon Museum, Berlin, 35.64 × 33.4 m.

Discussions of architectural form demonstrate how disability is negatively imprinted into the field of architecture. In architectural theory and the history of architecture, "form" typically refers to the physical essence and shape of a work of architecture. In the modern idea of form, it is a quality that arises from the activity of design and in ways that can be transmitted into the perceptions of a beholder of architecture. Form provides a link between an architect's physical creations and the aesthetic reception of these works. It occupies a central place within a general understanding of architecture: the idea of the architect as "form-giver," among many other turns of phrase, conveys the sense of some fundamental activity and aesthetic role of form within architecture, what architects create, and how people perceive works of architecture.

Recent writing on the topic of disability and architectural form focuses on the manner in which a building becomes alienating to disabled people by aestheticizing its inaccessibility. Critics of Thomas Heatherwick's Vessel building in New York or the Hunters Point Library by Steven Holl Architects disparage these works because they express their inaccessible elements (in both cases, stairs) as central aspects of their formal meaning.[1] By contrast, proponents of disability rights in architecture laud buildings such as the Ed Roberts Campus in Berkeley by Leddy Maytum Stacy Architects, or OMA's Maison à Bordeaux.[2] These buildings aestheticize tools of disabled access into powerful visual statements.

As examples they suggest that form has self-evident qualities and relationships to disabled people. Presumably, Vessel is alienating to someone like me, an amputee, because its form consists of interconnected and monumental staircases, while the Ed Roberts Campus affirms disabled experiences because its atrium contains a visually powerful tool and symbol of architectural accessibility: an enormous red ramp. This way of thinking about form and impairment can be compared to late nineteenth- and early twentieth-century writings on the aesthetics of form. These writings demonstrate how the concept of form contains more invidious ideas about human capacities and their relationship to architecture—ones that cannot be addressed through the concept of accessibility alone.

Bodies of Form

The modern aesthetics of architectural form begins with the writing of the Swiss art historian Heinrich Wölfflin. In the late nineteenth century, Wölfflin concocted a concept of form tied to an anthropomorphic referent but in a way distinct from earlier classical paradigms. In classical aesthetics, abstract human physical ideals such as the symmetry and geometry of the "Vitruvian" man guided the physical properties of architectural beauty. By contrast, Wölfflin argued that the "form" of architecture is an experiential sensation that emerges from the "empathy" that arises between the body and mind of an individual and that person's perception of a building. The kernel of this concept regards the way knowledge of one's own body becomes projected onto the particular expressive, psychological, and aesthetic power of architecture. For Wölfflin, such knowledge was attained in a totally physical and psychological manner.[3] He argued that because human beings must resist the effects of gravity to rise onto their own feet, they understand the same operative forces of resistance that keep a building from falling. This is the essential quality of "form" that can be perceived by a beholder and manipulated by an architect to some aesthetic effect: the building that rises, or resists gravity in an appealing manner—as in the "springing" stones of an arched space, or the "swelling" entasis of a column—does so because it causes a sensation within the observer. Put differently, one of the ways that matter—such as stone—is given expressive life in architecture is through the design and experience of its "form." A person's ability to rise and stand gives the body form analogously.[4]

Wölfflin's aesthetic ideas were foundational to the practice and teaching of art history, and they entered into concepts about the education of architects in numerous ways that continue to this day. His idea of empathy and physiological resonance provided a framework and language through which to interpret the architectural past. In his own discussion of Gothic ecclesiastical architecture, he described how the "body" of a Gothic building "stiffens and pulls itself together."[5] By comparison, baroque architecture "swells" in a "muscular" and "open" manner. The aesthetic differences in architecture across history become differences in physical moods and comportment.

Those educated in the United States in the latter half of the twentieth century were often exposed to this way of thinking about architecture, even if the particular concepts and theories behind it were little discussed. In architectural history classes, for example, professors spoke about form in lecture halls while standing beneath large projected images of buildings. One of the more celebrated architectural historians in the United States, Vincent Scully, described buildings to his students through a language of physiology while enacting various physical movements: works of architecture "stood" and "extended" into a surrounding space; they "looked"—out or down—onto landscapes; vast interiors "expanded" like the chest of someone breathing; columns were "planted" like a foot into the ground.[6] This way of understanding, seeing, and interpreting architecture also affected (and continues to affect) how students imagine experiencing buildings outside lecture halls and classrooms. One experiences the "rising" of a cathedral interior, the "leaping" components in a Renaissance facade, the "springing" of a floor or step underfoot as one climbs the stairs of a building.

The animated and physiological language of formalism has also dominated discussions of student and professional design work in the United States.[7] Within a formalist vocabulary, the designer of a building expands and contracts space, manipulating the building's mass and weight; their work could be animated with life, or held down by a sense of heaviness. Wölfflinian concepts of architecture encourage physicality as central to the activity of design not just in metaphoric ways, but also more directly. When I was a graduate student at Columbia University, for instance, a professor would have us pin to the wall pieces of drawing paper as wide as each of us could reach with both hands extended. Then, standing with our papers attached to the wall in front of us and pieces of charcoal in our hands, we were encouraged to express our bodies into drawings of imagined architectural spaces.[8]

In addition to such expressive exercises, the tools of design—formal analysis, abstracted diagrams, figure/ground drawings, and so on—drew out the shapes and interactions of architectural works. The physical way of thinking about design has not disappeared with the use of digital tools. A visitor to any architecture school in the United States today is likely to encounter people who use physiological language about form, although the words have changed. Today, one hears about "posture," "slouching" form, or the "fat folds" of a student's architectural design. The type of physicality, but also aesthetic judgment of bodies and their character—inherent in a Wölfflinian idea of aesthetic experience and history—permeate the work of apprehending and designing architecture.

The Aberrations of Form

If the forms of architecture were experienced, narrated, and designed through processes of physiological empathy, then Wölfflin and his followers also accounted for the manner in which a range of human physiological factors might be projected into architectural aesthetic experiences. In his first writings on empathy, Wölfflin discussed the way that formal symmetries and tensions within architecture recall physical normality, differentiation, and disfigurement of the human body.[9] The empathy one feels and that enables one to sense and appreciate architectural form extends from the gravitational forces acting

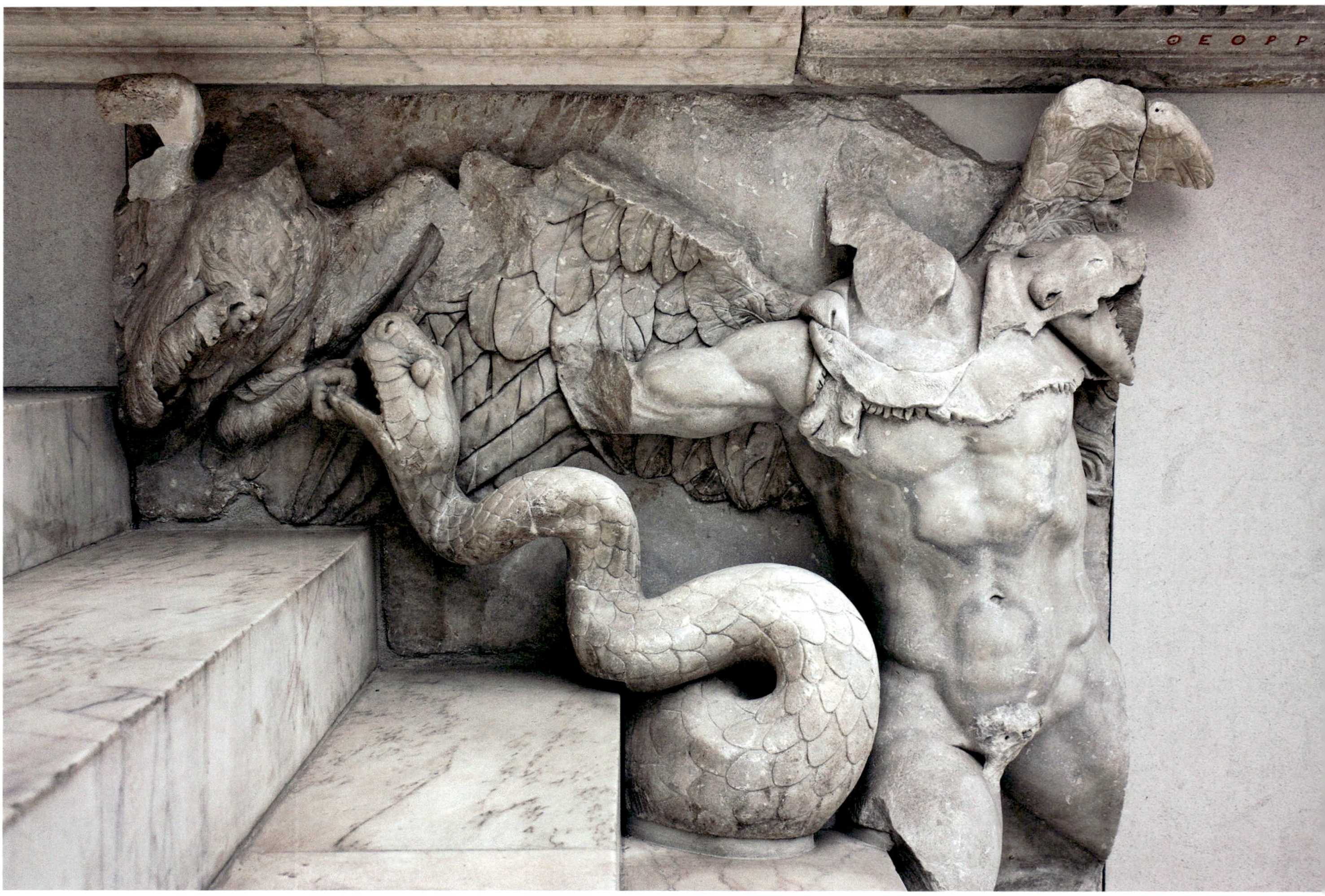

↑ The eagle of Zeus battles a snake and a giant on the west frieze of the Great Altar of Pergamon.

on both buildings and human beings to the corporeal makeup of individual human bodies. For example, Wölfflin argued that slender people tend to prefer buildings with slender proportions, while stocky people are drawn to buildings with greater mass.

His discussion of the corporeality of architecture also extended to physiognomic concepts—in which one sees features of human faces within built forms, such as the windows and doorway of a house.[10] Wölfflin argued that the appeal of architectural symmetry is due to the inherent symmetrical structure of the beholder, who "expect[s] to find symmetry in every structural body." He speculated that deviations from symmetry in architecture create unease because they evoke disfigurements of the human body—such as amputations and "mutilated" limbs. Wölfflin's language of empathy, with its roots in medical science, was entangled with ideas regarding normativity and deviance.[11]

The resonances between physical aberrations and architectural aesthetics were also explored in provocative thought experiments by Wölfflin's contemporary Adolf Göller. In examining his own concept of resonance, Göller argued that human physicality is elaborately and mechanically entangled with aesthetic perceptions. To emphasize this, he turned to an elaborate (and overwrought) thought experiment in which he imagined beings with fantastical physiologies that would engender entirely unique aesthetic sensibilities. For example, he wondered if creators and beholders of artistic works with "the legs of a stork" or abnormally "long forearms" would create works that resonated with their physical perceptions and physiology. In turn, these characteristics would be appreciated by similarly endowed beholders, because they would see their bodies projected into the artistic world.[12] Beauty is ultimately a type of innate knowledge of the physique carried by the beholder.

What was a thought experiment for Göller evolved into far more controversial aesthetic theories linking physical aberrance, environment, and race to the visual quality of art and architecture. The belief that human beings have different physicalities related to racial difference and tied to geography and environment inspired a racialized concept of architectural aesthetics. Wölfflin himself provided a pathway into this way of thinking within his earliest writings on architectural aesthetics. For example, he argued that the decorative features of North African ornamentation reflect the "hot-blooded breath" of their makers. Rhetorically, he used language that blurred the line between anthropomorphic and architectural description. He wrote about the Gothic "pointed nose" and "broad forehead" evident in cathedrals, further blurring the description between a person and building. His concepts regarding the physiological transference of human experience—and dress—and its connection to architectural aesthetics would inevitably be connected to art histories with a more overt racialist direction.[13]

One of the more infamous proponents of this type of writing was the German architect and art critic Paul Schultze-Naumburg. His 1928 book *Kunst und Rasse* (*Art and Race*) explored how the aesthetic sensibilities of a work are ultimately the product of the mentality and physicality of its maker.[14] For Schultze-Naumburg, biology, mentality, climate, environment, and personhood combined to create an advantageous or disadvantageous aesthetic culture. In a comparison of farmhouses in the German countryside, he extended Wölfflin's ideas into physiognomic interpretations of the buildings' formal composition. One farmhouse that appeared to have been built all at once by one builder and well integrated into its surroundings was judged to be the product of a single and good race. Another farmhouse that appeared more modern, more ad hoc, and was inspired by Mediterranean architecture was said to be lacking in "noble physique."[15] In his writing, Schultze-Naumburg gave Wölfflinian ideas of empathy an extraordinary role: modernist art and architectural forms became the expressions of the "degeneracy" of their makers—what he referred to generally as "human mush," and more specifically as "the downfallen, the sick, and the physically deformed."[16] More disturbing, Schultze-Naumburg ended his book with a call to eliminate from a transforming and threatened Germanic culture all those "devoid of physiognomy" and "incapable of giving shape."[17]

Disability against Form

Architectural forms can evoke ideas about capacity, disfigurement, and impairment, but the idea of architectural form itself was also defined in opposition to disability. This feature, central to a Wölfflinian aesthetics, remains largely unexplored. The idea of form relies on the potential human physiological and psychic resonance and tension that exists between a work of architecture and its beholder. "Form" describes more than a building's shape or any essential architectural quality. Form is an aesthetic concept—an experience and relationship—inspired by psychology and physiology, regarding how human beings relate to architecture and art. For Wölfflin, architectural form draws its experiential power from human beings' understanding that they also have physical capacities—in this case, giving life to their bones and flesh by standing and moving. Form is basically matter that has come alive and is "formed" into some figure.

In addition to this way of equating form with a type of physical capacity, Wölfflin hypothesized an opposite to form, which he called "formlessness" (in German, *Formlos*).[18] This physical state of being without form is not the same as simply lacking physical definition. Formlessness is analogous to incapacity. Wölfflin argued that it is a quality of being physically unanimated and/or exhausted of energy. He described it as the depletion of the human body's "vital energy," "irregular" breath and "wheezing," as well as an "imbalance" that potentially "collapses" the body into a state of "depressed" "formlessness."[19] Formlessness, in Wölfflin's logic, is an affliction of musculature, lungs, and artifacts.

Since Wölfflin, "formlessness" has gained additional meanings within fine arts and architectural aesthetics. Schultze-Naumburg, Georges Bataille, Rosalind Krauss, and Yve-Alain Bois have used the term in their aesthetic theories.[20] Wölfflin's concept of formlessness relates to these more contemporary usages, but it is ultimately more physiological: formlessness is essentially a type of exhaustion that keeps figures from rising. In Wölfflin's language, a person rendered formless is a person attempting but unable to give their body individuality and life. Formless architecture is architecture unanimated with this will and desire to confront gravity. For Wölfflin, formlessness is matter without the qualities of life, and thus without aesthetically desirable quality.

From Wölfflin on, the idea of form and its perception has involved a type of collective visual, physical, and mobile means of comprehension that brings vitality into human beings and inanimate artifacts. The language of formalism affirms these qualities of human life and aesthetics: buildings rise and ascend into space; they breathe with life; they twist and flex with physical forces; they stand firm against their surroundings. Statements such as these illustrate the language of any number of architects today who represent a diverse range of approaches and aesthetic beliefs. Curiously, such architects likely concentrate more on the differences among themselves than on their shared embrace of what I would call an "aesthetics of capacitation." In Wölfflin's logic, an incapacitated ("formless") person is not only a person who lacks form in their own body, but also a person lacking in capacities to create and experience form. Thus, formlessness is a potential quality of both sickened and weakened artifacts and comparatively sick and weak methods of aesthetic production and apprehension. For Wölfflin, all of this is cause for despair, because form is presumably an immensely desirable and enviable way of experiencing humanness through artifacts.

Wölfflin's concepts of form haunt discussions of architectural aesthetics. Many architects and authors writing about disability and the experience of architecture sense the tensions within formalist aesthetics, even if the theory behind form is less analyzed in their work. Disability activists call on architects to make formal aspects of architecture more relatable or accessible, or to make accessible elements more robust and formal. Such work transforms accessibility strategies such as ramps and elevators into striking sculptural elements. But this simply provides access to the experience, and therefore the concept, of architectural form. By contrast, a disability critique of formalism would extend beyond questions of access to the sculptural power of accessible forms. A disability critique of formalism would question the values instilled into the concept of form itself as a type of experience.

I want to embrace formlessness as a quality opposed to the physical power of form, but I have no idea what formlessness looks like, formally, nor do I think that it is an important speculation. More significant than its appearance, the presumably pejorative aesthetic experience that is tied to impairment opens a consideration of disabled ways of interpreting and creating aesthetic knowledge. This includes understanding how experiences of impairment have been conceptualized into architectural theory, sensing and working with architecture that embraces relatively "weak" methods of apprehension and production, and establishing an idea of architectural apprehension that devalorizes physical athleticism. All of this can open the study and practice of architecture to those of us alienated by the discipline's disparaging engagements with human weakness and incapacity.

Ultimately, these pursuits offer an alternative architectural aesthetics informed by impairment that extends past explorations of how form monumentalizes disabled access or represents disfigurement as formal aberrance, or any other representation of formalist impairment. They also challenge many of the qualities theorized as central to architectural aesthetics: an expressive overcoming of gravity and physical force, optical and mobile perception, and the kinesthetic production of architectural ideas and spaces. In total, this rethinking of form—rooted in impairment, describing both the weakness of form and the weakness of apprehension—offers a critique of form, for formalism embraces a narrow concept of humanness.

1. Critiques of the Vessel and Queens Library can be found in Kevin Gotkin, "Stair Worship," *Avery Review*, 2018, https://www.averyreview.com/issues/33/stair-worship; Sharon Otterman, "New Library Is a $41.5 Million Masterpiece. But about Those Stairs," *New York Times*, November 5, 2019.
2. On discussions of the Ed Roberts Campus, see Aimi Hamraie, *Building Access: Universal Design and the Politics of Accessibility* (Minneapolis: University of Minnesota Press, 2017); and on the Maison à Bordeaux, see Jos Boys, *Doing Disability Differently: An Alternative Handbook on Architecture* (London: Routledge, 2014).
3. Heinrich Wölfflin, "Prolegomena to a Psychology of Architecture," in *Empathy, Form, and Space: Problems in German Aesthetics*, ed. Harry Francis Mallgrave and Eleftherios Ikonomou (Los Angeles: Getty Center Papers, 1993), 149–192. The writing on Wölfflin's concepts of form, empathy, and style is vast. Good entry points on the emergence of these ideas within Wölfflin's thinking are Mallgrave and Ikonomou, *Empathy, Form and Space*; Alina Payne, "Portable Ruins: The Pergamon Altar, Heinrich Wölfflin, and German Art History at the Fin de Siècle," *RES: Anthropology and Aesthetics* 53, no. 1 (2008): 168–189; Alina Payne, "Wölfflin, Architecture and the Problem of Stilwandlung," *Journal of Art Historiography*, no. 7 (December 2012); and Zeynep Çelik Alexander, *Kinaesthetic Knowing: Aesthetics, Epistemology, Modern Design* (Chicago: University of Chicago Press, 2017). For an exploration of Wölfflin's idea of "vitality," see Vlad Ionescu, "Architectural Symbolism: Body and Space in Heinrich Wölfflin and Wilhelm Worringer," *Architectural Histories* 4, no. 1 (2016). Wölfflin discounted earlier aesthetics as limited to a "reckoning by the eye" and argued that aesthetic sensibilities involve a total psychological and physiological form of perception related to people's senses of their own bodies. Interestingly, he also used the example of blindness to elaborate on his point. Wölfflin, "Prolegomena," 155.
4. Wölfflin, "Prolegomena," 159–160.
5. Wölfflin, "Prolegomena," 183.
6. On the influence of Wölfflin in the work of postwar formalists such as Rowe, see Anthony Vidler, *Histories of the Immediate Present* (Cambridge, MA: MIT Press, 2011), 61–63. See also Mark Jarzombek, "De-scribing the Language of Looking: Wölfflin and the History of Aesthetic Experientialism," *Assemblage*, no. 23 (1994): 29–69.
7. This section on pedagogy is directly inspired by Zeynep Çelik Alexander's work. See Alexander, *Kinaesthetic Knowing*.
8. As someone who had only recently learned how to walk and stand on an artificial limb that extended up to my hip, I found this activity absurd at best.
9. "The effect of asymmetry, as has already been noted in passing, makes the relation clear: it gives us physical discomfort. This is because, in our anthropomorphic perception of the object, we identify with it just as if the symmetry of our own body were disturbed or a limb were mutilated." Wölfflin, "Prolegomena," 164.
10. "Even if a house has little resemblance with the human figure, we recognize in the windows organs which resemble our eyes. ... The part above the windows becomes a forehead. ... If the windows are shaded by a projecting cornice, we gain the impression that the eyebrows are knitted to form a protective roof over the eyes." Wölfflin, quoted in Daniela Bohde, "The Physiognomics of Architecture: Heinrich Wölfflin, Hans Sedlmayr, and Paul Schultze-Naumburg," in *German Art History and Scientific Thought: Beyond Formalism*, ed. Daniel Adler and Mitchell Frank (London: Routledge, 2012), 126.
11. Wölfflin, "Prolegomena," 164.
12. Mallgrave and Ikonomou, introduction to *Empathy, Form, and Space*, 53.
13. The key essay on race in architectural aesthetic theory is Irene Cheng, "Structural Racialism in Architecture," in *Race in Modern Architecture*, ed. Irene Cheng, Charles Davis, and Mabel Wilson (Pittsburgh: University of Pittsburgh Press, 2020), 134–152.
14. Schultze-Naumburg wrote: "To this end, it will be initially demonstrated how the relation between the physicality of the artist and his work is one of inextricable dependence, and how impossible it is for him to surpass the conditions of his own corporeality. A recognition, however, of this close relation simultaneously establishes the contrary procedure, which allows us to draw inferences from the artwork (or the judgment of such) to the artist (or the one making the judgment). Thus is it possible to gain information about the racial basis of the population not only from works of the past; rather in regard to the present, too, it is possible to arrive at interpretations of artistic products which explain certain things that would otherwise remain enigmatic." Paul Schultze-Naumburg, *Kunst und Rasse* (Munich: J. F. Lehmans Verlag, 1928), excerpted as *Art and Race* in *The Weimar Republic Sourcebook*, ed. Anton Kaes, Martin Jay, and Edward Dimendberg (Berkeley: University of California Press, 1994), 496.
15. Schultze-Naumburg wrote: "Houses have faces like human beings and they exhibit a certain expression by which one can recognize them and infer their inner state, provided one is able to understand the clear language of physiognomy, at least to a degree. On the basis of the expression of the two houses juxtaposed ... it is not difficult to imagine the person which corresponds to the buildings. The image at the top seems to bear the features which are to be expected in the face of a down-to-earth, loyal and friendly farmer of good race. ... The house at the bottom ... has no expression at all. Its face is swollen and, in its sheer dullness, it is vividly reminiscent of the human mush which has spread through the land and which has neither a clear face nor a noble physique." Quoted in Bohde, "Physiognomics of Architecture," 126. See also Paul Schultze-Naumburg, "Die Physiognomie der Industriearchitektur," *Die Umschau: Illustrierte Wochenschrift über die Fortschritte in Wissenschaft und Technik* 27 (1923): 673–678; Paul Schultze-Naumburg, *Das Gesicht des deutschen Hauses* (Munich: Callwey, 1929). Both of the latter works are cited in Bohde, "Physiognomics of Architecture."
16. Schultze-Naumburg, *Art and Race*, 498.
17. Schultze-Naumburg, quoted in Bohde, "Physiognomics of Architecture," 126. The scholar of disability Tobin Siebers has written on Schultze-Naumburg's theories of art in *Disability Aesthetics* (Ann Arbor: University of Michigan Press, 2008).
18. Wölfflin, "Prolegomena," 160.
19. This is a striking image in the time of Covid-19. Further, Wölfflin wrote: "Everything living tries to escape from this and to achieve the natural posture of regularity and balance. The relation of form to matter is conveyed in this effort of organic will to penetrate the body." Wölfflin, "Prolegomena," 160.
20. Schultze-Naumburg, *Art and Race*; Georges Batailles, "L'informe," *Documents* 1 (1929): 382; Yve-Alain Bois and Rosalind E. Krauss, *Formless: A User's Guide* (New York: Zone Books, 1997).

An earlier version of this essay was originally published by e-flux Architecture in 2022, and is adapted from David Gissen, "A Form of Impairment," in *The Architecture of Disability: Buildings, Cities, and Landscapes beyond Access* (Minneapolis: University of Minnesota Press, 2023). The author would like to thank Judy Selhorst for the edits to this version of the work.

p126 Kuttig—Archival / Alamy Stock Photo.
p128 Erin Babnik / Alamy Stock Photo.

CARE BEYOND BIOPOLITICS

MEREDITH TENHOOR

The welfare state institutions of architect Nicole Sonolet—mental hospitals, public housing complexes, and new village typologies built mainly in France and postcolonial Algeria from the 1950s to the 1980s—argued for a design practice that offered care for its own sake. Indeed, when Michel Foucault conceptualized the term "biopolitics" as a critical description of the economization of life, he was part of a constellation of researchers and architects including Sonolet who developed care praxes that defined the value of life otherwise. Sonolet's buildings, particularly the mental health care complexes she designed for residents of Paris's 13th arrondissement, were designed not only to support but to center the needs of people often excluded from design processes. They exceed the economic accountings of the liberal biopolitics Foucault described.

Although her work is formally sophisticated and theoretically rich, the work of Nicole Sonolet is not well known. In 1944 she was admitted to the École des Beaux-Arts in Paris to study architecture, but her education was interrupted by the Second World War; she completed her thesis project for a psychiatric hospital in 1954. During the postwar years and into the 1960s, she designed mid-sized subsidized housing complexes in Parisian suburbs. Commissions for private houses helped fund her practice. In those years she also returned to the subject of her thesis and began to design mental health care facilities. Her first major mental hospital was l'Eau Vive, located in the Parisian suburb of Soisy-sur-Seine, which she began to work on in conversation with the psychiatrist Philippe Paumelle starting in 1958.

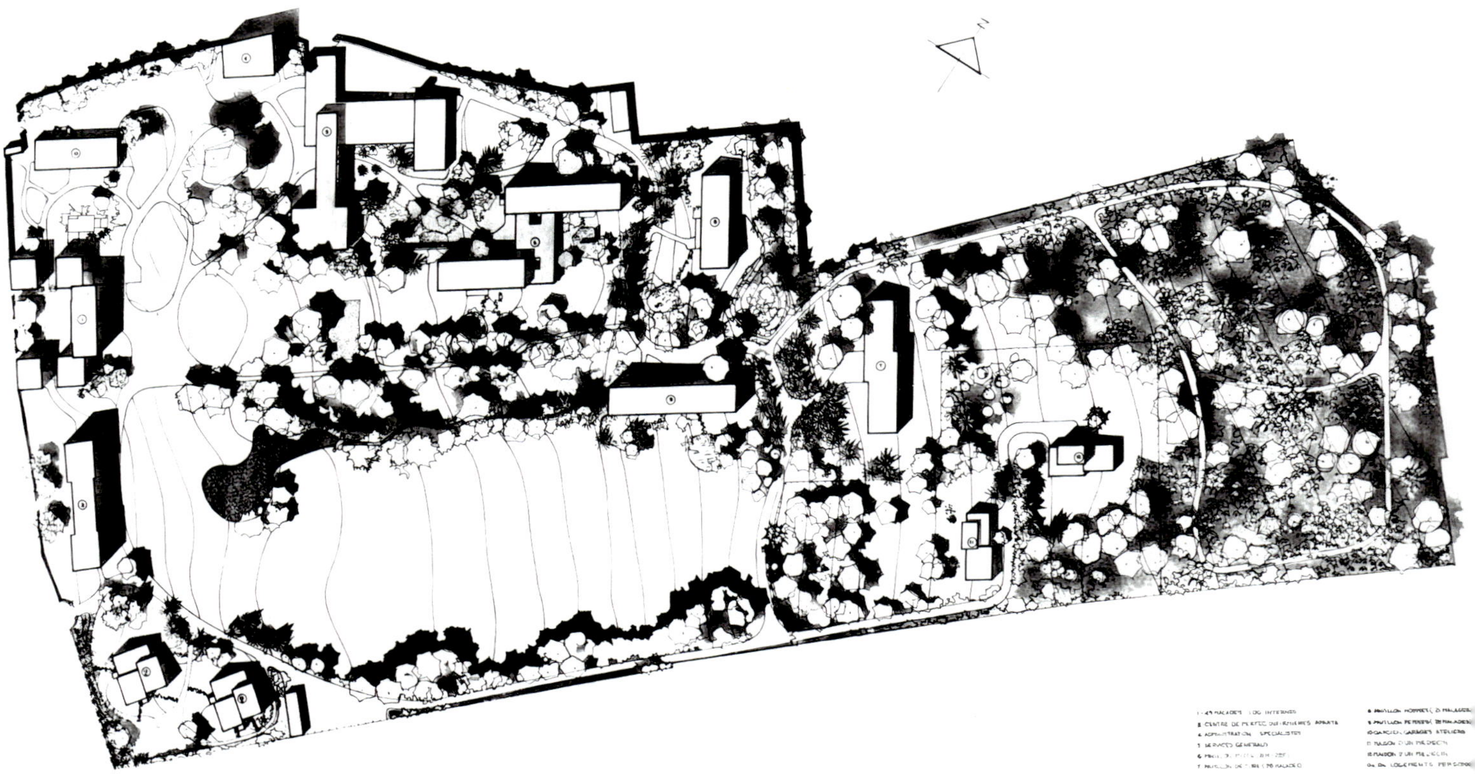

↑ Nicole Sonolet, plan of the grounds and buildings of l'Eau Vive hospital, Soisy-sur-Seine, 1960s.

↗ Exterior view of l'Eau Vive hospital, Soisy-sur-Seine, 1960s.

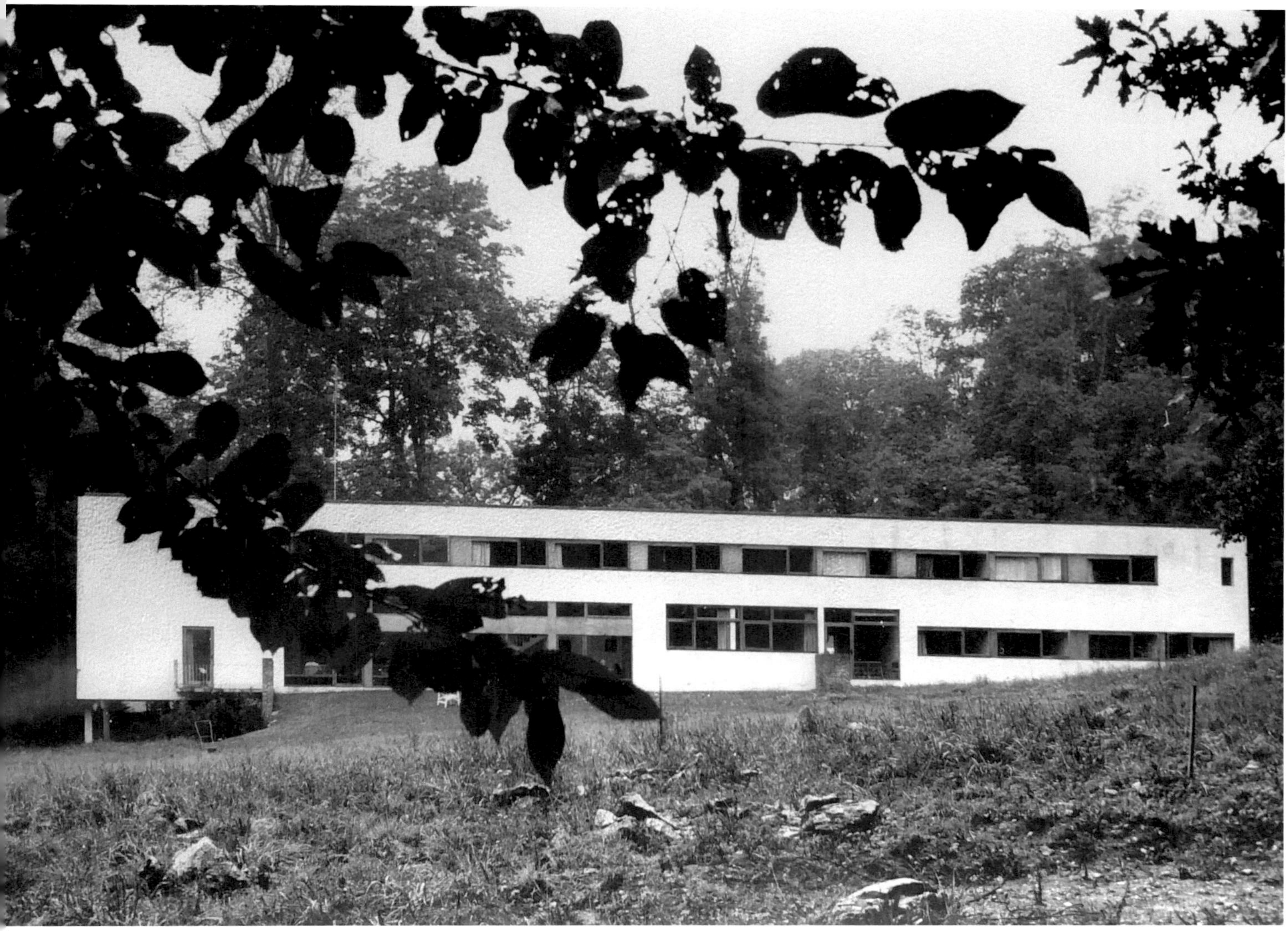

In the late 1960s and early 1970s, she and Paumelle collaborated again to build the Center for Mental Health of the Association de Santé Mentale 13 (or ASM 13) in Paris, a complement to l'Eau Vive which was focused on outpatient care. In these years, Sonolet also published articles on social housing and the architecture of mental health, conducted research on environmental psychology, and taught at the École Spéciale d'Architecture and the École des Beaux-Arts, sheltering students at her apartment during the events of May 1968.

Sonolet's interest in mental health care was intellectual as well as personal (a close relative had been hospitalized), and she was dedicated to advocating for more humane treatment for depressive, psychotic, and schizophrenic patients. In the course of her thesis research, she met with leading thinkers in the institutional psychotherapy (IP) movement, including Paumelle. IP practitioners sought to treat patients within their social and political contexts, and to use all of the interactions around psychotherapeutic care (including the space of the hospital or clinic, the exchanges a patient might have with a physical therapist, a housekeeper, or an art teacher) as a means of rebuilding damaged social and relational bonds, empowering patients to develop their own courses of healing in collaboration with their doctors.[1]

Following IP innovators François Tosquelles and Frantz Fanon, Paumelle was particularly dedicated to offering community-based care. He saw it as an alternative to the isolation and neglect patients too often endured in French asylums whose rural locations forced patients to leave their communities and families, only to then receive inconsistent treatment from rotating teams of doctors and nurses. Paumelle hoped to set up free clinics, as well as to provide patients with consistent medical teams, outpatient psychotherapy, and occupational therapies in order to limit hospitalizations. He argued that this would reduce national health expenditure, since local outpatient care was far less expensive than hospitalization, while at the same time increasing the availability of services. While the French state did eventually develop a policy to distribute care facilities throughout geographic "sectors" in the 1960s, Paumelle's plans predated this, and he was only able to begin to set up this system with private support. In 1958, with assistance from a donor who wanted to improve treatments for alcoholics, he founded the Association de Santé Mentale 13, a nonprofit organization intended to serve the mental health care needs of the population of the 13th arrondissement in Paris. This enabled Sonolet and Paumelle to plan l'Eau Vive, which would be the ASM 13's first hospital, and would serve as a kind of testing ground for community care typologies.

Paumelle had hoped to situate the ASM 13's hospital in Paris close to the population it would serve. But when land became available in the verdant park-like landscape of a former theological center in Soisy-sur-Seine, a suburban town just south of Paris, the ASM 13 accepted the opportunity to create a hospital outside the city. On this plot, Sonolet designed l'Eau Vive hospital, a campus with ten new buildings intended to serve 175 patients. A series of low, rectilinear pavilions housed a welcome center, housing for doctors and staff, a social center and cafeteria (which would allow doctors a chance to casually exchange ideas), an administration building, and five separate residential treatment buildings, each overseen by a different team of doctors and nurses.[2] Within the residential treatment buildings, patients were organized into groups of seven and monitored by one consistent nurse rather than a rotating team of staff, which the care team hoped would foster deeper and more therapeutic relations. In order to design the complex, Sonolet interviewed doctors, nurses, and staff working in the hospital to understand the particular burdens of caregiving. She intended for the design to offer them opportunities to recharge from care and even escape from patients when necessary, which would counterbalance the fact that IP practices meant that they would also be available to interact with patients outside of structured treatment times.

This clinic would not be "closed" in the carceral manner of old asylums, where patients were primarily confined to their rooms, but rather would encourage movement both within the buildings and on the grounds, a kind of healing circulation that echoes that of post–miasma theory hospital design. This decision was not made out of a fetishization of movement, but rather because Sonolet and Paumelle believed that patients had the right to evolve emotionally in the course of their treatment; if they were not fixed in one space within the confines of the hospital, they also could evolve beyond a fixed mental state or diagnosis. This idea of movement drove the design of the hospital. Sonolet theorized that architectural and interior design could "condition" spaces and provide a variety of experiences: of openness to the world or of enclosure; of stimulation or repose; of warmth or coolness. In the course of her design research, doctors would explain the kinds of phenomenological qualities they hoped to offer. Sonolet would then develop designs for these spaces, and

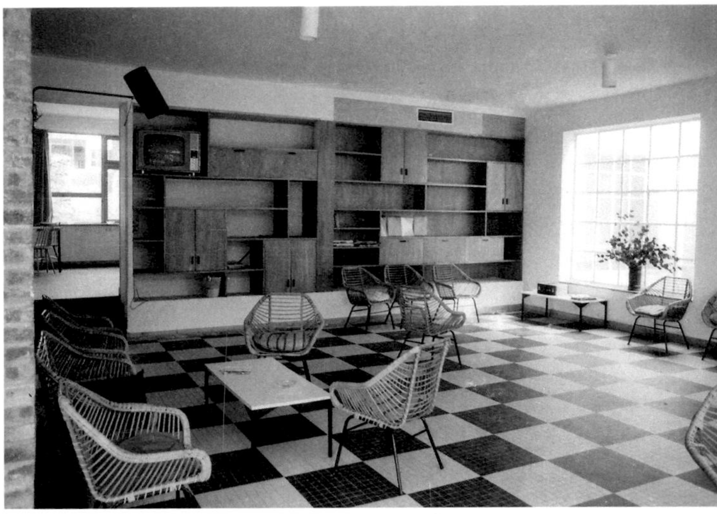

once built, patients would move through the hospital to spend time in places with the qualities they desired. Different materials, configurations of light, visual privacy, noise levels, and activities would all contribute to patients' emerging understanding of how they could use space in the course of their own treatment. Moving from an isolated state to a more socially engaged space would, in theory, help prepare patients to reintegrate into their communities.

Sonolet rendered all of these "conditions" in a largely modernist architectural vocabulary. In break rooms, for example, chairs could be grouped and regrouped to offer flexible possibilities for socialization; bedrooms were set up so that patients could keep the door open to be "open" to others while still maintaining some visual and aural privacy; windows could be opened or closed to allow for connection to the landscape; common bathrooms allowed both for larger, sunnier bedrooms and bringing patients into contact with others. Even though Soisy was far from Paris, Paumelle and Sonolet hoped that on its insides and between its pavilions, l'Eau Vive could model the forms of community immersion that would be possible in an urban mental health center. Even though bucolic, it was urban, and urbanity was healing.

After the initial phase of construction was complete in 1963, Sonolet began to publish conclusions from her experience constructing Soisy and her conversations with IP practitioners in journals of architecture and psychology.[3] She became known as an expert in the architecture of these new practices of mental health, and frequently consulted with international researchers interested in the intersections of architecture and mental health care. Her expertise was well-known to Félix Guattari, who a few years after the opening of l'Eau Vive founded a group called CERFI, or the Centre d'études, de recherches et de formation institutionnelles (Center for Institutional Studies, Research, and Training). Guattari's analytic beliefs were slightly more radical than Paumelle's, but he considered Sonolet a friend and admired colleague, exchanging letters with her

↑ Patient lounge at l'Eau Vive hospital, Soisy-sur-Seine, France, 1960s.

→ Exterior of the Center for Mental Health, Paris.

about various CERFI projects and drawing on her knowledge to organize an early issue of the group's journal, *Recherches*, on architecture, programming, and psychiatry.[4]

Programming Collective Facilities

The 1967 issue of *Recherches* was one of CERFI's first deep investigations of "programming," a special term for the group that encompassed architectural as well as other forms of planning.[5] As part of a discussion about how mental health infrastructure should be incorporated into the city, the issue put Sonolet in dialogue with psychiatrists and practitioners of institutional psychotherapy, as well as the architects Aymeric Zublena, Alain Schmied, Alain Fabre, and Albert Schwartz. Sonolet's contribution reprised material she had previously published based on her work at l'Eau Vive, outlining challenges, processes, and formal considerations that would be necessary when programming hospitals, along with a menu of programmatic possibilities and several charts schematizing how such a scheme could work with different population densities.[6] She stressed that long-term success could only be achieved after considerable research and conversation. While she was knowledgeable about mental health design, geographies, and care strategies across France, she was clear that a fixed program or typology could not be derived without deep conversation with doctors and staff. From this publication, Sonolet's insights about programming became part of a much larger conversation within CERFI.

While CERFI was started by Guattari, it was led by a large interdisciplinary group of militants, activists, sociologists, historians, writers, and psychoanalysts. They shared a desire to reform the instruments of the French state via new combinations of institutional, historical, sociological, and psychoanalysis, as well as through philosophy, critique, conversation, and design. The group received significant funding from the French government to develop projects and research—somewhat surprising given that they interrogated the state's projects of normalization and alienation. Nonetheless, a funder at the Ministry of Public Works was intrigued by CERFI's work on *équipements collectifs* (collective facilities, or infrastructures).[7] The Ministry wanted to build evidence for developing this infrastructure and to understand its forms, lifecycles, and potential impact on everyday life. CERFI hoped to use this funding to rethink the relationship between infrastructure and power through emerging critical discourses, rethinking Althusserian and Lacanian theories of subject formation in the context of praxis.

CERFI's first research contract from the Ministry of Public Works in 1971, Programmation des équipements collectifs dans les villes nouvelles—les équipements d'hygiène mentale (Programming Collective Facilities in New Towns—Facilities for Mental Health), offered a significant opportunity to develop architectural ideas about mental health.[8] The goal was to discuss how to plan community care facilities not just as pilot projects, as Sonolet and Paumelle had done at l'Eau Vive, but on a national scale. As part of this project, Sonolet was asked to share insights from her research. She discussed the necessity for private spaces, access to greenery and light, and the scale of patient-doctor units. However, she and another architect-interlocutor, Alain Schmied, both argued against the idea of mental health typologies: there was no architectural formula that could translate health into space. Rather, Sonolet explained, spaces had to be developed through a conversational programming process, one that would elicit the desires of both clinicians and patients, and whose outcome was not known in advance. In other words, the design of mental health architecture had to be akin to the open-ended practices of institutional psychotherapy itself.

CERFI's subsequent work on other kinds of collective infrastructures drew from this early work on community mental health. From 1971 to 1976, they organized an integrated childcare center in the new town of Melun-Sénart, which combined day care facilities, leisure facilities for children, a school, child

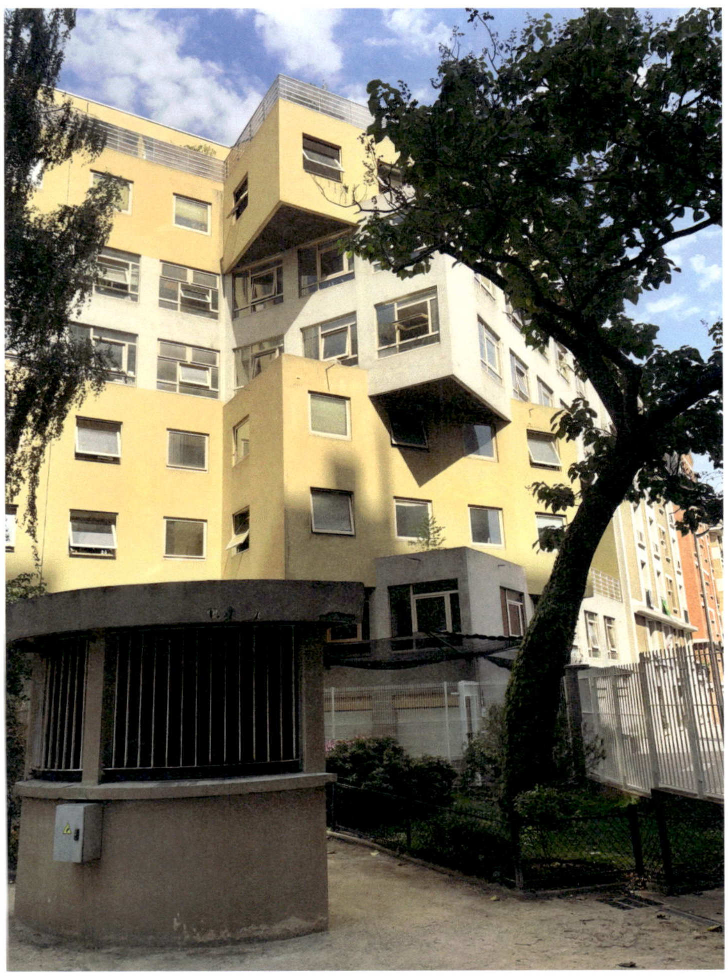

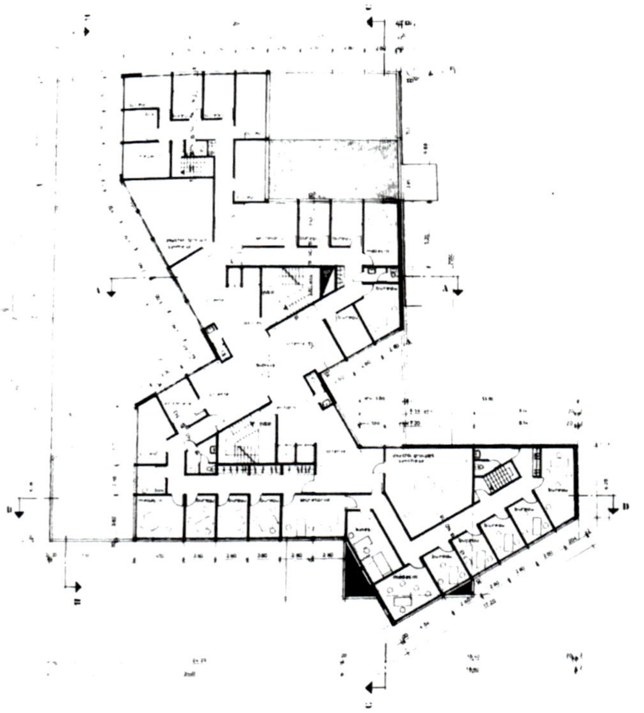

4ème étage : 4 équipes médico-sociales

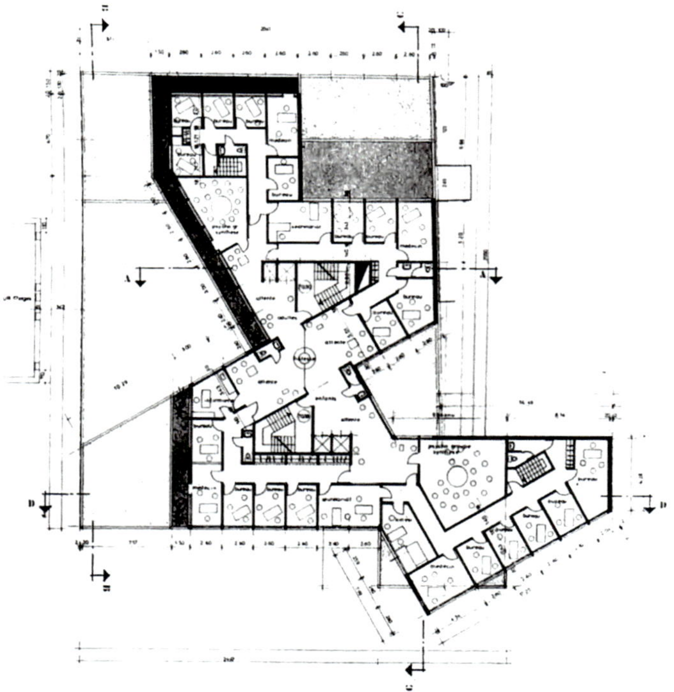

5ème étage : 4 équipes médico-sociales

↑ Nicole Sonolet and Maria Baran, plan of the Center for Mental Health of the ASM 13, Paris, 1971.

↗ Nicole Sonolet and Maria Baran, facade drawings of the Center for Mental Health of the ASM 13, Paris, 1971.

protection services, and after-school care; they studied Alma-Gare, a neighborhood of worker housing in Roubaix, and proposed programmatic and architectural strategies for improvement; they planned mental health facilities in new towns (which influenced the development of similar services in Paris); and they helped preserve a workers' retreat and establish a cultural center at the farm at Buisson outside the former Menier Chocolate Factory in Noisiel. In all of these projects, CERFIstes sought to understand how shared infrastructures might structure different practices of liberation, remaking the family, the neighborhood, and the clinic. All of this work was interdisciplinary, with architects participating on research teams alongside historians, philosophers, doctors, artists, urbanists, and many others.

Some of CERFI's funding was also funneled to Michel Foucault. His 1973–1974 research seminar "Recherche sur l'institution hospitalière à la fin du XVIIIe siècle, généalogie des équipements collectifs" ("Research on the Institution of the Hospital at the End of the Eighteenth Century: Genealogy of Public Amenities") was partially funded by the group, and it was in the course of this seminar—and conversations with architects and architectural historians (though not Sonolet)—that he developed the term "biopolitics." Seminar participants—Blandine Barret-Kriegel, the architects Bruno Fortier and François Béguin, and Foucault's niece Anne Thalamy—analyzed architectural plans, medical proclamations, and state records in order to elaborate a history of the belief that architecture was one of several *dispositifs* or apparatuses capable of producing health effects in the body of the population. The results of this research were published as a book, *Les machines à guérir: aux origines de l'hôpital moderne* (*Curing Machines: On the Origins of the Modern Hospital*) in 1976.[9] Foucault's essay, "The Politics of Health in the Eighteenth Century," introduced the research and argued that biopolitics particular to the late eighteenth century were elaborated through the medicalization of space and the subsequent creation of spatial-medical *dispositifs*, or material and institutional instruments. Once life was capable of being prolonged through the eighteenth-century hospital, he claimed, life itself it could be conceived of as a controllable value capable of being modulated across a population.

Bruno Fortier, a co-organizer of the seminar, developed conclusions related to the discipline of architecture out of the group's research. In his chapter "The Architecture of the Hospital," he described the process by which the design of hospitals was standardized, showing how control over hospital design shifted from being the purview of architectural professionals to becoming a medical concern, and then, once deemed important enough, again the purview of architects.[10] Fortier made an implicit

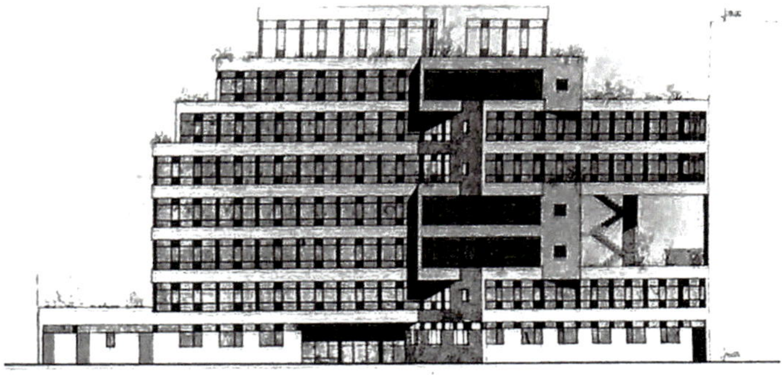

façade avenue edison et jardin

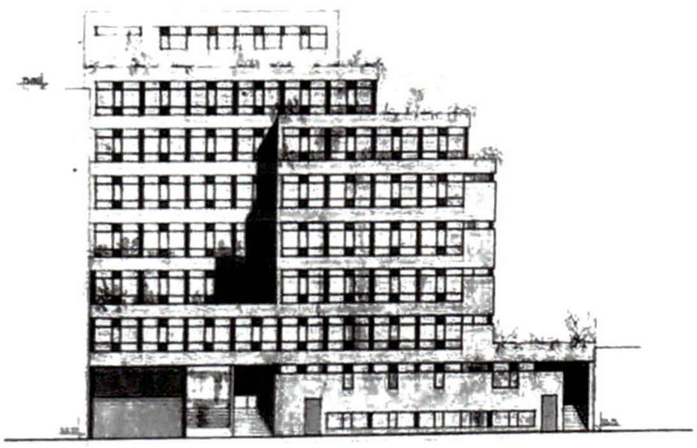

façade rue albert bayet

connection between understandings of the social effects of architecture in the eighteenth century and understandings of these effects in twentieth-century modern architecture, arguing that architectural standardization in the eighteenth century produced the idea of a perfectible architectural type.[11] Fortier argued that this allowed for a conceptualization of program and organization as something separate from previously "architectural" concepts of order or decoration. Thus, the political importance of the hospital's health effects did not just extend to the bodies of citizens, as Foucault had elucidated in his essay, but also helped eighteenth-century architects make a claim that there was an ideal form for a particular program, the very idea which Sonolet and Schmied had countered in CERFI's 1971 research project on mental health in new towns. Foucault and Fortier explained that there had been an eighteenth-century fantasy of a spatial "curing machine," which created a belief that there was a cause-and-effect relationship between health outcomes and architectural design. But their analyses make clear that rather than a reality, this was an idealized discourse about the design of the operation of government. Architecture was not a machine, and architecture alone could not produce forms of behavior or new political realities. Fortier left out the colonial dimensions of this fantasy of machinic control—ones essential for extracting value from land and life, and particularly Black lives, from a distance.[12]

Fortier's analyses complemented and intensified Sonolet and Schmied's conclusions about programming. Fortier's genealogy shows that the idea of programming had a long history of being reclaimed by practitioners of various disciplinary backgrounds, and that architecture in France had long been open to concerns that seemed to be outside of its disciplinary purview. CERFI's research project on mental hospitals in new towns anticipated and contributed to Foucault's first theorization of the term "biopolitics." While Guattari, Schmied, Sonolet, and the doctors they collaborated with did not coin this term, from the beginnings of their conversations it is clear that Sonolet and the CERFIstes were trying to produce alternatives to a neoliberal biopolitical calculus where decisions about governance were made according to monetary value assigned to life. This valuing of life justified the French state's construction of infrastructure like the eighteenth-century hospitals Foucault and Fortier described, as well as the twentieth-century research contracts that CERFI received to install mental health services in new towns. In contrast, Sonolet's hospitals and CERFI's *équipements collectifs* were organized around the provision of care for its own sake, demonstrating that another rationale for care was possible.

The Center for Mental Health

CERFI did not ultimately manage to create nationwide programs for mental health services. Their funding decreased precipitously alongside French state funds for mental health care in the early 1970s. However, around this time, private philanthropy allowed Sonolet and Paumelle to build a Paris-based mental health complex for the ASM 13 that they had also hoped to construct in the late 1950s: the Center for Mental Health, located on Avenue Edison near the Place d'Italie.[13] Sonolet had long worked on conceptual plans for an urban counterpart for l'Eau Vive. With a site and a sponsor secured, she and a design collaborator, Maria Baran, drew up detailed plans, and construction permits were granted in 1972. The Center for Mental Health both inspired and bears traces of CERFI's work on collective facilities: it offered outpatient and emergency residential services for residents of the 13th arrondissement, allowing patients the ability to remain in their communities while receiving care. The complex combined two treatment centers, one for adults and the other for children (named respectively for Albert Binet and Philippe Paumelle, after his premature death in 1974), as well as a psychoanalytic institute and family support clinic. Even though the Center for Mental Health was supposed to make up for the lack of urbanity at l'Eau Vive, it also attempted to import a trace of pastoral aesthetics into an urban setting: as part of the project, a new public park was built on an adjoining parcel of land in 1973. The park made the project more appealing to neighbors, who received a much-needed green space, and allowed Sonolet and Baran to open the building to light and air on an urban scale.

The geometry of the Center for Mental Health is much more complex than l'Eau Vive's rectilinear pavilions. Treatment spaces and offices rotate around two central stair cores, and the building steps back as it rises, allowing light to fall on terraces and outdoor planted spaces that line the building and buffer the offices, waiting rooms, and treatment areas from the street. Triangular forms jut toward the street to create a variegated and lively facade, one that perhaps signified the particularity and unpredictability of treatment paths espoused by practitioners at ASM 13. On the interior, waiting rooms fill the negative space of the exterior angles, offering patients semiprivate corners with views to terraces or the public gardens. The complex also featured spaces for teaching, including an auditorium, library, classrooms, and meeting rooms, as well as several spaces for group psychotherapy on each floor. The top floor housed a restaurant and cafeteria for staff, facilitating interaction between the many doctors on site.

Much of the treatment at the Center for Mental Health was done in private offices, which, despite the angular facades, were mostly rectilinear and set along the street-facing sides of the buildings. Patients would have been able to enjoy vegetal views onto planted terraces during therapy sessions and perhaps in some cases access them from an office. As she had at l'Eau Vive, Sonolet tried to ensure that staff needs were met in the design. The terraces were planned to offer doctors and staff visual repose for times when the psychic interiors they inhabited became too overpowering. The presence of planted terraces at street level not only buffers the hospital, but also suggests that spaces for mental health can offer amenities even to residents who didn't directly partake of them. The gardens themselves helped to ease and normalize the provision of care.

Because of its condensed footprint, and because treatment was largely done in single rooms, as well as over short durations, the Center for Mental Health did not offer patients the healing circulation that was a key part of residential treatment at l'Eau Vive. This was in part because the patients who used the Center for Mental Health were less sick and could manage with only outpatient treatment; spending less time in the building meant that it would not need to offer as many treatment resources. The clinic therefore did not present itself as a *dispositif* for healing, a space that would be activated through creative use and misuse. A patient could not write her own treatment path through the building. If she wanted to do so, she would need to leave the clinic to experience the city itself, to use *it* as a form of treatment. *Équipements* did not just support the city; they were the city.

Sonolet, Foucault, and the CERFIstes connected architecture and infrastructure to health and subjectivity. While it is well established that late twentieth-century architects learned from and adapted so-called "French theory" into design paradigms, Sonolet's work reveals the extent to which architectural thought and practice contributed to its theories of power, and how much a preoccupation with illness fueled these inquiries. Sonolet's spaces of care, along with CERFI's work on *équipements collectifs*, helped generate a theory of infrastructure that was not biopolitical but instead based on both care and desire. This architectural practice beyond biopolitics likely shaped Foucault and Fortier's historic work about hospitals, sharpening their critique of emerging neoliberalism in France. It may have informed Foucault's theories of biopolitics.

These feedback loops between critique, analysis, programming, and design had parallels with the patient-specific treatment protocols that IP practitioners developed as they worked against the idea of a uniform and standardized formula for treating different illnesses. Sonolet modified the psychoanalytic practice of providing care to derive a process for designing hospitals. Following the principles of IP, this would yield designs that in turn were guided by a set of common principles, but ones specific to each situation and team of staff members as well as the community from which they issued. Designing these spaces required close collaboration. Acknowledging this helps to account for the formal variations in Sonolet's work, and the careful intentionality of her designs. In an ideal scenario, implied Sonolet, care could be designed for all collective facilities.[14]

An earlier version of this essay was originally published by e-flux Architecture in 2022.

1. For more on the theories and politics of institutional psychotherapy, see Valentin Schaepelynck, *L'institution renversée: Folie, analyse institutionnelle et champ social* (Paris: Eterotopia, 2018), and Camille Robcis, *Disalienation: Politics, Philosophy, and Radical Psychiatry in Postwar France* (Chicago: University of Chicago Press, 2021).
2. For more detail on the design of l'Eau Vive, see Meredith TenHoor, "The Design of Community Mental Health Care: Nicole Sonolet in Postwar France," in *gta papers* 7, "Care," ed. Torsten Lange and Gabrielle Schaad (Zurich: gta Verlag 2022); and Julie Mareuil, "Une clinique-pilote de la sectorisation psychiatrique: L'hôpital de l'Eau Vive et son évolution de 1959 à 1977" (MA diss., ENSA Paris-La Villette, 2020).
3. Nicole Sonolet, "Un centre de santé mentale. Point de vue et proposition d'un architecte," *Information Psychiatrique*, no. 6 (June 1966): 527–532; Nicole Sonolet, "An Urban Mental Health Center: Proposal for an Experimental Design," *Social Psychiatry* 2, no. 3 (1967): 137–143.
4. CERFI, "Programmation, Architecture et Psychiatrie," *Recherches* 6 (1967).
5. Susana Caló and Godofredo Pereira offer a helpful analysis of this issue of *Recherches*, focusing on how CERFI modified ideas about mental health and its place in urban design and planning in France. See Susana Caló and Godofredo Pereira, "CERFI: From the Hospital to the City," *London Journal of Critical Theory* 1, no. 2 (May 2017): 83–100.
6. Nicole Sonolet, "Un centre de santé mentale urbain: proposition d'une experience," *Recherches* 6 (1967).
7. CERFI's work on this topic caught the attention of the landscape historian Michel Conan, who was in charge of urban research at the Ministry of Public Works. Conan arranged funding for CERFI to undertake projects to plan mental health facilities in the New Towns of Évry and Melun-Sénart. For more detail, see Meredith TenHoor, "State-Funded Militant Infrastructure? CERFI's *équipements collectifs* in the Intellectual History of Architecture," *Journal of Architecture* 24, no. 7 (2019): 999–1019.
8. CERFI had to submit official reports of the work completed for its various research contracts, and did so in this case by publishing a small booklet: CERFI, *La programmation des équipements collectifs dans les villes nouvelles (Les équipements d'hygiène mentale): Rapport sur l'exécution de la convention d'études entre le CERFI et le Ministère d'équipement et du logement (Direction de l'aménagement foncier et de l'urbanisme) du 4 mai 1971* (Paris: Centre d'études, de recherches et de formation institutionnelles, 1972).
9. Michel Foucault, ed., *Les Machines à guérir: aux origines de l'hôpital moderne* (Paris: Institut de l'environnement, 1976). Foucault's essay has been translated into English as Michel Foucault, "The Politics of Health in the Eighteenth Century," in *Power/Knowledge : Selected Interviews and Other Writings, 1972–1977*, trans. Colin Gordon (New York: Pantheon Books, 1980). A translation of the entire text, edited and introduced by Anne Kockelkorn and Moritz Gleich, is forthcoming and eagerly anticipated.
10. Bruno Fortier, "Architecture de l'hôpital," in Foucault, *Les machines à guérir*.
11. Fortier, "Architecture de l'hôpital," 72.
12. This is equally true of Foucault's theories of biopolitics, which miss many of the most crucial sites of eighteenth-century biopolitical formation, particularly those of extractive economies and enslavement, as Alexander Wehilye, Simone Brown, and many others have documented. See Simone Browne, *Dark Matters: On the Surveillance of Blackness* (Durham: Duke University Press, 2015); Alexander G. Weheliye, *Habeas Viscus: Racializing Assemblages, Biopolitics, and Black Feminist Theories of the Human* (Durham: Duke University Press, 2014). However, CERFI's and Sonolet's resistance to theories of machinic governance aligned with their anticolonial stances more generally.
13. Sonolet collaborated with architect Maria Baran on the project; later they were joined by Olek Kujawski and Tristan Darros who oversaw construction. Permits for the project were approved in 1972, but because of funding and other challenges, it took nearly nine years to be completed.
14. This chapter condenses arguments and analysis from several lectures given from 2018 to 2020, as well as previously published texts: Meredith TenHoor, "State-Funded Militant Infrastructure? CERFI's Équipements Collectifs in the Intellectual History of Architecture," *Journal of Architecture* 24, no. 7 (October 3, 2019): 999–1019; Meredith TenHoor, "Des architectures du soin: Philippe Paumelle et Nicole Sonolet," ed. Christine Langlois and Baptiste Moutaud, *Terrain* 76 (Spring 2022); Meredith TenHoor, "Architecture and Biopolitics at Les Halles," *French Politics, Culture and Society* 25, no. 2 (2007): 73–92. I am grateful to the editors of these publications for permission to summarize them here, and to Christine de Bremond d'Ars for sharing her insights and Sonolet's archives with me.

p132, 133, 134, 136, 137 Archives of Nicole Sonolet, collection of Christine de Bremond d'Ars.
p135 Photo: author.

THE RIGHT TO TERRITORIALITY AS A MODEL OF INCLUSION

GIDEON BOIE

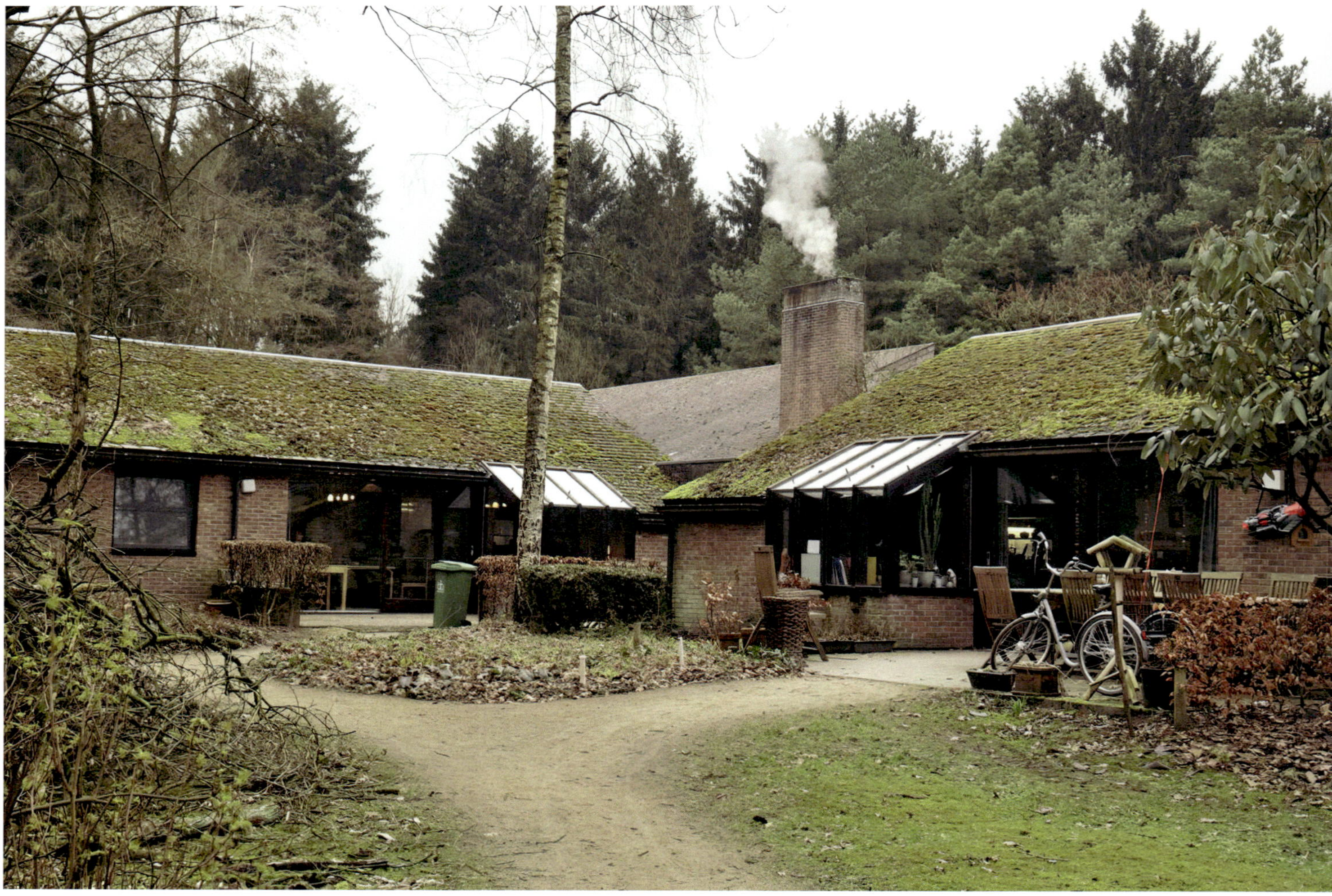

↑ Luk Van den Broeck, Monnikenbos (1980).

Contemporary conceptions of care in architecture are often indebted to the well-meaning goal of repairing the historical damage done by the separation of sick and disabled persons from society. In 1970s in the Netherlands, the call for a "return to the city" led to a process where psychiatric institutions and asylums were abandoned, only to be later redeveloped as housing estates.[1] In Belgium today, these ideas translate into calls for "invisible care," which aim to recreate a sense of homeliness in hospital facilities, and "caring neighborhoods," which embed healthcare facilities within the urban fabric.[2] These models foster certain principles about what it means to be normal today—to live and work in the city, to live independently, etc.—and inadvertently repeat the "moral treatment" of psychiatric patients in the late eighteenth century at the Retreat run by Samuel Tuke, where patients lived in an idyllic spatial setting in the countryside close to the modern city and participated in everyday homely activities such as tea parties.[3]

The history of Monnikenheide, a residential care complex for persons with mental and physical disabilities in Zoersel, Belgium, allows for a more nuanced and differentiated vision of what inclusion means, both spatially and architecturally. Monnikenheide was founded in 1972 by Wivina Demeester-De Meyer and her husband Paul.[4] As a member of the Flemish Christian-Democrat party, Wivina was state secretary in several federal and regional governments in Belgium from 1985 to 1999, during which time she held roles in healthcare, welfare, and public administration.[5] She has also been a decisive figure in the landscape of architecture in Flanders, playing a foundational part in the development of both the position of the Flemish Government Architect and the Flanders Architecture Institute.[6] Her interests in politics, care, and architecture culminated in the charity for persons with mental and physical disabilities.

The Demeester couple was first confronted with the issue of housing for persons with disabilities in 1969, following the birth of their son Steven, who has Down's syndrome. Soon, their desire grew not only to adapt housing for their own family, but to develop alternative forms of accommodation for persons with mental and physical disabilities. Although far from sick, in the 1970s disabled persons were often confined to living either in or at the margins of psychiatric institutions.[7] According to Wivina, she and her husband reached a breaking point in a visit to the well-known Stropstraat in Ghent, the main campus of the Brothers of Charity, which then provided care services for all sort of sick, mentally ill, and disabled persons.[8] After the visit, the Demeesters began their endeavor to provide alternative housing that includes mentally and physically disabled people in society.

Inclusion at Monnikenheide did not mean "returning to the city," but rather the opposite: moving to the village, and in particular Zoersel, which at the time was an expanding suburb in the Kempen region, east of Antwerp. The Demeesters owned a piece of land in the vast Zoerselbos nature reserve, which was chosen as the site. This choice was also motivated by the theories of environmental psychologists Cornelis B. Bakker and Marianne K. Bakker-Rabdau, who demonstrated how people, especially children, build their identity through dealing with territory.[9] As a low-stimulus environment located within walking distance of the village center, the location at Zoerselbos was considered suitable for housing people with mental and physical disabilities. The idea was to accommodate the specific territorial needs and desires of the residents, allowing them to roam around and transgress borders, while at the same time offering feelings of homeliness, safety, belonging, and even pride.

Monnikenheide was designed to free disabled persons from the logic of asylums by situating them in a normal urban and social tissue, which in this case is the housing idyll of Flemish suburbia. The exceptional location marks a distinction from the world of the traditional mental asylum. The name was inspired by the indication on the Ferraris map (1771–1778) where *Monincken Heijde* (Old Dutch for Monk's Heath) refers to the reclamation of the land by Cistercian monks. Pavilions are scattered around the estate, mimicking the surrounding suburban context. Each has its own distinct street address. Residents are encouraged not just to use their units, but also to roam around in the woods, the neighborhood, and even in the village center—all without, if possible, being accompanied by staff.

The recognition of the right to territoriality for disabled persons has translated into a continuous effort to understand what inclusion means with respect to the very different territorial needs and desires of residents and how to spatially facilitate it. Today Monnikenheide comprises a series of residential facilities spread out on the wooded terrain in the back of the Demeester family villa. Merging with the suburban village, the various projects differ from one another in the relationships they establish with the environment, public services, and neighbors. This differentiation has also resulted thanks in part to the deliberate choice to involve new architects for each project. Monnikenheide was therefore created out of a design intelligence that combines everyday conversations and situated knowledge with typological experimentation.[10] A tour through Monnikenheide today presents an evolution of care, following progressive insights on how architecture can support the inclusion of disabled people.

At Monnikenheide, the traditional logic of asylums with large "bed houses" was replaced with an open setting of small-scale facilities that operate as substitute families, which allow for small groups of

→ UR architects, De Eiken (2016), ground-floor plan.

↓ UR architects, De Eiken (2016).

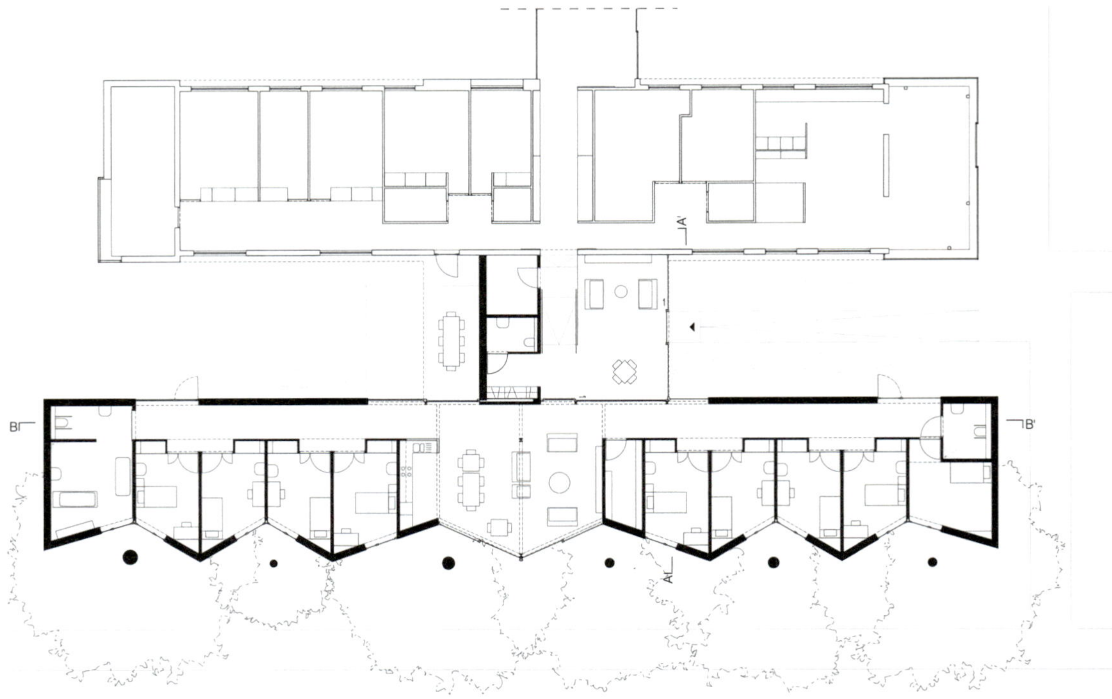

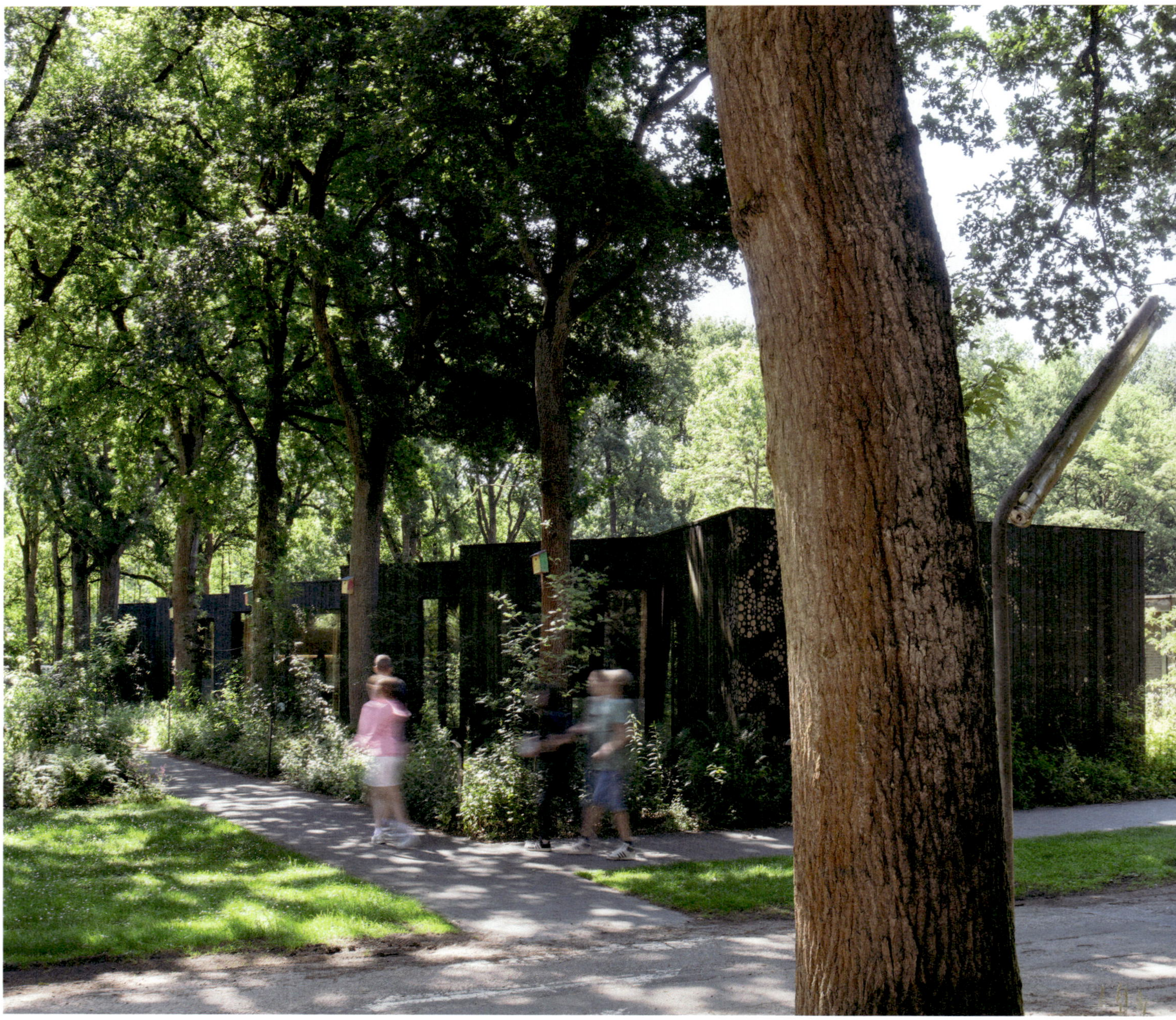

→ UR architects, Monniken-
bos Renovation (2020).

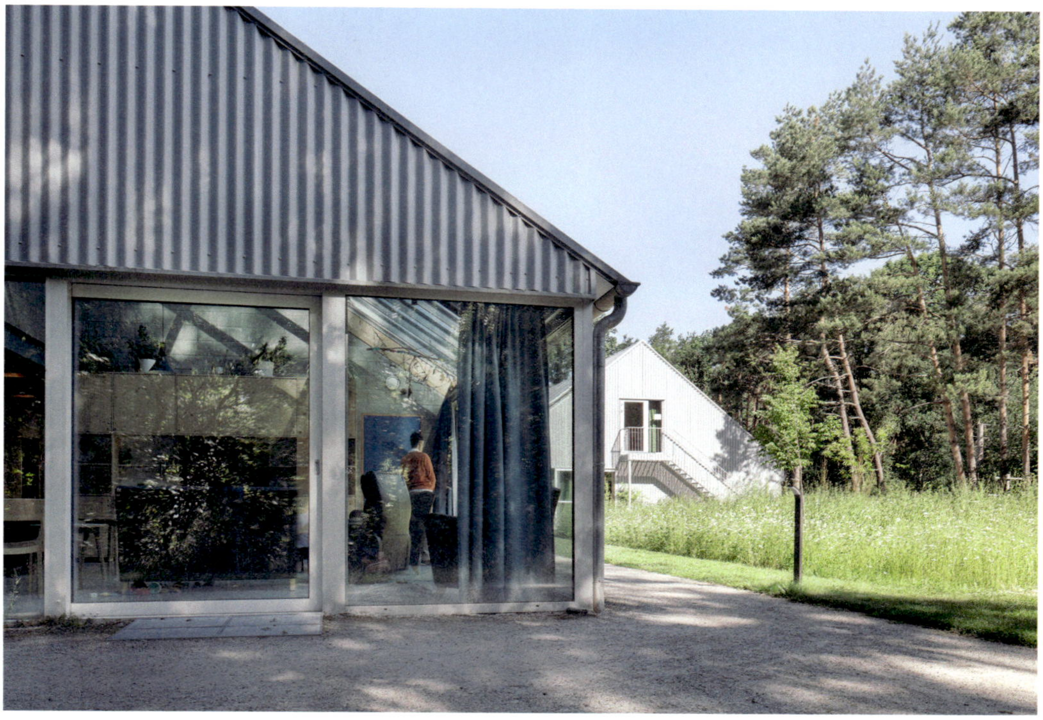

residents to function quasi-independently.[11] These facilities show how the right to territoriality was not just an element of spatial planning and landscaping, but also translated into the interior of the facilities and the intimacy of the bedroom. The first "short-stay home" for children, which was designed by Bruno Boulanger in 1973 and today functions as the central service building, originally consisted of four identical pavilions. Built using the Danilith prefab system, a single corridor connected two common services pavilions in the middle, with boys and girls pavilions on either side. Each pavilion has two living groups of seven beds. Although the short-stay home is still equipped with collective sleeping rooms, the repetition of pavilions sharply contrasts the classical dormitory typology used in hospitals. This focus on small-scale units is recognizable in all other later buildings on the site.

More recent architectural production at Monnikenheide is defined by an evolving typology of the "family replacement" unit. In its 2003 renovation by Jo Peeters, the capacity of Boulanger's short-stay home was reduced to one resident group per pavilion, with living rooms placed on one side of the corridor and individual sleeping rooms on the other. The central corridor was also extended and a fifth pavilion added in the row. The spine knitting all pavilions together was transformed by large glass windows, creating a stronger connection to the exterior and removing any connotation of the space as a hospital corridor. A laundry and therapy pool were built opposite the building's new entrance. These separate facilities are meant to stimulate the use of the exterior and enhance the dynamic of going inside and out. UR architects recently added a sixth pavilion to the spine, De Eiken (2016), with a facade that suggests it is the end of the line.

The second building at Monnikenheide, the Monnikenbos (1980), was designed as clustered housing for permanent residency by Luc Van den Broeck. Made out of brick with sloped roofs, the complex brings together three houses, each accommodating eight people, around a shared entry hall. The central space was meant to function as a place for work, but after the construction of another building, the Workshop (1985, designed by Mark Depreeuw), it was converted into a polyvalent space for sports and social activities. In 2020, as part of an overall renovation of Monnikenbos by UR architects, the central entrance pavilion that once provided access to the three pavilions was removed, thus turning the circulation logic inside-out and resulting in a new central space that functions as a shared open courtyard for the different residents.

Through these incremental experiments, Monnikenheide has pioneered the architectural typology of sheltered housing that offers mentally disabled persons the opportunity of independent living. Yet the inclusive location in a suburban area limits the possibilities for some guests, especially those seeking more self-dependence. The House at the Voorne (2003), designed by Dirk Somers, was therefore located not on the Monnikenheide campus, but along the main street just outside the village center of Zoersel. This provides its residents with direct proximity to social services (bakeries, grocery stores, bus stops, etc.) while supporting their participation in the village community. The house has a capacity for eight residents, who are expected to organize their work and living independently. Nursing staff is available only for help with breakfast and in the evening.

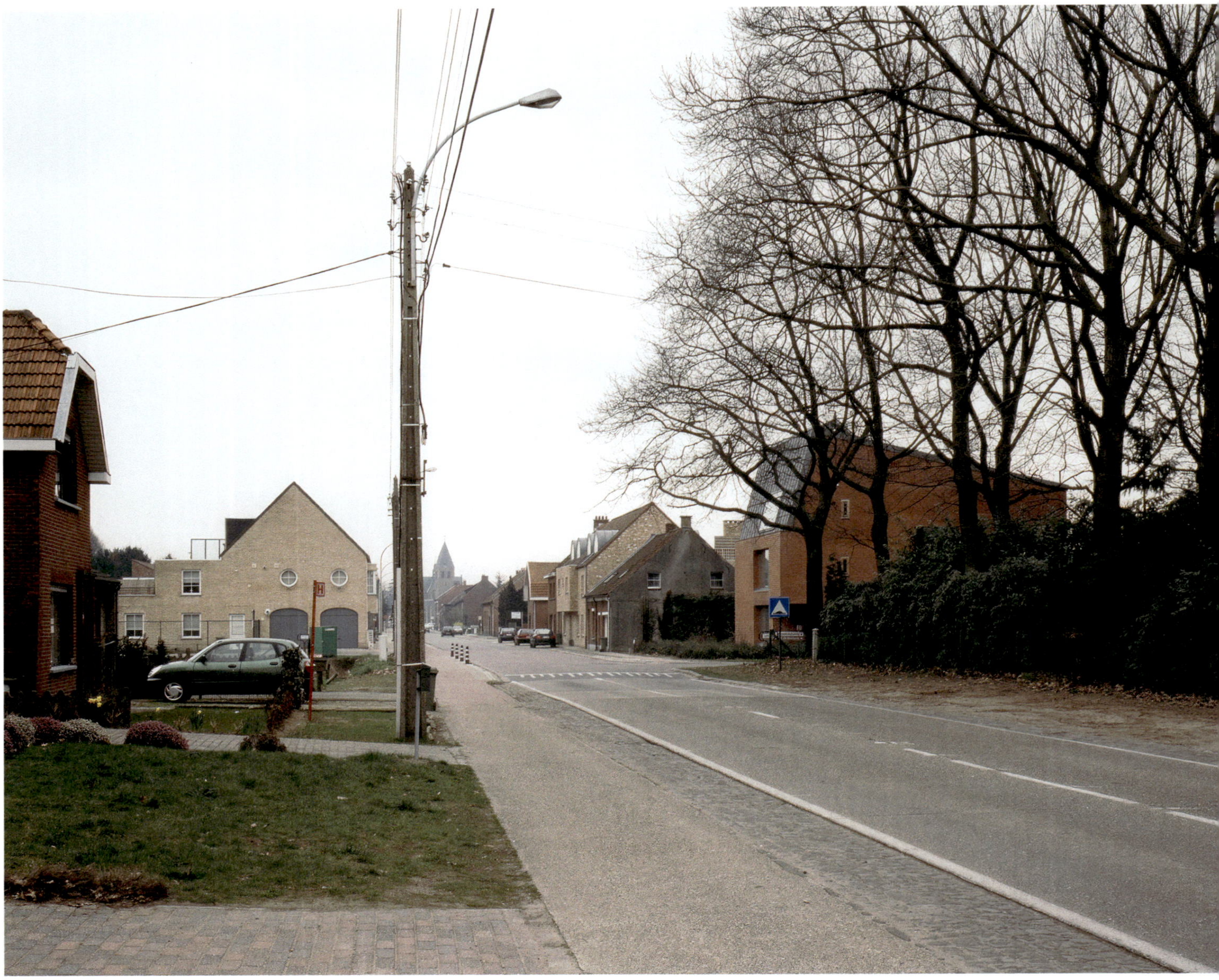

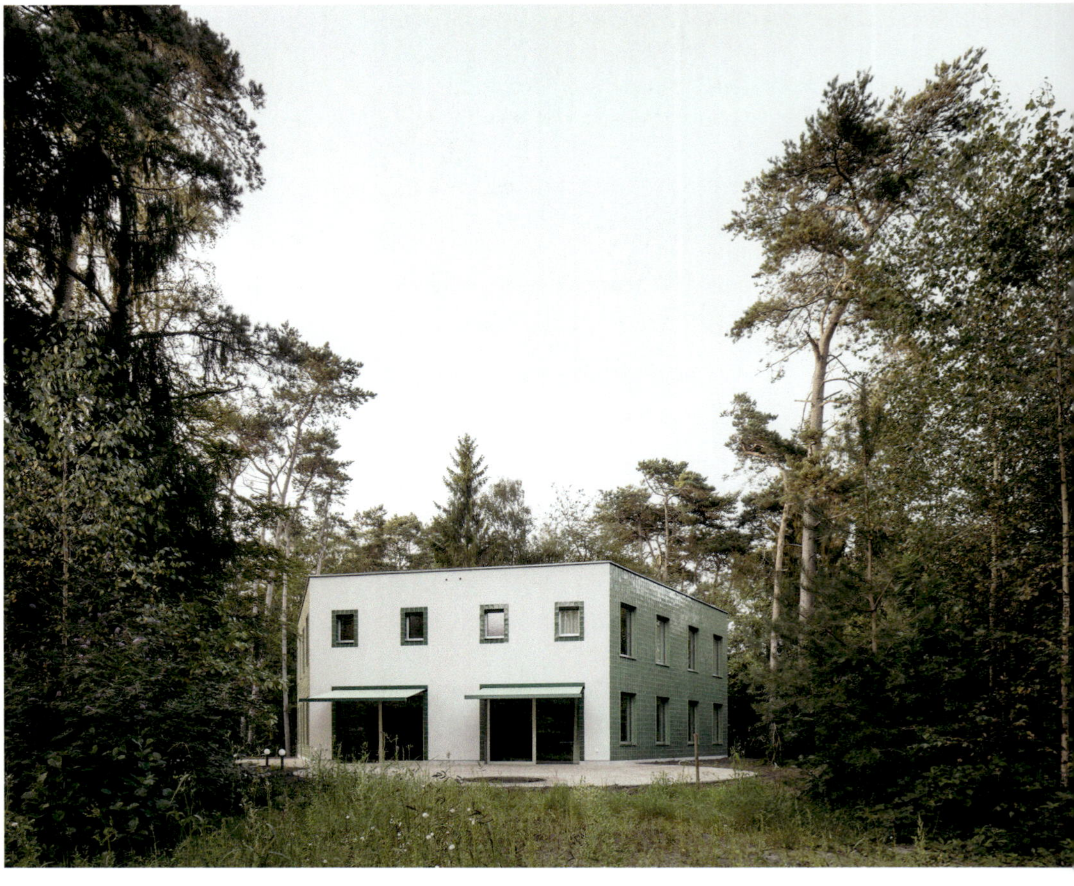

↑ Dirk Somers (Huiswerk, now Bovenbouw), Huis aan de Voorne (2002).

→ FELT, Villa Kameleon (2021).

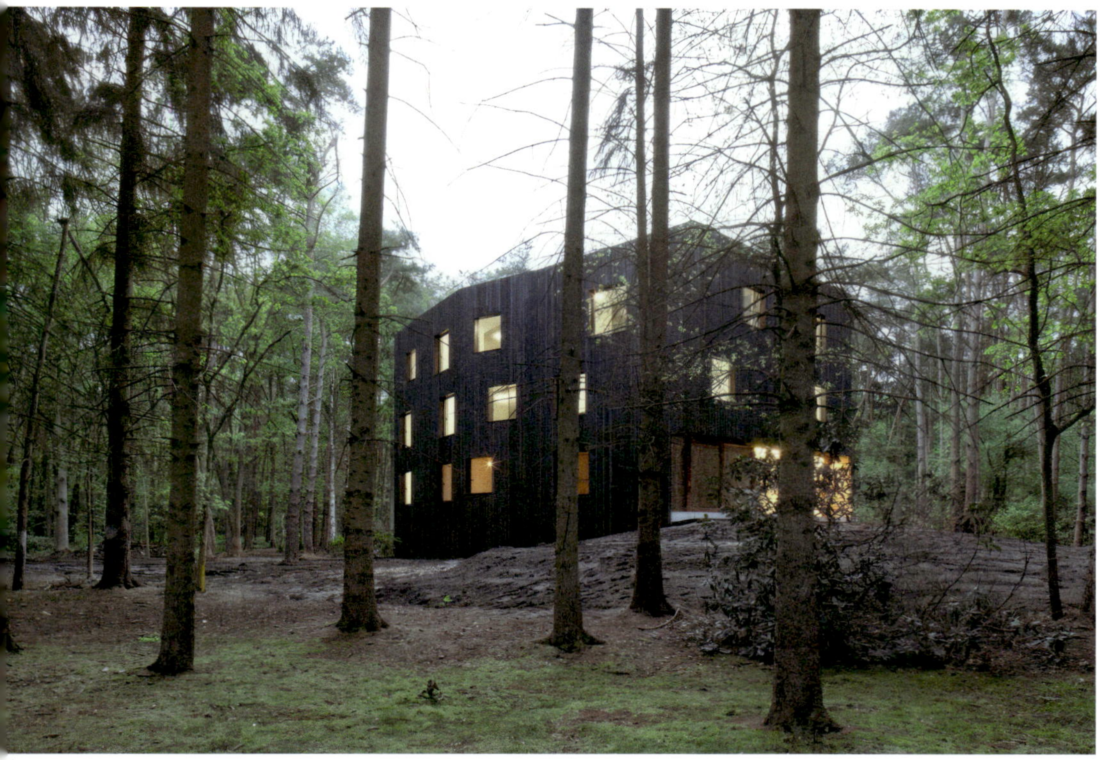

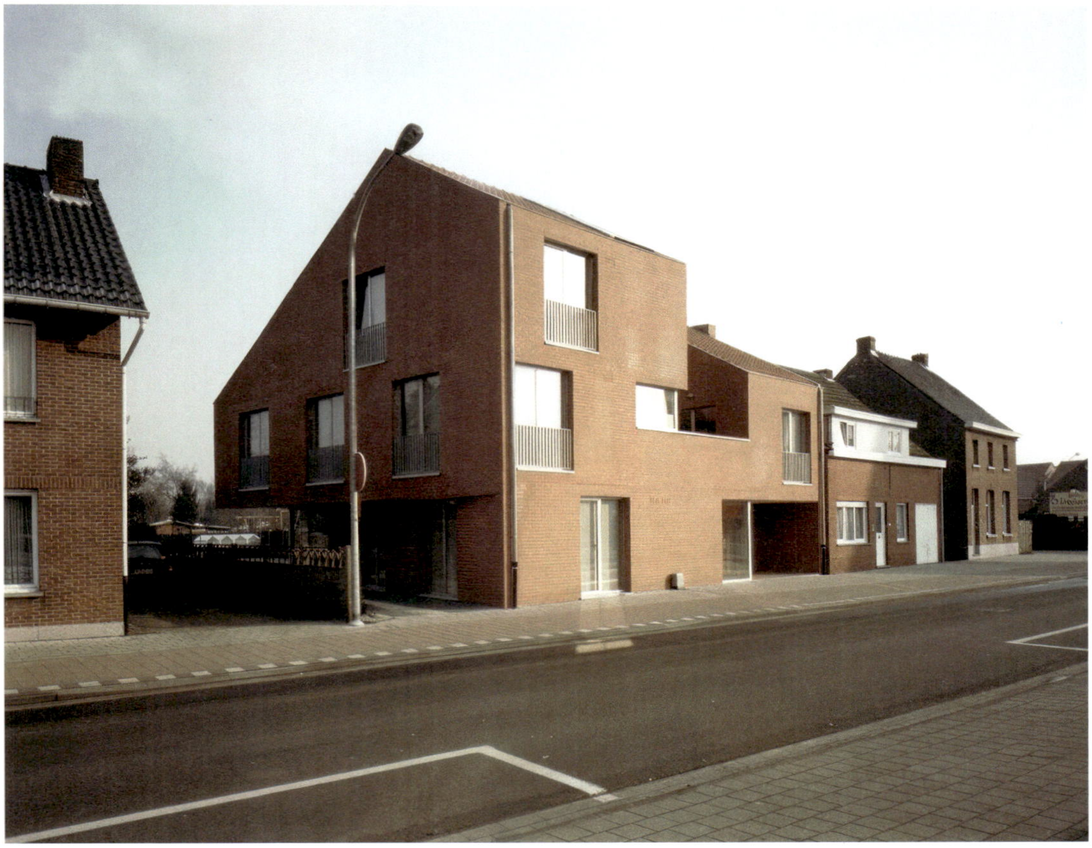

↑ 51N4E, Huis at the Laar (2012).

↓ Johan De Coster (VDC architects), House at the Church (2004).

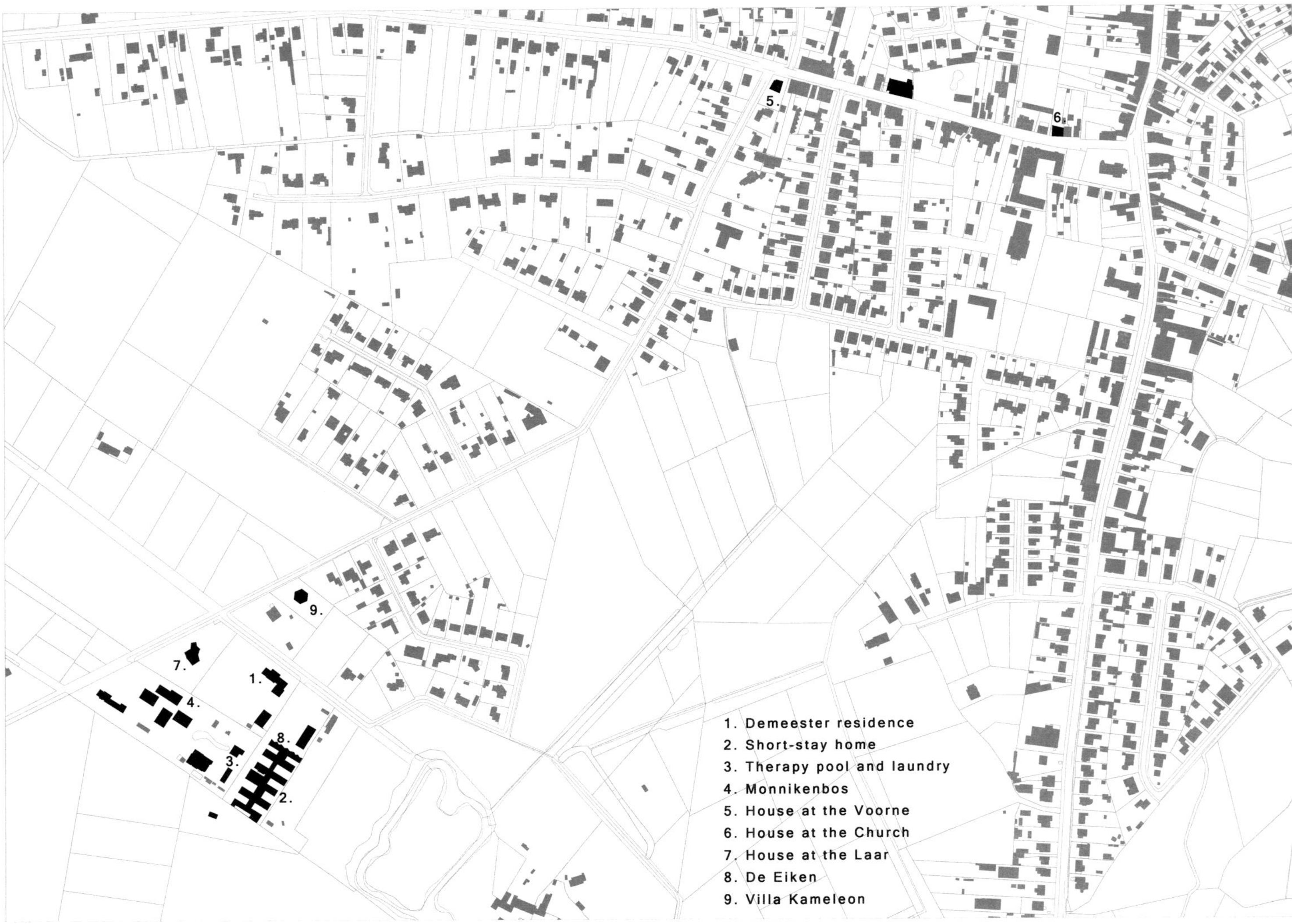

The House at the Church (2004), designed by Johan De Coster, follows the same logic but is located in the heart of the village, right in front of the main church and the elementary school. Wivina Demeester calls the position an intentional provocation, allowing the residents to establish a relational network and in turn allows villagers to unwittingly care for the persons with disabilities—whether by helping them cross the street or giving them change when checking out at the grocery store, etc. According to Heleen Verheyden, this building is a prime example of an architecture that goes beyond the special needs of disabled persons and addresses the public in the first place. It is what she calls an "architecture of presence."[12]

Again, territoriality is not just about spatial planning but is reflected in the interior and the intimacy of the bedroom. The typologies of these two sheltered housing units differ from one another. In the House at the Voorne, the communal space remains rather limited and bare, as the living room is simultaneously the dining room, kitchen, and atrium, while individual rooms are designed as studios and equipped with their own kitchenettes. The internal logic of the House at the Church, however, is designed more like that of a typical house, with a living room and kitchen functioning as cozy and familiar communal spaces, and an open staircase leading to individual bedrooms.

These typological experiments have been incorporated back into new buildings on the main Monnikenheide campus. Huis at the Laar (2013), designed by Peter Swinnen, transposes the typology of the sheltered house into a freestanding house in the woods. Huis at the Laar is meant for persons with higher care needs but who are still able to live independently. The house brings two groups of eight people together via a helical staircase, around which the groups can relate to each other but never come into physical contact. The rooms are conceptualized as small L-shaped studios with two windows, giving each room multiple viewpoints.

The same logic appears in Villa Kameleon (2021), designed by FELT architecture & design, a sheltered house situated a stone's throw away from the Demeester estate. The house presents itself as a freestanding villa, blending into the suburban plan. Despite this, a special permit was needed to change the land use of the plot from housing to care facility. Eight L-shaped rooms come together in a

↑ Location of different Monnikenheide buildings in the village of Zoersel.

hexagonal-shaped floor plan. The central lobby is a rather bare circulation space that allows residents to reach their private rooms without needing to pass common living or dining areas, thus enjoying privacy and independence in their daily comings and goings.

Monnikenheide testifies to the dynamic logic of inclusion for persons with mental and physical disabilities, going beyond the usual story of first retreating from the city and next turning back. Slavoj Žižek argues that Hegelian synthesis is not so much a peaceful reconciliation of opposites, but the "negation of (the first) negation."[13] While its initial establishment and early building projects sought to negate the old logic of separation underlying the asylum and its stigmatizing housing models,[14] the subsequent development of diverse facilities have continuously stretched and rethought the territorial reach of the residents. The architecture caters to the different needs of persons with mental and physical abilities. It also adapts to changing needs in the span of a lifetime, making it possible for residents to move from one house to another within the familiar environment. Steven Demeester, for instance, who inspired the whole project and lived independently in House at the Church, returned to a family unit on the main campus after developing dementia before passing away in 2024.

An earlier version of this essay was originally published by e-flux Architecture in 2022.

1. Noor Mens and Cor Wagenaar, *Health Care Architecture in the Netherlands* (Rotterdam: NAi Publishers, 2010).
2. Peter Swinnen, "Onzichtbare zorg," in *Pilootprojecten Onzichtbare Zorg: Innoverende Zorgarchitectuur*, ed. Joeri De Bruyn and Stijn De Vleeschouwer (Brussels: Team Flemish Government Architect, 2014), 6. Lisa De Visscher, "Take Care!," *A+ Architecture in Belgium* 283 (April-May 2020): 15. See also the entry on "Caring Neighbourhoods," in the "The Great Transformation 2020–2030" project, organized by Architecture Workroom Brussels.
3. Samuel Tuke, *Description of the Retreat: An Institution Near York for Insane Persons of the Society of Friends* (York, 1813). See Michel Foucault, *Madness and Civilization: A History of Insanity in the Age of Reason* (Abingdon: Routledge, 2001), 229–264.
4. This chapter draws on research conducted together with Vjera Sleutel (BAVO). See Gideon Boie, ed., *Living in Monnikenheide: Care, Inclusion and Architecture* (Antwerp: Flanders Architecture Institute, 2023).
5. The history of Monnikenheide is documented in Wivina Demeester-De Meyer, Kris De Koninck, and Johan Vermeeren, eds., *Monnikenheide 40* (Zoersel: Monnikenheide, 2014).
6. The history of the Vlaams Bouwmeester (Flemish Government Architect) is documented in Marc Santens and Jan De Zutter, *Het Vlaams Bouwmeesterschap 1999–2005* (Antwerp: Houtekiet, 2008).
7. Foucault, *Madness and Civilization*, 35–60.
8. "Adieu to the Bed House: Design Challenges in Residential Care," lecture, organized by the Dr. Guislain Museum and others, Ghent, September 24, 2019. See the report: Vjera Sleutel, "Adieu aan het Beddenhuis: verslag," Flanders Architecture Institute, September 2019, https://www.vai.be/nieuws/verslag-studienamiddag-adieu-aan-het-beddenhuis. An abridged version of the address was published in the *A+* issue on care architecture: Wivina Demeester, "Opinie," *A+ Architecture in Belgium* 283 (April-May 2020): 7.
9. Cornelis B. Bakker and Marianne K. Bakker-Rabdau, *No Trespassing! Explorations in Human Territoriality* (San Francisco: Chandler & Sharp, 1973).
10. Michael Speaks argued that design intelligence is constructed through daily chatter rather than fixed typologies and heroic forms. See Michael Speaks, "Design Intelligence," in *Constructing a New Agenda*, ed. A. K. Sykes (New York: Princeton Architectural Press, 2010), 204–215.
11. The "bed house" is a neologism, first used by a patient at the Karus Psychiatric Hospital, who added the prefix "bed" (i.e., the calculation unit for government funding of hospitals in Belgium) to *ziekenhuizen* (hospitals). It is used as a name for the large-scale hospital facilities mainly consisting of bedrooms, stripped bare of other necessities of life. See Gideon Boie, "Design Your Symptom," in BAVO and architecten De Vylder Vinck Taillieu, *Unless Ever People* (Antwerp: Flanders Architecture Institute, 2018), 186–223.
12. Heleen Verheyden, "Architecture of Presence," in *Living in Monnikenheide: Care, Inclusion and Architecture*, ed. Gideon Boie (Antwerp: Flanders Architecture Institute, 2023).
13. Slavoj Žižek, *The Ticklish Subject* (London: Verso, 1999), 72.
14. Michel Foucault argued that the program of resocialization was, after all, a strange thing considering the fact that we first separate these people. Although justified as critique, the argument does not take into account that separation might be necessary in some delicate care programs. Foucault, *Madness and Civilization*, 229–264.

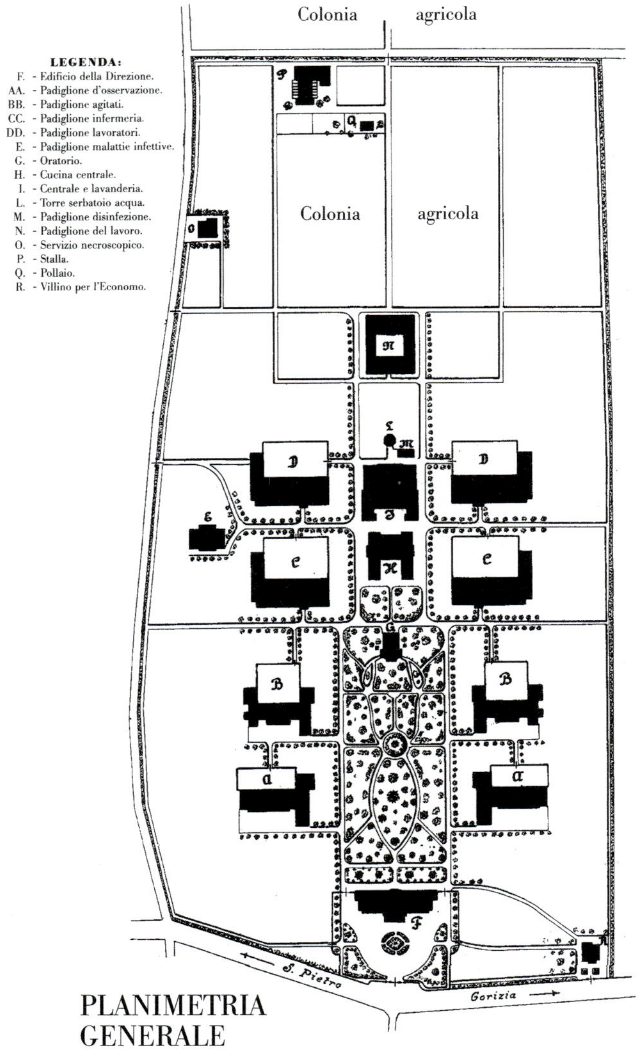

↑ Site plan of the provincial asylum Franz Joseph I, Görz, 1913.

NEGATION AND DEINSTITUTIONALIZATION

GIUSEPPINA SCAVUZZO

In 1978 all psychiatric hospitals in Italy were closed under the newly enacted Law 180, or the "Basaglia Law." Its namesake, the psychiatrist Franco Basaglia, was a decisive figure in the medical and political-cultural movement to reform the treatment of mental illness that emerged in Italy in the 1960s and 1970s. Thanks to the participation of doctors, intellectuals, politicians, photographers, and journalists, the movement helped change representations of the mentally ill and the function of internment, which until then had been anchored in nineteenth-century cultural and scientific models. Their actions led to the closure of asylums and a new approach that involved the community as a whole in the treatment of patients, ushering in so-called "deinstitutionalization."[1] Law 180 regulated compulsory medical treatment by guaranteeing psychiatric patients civil and political rights as much as possible, including the right to choose the place of treatment. The Italian process of deinstitutionalizing psychiatric hospitals is a unique case, which, even before the adoption of Law 180, placed Italy at the center of an international dialogue on managing and treating mental distress.[2]

Article 7 of Law 180 states: "It is in any case forbidden to build new psychiatric hospitals, [and] to use existing ones as specialist psychiatric divisions of general hospitals."[3] Acknowledging the profound impact that architectural environments exert on psychiatric care practices, this is the only case in Italian history in which a law has prohibited an architectural typology. Basaglia's intention was to replace psychiatric hospitals with community-integrated care systems, an approach that was grounded in his recognition of the social dimensions of psychiatric suffering. He posited that societal factors contributed to the onset and perpetuation of mental illness, with institutionalization serving to exacerbate rather than alleviate such conditions. However, this replacement was undermined by the hasty and incomplete application of the law. As a result, the law effectively interrupted the dialogue that had been ongoing between practitioners in the fields of architecture and psychiatry, which had in fact contributed to the development and approval of this new legislation.[4]

Gorizia: A Border Asylum

Basaglia's efforts to change psychiatric practice began many years before the adoption of Law 180, as director of the Provincial Psychiatric Hospital of Gorizia from 1961 to 1969. Together with a team of doctors and nurses, Basaglia confronted the inherent contradictions of institutionalized care, with the overarching goal of transcending and ultimately dismantling the very institution in which they operated.[5]

Gorizia is a small city on the border between Italy and Slovenia with a long history of territorial disputes and an interweaving of different cultures, identities, and languages. When its first asylum, named for Emperor Franz Joseph I, was built in 1911, the town was called Görz and was still part of the Austro-Hungarian Empire. The asylum was one of seven built between 1890 and the outbreak of World War I in various regions under the Hapsburg crown.[6] Steinhof, designed by Otto Wagner in Vienna, was the largest asylum in Europe at the time, and had been the model for the other six, almost all of which were designed by Viennese architects.[7]

The asylum in Görz was the smallest of the seven but followed the same layout as the rest, with a central axis containing services and administration dividing a symmetrical series of pavilions into male- and female-only areas. The spaces reflected a wider debate in Vienna on the balance between freedom, privacy, and control in psychiatric institutions:[8] the gardens were richly designed, with fences disguised as hedges, while the interiors were divided into first-class rooms that resembled hotel suites, second-class dormitories, and restraining cells.[9]

The outbreak of World War I prompted the evacuation of inmates from Görz—which was located on the front lines—to Kremsier, in Moravia, another region of the Austro-Hungarian Empire (now Kroměříž, Czechia). At the end of the war, Görz transitioned to Italian sovereignty, and its name changed to Gorizia. The asylum had also been destroyed, so the inmates—who were no longer Hapsburg subjects nor Czech—were transferred first to Siena and then to Venice.[10] They never made it back to Gorizia.

The Provincial Psychiatric Hospital of Gorizia was built in Fascist Italy in 1933 and was modeled on the plan of the original Austro-Hungarian asylum. However, the first-class pavilions were not rebuilt, and because private clinics proliferated elsewhere in the region for affluent patients, the hospital became a refuge for the economically disadvantaged. Proponents of the deinstitutionalization movement gave it the epithet "asylum of the poor," which underscored the facility's transformation into a repository for society's marginalized, extending beyond the mentally ill.

In place of the original asylum's first-class pavilions, a new pavilion was built, the small "villino dell'economo" ("treasurer's cottage"), which was located directly on the street but connected to the hospital entrance, the administration building, and the area of the pavilions by way of three private paths. At the center of the asylum, then, was not the psychiatrist but the treasurer. The prosperous agricultural colony that had been annexed to the institute—and for which inmates performed free labor—made the asylum "a convenient place to get rid of inconvenient people."[11]

In 1947, the borders around Gorizia shifted again with the American soldiers' delineation of the "Iron Curtain" that cut directly through the city. An existing wall—that of the asylum, which already seemingly divided the world into two—was used to guide its path. Inmates from territories that had been cut away and given to Yugoslavia were declared *a-polidi* ("stateless," literally "without a city," a *polis*), only further emphasizing the extraterritoriality of madness.[12] This intersection of madness and borders formed the crux of Basaglia's anti-institutional psychiatry movement, wherein psychiatric care extended beyond treatment to encompass broader questions of otherness and identity—Italians becoming Yugoslavs, or a sane person becoming, or being declared, insane. Not only was the hospital itself a site of alienation—from the Latin word *alius*, meaning "the other"—Gorizia was also a place where Slovenian-speaking Italian people were linguistically othered by being referred to as "allophone." These conditions were often incarnated in the same bodies that the hospital treated.

Basaglia contested the reduction of individuals deemed mentally ill to mere objects, advocating instead for the recognition of their inherent humanity and agency within society. This perspective acknowledged the intertwined nature of insanity and societal marginalization, urging a reevaluation of prevailing attitudes toward mental health and otherness.

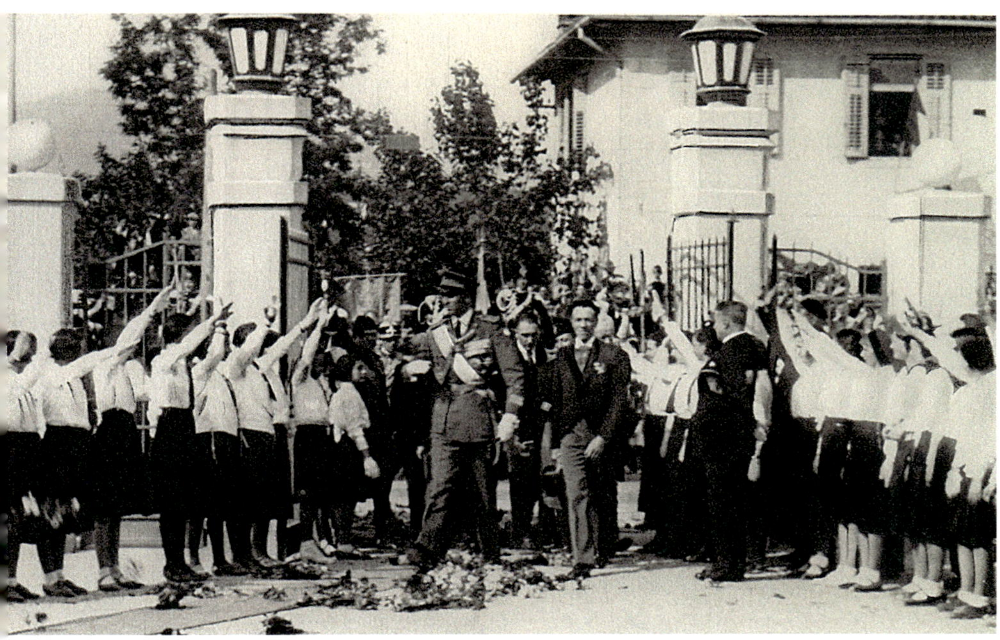

← The Duke of Aosta inaugurates the Provincial Psychiatric Hospital, 1933.

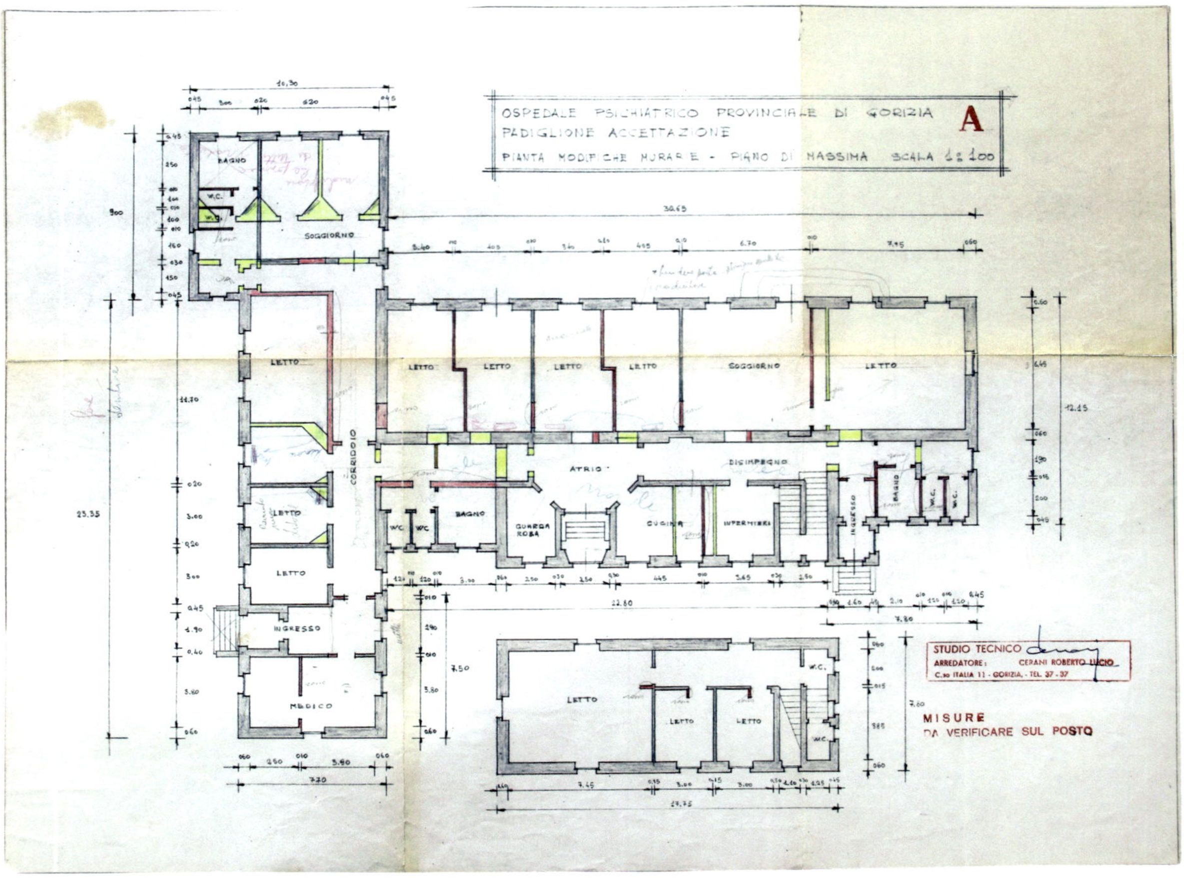

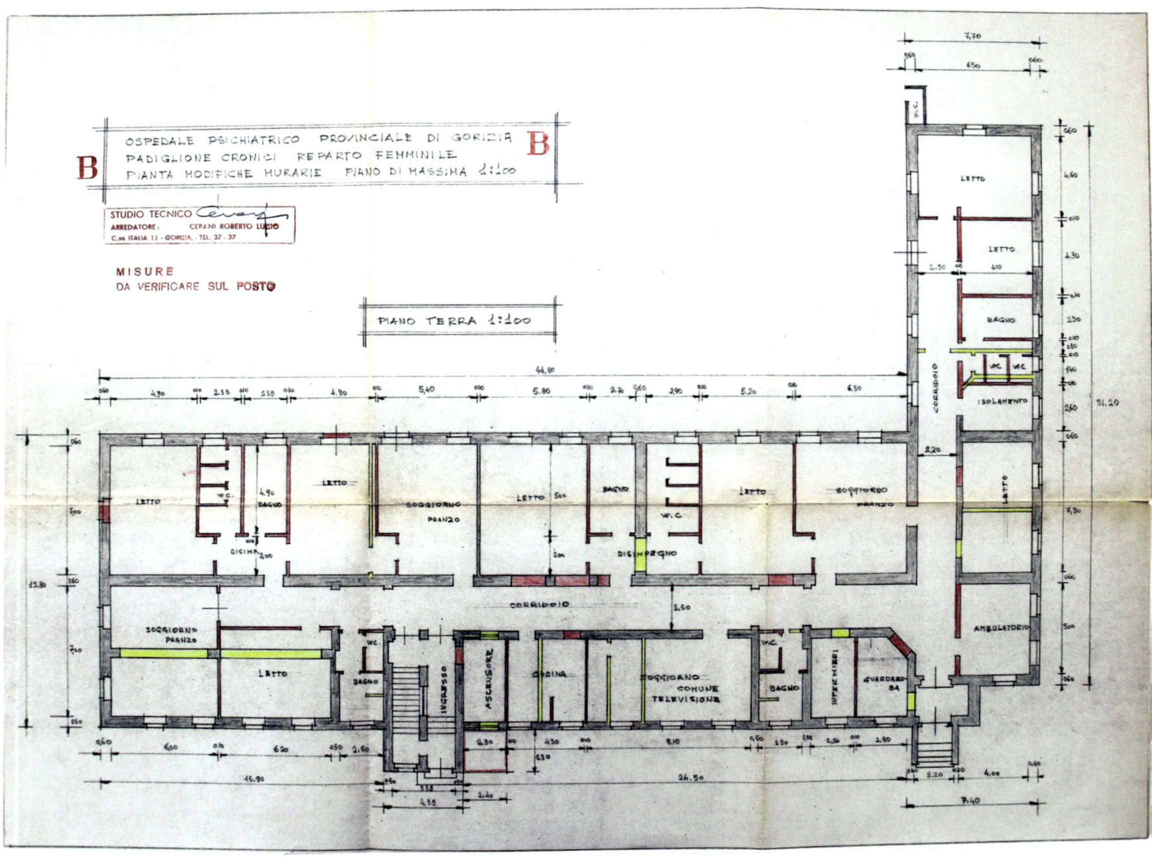

↑ Plan of the women's admissions pavilion of the psychiatric hospital in Gorizia, with indications of demolitions and new constructions according to Basaglia's project, 1964.

↓ Plan of the women's chronic pavilion of the psychiatric hospital in Gorizia, with indications of demolitions and new constructions according to Basaglia's project, 1964.

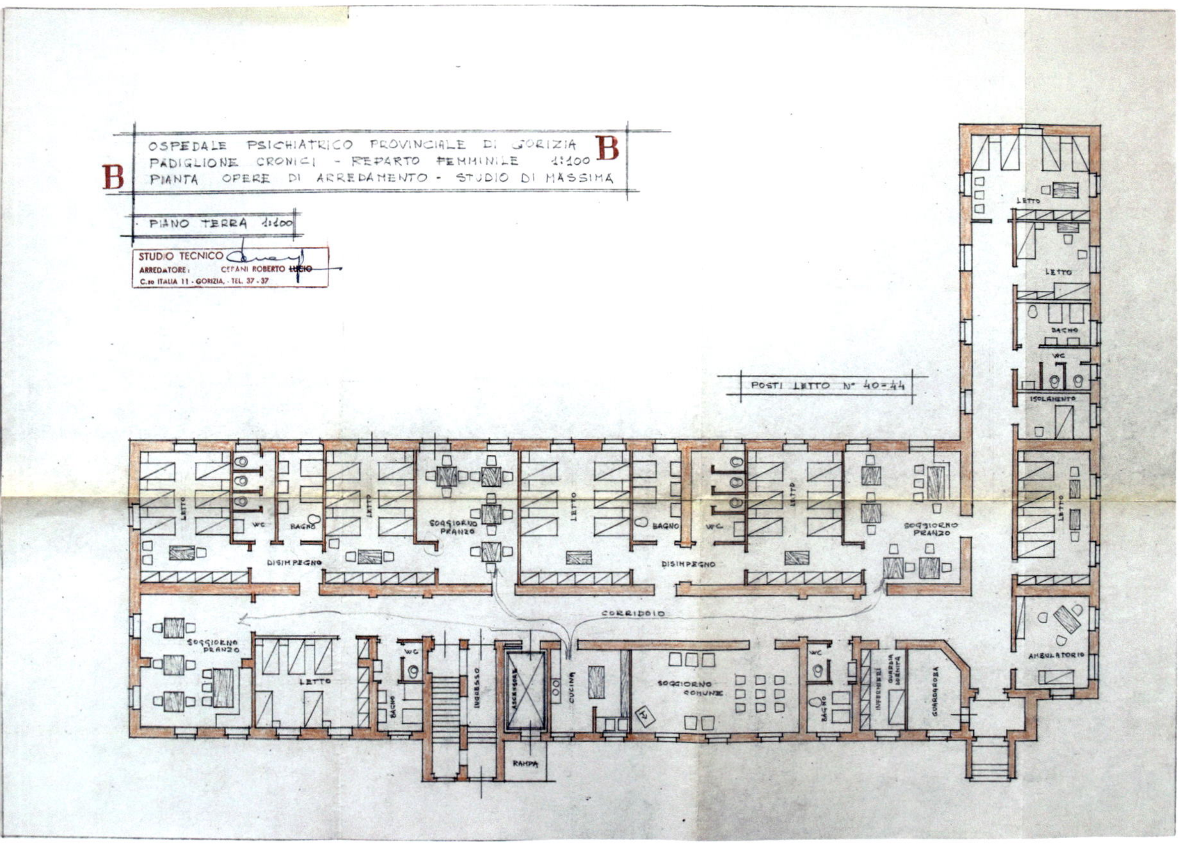

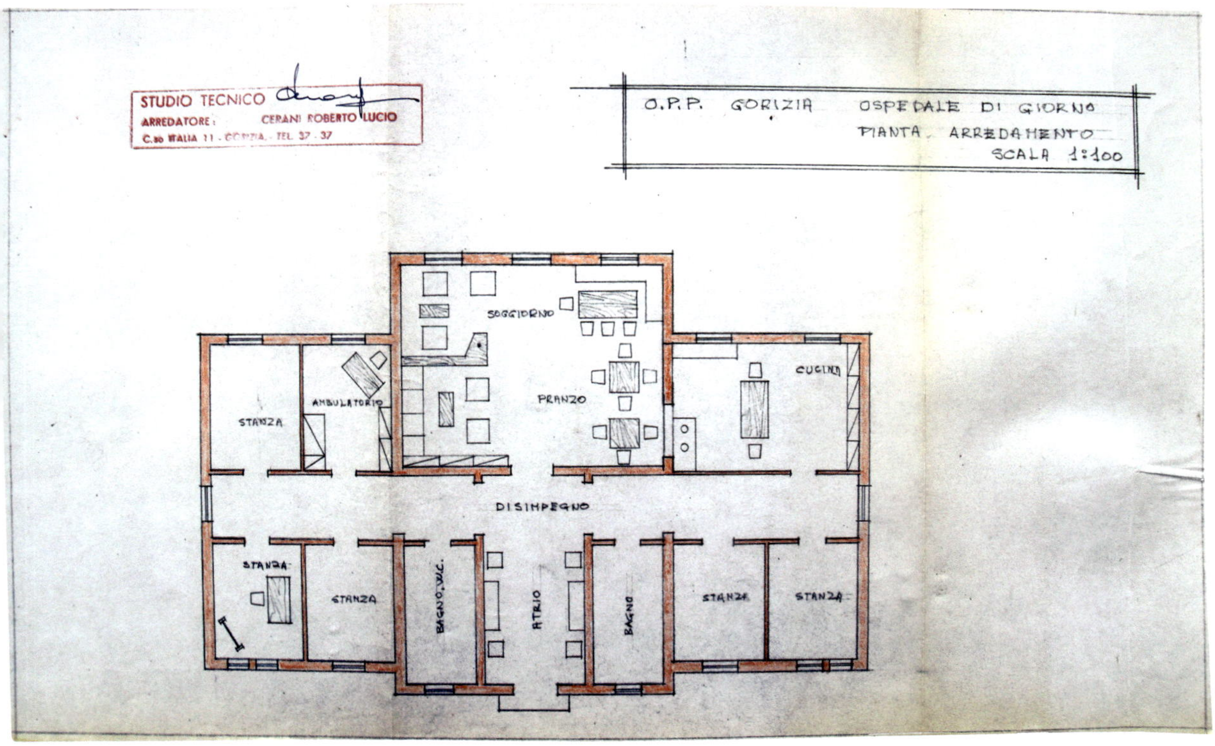

↑ Furnished plan of the women's chronic pavilion of the psychiatric hospital in Gorizia, demonstrating the results of the demolitions and new constructions according to Basaglia's project, 1964.

↓ Furnished plan of the new day clinic typology according to Basaglia's project, 1964.

Negating an Institution

When Basaglia arrived in Gorizia in 1961, people like Jean-Paul Sartre and Michel Foucault viewed mental health treatment as a measure of society's democratic health.[13] The hospital of Gorizia emblematically exemplified a "heterotopic" condition, surrounded as it was by a real border which the inmates carried with them as a sign of exclusion.[14] This did not escape the notice of Foucault, who closely observed Basaglia's endeavors in Gorizia and acknowledged the impact of psychiatric deinstitutionalization on his own advocacy, particularly regarding prison reform.[15] Both Foucault and Basaglia shared the conviction that for every manifestation of deviance—whether criminal or psychiatric—the social marginalization that generated it must be taken into account. For both, madness only begins to claim its part in history when it emerges from the silence of exclusion.[16]

Basaglia's process of negating institutionalization extended to physical reforms within psychiatric hospital settings.[17] At Gorizia, he initiated changes to address the contradictory nature of asylum boundaries, which imposed confinement while disregarding personal space and privacy. Even before abolishing the use of electroshock therapy, straitjackets, and cages, one of Basaglia's first acts as director in Gorizia was to give inmates, who had been deprived of all personal belongings on hospital admission, bedside tables. These small pieces of furniture provided a personal space in which to keep objects and memories, facilitating the reconstruction of their denied subjectivity.

At Gorizia, Basaglia sought to create an architecture that would support the process of liberation from institutional life. In 1962, together with Daniele Calabi, architect and professor at the IUAV University of Venice, Basaglia wrote a "Preliminary Study for the Reorganization of the Psychiatric Hospital of Gorizia."[18] This text, devoid of illustrations, criticized the idea of compulsory internment as therapy and proposed a new diagnostic center alongside the conversion of pavilions into residential spaces termed "homes for the patients." Pavilions would thus cease to be therapeutic environments associated with institutional life.

The death of Calabi and the slowness in acquiring funding for the proposed reorganization led Basaglia to start modifying the interiors of the

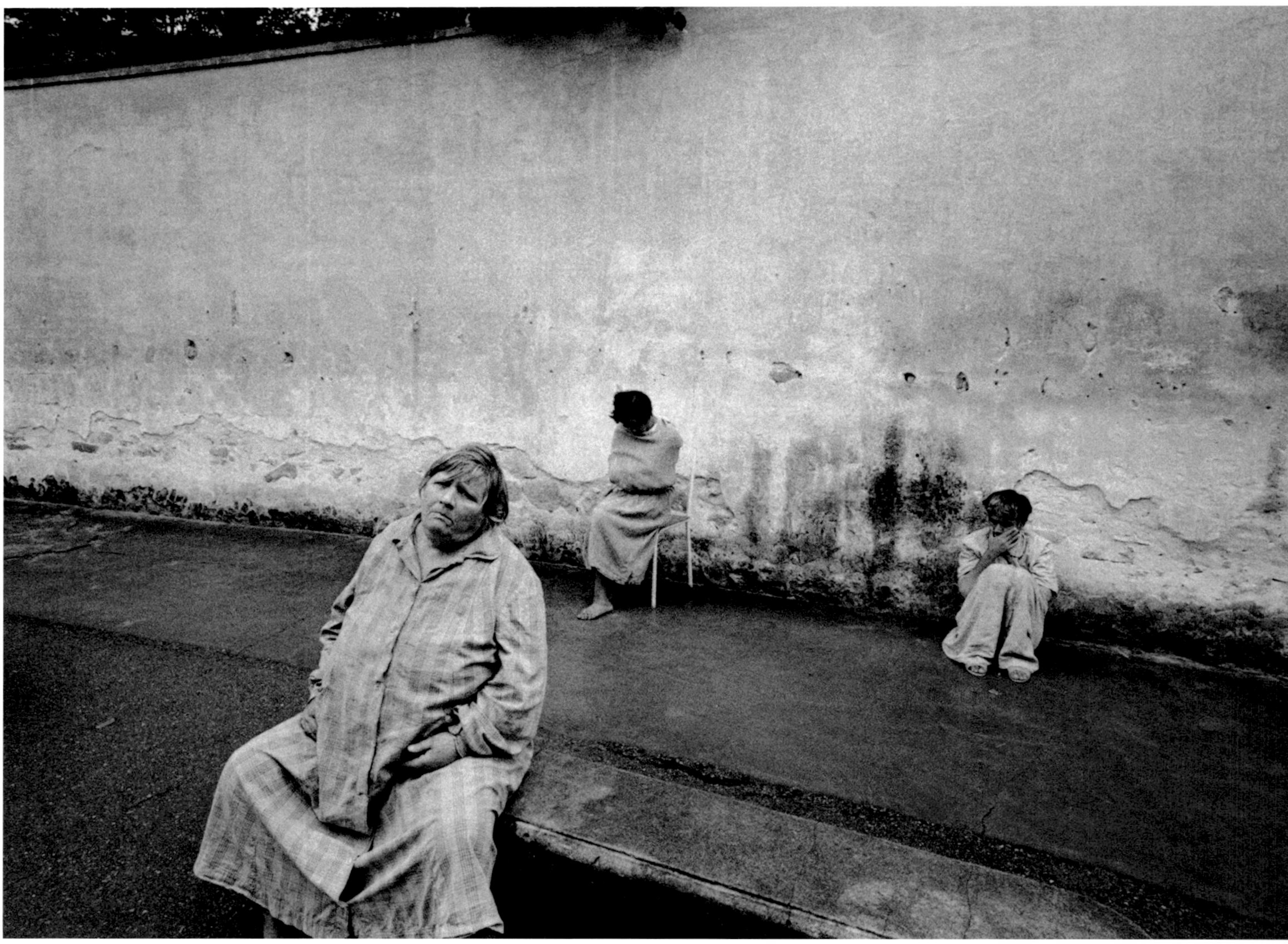

↑ Photo included within *Morire di classe* (Turin: Giulio Einaudi, 1969).

pavilions and transforming the infectious disease pavilion into a day hospital, a smaller version of the diagnostic center, which he had designed together with Calabi. Drawings for this project were commissioned to a local interior designer, while Basaglia wrote the project report.[19] The drawings show the proposed demolition of isolation cells and the reconfiguration of dormitories through a process termed "nucleation," in which "nuclei" rooms accommodating small groups of patients were to be equipped with new service blocks and living and dining spaces. Transitional spaces were conceived to balance privacy and social interaction, countering the rigid surveillance architecture of the Fascist era. Additional communal areas were designated for general assemblies, which allowed doctors, nurses, and patients to engage in dialogue and restore patients' right to speak.[20]

In 1967, Basaglia drafted an article for the special issue on "Programmation, Architecture, and Psychiatry" of *Recherches*, published by the Center for Institutional Studies, Research, and Training (CERFI), under the direction of Félix Guattari.[21] The article advanced his radical criticism of the psychiatric institution as a form of social exclusion and segregation, denouncing how the mentally ill person embodied the contradictions of a society based on myths of well-being, competitiveness, and productivity. Basaglia argued that traditional psychiatric hospitals primarily served to conceal and deny aspects of society deemed undesirable, rather than providing genuine treatment. To escape this form of removal, psychiatry needed to devise new therapeutic forms, such as the "Therapeutic Community," alongside architectural designs that facilitated personal meaning-making rather than imposing spaces onto patients.[22]

This call for transformative architecture was reiterated in Basaglia's report for the 1968 Ministerial Committee for the Transformation of Hospital Facilities, established by the Italian National Health Ministry and to which Basaglia was nominated to be a member. Here he emphasized the need for psychiatric architecture to acknowledge the transient nature of patients' conditions. He proposed integrating care facilities into urban contexts, including day, night, and weekend hospitals, to counteract the perception of psychiatric institutions as the ultimate and definitive destinations for mental health treatment.[23]

Recognizing psychiatry as both a medical and sociopolitical issue, Basaglia employed a "narrative machine" to raise social awareness and used both media-based and spatial tools to communicate the reality of the asylum.[24] For example, the photo book *Morire di classe* (*Dying Because of Your Class*), made in Gorizia in 1968, depicted the dehumanizing reality of the asylum through stark images of patients' bodies in desolate spaces.[25] These photographs could only be published because the patients they portrayed lacked all civil rights that would protect their image and dignity. Meanwhile, the film *I giardini di Abele* (*Abel's Gardens*), produced by Italian public television the same year, showcased the positive transformations occurring under Basaglia's direction, with patients sharing their stories amidst more dignified surroundings.[26] In the documentary, the insane are identified with Abel, the nomadic shepherd and weak brother of the elder Cain, the farmer, settler, and builder of cities and borders, who eventually kills his younger sibling. Another documentary, *La favola del serpente* (*The Snake's Tale*), by the Finnish journalist Pirkko Peltonen, depicted the development and evolution of hospital facilities in Gorizia, including new amenities like a bar and a hair salon, alongside abstract murals in communal areas where assemblies were held.[27] The film captured patients participating in decisions about their representation in the documentary, highlighting debates over payment and their portrayal to external audiences. Some patients argue that new methods of treatment improved their lives and should be shared for free, "like penicillin." Another patient, with extraordinary awareness, argues that the sick must receive payment as actors, because those who will watch the film outside the hospital will see them as characters of a comedy: the mask of depression, the mask of schizophrenia, the mask of dementia, etc. The snake of the title refers to an apologue told by Basaglia, in which a snake enters the mouth of a man and begins to dominate him, preventing him from desiring and having a will of his own. One morning, the man feels that the snake has left but realizes he no longer knows what to do with this freedom. Basaglia's parable underscored the journey of patients reclaiming their autonomy after institutionalization, signifying the transformative potential of space in community-building and advocacy for mental health rights.

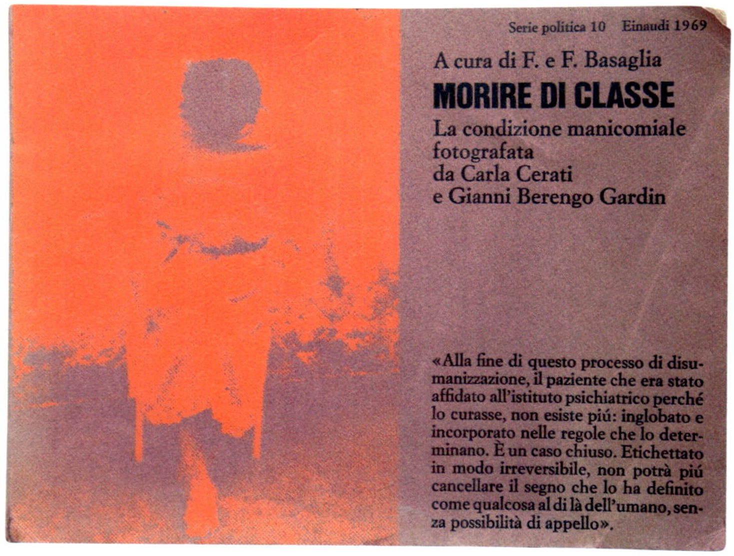

↑ Cover of *Morire di classe* (Turin: Giulio Einaudi, 1969).

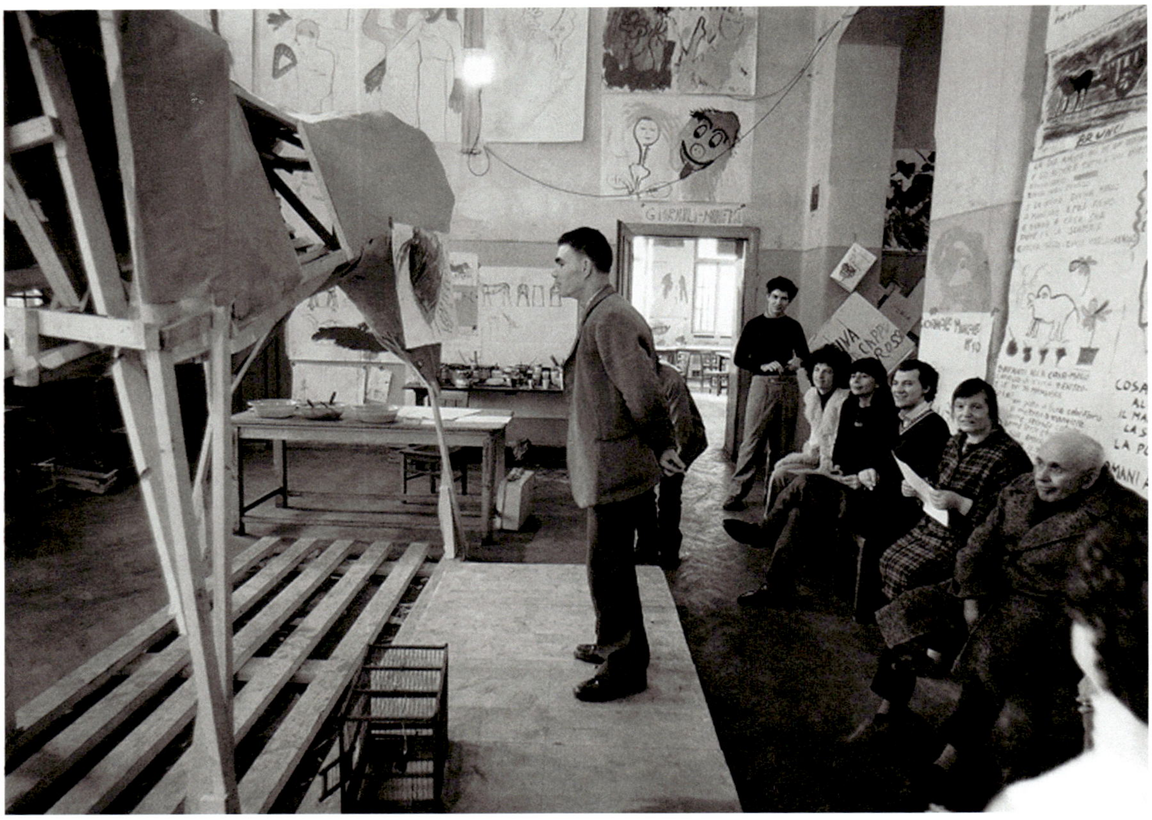

← Patients building Marco Cavallo in the psychiatric hospital of Trieste, 1973.

→ Marco Cavallo in the streets of Trieste, 1973.

Trieste: Deinstitutionalization

Basaglia's experience in Gorizia ended in 1968, when a murder committed by a patient on leave resulted in legal proceedings, a hostile climate in the city, and ultimately his resignation. In 1971, he assumed the directorship of the Trieste Psychiatric Hospital, another institution dating back to the Austro-Hungarian Empire. Here, Basaglia continued his efforts to deinstitutionalize psychiatry while further garnering international attention. Trieste was selected in 1973 as Italy's "pilot zone" for the World Health Organization's research on mental health services. This allowed Basaglia and his team to advance their work restoring patients' subjectivity and rights. By 1977, the Trieste Psychiatric Hospital was officially closed and replaced by a therapeutic community, laying the groundwork for the enactment of Law 180 the following year.

Upon his arrival in Trieste, Basaglia engaged the Venetian architectural firm Bellavitis & Valle to devise a comprehensive plan for the redevelopment and urban integration of the psychiatric hospital. Over five years, the firm proposed various interventions, including the redesign of internal roads, the restoration of pavilions for residential and hospital use, and interior refurbishments. For Basaglia, these modifications represented a temporary and transitional arrangement before the hospital's definitive closure. Like the interventions carried out in Gorizia, they aimed to eliminate the institutional character of the pavilions and transform them into residential spaces. The overarching goal was for patients to leave the institution, live independently, and only come to the hospital—or other community-based care centers decentralized across the city—for treatment. These architectural transformations faced administrative delays and funding issues, yet the process of deinstitutionalization continued. While permits for construction work were still pending, thanks to the establishment of the "pilot zone," patients were allowed to move out of the institution and find housing in the city. They did this with the help of doctors and nurses, who often acted as guarantors for rental contracts.

Once patients were allowed to move out of the institution, the Bellavitis & Valle project became obsolete. In 1976, Basaglia drafted an article for *Casabella* entitled "Psychiatry and Architecture," reflecting on the unrealized Trieste project.[28] This epilogue revealed a crisis in the relationship between architecture and psychiatric institutions, particularly concerning the transition from institutional to community-based care. While institutional psychiatry provided technical directives to architects, wrote Basaglia, deinstitutionalization challenged the profession to support the significance of the individual and collective well-being without predefined typologies.

Basaglia's last narrative tool, which he developed at Trieste, was known as Marco Cavallo (Mark the Horse), a blue papier-mâché horse created by patients in 1973, who carried it out of the hospital and marched in a procession through the streets of the city. As opposed to a Trojan horse, Marco Cavallo

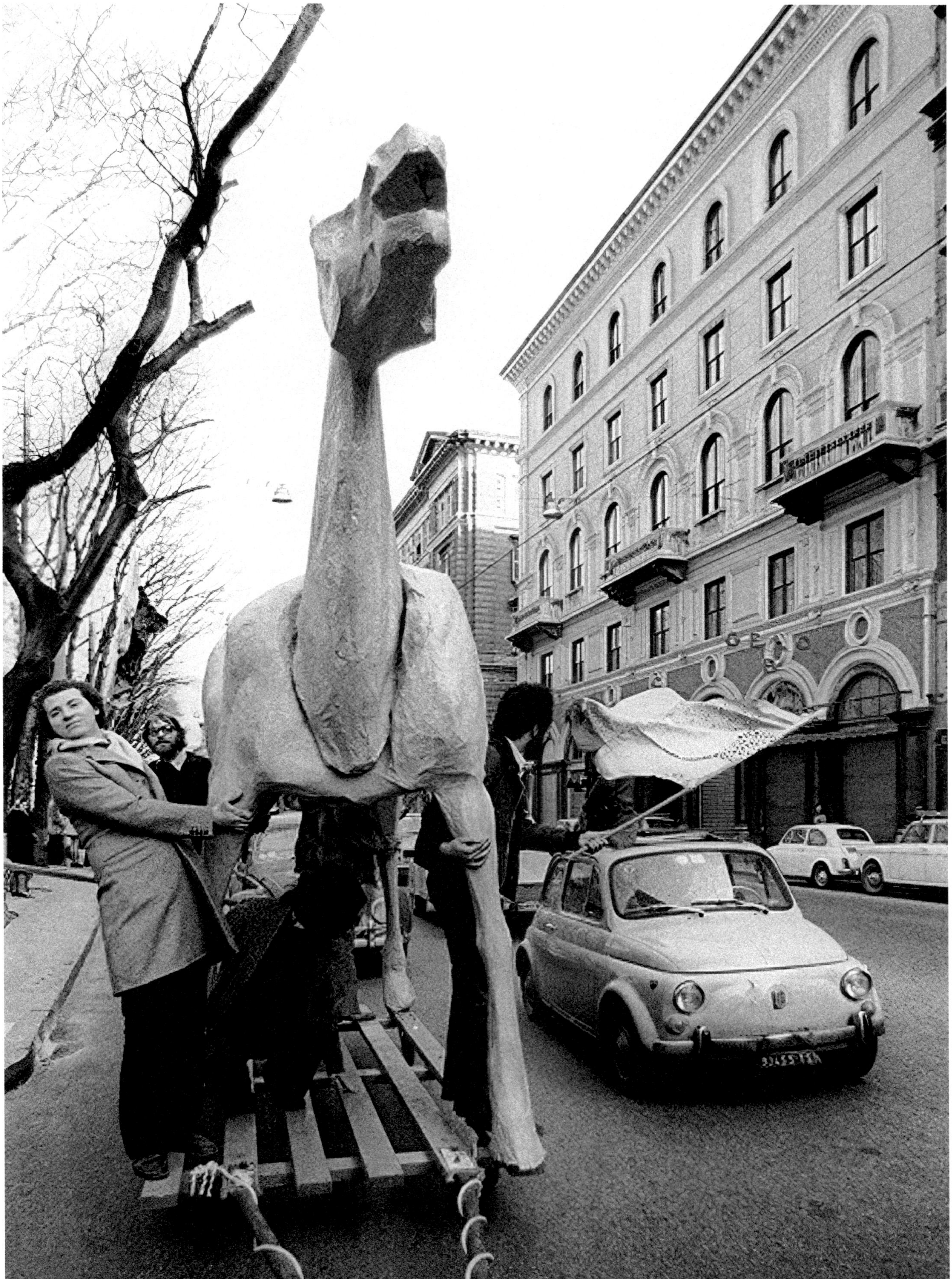

came out of the walls of the fortified city—the boundaries of the asylum—with its belly full of desires written by the inmates. Marco Cavallo symbolized the patients' emergence from institutional confines with aspirations for life beyond the hospital's walls, setting a stark contrast with the void left by institutional departure depicted in Basaglia's parable of the snake.

Law 180 was enacted in 1978, marking both the closure of psychiatric hospitals and the conclusion of research into mental health architecture in Italy. Many questions were left unanswered regarding architecture's role in anti-institutional psychiatry. Basaglia, who had become seriously ill, asked the architect to "open his eyes and ears to see and hear, beyond the claims of prevailing reason, the demands of the dispossessed."[29] Instead, however, architecture seems to respond only to the power of reason, which for both Basaglia and Foucault silences madness. Basaglia died two years later.

The history of the Gorizia and Trieste hospitals prompts reflection on architecture's relationship to psychiatric institutions and advocates for a transfer of imaginative power to support inhabitants' projects rather than reinforcing institutional or societal structures. Ultimately, this demand for architectural activism echoes the call to militancy that Foucault heard coming from the Gorizian Revolution and that Marco Cavallo proclaimed on Trieste's streets.

In 1973, the movement became more structured by taking the name Psichiatria Democratica (democratic psychiatry) and included several psychiatrists and intellectuals who shared the need for a social and political approach to psychiatric care.
2. The Italian case has been the focus of many studies carried out both nationally (Valeria Babini, *Liberi tutti. Manicomi e psichiatri in Italia: una storia del Novecento* [Bologna: Il Mulino, 2009]) and internationally (John Foot, *The Man Who Closed the Asylums: Franco Basaglia and the Revolution in Mental Health Care* [New York: Verso Books, 2015]).
3. Law no. 180 of the Italian Republic dated May 13, 1978, "Accertamenti e trattamenti sanitari volontari e obbligatori," Article 7.
4. This article draws on research conducted at the University of Trieste, which is documented in Giuseppina Scavuzzo, *Il parco della guarigione infinita. Un dialogo tra architettura e psichiatria* (Syracuse: LetteraVentidue Edizioni 2020).
5. This is chronicled in Basaglia's seminal work, Franco Basaglia, ed., *L'istituzione negata. Rapporto da un ospedale psichiatrico* (Turin: Einaudi, 1968).
6. The institutions were the following: the Franz Josef Regional Asylum in Mauer-Öhling, Austria (1898–1902); Otto Wagner's hospital of Steinhof in Vienna, Austria (1904–1907); Franz Josef I Sanatorium of Kremsier, Moravia, today Kroměříž, Czech Republic (1905–1908); Andrea di Sergio Galatti Civic Asylum, Trieste, Austria, today Italy (1904–1908); Francesco Giuseppe I Provincial Asylum, Görz, Austria, today Gorizia, Italy (1905–1908); Royal Asylum of Prague, Bohemia, now the Czech Republic (1905–1924); Institute for Mental and Nervous Diseases of Kobierzyn, Galicia, today Poland (1910–1924).
7. Leslie Topp, *Freedom and the Cage: Modern Architecture and Psychiatry in Central Europe, 1890–1914* (University Park, PA: Penn State University Press, 2017).
8. In Vienna at the time, there was no lack of attacks on the psychiatric institution in relation to the conflict between the protection of individual freedom and the demands of social control. Among the most famous and pointed critiques were those of Karl Kraus. See Karl Kraus, *Sittlichkeit und Kriminalität* (Vienna: Rosner, 1908).
9. Leslie Topp, "Isolation, Privacy, Control and Privilege: Psychiatric Architecture and the Single Room," in *Healing Spaces, Modern Architecture and the Body*, ed. S. Schrank and D. Ekici (Abingdon: Routledge, 2016), 85–102.
10. This wandering around Europe bears resemblance to Michel Foucault's depiction of the *Stultifera Navis*, or ship of fools, evoking the displacement experienced by individuals marginalized due to their mental health, sometimes entrusted to "boats that conveyed their insane cargo from town to town." Michel Foucault, *Madness and Civilization: A History of Insanity in the Age of Reason* (New York: Random House, 1965), 8.
11. Andrew T. Scull, "A Convenient Place to Get Rid of Inconvenient People: The Victorian Lunatic Asylum," in *Buildings and Society: Essays on the Social Development of the Built Environment*, ed. Anthony D. King (London: Routledge & Kegan Paul, 1980).
12. Antonio Slavich, *All'ombra dei ciliegi giapponesi. Gorizia 1961* (Merano: Edizioni Alpha Beta Verlag, 2018), 22.
13. In 1967, Jean-Paul Sartre wrote: "If you want to see a reality where practical knowledge is developed, go to Gorizia." Cited by Babini, *Liberi tutti*, 178. Michel Foucault, who authored an essay titled "La casa della follia" ("The House of Madness") for Basaglia's book *Crimini di pace* (*Crimes of Peace*), was interested in what was being attempted in Gorizia, to the extent that he was "jealous" of what Basaglia and other psychiatrists were putting into practice from his book *History of Madness,* which he claimed gave his theoretical work a concrete, militant outcome. Michel Foucault, "La casa della follia," in *Crimini di pace. Ricerche sugli intellettuali e sui tecnici come addetti all'oppressione*, ed. Franco Basaglia and Franca Ongaro Basaglia (Turin: Einaudi, 1975). Michel Foucault, "Un problème m'intéresse depuis longtemps, c'est celui du système pénal," in conversation with J. Hafsia, in *La Presse de Tunisie*, August 12, 1971, 3; and subsequently in *Dits et* écrits. *1954–1988*, vol. 2, ed. D. Defert and F. Ewald (Paris: Gallimard, 1994), 209. "In recent years there has been a movement in Italy around Basaglia, and also in Britain, known as 'anti-psychiatry'. Of course, these people developed their movement from their own ideas and experiences as psychiatrists, but they saw in the book I had written a kind of historical justification and somehow made it their own; they have, to a certain extent, recognized themselves in it and behold, this historical book is having a kind of practical outcome. So let's say that I am a little jealous and that I would now like to do these things by myself. Rather than writing a book on the history of justice, which would then be taken up by people who actually question justice, I would like to begin practically by questioning justice." Translated by the author. Michel Foucault, *Folie et déraison—Histoire de la folie* à *l'âge classique* (Paris: Librairie Plon, 1961).
14. Michel Foucault, "Des espaces autres," in *Dits et* écrits. *1954–1988*, vol. 4, ed. D. Defert and F. Ewald (Paris, Gallimard, 1994).
15. Foucault, *Dits et* écrits, vol. 2, 209.
16. Pierangelo Di Vittorio, *Foucault e Basaglia. L'incontro tra genealogie e movimenti di base* (Verona: Ombre Corte, 1999), 161.
17. Basaglia, *L'istituzione negata*.
18. "Studio preliminare per il riordinamento dell'ospedale psichiatrico di Gorizia," June 1, 1962, signed by Daniele Calabi and Franco Basaglia. Archives of the Friuli Venezia Giulia Region, files 1955–1990.
19. This material was only recently discovered by the author—along with the program written with Calabi—among the documents related to the hospital of Gorizia, all of which were transferred to Trieste in the 1990s, after the management of the hospital was transferred from the Province of Gorizia to the Friuli Venezia Giulia Region, of which Trieste is the capital. It consists of four plans: a furnished plan of the day hospital, obtained from the transformation of the infectious diseases pavilion; a plan of the women's admissions pavilion with indications of demolitions and new constructions; two plans of the women's chronic pavilion, one with indications of demolitions and new constructions, and the other with furnishings. The drawings are not numbered but can be found in the folder "Expansion and renovation of the Provincial Psychiatric Hospital of Gorizia. Project and state contribution," Archives of the Friuli Venezia Giulia Region, files 1955–1990.
20. In these Gorizia assemblies, Foucault saw the possibility that, finally, "the victims of the asylum could begin a political struggle against the social structure which had denounced them as insane." "Basaglia tried experiments of this kind in Italy: he brought together the patients, the doctors, and the hospital staff. It was not a matter of repeating a socio-drama during which everyone could bring out his or her ghosts, but of asking this question: would the victims of the asylum launch a political struggle against a social structure that denounced them as insane?" Michel Foucault, *Microfisica del potere: interventi politici* (Turin: Einaudi, 1977), 66. Translated by the author.
21. The article was considered too theoretical and political to be included in the special issue, whose goal was to provide institutions with useful proposals for renewal actions. It was therefore published in another issue of the magazine: Gian Franco Minguzzi, Franco Basaglia, and Franca Ongaro Basaglia, "Exclusion, programmation et intégration," *Recherches*, no. 5 (1967): 75–84.
22. Minguzzi, Basaglia, and Basaglia, "Exclusion, programmation et intégration," 82.
23. Franco Basaglia, "Relazione alla Commissione di studio per l'aggiornamento delle vigenti istruzioni per le costruzioni ospedaliere del Ministero della Sanità," in Franco Basaglia, *Scritti, 1953–1980* (Milan: Il Saggiatore 2017), 517.
24. See Marina Guglielmi, *Raccontare il manicomio. La macchina narrativa di Basaglia fra parole e immagini* (Florence: Franco Cesati Editore, 2018).
25. Franco Basaglia and Franca Ongaro Basaglia, eds., *Morire di classe. La condizione manicomiale fotografata da Carla Cerati e Gianni Berengo Gardin* (Turin: Einaudi, 1969).
26. *I giardini di Abele*, directed by Sergio Zavoli, produced by RAI, 1968, https://archive.org/details/i-giardini-di-abele.
27. *La favola del serpente*, directed by Pirkko Peltonen, produced by the Finnish Broadcasting Company (Yleisradio Oy), 1968, https://www.youtube.com/watch?v=0iNUax7sTKA.
28. The essay was drafted together with his wife, Franca Ongaro—who coauthored many of his writings—and the two architects Giorgio Bellavitis and Nani Valle. "Schema di un articolo per *Casabella*," with annotation: [Provisional Title] "Psichiatria e architettura," to be drafted in collaboration with Franca Ongaro Basaglia, Giorgio Bellavitis, and Nani Valle, typescript, seven copies; Basaglia Archive, Series 9 Works, Subseries 9.1, file. 5, 1972–1980.
29. Franco Basaglia, "Introduzione," in S. Santiano, *B come architetture, z come salute* (Perugia: Bertoni, 1980), 5.

p148, 149 Reproduced from *L'Ospedale psichiatrico provinciale di Gorizia*, 1933.
p150–151, 152 Archives of the Friuli Venezia Giulia Region.
p154, 155 Photo © Claudio Ernè.

PROSTHETIC VILLAGE

VICTORIA BERGBAUER

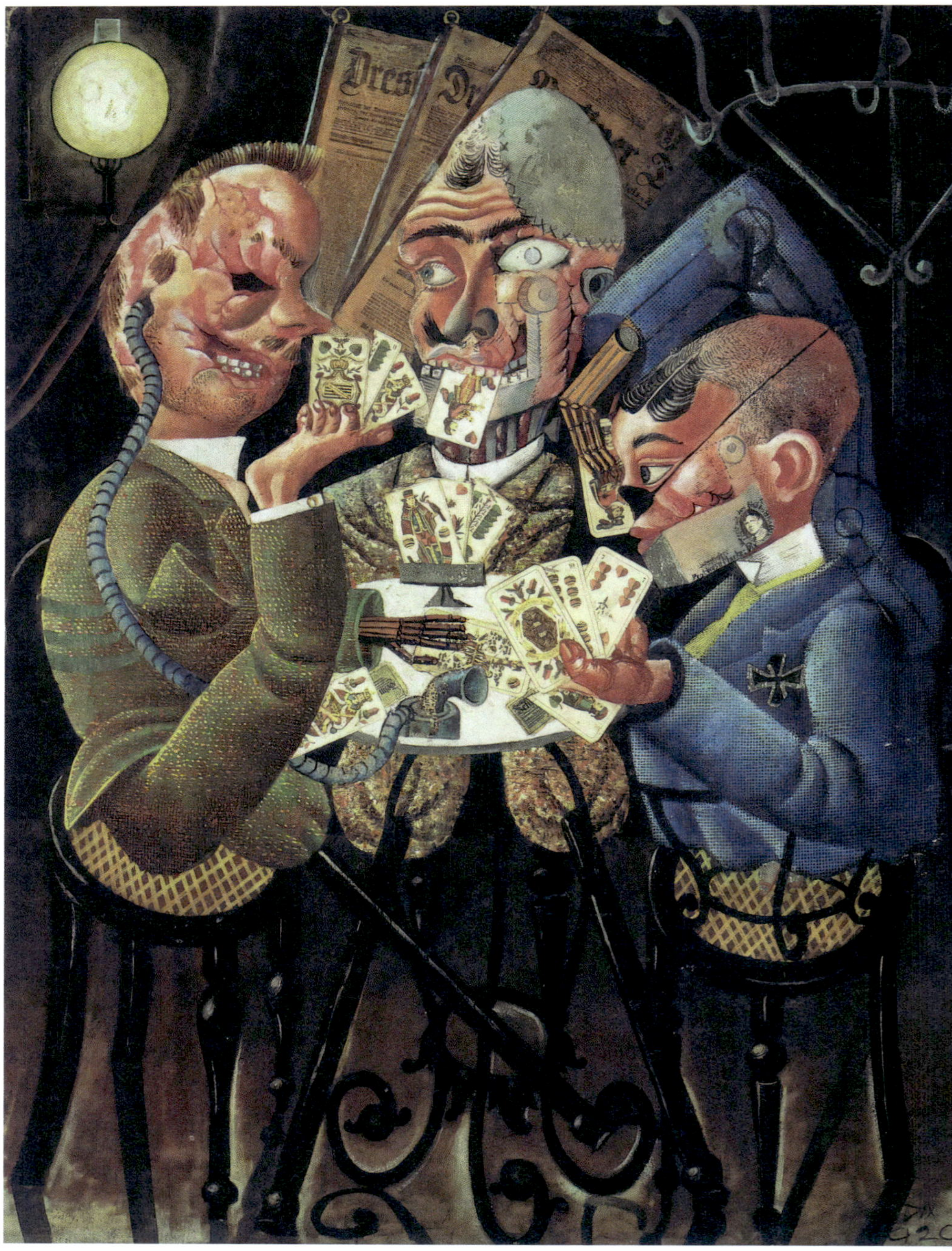

↗ Otto Dix, *Die Skatspieler* (*The Skat Players*), 1920.

Otto Dix's *Die Skatspieler* depicts three men playing cards in a room. Staged at the center of the work, their bodies and faces seem fragmented. Newspapers and a coatrack are positioned in the dimly lit background. A collage of different materials evokes the presence of wounds. The painting was completed in 1920, two years after the end of World War I. Read in its wartime context, the men appear as former soldiers: men whose bodies recall the recent fighting. Yet there is more. Does the table have two or three legs? Is the blue horn reaching out of the tabletop? What image emerges from the lamp? This blurriness, so present in Dix's painting, also marks the built environment of Europe in the aftermath of World War I.

The physical legacies of the war impacted the collective European psyche and landscape. They also affected its cities and architecture. One such imprint lies in the writings of British landscape architect Thomas Mawson and his *An Imperial Obligation: Industrial Villages for Partially Disabled Soldiers and Sailors*. Dedicated to his youngest son, who died in the Battle of Ypres in August 1917, Mawson's book proposed to create special surroundings for "the partially disabled soldier; for the new and strange conditions under which he must, from the nature of his infirmity, live and work in the future."[1] New surroundings would give the man, "with eyes more troubled than when he looked over the stricken fields of France," a new perspective on his future.[2] The adapted built environment could restore "peace of mind where we are unable to rebuild the shattered body."[3]

Mawson's plan did not arise in isolation. The Great War left "more than 750,000 ex-servicemen permanently disabled" in Britain alone, and specialized institutions were established to accommodate them.[4] If, as historian Annette Becker concludes, World War I was "a laboratory for the twentieth century: a field experiment or test site where violence could be carried out," it also produced architectural experiments when the battle was supposedly over.[5] Architecture was enlisted in Britain's postwar reconstruction effort, and Mawson's plans became part of this collective endeavor. One year after the publication of *Imperial Obligation*, they materialized in Lancashire, whose residents undertook the creation of two memorials: one conceived to be a commemorative stone monument, the other an entire village.

Westfield Memorial Village was built to accommodate war veterans returning from battle with disabilities, in recognition of their service. Designed by Mawson and supported by local industrialist and philanthropist Herbert Lushington Storey, the village's foundation stone was unveiled in 1919.[6] By then Mawson's project had received wide acclaim. In 1918, politician Sir Alfred Hopkinson praised Storey's action and called "the development of industrial villages ... one of the most hopeful things to look

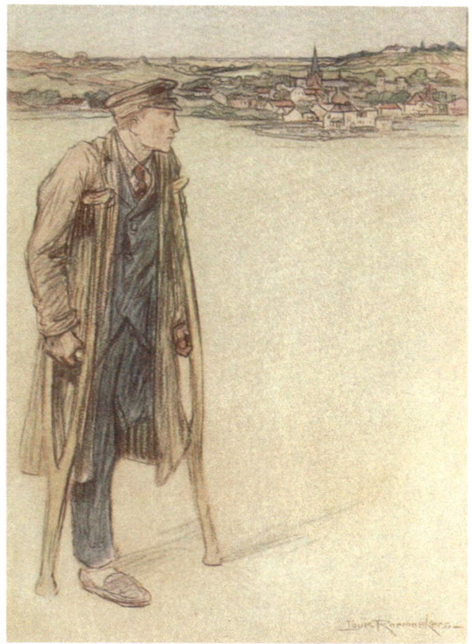

← Louis Raemeker, "Looking Forward into the Future with Eyes More Troubled Than When He Looked over the Stricken Fields of France."

forward to in the rebuilding of Britain."[7] American journals equally lauded Mawson's sketches.[8] The project also elicited critical reactions. In the Inter-Allied Conference on the Aftercare of Disabled Men of 1918, Mawson recalled views that found his scheme "impractical and uneconomical."[9] The director of the Red Cross Institute for Crippled and Disabled Men in New York, Douglas McMurtrie, thought that these villages would nourish "a segregation of the disabled."[10]

Westfield was founded at a time when, as Stefanos Geroulanos and Todd Meyers point out, new kinds of injuries reshaped the thinking of soldiers, doctors, theorists, and policymakers alike, leading to "the rise of a new conceptual architecture that offered a new epistemology of the body, a new ontology, notably of patienthood."[11] The village was a manifestation of the wide-ranging effects of these medical ideas at the scale of the built environment. Five years after discussions on Mawson's designs had seen print, a committee responsible for the selection process of applicants and for general administrative decisions had been installed, and the first veterans—primarily men that had served with the city's local regiment (the King's Own Royal Lancasters) and Lancastrians who had been left with a disability—arrived at the twenty-six completed cottages.[12]

The village was based on Mawson's sketches, and components of the original plan from *Imperial Obligation* became its central aspects. The presence of banks, shops, a cinema, schools, churches, hotels, libraries, and a post office recalls the structure of a "normal" village. Indeed, normality was a structuring force in Mawson's writings, and was essential to Westfield's design. Although meant to constitute a space for those whose bodies and lives were irreversibly transfigured by war, it resembled environments surrounding people who did not have a disability. A factory, warehouses, and workshops contributed an industrial nature to the area, while

→ Architectural plan of Westfield Memorial Village, 1917.

↘ Memorial for Westfield War Memorial Village, Storey Institute.

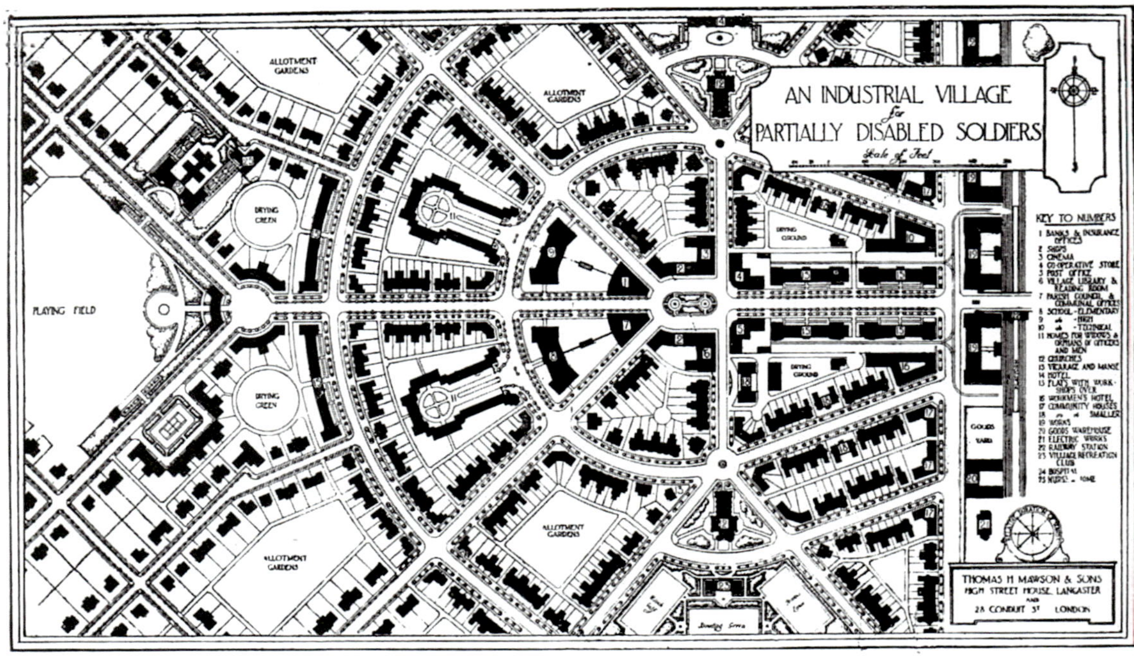

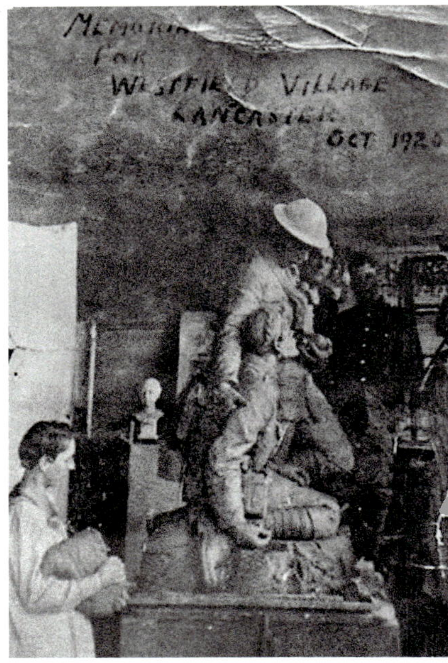

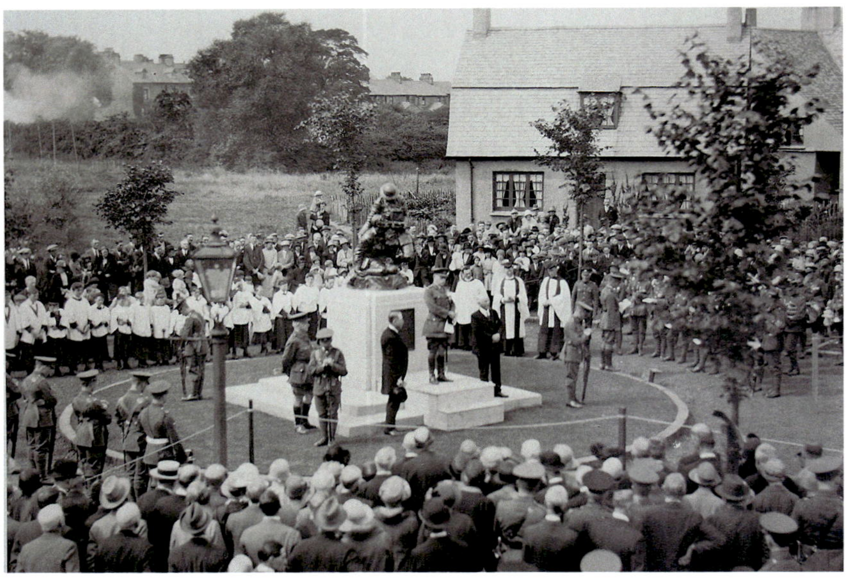

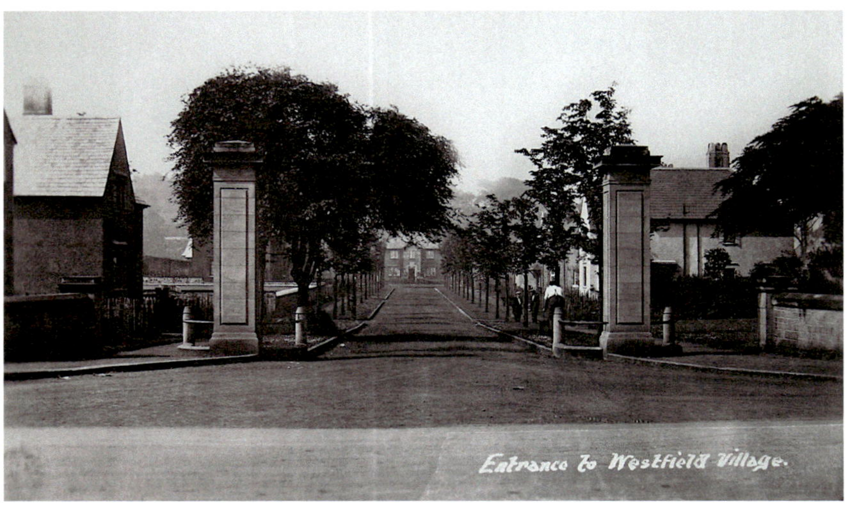

↖ Official unveiling of the Westfield War Memorial, 1924.

← View of the entrance to Westfield War Memorial Village, Lancaster, down to the first house constructed, 1924–1926. Photographer unknown.

→ Blocks of flats with workshops for small trades above, 1917. Reproduced from Thomas Mawson, *An Imperial Obligation: Industrial Villages for Partially Disabled Soldiers and Sailors* (London: Grant Richards, 1917), 52.

extensive space for gardens, fields, greens, and orderly cottages concretized Mawson's aim of maintaining a rural character. These elements contributed to the making of a space that was to normalize rather than center individuals and their disabilities.

For the memorial monument at the village's center, Storey commissioned the local sculptor Jennie Delahunt to create a model that represented a soldier handing water to his wounded comrade. "[Gracing] the small formal garden with its bright-hued flowers occupying the middle of the Town Square," the sculpture was placed on top of two platform-like steps and a plinth—an elevation that did not evoke accessibility, as to be expected in a village that responded to its residents' individual bodies.[13] For those for whom Westfield was built, Delahunt's sculpture was only meant to be looked at from a distance; a constant "reminder to passers-by of those who have gone west during these fateful years."[14] Cottages, gardens, and factories only furthered this distance by prioritizing societal norms over accessibility.

The Cottages

Mawson considered "self-contained cottages" to be key in creating a sense of normality.[15] "Our dream is to consist of a village and not a barracks," Mawson wrote.[16] As "the majority of the initial intake of Westfield tenants were men who lost lower limbs,"[17] Mawson sketched out "broadened doorways, aisles, and gangways for the accommodation of bath-chairs and wheeled litters."[18] Many of these measures, however, were not implemented upon construction. As Martin Purdy points out, despite "the clear demand for single-storey housing, all of the properties constructed in the mid-1920s ... were two-storey cottages," thus presenting an obstacle to anyone who, for example, had suffered a leg amputation from the war.[19]

This idea of "normality"—of constructing accommodation in the same way as outside of the village—not only influenced the design of the cottages, but also impacted the criteria for who could ultimately live there. The "26 families made up of 72 adults and 51 children" who would be given a house not only had to have carried disabilities from the war, but also had to have a local background, be married, and generally be clean and respectable.[20] Veterans, often fathers, lived with their unwounded families in these cottages. A "working-man's hotel" was installed near the recreation ground to house relatives.[21]

While interactions between former soldiers and unwounded residents were part of daily life in Westfield, the landscape architect located the village's success in creating a context that allowed the veterans to share experiences of disability with each other. Arguing against criticisms of segregation, of "herding together the disabled," Mawson insisted on the village's communal character.[22] He claimed that the "crippled hero" was "most painfully reminded of his disablement" when "surrounded by and competing with the able-bodied and struggling all the time in competition with them."[23] Mawson emphasized the possibility of creating an environment that enabled a collective experience of disability. Considering the pervasiveness of multistory cottages alongside Mawson's aim of avoiding "competition" exposes how binaries, such as "disabled" and "able," or "abnormal" and "normal," result from a construction process that is ever formed and distorted by individual and collective ambitions, preconceptions, and experiences.

The Factory

According to Mawson, Westfield Memorial Village was designed to "chase away ... the veil which shrouds a future overcast by the burden of a lifelong physical disability."[24] He argued that "real villages" would lead to a new future, one "grow[ing] from their own root, in which the children of [the] protégés would grow up and take place in factory, office, shop, or husbandry."[25] Toward these ends, Mawson's plan for Westfield included "elementary and high schools," as well as a

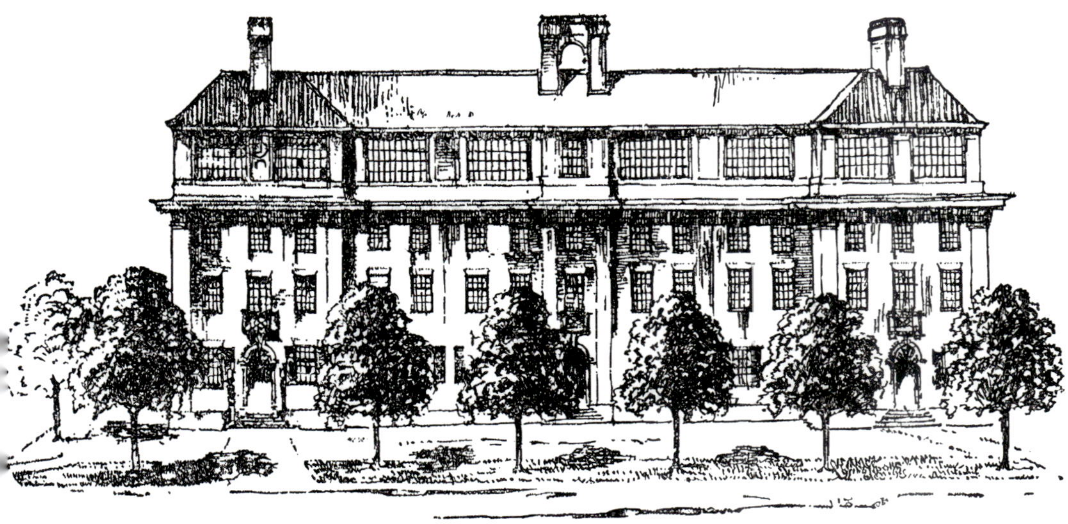

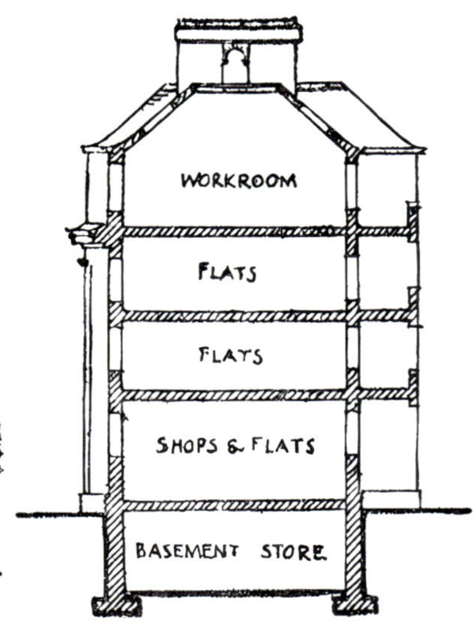

factory.[26] Mawson was interested in recovering a body's productivity. His sketches evoked the then commonly held idea of the worker as "a machine capable of infinite productivity."[27] He stated that postwar Britain could not afford to let "all the energy remaining to the partially disabled run to waste or be used inefficiently."[28] He considered "the creation of an exceptionally favorable environment" essential to the efficient use of this energy, thereby preserving "a spirit of sterling independence and self-helpfulness."[29]

This idea of energy efficiency ran from Mawson's treatment of individual bodies to the environment in which they were positioned. Already in earlier writings, Mawson had argued for the need to group buildings "economically and practically to ensure the smallest amount of unremunerative labor and running to and fro."[30] In Westfield, units were "part of a larger composition embracing everything within sight," all surrounding the Central Square, "the administrative center of the village," which held banks, the post office, large shops, a cinema, and the offices of the committee.[31] "The electric generating station ... supplies the village not only with light for public and private uses, but also with power for its various industries,"[32] and industries were placed "in relation to railway facilities" to speed the arrival of raw materials and dispatch finished products.[33]

Centralization would, according to the architect's plans, increase efficiency and ensure rentability. It would further allow for "the arrangement of special conditions of work to meet special needs."[34] Spaces that were adaptable to veterans' individual skills would equally encourage efficiency and self-sufficiency. Mawson warned that "every man must be seen following the occupation he is best fitted for mentally, temperamentally, and physically."[35] This reflected the wider views of *The Disabled Soldier's Handbook*, which was published by the Ministry of Pensions in 1918 and claimed that "the first thing to do" as a veteran with disabilities "is to get as well and to keep as well as you can. The next thing is to get back to work of a kind that you can stick to."[36]

Factory workers, craftsmen, writers, composers, agriculturists, and shopkeepers were meant to interact with one another at Westfield. Alongside the main avenue, Mawson designed buildings "containing shops on the ground floor with flats behind and over," with workshops placed on the top floor. Goods produced on the upper floors could thus be "sold or dealt on the ground floor." An elevator was also provided within these buildings, "for the easier conveyance of materials and articles of trade, but also for the use by those employees too crippled for the safe or easy climbing of stairs."[37] The built environment heightened an efficient transport of both goods and men, assimilating the body to a machine.[38]

The Gardens

Influenced by Ebenezer Howard's Garden City concept and the Arts and Crafts movement, the soldiers' village was to be a "product of English rural life."[39] Mawson's plans called for "more open-air life" through the installation of market gardens, bulb farms, agriculture, and animal husbandry at the outskirts of the village.[40] Echoing Raymond Unwin's and Richard Parker's focus on the union of craft and intellectual work through cottage homes, the village was to be as "artistic as it is practical," and bound together by "present activities and surroundings, all working together in happy collaboration."[41]

Mawson considered gardens to be essential to this harmonious framework. Each property was meant to have a large garden. Westfield's committee members, however, focused on their maintenance and chose tenants according to their capacity to garden.[42] Worries about the effects "on the wider aesthetic," or "the community's natural facade" even led to the introduction of a tenancy condition to keep one's house and gardens "clean and tidy," threatening those who failed with eviction. This echoed the conclusions of the 1918 National Conference on Housing after the War, which recommended that "when such garden land is provided, town planning schemes should include adequate power for the responsible authority to enforce upon the occupier its use for the purpose."[43]

Though conceived to respond to soldiers' bodies that carried wounds and disabilities from the war, the gardens of Mawson's village were part of an architecture created to evoke "normality." The village's "Playing Field [was] designed on simple and harmonious, but nevertheless dignified lines."[44] And the workshops, which were designed with "strongly marked horizontal lines, leading the eye forward to the more ordered architecture of important buildings surrounding the Town Square," further contributed to the tidy appearance of Westfield.[45] Even the village hospital was set to be "facing pleasantly across the open field."[46] These "vistas," as Mawson referred to them, were meant to create impressions of pleasantness, dignity, and harmony.[47] These conceptions of an idyllic rurality blurred the lines between individuals and the spaces they lived in.

Crutch or Prosthesis?

Westfield's architecture was designed to establish a distance from past wars and their effects on veterans. Mawson called "the maimed soldier of the Napoleonic wars stumping the Country from village to village ... a sight too humiliating alike to our self-respect and our sense of fitness."[48] The architect sought instead to create "a real village ... far even from appearing to be a village of cripples, especially as we have every reason to believe we shall be able to clothe it with a general air of well-being and industrious

→ A man wearing a leg prosthesis aided by a nurse who kneels to adjust the straps. Photo 1914/1918, author unknown.

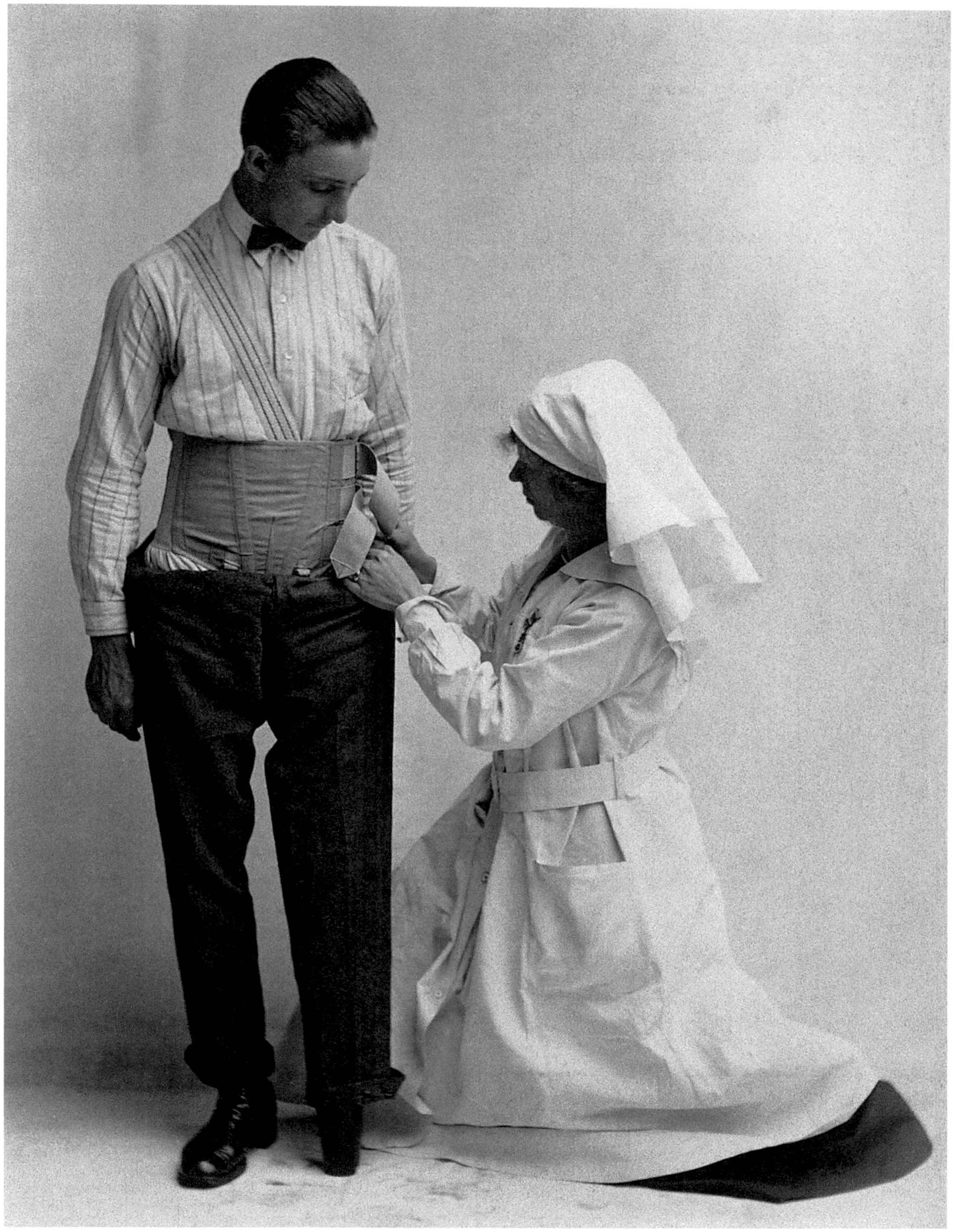

contentment."[49] Distance arose as both a temporal and spatial tool in this context. While dissociating from past conflicts through the built environment, the village's architectural components also pushed the bodies of individual veterans and their disabilities into the background. Concretizing a juxtaposition between Westfield's residents and outside communities, which Mawson called "normal," the aim of creating specialized surroundings subsided to a construction that imitated the logics of these "normal" spaces.

An Imperial Obligation forewarned those who might imagine themselves meeting "draggled, haggard, and miserable objects, painfully conscious and even ashamed of a disablement which cannot be hid," upon entering the memorial village.[50] Mawson's writings open with a call to dream collectively: "I have dreamed a dream, and I want you to dream it with me, and perhaps when you and I have dreamed the dream together, you may be, as I am, filled with a great desire for its realization."[51] If he dreamt of surroundings for returning soldiers specifically, its concrete realization in the architecture of Westfield also reflected the wider society. Architecture was conceived to clothe at Westfield. Normalizing logics marked its walls, roads, and constructions. Reflecting the appearance of buildings across Britain,

↓ Manufacture of artificial limbs in Glasgow for Scottish servicemen injured in World War I, 1917.

Westfield was shaped by collective and societal norms rather than by a response to individual bodies and their realities.

A world of normality structured the cottages, the central space, and the ordered gardens of Lancaster's memorial village. The seemingly stable lines of its architecture break apart, however, when one ceases to perceive the "disabled war veteran" as a given entity. Behind the veil of neat gardens and orderly cottages stand dismembered bodies, bodies taken apart by designers and the committee's selection process, bodies reconstituted to a wholeness in a "pleasant" rurality, re-membered in a memorial space.[52] As views about disability shaped Westfield's architecture, the built environment shaped experiences of disability. Though the village was conceived to adapt to the individual needs of its residents, its structure continued to evoke elements of "normality" that were common to spaces outside of Westfield. Lines between design and the veterans' war-torn bodies were blurred. It is unclear who wore Westfield; whether its structures responded to the needs of veterans or their families, the village committee, its architect, or donors. Yet this blurriness is telling: it reveals an environment that became prosthetic.

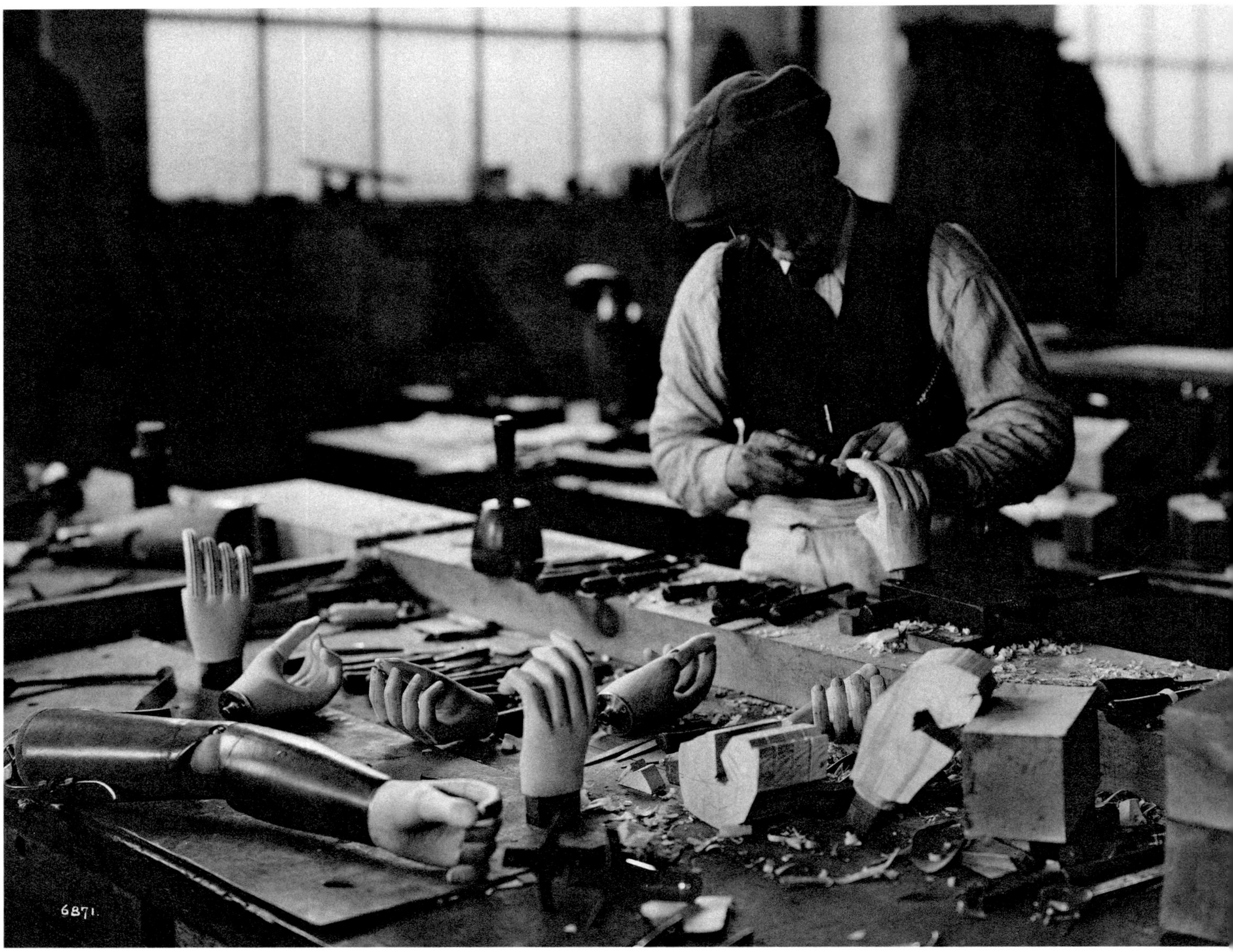

An earlier version of this essay was originally published by e-flux Architecture in 2020.

1. Thomas Mawson, *An Imperial Obligation: Industrial Villages for Partially Disabled Soldiers* (London: Grant Richards, 1917), xx.
2. Mawson, *An Imperial Obligation*, 5.
3. Mawson, *An Imperial Obligation*, 5.
4. For overviews of these organizations, see Deborah Cohen, *The War Come Home: Disabled Veterans in Britain and Germany, 1914–1939* (Berkeley: University of California Press, 2001), 2; and Julie Anderson, *War, Disability and Rehabilitation in Britain: "The Soul of a Nation"* (Manchester: Manchester University Press, 2011).
5. Annette Becker, "The Great War: World War, Total War," *International Review of the Red Cross* 97, no. 900 (2015): 1032.
6. Martin Purdy, "Westfield War Memorial Village: Disability, Paternalism and Philanthropy, 1915–2015" (PhD diss., University of Lancaster, 2017), 14. Purdy's thesis manifests a detailed reading of the village's institutional files.
7. Alfred Hopkinson, *Rebuilding Britain: A Survey of Problems of Reconstruction after the World War* (London: Cassell, 1918), 145.
8. A book review of the *American Architect and Architecture* found "Mr. Mawson's dream well worth our serious conservation 'over here,'" while an editorial in *Landscape Architecture*, the magazine of the American Society of Landscape Architects, considered it "fortunate that Mr. Mawson's plans will be given an opportunity to prove their practicability." T.K., "Industrial Villages for Disabled Soldiers," *Landscape Architecture* 9, no. 1 (1918): 32–34. Mawson's project also appeared in Theodora Kimball, "Our British Allies and Reconstruction," *Landscape Architecture* 8, no. 4 (1918): 169–174. One year later, the same magazine referred to the village: "Editorials: Industrial Villages for Disabled Soldiers," *Landscape Architecture* 9, no. 11 (1919). *An Imperial Obligation* further made its way into a range of American libraries and organizations, such as the National Housing Association, the Department of Labor, and the US Army War College. Federal Board for Vocational Education, "Vocational Rehabilitation of Disabled Soldiers and Sailors: Letter from the Federal Board for Vocational Education, Transmitting, in Response to a Senate Resolution of Jan. 27" (Washington, DC, 1918); National Housing Association, *National Housing Association, Proceedings of the Seventh National Conference on Housing Boston November 25, 26, and 27, 1918* (New York: National Housing Association, 1918), 405. See also Army War College Library, *Monthly List of Military Information Carded from Books, Periodicals, and Other Sources* (Fort Leavenworth, KS: Army Service Schools Press, 1917–1918); Laura Thompson, *Reconstruction: A Preliminary Bibliography* (Washington, DC: Department of Labor, 1918).
It continued to be filed in bibliographies under section titles as "Refitting Men into Normal Family and Community Life." Paul Moore Strayer and Committee, *Outline Studies on the Problems of the Reconstruction Period* (New York: Association Press, 1918), 16.
9. John Galsworthy, *The Inter-Allied Conference on the Aftercare of Disabled Men. Second Annual Meeting held in London, May 20 to 25, 1918. Reports Presented to the Conference* (London: H.M. Stationery Office, 1918), 83.
10. T.K., "Industrial Villages for Disabled Soldiers."
11. Stefanos Geroulanos and Todd Meyers, *The Human Body in the Age of Catastrophe: Brittleness, Integration, Science, and the Great War* (Chicago: University of Chicago Press, 2018), 318. For the connection between design and the human body, see Beatriz Colomina and Mark Wigley, *Are We Human? Notes on an Archaeology of Design* (Zurich: Lars Müller, 2016).
12. Mawson, *An Imperial Obligation*, 61.
13. Mawson, *An Imperial Obligation*, 43.
14. Lancaster Corporation, "Minutes of the Members of the Council in Committee," February 12, 1919, cited in Purdy, "Westfield War Memorial Village," 137.
15. Mawson, *An Imperial Obligation*, 18.
16. Mawson, *An Imperial Obligation*, 8.
17. Purdy, "Westfield War Memorial Village," 103.
18. Mawson, *An Imperial Obligation*, 103.
19. Purdy, "Westfield War Memorial Village," 104.
20. See Westfield Memorial Village, http://westfieldmemorialvillage.co.uk/the-early-years/. Purdy, "Westfield War Memorial Village," 164. Some of the first tenants included Mr. T. Cragg, "a father of two, whose left leg had been amputated; Mr. J. Rumley, another father of two who had a one hundred percent disablement (paralysis) as the result of several 'severe' wounds, and Mr. C. Howse, a father of five with a severe leg injury." Purdy, "Westfield War Memorial Village," 98.
21. Mawson, *An Imperial Obligation*, 46.
22. Mawson, *An Imperial Obligation*, 83.
23. Mawson, *An Imperial Obligation*, 83.
24. Mawson, *An Imperial Obligation*, 5.
25. Mawson, *An Imperial Obligation*, 89.
26. Mawson, *An Imperial Obligation*, 43.
27. Anson Rabinbach, *The Human Motor: Energy, Fatigue, and the Origins of Modernity* (New York: Basic Books, 1990), 2.
28. Mawson, *An Imperial Obligation*, 89.
29. Mawson, *An Imperial Obligation*, xxi, 49.
30. Thomas Mawson, *The Art and Craft of Garden Making*, 5th ed. (New York: Charles Scribner's Sons, 1926), 29.
31. Mawson, *An Imperial Obligation*, 38.
32. Mawson, *An Imperial Obligation*, 46.
33. Mawson, *An Imperial Obligation*, 102.
34. Mawson, *An Imperial Obligation*, 102.
35. Mawson, *An Imperial Obligation*, 8.
36. Ministry of Pensions, *The Disabled Soldier's Handbook* (Wiltshire: Ministry of Pensions, 1918), 3.
37. Ministry of Pensions, *The Disabled Soldier's Handbook*, 37.
38. A connection that becomes more apparent as we follow historian Annette Becker's insight that prosthetics used for amputees often looked "more like working tools than hands." Annette Becker, *Voir la Grande Guerre. Un autre récit (1914–2014)* (Paris: A. Colin, 2014), 60: "les prothèses sophistiquées des membres ressemblent souvent plus à des outils qu'à des mains."
39. Mawson, *An Imperial Obligation*, 47, 49. Mawson cites the promoters of the Garden City and Garden Suburb schemes once, 25.
40. Mawson, *An Imperial Obligation*, 46.
41. Mawson, *An Imperial Obligation*, 11.
42. Purdy, "Westfield War Memorial Village," 113.
43. *The National Conference on Housing after the War, Report of the Organizing Committee* (Manchester: Kirkham & Pratt, 1918), 78.
44. Mawson, *An Imperial Obligation*, 44.
45. Mawson, *An Imperial Obligation*, 38.
46. Mawson, *An Imperial Obligation*, 44.
47. Mawson, *An Imperial Obligation*, 41.
48. Mawson, *An Imperial Obligation*, 70.
49. Mawson, *An Imperial Obligation*, 82–83.
50. Mawson, *An Imperial Obligation*, 81.
51. Mawson, *An Imperial Obligation*, 3.
52. On the connection between dis- and re-membered bodies, see further Joanne Bourke, *Dismembering the Male: Men's Bodies, Britain and the Great War* (Chicago: University of Chicago Press, 1996), 210.

p158 © 2024 Artists Rights Society (ARS), New York / VG Bild-Kunst, Bonn.
p159, 160 (top), 161 Reproduced from Thomas Mawson, *An Imperial Obligation: Industrial Villages for Partially Disabled Soldiers and Sailors* (London: Grant Richards, 1917), frontispiece (159), 16 (160 top), 52 (161).
p160 (middle right, middle left, bottom) Courtesy of King's Own Royal Regiment Museum.
p163 Courtesy of The Wellcome Collection.
p164 Photo Yarrow & Co Ltd. Courtesy of The Wellcome Collection.

→ Nazi Propaganda Minister Joseph Goebbels opening the exhibition *Die Frau in Haus, Familie, und Beruf*, March 18, 1933.

REGEL-ATED BODIES

HOLLY BUSHMAN

> We do not see the woman as inferior, but rather as having a different mission, a different value, than that of the man. Therefore we believed that the German woman, who more than any other in the world is a woman in the best sense of the word, should use her strength and abilities in other areas than the man. ... At the risk of sounding reactionary and outdated, let me say this clearly: The first, best, and most suitable place for the woman is in the family, and her most glorious duty is to give children to her people and nation, children who can continue the line of generations and who guarantee the immortality of the nation.[1]
> —Joseph Goebbels

On March 18, 1933, just four days after his appointment and in his first public appearance as Reichsminister of Public Enlightenment and Propaganda, Joseph Goebbels spoke at the opening of the exhibition *Die Frau in Familie, Haus und Beruf* (*The Woman in Family, Home, and Workplace*). His deeply sinister statements on the role of women in the National Socialist party's vision for society signaled the violently misogynistic rhetoric that was to be legally codified in the coming months, and to remain a pillar of Nazi ideology for the entirety of its time in power. "As long as a nation has such a proud and noble womanhood, it cannot perish," Goebbels declared. "These women are the foundation of our race, of its blood, and of its future."

In opening an exhibition devoted to women's lifestyles and livelihoods, the Nazis were initiating a series of policies that would ultimately limit women's access to university education, restrict professional opportunities, and determine who could and could not have children. By naming "our race, our blood, and its future" in his opening remarks, Goebbels underscored the central aim of the exhibition: to didactically display a vision of femininity centered around the woman's reproductive potential. Nazi rhetoric famously heralded the connection between *Blut und Boden* (blood and soil) as rationale for its racist and nationalist foundations. *Die Frau in Familie, Haus und Beruf* presented visitors with one form of the "blood" integral to the development of a German *Herrenrasse*, yet one that was deeply discomfiting to the misogynistic, hygiene-obsessed Nazis: menses. As National Socialist policies sought to reverse falling birthrates, a series of posters describing menstrual hygiene featured prominently in the exhibition's section on women's health and wellness. The way in which the topic was discussed and depicted had profound implications for the role of women in Nazi society, an inchoate expression of the repressive policies to come.

The didactic posters used both quantitative diagrams and illustrations to describe the importance of proper menstrual care, the imperatives of maintaining a "regular" menstrual cycle, and the significance of menstrual health for the future of the *Herrenrasse*. While the larger exhibition contained a wealth of information on Nazi conceptions of womanhood and femininity, its materials attending to menstruation in particular offer an opportunity to scrutinize engagements between the Nazi political apparatus and the members of the society it sought to perfect and

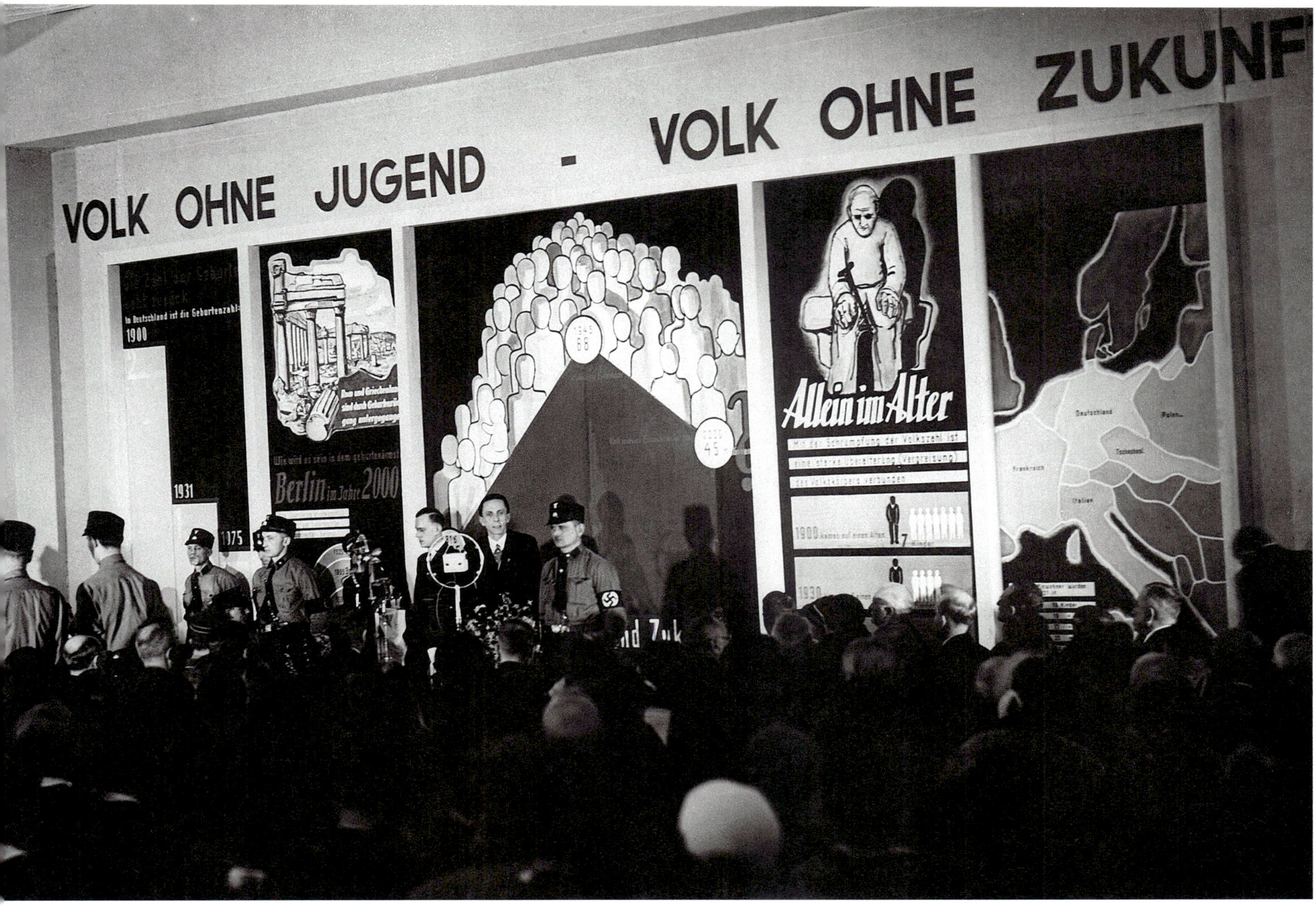

control. The timing, content, and visual program of the exhibition reveal the complex nature of the ways in which these shifts were felt in German society.

Die Frau was instrumental in constructing the image of the "Aryan" woman. The violence that this construct inflicts, both rhetorically and directly, cannot be overstated.[2] As Wilfried van der Will has written, the oppressive practices of representation particularly evinced in depictions of the human body followed a deliberate shift away from the more heterogeneous social structure of the Weimar era toward a broader ideology of control and a political grammar "based on the symbolism of hierarchical integration."[3] Nazi depictions of the female form attempted to restore women to a preindustrial (and clearly fictitious) idea of German femininity, to an idyllic destiny corrupted by the onset of the discursive practices of industrial modernity.[4] Yet in embarking on a project of ostensibly "idyllizing" the German female form, early Nazi propaganda paradoxically drew on the aesthetic logic of the avant-garde and the very heterogeneity of Weimar visual culture it was soon to renounce. Photomontage, collage, caricature, and cautious cubism were used to depict a conservative and accessible image of the woman, one that is solely organized around her childbearing and homemaking potential.

Exhibiting Femininity

Die Frau in Familie, Haus, und Beruf was staged at the Funkturm exhibition center in the Westend neighborhood of Berlin. Despite its short history, the site had already hosted multiple important public attractions which aimed to convey the promises and practices of a "modernizing" society. From the radio technology exhibits that inaugurated its opening in 1926 to a series of trade fairs promoting new and innovative German products, the exhibition center was inscribed in public consciousness as the venue par excellence for modern, future-oriented public programming. Convened as a joint effort of the city of Berlin, the Deutsches Hygiene-Museum in Dresden, and several Nazi-affiliated women's organizations known as *Frauenverbänden*, *Die Frau* was initially conceived as a successor to an expo of the same name originally staged by the woman's group Lyceum in 1912 at Berlin's botanical garden.[5] While the 1912 exhibition was praised for foregrounding women's autonomy (thanks in large part to the work of Gertrude Bäumer, a women's rights activist and Lyceum member), the 1933 exhibition received acclaim for the centrality of *motherhood* as a driving force behind its design.

Bruno Gebhard, the newly appointed scientific director of the Berlin Trade Show Commission and director of *Die Frau*, had trained as a doctor in Rostock and Leipzig before beginning a medical career in Dortmund. But it was a visit to the 1926 *GeSoLei* expo in Düsseldorf, the largest trade fair staged in the Weimar Republic, that convinced him to seek work in exhibition design. Between 1927 and 1932 Gebhard worked as a scientific assistant at the Deutsches Hygiene-Museum in Dresden, and his experiences at that institution—itself founded following the success of the 1911 Dresden Hygiene Exhibition—provided formative experience in tailoring medical knowledge for public consumption.[6] The Deutsches Hygiene-Museum contributed significant materials to three subsections in *Die Frau* dedicated to women's health—"The Woman as Wife and Mother," "The Woman as Mother (the Child)," and "What Should the Woman Know about Food?"—covering topics such as livelihood, housekeeping, sexual wellness, reproductive health, common children's diseases, other childrearing considerations, nutrition, and lifestyle. Most of the posters and physiological models were retained by the Deutsches Hygiene-Museum following the closure of the exhibition, but 1945 Allied bombing campaigns destroyed much of the collection. What survived, however, is a series of photographs which document individual

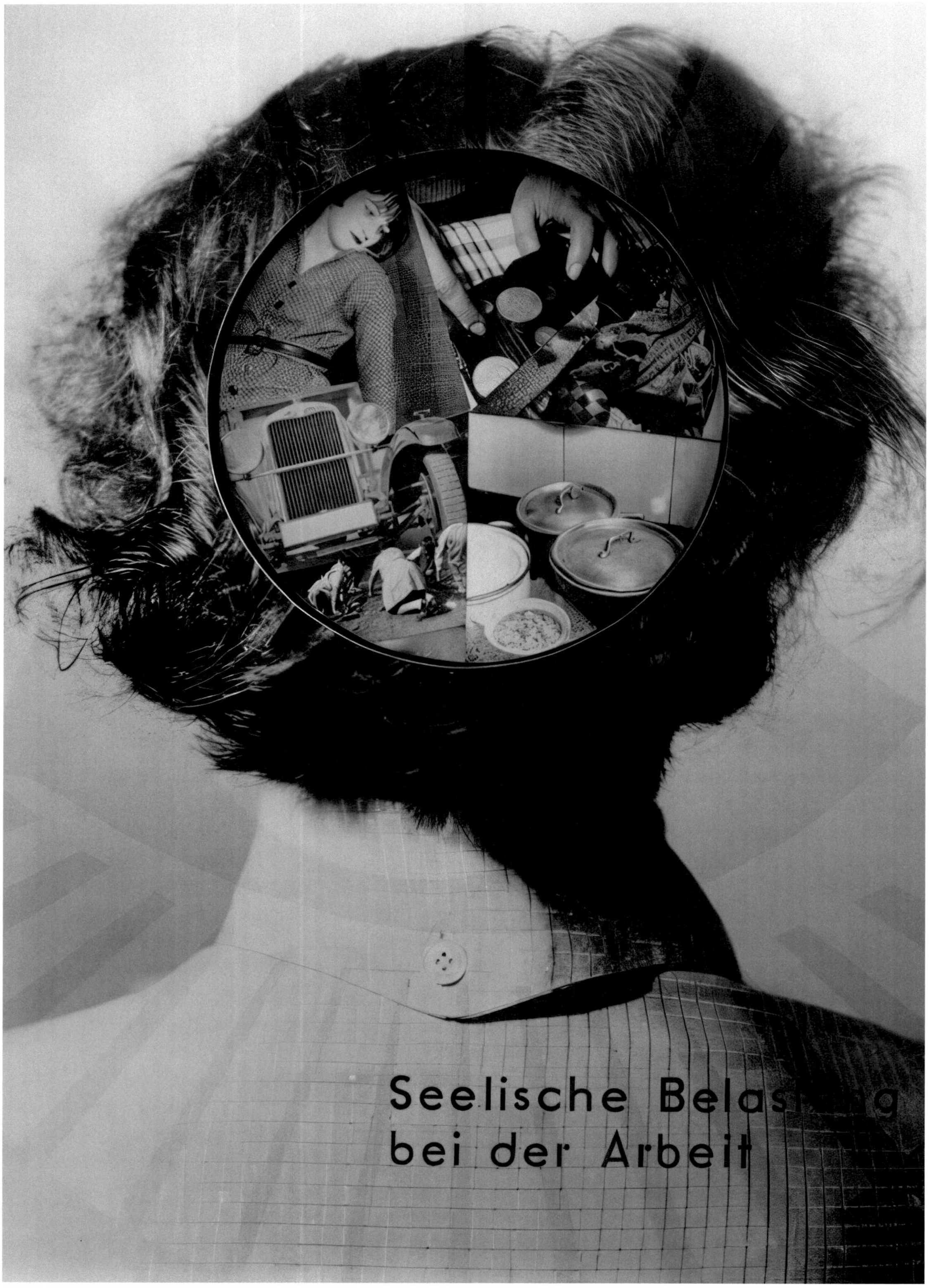

↙ Poster included in *Die Frau in Familie, Haus, und Beruf*, in the subsection "The Woman as Wife and Mother." "Seelische Belastung bei der Arbeit" ("Emotional Stress at Work"), 1933.

→ John Heartfield, *Wer Bürgerblätter liest wird blind und taub. Weg mit den Verdummungsbandagen!* (*Whoever reads bourgeois newspapers becomes blind and deaf: away with the stultifying bandages!*), 1930.

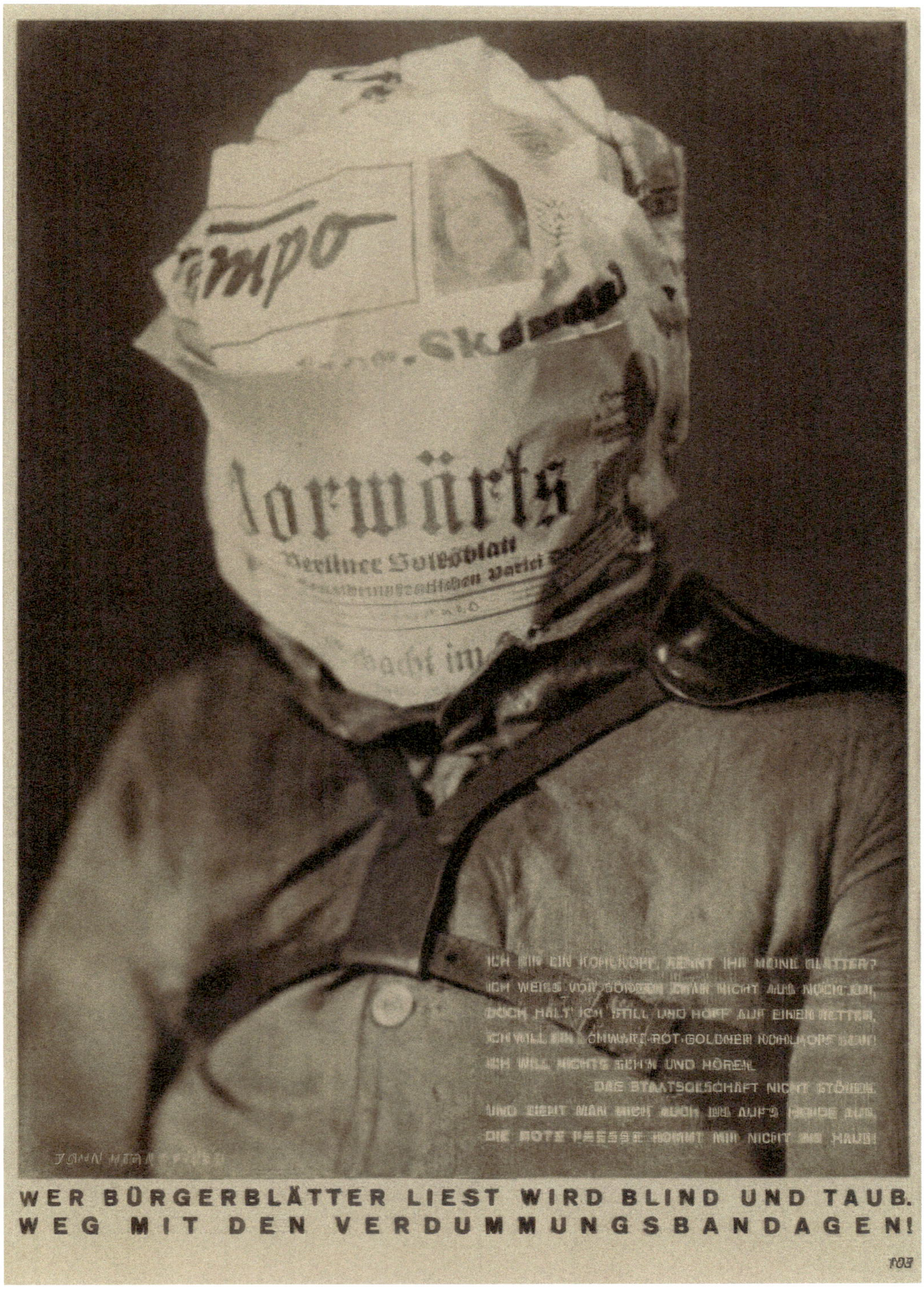

objects from the women's health subsections. While no comprehensive plan of the exhibition survived, its aesthetic program is still abundantly clear thanks to this documentation.

One poster included in "The Woman as Wife and Mother" depicts a woman's head, photographed from behind. We cannot see the woman's face, but the visual clues as to her mental state are collaged into a circle in the middle of her head. In what appears to represent a literal look into her skull, we see a photomontage which includes pots on a stove, children playing precariously close to the wheels of an automobile, a reclining woman who appears exhausted, and a wallet with only a few coins left in its folds. The resemblance of this poster to techniques of Dada photomontage is striking. John Heartfield's *Whoever reads bourgeois newspapers becomes blind and deaf: away with the stultifying bandages!* (1932) not only uses a similar graphic language but does so in order to make a shockingly similar argument about mental precarity in the face of modern life. Yet while Heartfield's slightly earlier photomontage is an affront on the stultifying potential of popular media, the poster from *Die Frau* suggests that it is a woman's commitments as a mother and housewife that are all-consuming. Taken alongside other material

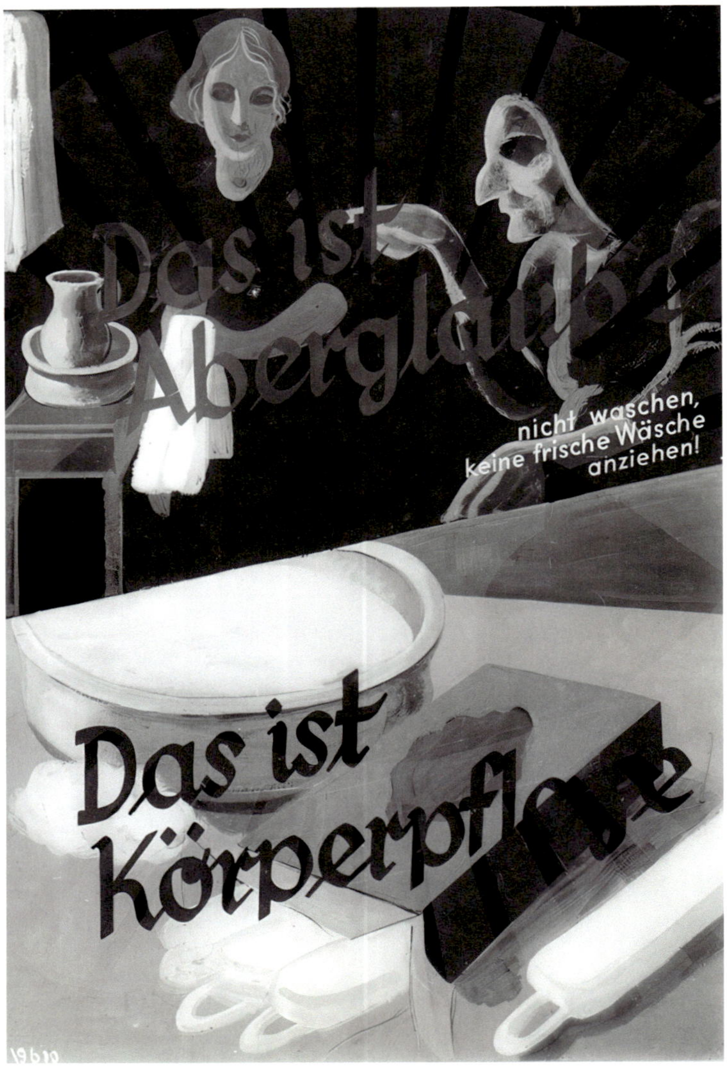

from the exhibition, it effectively cautions against pursuing responsibilities outside of the home. Within a month of the exhibition's opening, on April 7, 1933, the Nazi parliament passed the Law for the Restoration of the Professional Civil Service (Gesetz zur Wiederherstellung des Berufsbeamtentums), which allowed party officials to cull anyone perceived as "politically threatening" from public employment and led to dozens of women being fired who had held jobs in the public sector for their leftist or feminist views.

The Menstrual Pad Two posters from "The Woman as Mother (The Child)" each include didactic messages about how a woman should conduct herself during menstruation. The first poster is a divided image, an illustration of an encounter between a young woman and an old woman contrasted with an illustration of modern sanitary products. At top, the young woman holds a towel and appears to hesitantly glance at a jug of water and a washbasin as the veiled older woman, whose profile is a racialized caricature, gestures toward these objects. The figures are simple illustrations that show a clear contrast between the young (represented as healthy, beautiful, and pure) and the old (portrayed as dark, unattractive, and unclean). At the bottom, an open box of sanitary pads sits next to a basin of water. Superimposed text over the figures reads "Das ist Aberglaube / nicht waschen, keine frische Wäsche anziehen!" ("That is superstition / no washing, no fresh undergarments!"), and over the sanitary products reads "Das ist Körperpflege" ("That is bodily care"). The message of the poster is obvious: the modern woman should reject outdated folk knowledge in favor of contemporary hygiene. What is striking, however, is not the contrast between light and dark in the two halves, but the surreal *whiteness* of the menstrual pad; an object so commonly associated with abjection, and a distinctly feminine abjection at that.

In *Männerphantasien* (*Male Fantasies*), his seminal 1977 psychoanalytic study of the rise of German Fascism, Klaus Theweleit advances a number of theses on the repression of the "soldier male," his term for misogynistic Freikorps members. Theweleit opens his study by addressing the relationship between soldier males and women, as depicted in literature written by Freikorpsmen: mother and wives, enemies in the form of communist fighters and nurses, as well as the abstracted conflation of both archetypes. Where the mother and wife are rendered "white"—angelic and benevolent, but also vacuous, empty, void of emotion—the "red woman" is a violent deluge: she is sexualized, wild, unclean, unrestrained, and often depicted as masculine. The "red woman" will attack the soldier male with sweat and spittle flying off of her unwashed body; she will seduce him only to drown him in blood—his own blood, or that of her menses. Theweleit's analysis allows him to advance the thesis that among the soldier male's greatest phobias was the "flood": the unchecked surge of an advancing army, of bodily fluid, and emotion. He summarizes this notion at the beginning of his study's second volume: "The most urgent task [of the soldier male] is to pursue, to dam in, and to subdue any force that threatens to transform him back into the horribly disorganized jumble of flesh, hair, skin, bones, intestines, and feelings that calls itself human—the human being of old."[7] The sanitary products poster in *Die Frau* demonstrates how the Nazi party sought to address the "flood" expelled from each woman's body, from her terrifying interior, every month. The only way sanitary hygiene could be depicted was through imagery which emphasized the order and organization of a given product, which was in turn rendered banal and nearly stripped of its relationship with abjection.

The sanitary pads depicted at the bottom of the poster are an unfamiliar design today. Self-adhesives were not used in the production of women's sanitary products until 1972. Instead, beginning in the late nineteenth century, women wore objects with hoops to be attached to belts and worn under clothing

← "Das ist Aberglaube ... Das
st Körperpflege" ("That is
superstition ... That is bodily
care"), 1933.

↘ Polish illustration, ca.
920s.

↓ Teufel's brand "Diana-Gür-
el," early twentieth century
ca. 1900).

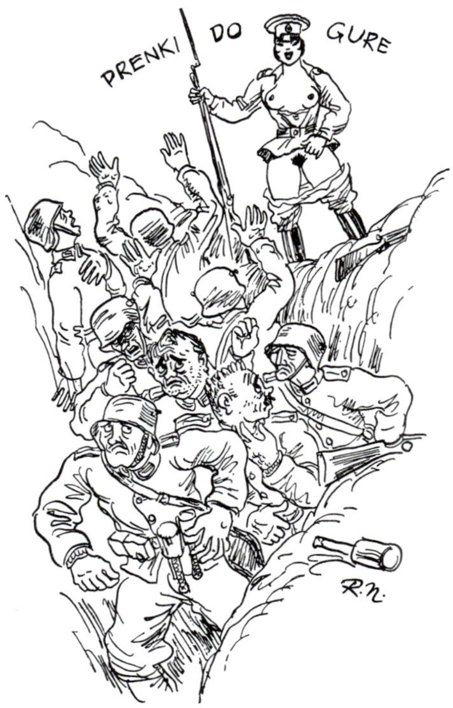

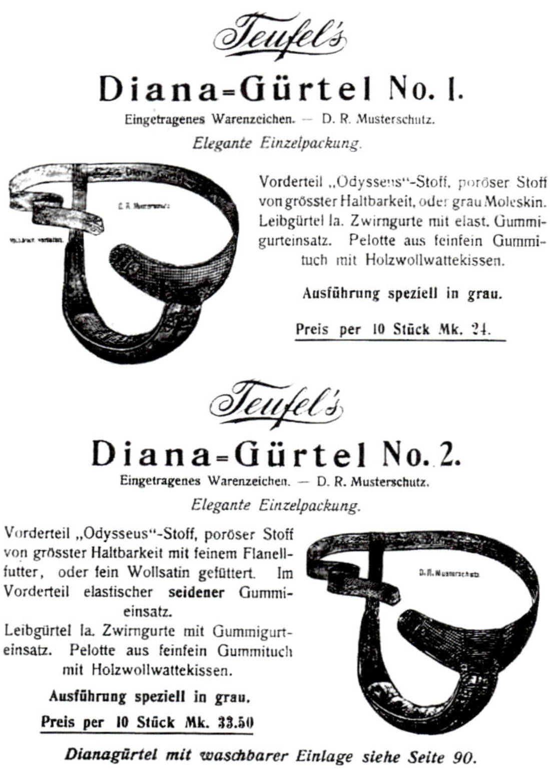

during menstruation. In 1926—the same year that the Funkturm exhibition grounds opened to the public—the Camelia company brought the very first disposable menstrual pad to market. Founded by the Jewish businessman Oskar Rosenfelder, the Camelia brand's previously washable pads were marketed toward women with a logic of discretion: the products were named for Alexandre Dumas's play *La Dame aux Camélias*, in which a prostitute wears a white flower when she can receive clients and a red flower when she is menstruating. Each Camelia box came with a removable card, which a woman could pass off to a shop clerk rather than voice her request directly.[8] The status of menstrual products in 1930s Germany, then, included secrecy, veiled allusions to sexuality, and the nature of "independence" and "mobility" still central to much sanitary product marketing today.

Women's menstrual care has always inscribed a logic of control on the female body. This also has a semantic dimension: in German, several words refer to menstruation, including *die Periode*, *die Menstruation*, and *die Regel*. While the first two of these words have obvious English cognates, *die Regel* does not—at least not commonly. Alternatively translated as "rule," "law," or "regulation," the term implies what is clearly at play in the visual rhetoric of menstrual garments: that menstruation should by its very nature adhere to a rule, a law, a regulation. The emphasis on order and regimentation in the poster's depiction of menstrual pads, alongside its overt rejection of folk knowledge and tradition, suggests a distinctly modern approach to menstrual hygiene. Here the modern menstrual pad can be read as a symbol for the Nazi formulation of the "normalized" woman: ordered and regular, white and sanitized, a corrective to the unpalatable figure of the aging, unhygienic symbol of an abject and infertile past.

The Menstruating Woman

The second poster, which also contains two images, insists on what women should avoid during menstruation. At top, heralded by the title "Was muss die Frau während der Periode vermeiden?" ("What must the woman avoid when on the period?"), abstracted female figures complete a series of activities: they bend over, lifting baskets and buckets; dressed in sports leotards, they hurdle; one figure is swimming. Messages correspond to each action: "Schwer heben, schwer tragen" ("Heavy lifting, heavy carrying"), "Rekordleistungen beim sport" ("Record-setting sports"), "kalt baden" ("cold bathing"). At the bottom of the poster is a more detailed illustration. In the foreground is a crude dwelling, where the silhouette of a crouching female is just discernible. In the middle ground, another series of dwellings and a group of figures (presumably male) sitting cross-legged on the ground. In the background is a landscape, with rolling hills and sparse suggestions of vegetation. The text which accompanies this image reads "Geschlechtsverkehr: Bei dem primitiven Völkern zogen sich die Frauen während dieser Zeit in abgesonderte Hütten zurück." ("Sexual intercourse: among primitive people, women were sent to isolated huts during this time.")

An operation similar to that of the first poster takes place here. The "primitive community" shown in the bottom half of the poster references alterity in emphasizing the contemporary conditions of Nazi society. The text included in the image makes no argument: the statement that women were "sent" or "sent back" (*zurück*) to isolated huts is not a commentary on antiquated practices so much as it is a display of difference, of primeval logic which might bear importance for the present. At top, the menstruating female figure is rendered faceless, nearly formless; performing tasks like lifting and hurdling, she is not a subject but an object, a lifeless automaton.

In his analysis of Nazi labor discourses, Anson Rabinbach describes the Amt Schönheit der Arbeit, or Bureau of Beauty of Labor, founded on November 27, 1933.[9] The Bureau's projects included incentivizing the beautification of factories and other industrial spaces, dissemination propaganda concerning "ideal workers," and the production of models for everything from workrooms to kitchenware and furniture. While the Bureau sought to develop a "plant community" foregrounding antiliberal ideals of work and masculinity, it also inherently drew on a "social aesthetic" which relied on prior discourses of rationalization and industrial modernization more commonly associated with leftist discourses on work and labor. In the context of the factory, the Nazi fantasy of a utopian space of labor was one where, as Nazi engineer Karl Arnhold put it, "the tempo of the machine [should] be brought into harmony with the rhythm of the blood."[10] The same logic undergirding Arnhold's impression of the laborer as automaton is at play in the poster depicting menstruating bodies. What is visible in the poster is both a mechanization of the woman's body and a fetishistic recapitulation of a natural process. This dualism would become increasingly prevalent in the broader context of Nazi theories of figurative representation, where the female form is rendered at once a machine and as something natural and unknowable. She is the idealized industrialization that the Nazis will bring to Germany and mother earth; revered and deeply sexualized just as she is exploited and appropriated.[11]

There are uncanny similarities between the figures in motion and the "primitive hut" rendered below. The shape of each woman's figure—in the peak of the elbow of the woman swimming, the spread legs of the hurdlers, and the bent back and extended arms of the carriers—mirrors the architectural form of the hut. These figures, then, instill this pseudo-historicist logic in another way: they literally *embody* the space of abjection, the hut for menstruation. Their forms reflect a primitive architecture, a distinct challenge to industrial and urban modernity. Here, perhaps, the construct of "blood and soil," the Nazi romanticization of a primordial, rural, and agrarian German identity, is compounded with the menstrual blood which informs this split scene: the harmony of the machine, be it in the factory or embodied in the machinic figures, is regimented by the repetitive nature of menstruation. There is no blood and soil, no advancing Nazi tide, without the blood of menses.

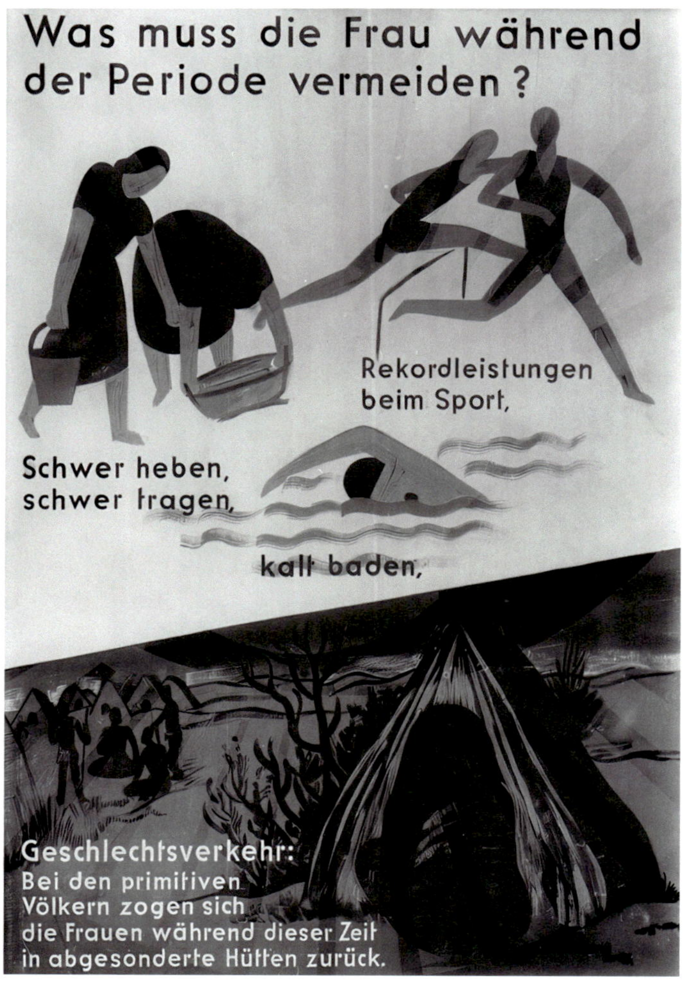

↑ "Was muss die Frau während der Periode vermeiden?" ("What must the woman avoid when on the period?"), 1933.

Regel-ated Representation

These posters were two objects in a much larger exhibition meant to display new conventions of femininity and womanhood. Yet "new" is the operative term. The "novelty" of women in Nazi society, understood in most readings as a repressive novelty, did not begin with the burning of the Reichstag. Such social transitions are embedded in imagery long before violent rhetoric becomes policy. Menstruation fit uncomfortably into the conventions of National Socialism, and the discomfort it instilled staged a figurative representation and visual field that was inflected to support its ideology. It also remains dominant today.

Violent policies continue to villainize women who do not menstruate: trans women cannot exist in contemporary society without seeing their bodies rendered political, while those cis women who cannot or do not menstruate still face stigma and rejection in a society still largely unable to separate the notion of womanhood from the notion of motherhood. The way society sees women is always already historically and politically contingent: to the fascist male imaginary, as to many conservative commentators today, menstruation evokes a fear of the abject—but the lack of menstruation is an even more fearful condition. In *Die Frau*, where women were represented with both the imperative to procreate and the uncomfortable acknowledgment of female sexuality and subjectivity, artistic forms which predate the neoclassical realism celebrated by Nazi cultural ideologues drew on the aesthetic logic of movements once considered "radical." We must continue to pay careful attention to the ways in which menstruation is represented, to the embedded logics of instruction, normalization, and regulation in such imagery. For just as the menstruation posters in *Die Frau* convey the complex ideology of early Nazi-era German society and intimate the murderous violence to come, we might find paradoxes which open up fraught dimensions of contemporary society's understanding and treatment of menstruation.

An earlier version of this essay was originally published by e-flux Architecture in 2022.

1. "German Women," speech by Joseph Goebbels, March 18, 1933, trans. Randall Bytwerk, German Propaganda Archive, Calvin University, https://research.calvin.edu/german-propaganda-archive/goeb55.htm.
2. Here my lack of consideration for Nazi perspectives on "non-Aryan" women should not be taken to mean that those formulations were any less complex or convoluted. Indeed, significant scholarship has examined femininity among communities persecuted by the Nazis: I point the reader toward work by Renate Bridenthal, Myrna Goldenburg, and Zoë Waxman as authors of various important studies which examine these themes. See Renate Bridenthal, Atina Grossman, and Marion Kaplan, eds., *When Biology Became Destiny: Women in Weimar and Nazi Germany* (New York: Monthly Review Press, 1984); Myrna Goldenberg, *Before All Is Lost: Women's Voices from the Holocaust* (Toronto: Azrieli Foundation, 2014); and Zoë Waxman, *Women in the Holocaust: A Feminist History* (Oxford: Oxford University Press, 2017). Some scholarship on the role of menstruation among concentration camp detainees has also been produced, which draws heavily on oral histories and ethnographic work compiled by the United States Holocaust Memorial Museum. Emily A. Wood, "Tracing the Destruction of Women's Bodies: Survivor Testimony of Menstruation in the Holocaust" (MA diss., University of New Brunswick, 2019).
3. Wilfried van der Will, "The Body and the Body Politic as Symptom and Metaphor in the Transition of German Culture to National Socialism," in *The Nazification of Art: Art, Design, Music, Architecture, and Film in the Third Reich*, ed. Brandon Taylor and Wilfried van der Will (Winchester, UK: Winchester Press, 1990), 14.
4. I say "discursive" here intentionally; it is very common in Nazi rhetoric that "industrialization" is made into some sort of vague boogeyman to which nearly any social ill can be attributed, and most frequently as a dog whistle for communism, which was characterized by fascists as antihumanist. For more see Jill Stephenson, *Women in Nazi Germany* (London: Routledge, 2001), 12.
5. Katherine Rossy, "Politicizing Pronatalism: Exploring the Nazi Ideology of Women through the Lens of Visual Propaganda, 1933–1939," *Graduate History Review* 3, no. 1 (2011): 58n48.
6. Bruno Gebhard, "The Health Museum," *Journal of Health Education* 6 (1948): 133 (biographical notes).
7. Klaus Theweleit, *Male Fantasies*, vol. 2: *Male Bodies: Psychoanalyzing the White Terror*, trans. Erica Carter and Chris Turner in collaboration with Stephen Conway (Minneapolis: University of Minnesota Press, 1989), 160.
8. Juliane Sander, "Camelia, oder der Beginn der 'Modernen' Monatshygiene?," Fränkisches Freilandmuseum Bad Windsheim, https://freilandmuseum.de/forschung/sammlung/die-objekte-des-monats/detail/camelia-oder-der-beginn-der-modernen-monatshygiene.
9. Anson Rabinbach, *The Human Motor: Energy, Fatigue, and the Origins of Modernity* (Berkeley: University of California Press, 1992), 286.
10. Rabinbach, *The Human Motor*, 287.
11. This is an argument put forth in slightly different ways by several different scholars. Annie Richardson's discussion of Nazi artworks and femininity, for example, reframes this duality. Citing the art historian Berthold Hinz, Richardson notes that one of the most critical dimensions of the representation of women in National Socialist visual culture was that of the potential for "distraction"—the ability of the image of the woman to serve as allegory for the war, promise of the aforementioned "return" to an idealized German society, and (most provocative) the attempt to directly "manipulate" the male's sexuality by centering imagery of the female form. Annie Richardson, "The Nazification of Women in Art," in Taylor and van der Will, *The Nazification of Art*, 54.

TOUCHING, DISEASE, AND THE SACRED ARTIFACT

AN TAIRAN

I As the plague smoldered in Milan in 1630, three French youths—a scholar, a painter, and an artisan—journeyed to the city from the north, in the hope of surveying famed Milanese monuments. Contemplating the bas-reliefs on the still-incomplete facade of the Duomo, the foreign admirers were seized with a sudden impulse to stroke the sculptural figures with their hands. In wordless awe, they rubbed the Candoglia marble as if sight alone could no longer suffice, unaware of a leery crowd of locals who distrustfully clustered around them. Scowling at the alleged evildoers, they quickly overwhelmed the young Frenchmen with furor and violence. Thought to be *untori*, or "plague greasers," a mythical group widely believed to have surreptitiously spread the contagious disease by daubing buildings with poisonous ointments, the visitors would have been lynched had magistrates not apprehended the three of them.[1]

This story was witnessed and noted down, in Latin, by the seventeenth-century Italian chronicler Giuseppe Ripamonti, and was immortalized nearly two centuries later by Alessandro Manzoni in his monumental *I promessi sposi* (*The Betrothed*, 1827), which uses Ripamonti's eyewitness accounts of the 1630 plague of Milan as its major historical source. With measured irony, Manzoni wrote: "As if to make sure that it was really marble, one of them reached out his hand to touch [*toccare*] the stone. That was enough."[2] To touch architecture—in this case, to ascertain its material—was enough to justify conviction. As if the novelistic reappraisal of the epidemic's social toxins of phobia and blame was inadequate, Manzoni strikingly appended to the second edition of *I promessi sposi* his now celebrated historical essay, "Storia della colonna infame" ("History of the Infamous Column," 1840), which directly took as its subject the crooked trials of the *untori*.[3] Indeed, at a moment when paranoid imputation and hysterical victimization pervaded the city, public buildings were deemed menacing, and to touch them was supposed to evince crime.

The transition (and translation) from Ripamonti's Latin documentation of the event to Manzoni's Italian reenactment is not as frictionless as it appears. In Ripamonti's original text, the French travelers invoked the sense of touch precisely not to certify vision (as in Manzoni's rewording, "per accertarsi ch'era marmo"—as if human sight alone was unreliable) but to complement it. In fact, Manzoni's word choice for touch—*toccare*—finds no Latin equivalent in the original; in Ripamonti's version, the sense of touch is anything but explicit:

> *atque pulcherrimum hauserant oculis, etiam altero hoc delibare sensu, & manum subinde admouebant.*
>
> They drew close what to their eyes most exquisite, enjoyed [*delibare*] with this other sense, and immediately moved their hands.[4]

In other words, the tactile, this "other sense," was only implied in the original source by Ripamonti; it was Manzoni himself who rendered the immensely ambiguous Latin *delibare* (which is derived from completely different roots; this hardly translatable verb really means to pluck, to scrape off, to detract, and, by extension, to nibble, or to enjoy by tasting) into its unequivocal nineteenth-century version as *toccare*. In this translation from *delibare* to *toccare*, the sense of touch is abstracted out of an indefinite matrix of human sensibility to serve as vision's verification.[5]

Strictly speaking, the three architectural pilgrims of 1630 did not "touch" the Duomo facade until two centuries later, when the novelist refigured the dead language of the chronicler and restaged their historic misfortune as fiction. The joined hands of a scholar, a painter, and an artisan (what story better allegorizes the perilous unification of the various departments—the scholarly, the artistic, and the technical—in the thing called "architecture"?) "touched" the foreign monument they admired only belatedly.[6] As multiple agents traveled through geography and time (just like the French youths), the fear of physical contact in the public space—largely induced by the fear of contagion (which is more contagious than the disease itself)—gradually arrived at its modern definition.[7]

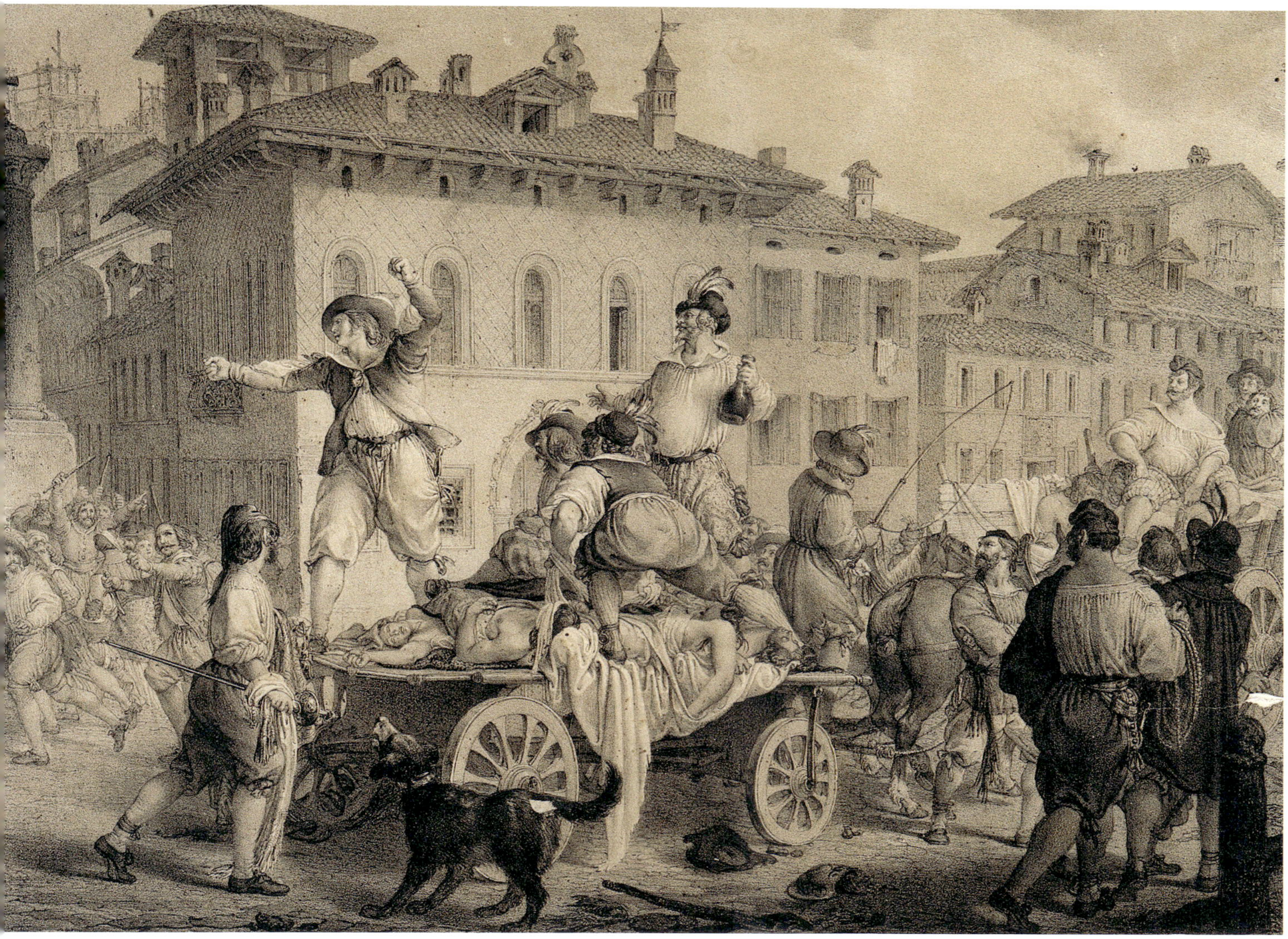

II The French travelers' fatal contiguity with architecture is complicated by the fact that the wall they touched did not belong to just any building, but to a shrine of a divine being, a monument that—in its sacredness—had already assumed an ambivalent admixture of repulsion and attraction, taboo and temptation (*mysterium tremendum et fascinans*).[8] The Latin word *sacer*, from which "sacred" is derived, is itself a well-known instance of a contronym that encompasses both holiness and impiety, adoration and abomination, or in spatial terms, embrace and forbiddance.[9]

In his essay "Touch," the literary theorist Gabriel Josipovici mulls over a significant distinction between two attitudes toward the sense of touch in Christianity: touching as antidote to incredulity, and touching as encounter across space and time.[10] According to Josipovici, the probative hand of Thomas the Apostle (more commonly known as Doubting Thomas for his suspicion of the resurrection of Jesus when first told of it) epitomizes the former, while the pilgrims' veneration of touchable relics exemplifies the latter. Poking his finger into Christ's piercing wounds of the Passion, Doubting

↑ Accusing the *untori* in the great plague of Milan in 1630; a scene from Manzoni's *I promessi sposi*. Renzo, the protagonist, having escaped the lynching of the crowd who have mistaken him for an *untore*, jumps on the chariot of corpses and from there shows his fists to the crowd that retreats to avoid any contact with the chariot. A *monatto* at the center of the pile of corpses on the chariot raises a flask of wine which he offers to Renzo as a reward for his daring. Lithograph by G. Gallina after A. Manzoni.

↓ A worker sanitizes the stones of the Western Wall in anticipation of the High Holidays in keeping with Covid-19 regulations.

Thomas made bodily contact so as to procure physical evidence, since for him vision alone would not suffice to authenticate the seemingly impossible.[11] In contrast, Josipovici claims that early medieval pilgrims—just like our French pilgrims of architecture—were not in the least doubting of the virtue laid in the sites and artifacts that were the goals of their journeys. "Contact relics" such as the *brandea* of Saint Peter (the strips of cloth that touched the saint's sarcophagus) were held to be as full of the saint's *praesentia* (the physical presence of the holy) as any physical remains, and could emanate the same healing power.[12] To touch the translated relic was therefore to converse with an invisible person of another spatiotemporal order. In Josipovici's words, "Thomas was, in effect, a *modern skeptic*, unwilling to trust anything he could not himself see and touch," while for the devout pilgrim, "the site of pilgrimage was not just the site of holiness and power, but rather the site of an *encounter*."[13]

Manzoni's retelling of Ripamonti's story translates one attitude of touching to the other, and converts the three architectural pilgrims into "modern skeptics." The heady adoration of the foreign travelers, as they felt with their fingers the grainy marbles of the Duomo facade to conjure up an invisible past and a possible future, was radically refashioned by the fiction writer into a suspicion of vision that was specific

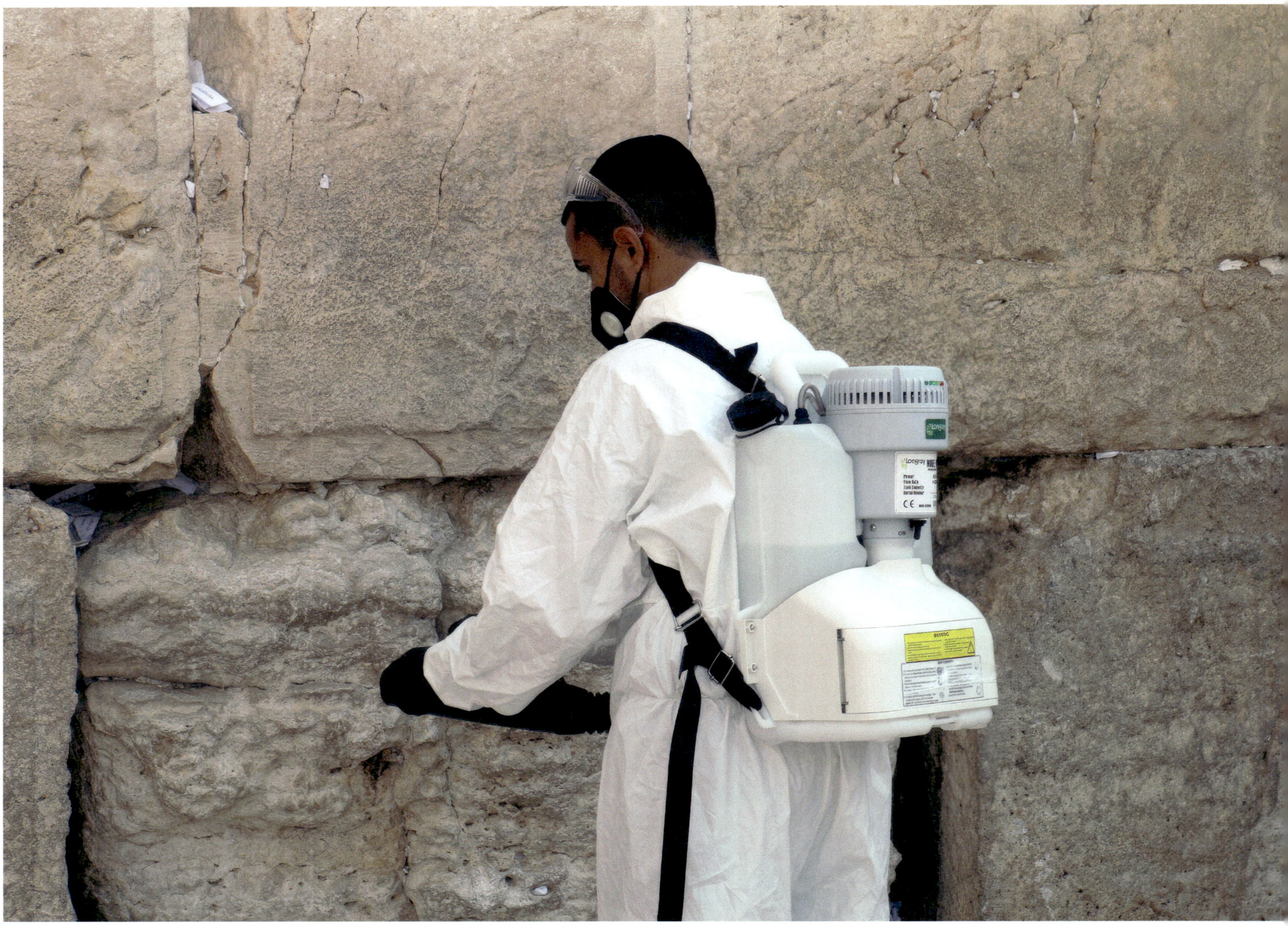

to its moment, stringently anchored to the visible (un)reality of the there and then.

Josipovici reminds us that only in the attitude of a devotee's touch could the holy person ever heal any malady, be it the therapeutic laying-on of hands in various religious traditions, the performance of anointing rituals, or the touch of *les Rois thaumaturges* that cured scrofula.[14] Probative, skeptical touch is exactly the opposite: it is to touch only as a redress of vision's inefficacy, as a sense of compensation and unbelief, as a supposedly contagious contact that might transmit infection. These two attitudes toward the sense of touch have collided, coalesced, and coevolved throughout history. Epidemics, in the most afflictive manner, lay bare their conflicts and contradictions.

III With the outbreak of Covid-19, worshipers in Jerusalem were urged not to kiss the Western Wall.[15] (To draw lips closer to hands, one could point to the clear gustatory connotation of *delibare*, not to mention the intimate derivation relationship between "taste" and "tactile.") While the pious osculatory contact was held in check, it was the "touch" of disinfectant that grazed the revered wall in the Old City of Jerusalem instead.[16] Similarly falling victim to the pandemic was the Spanish pre-Easter tradition in which Catholics line up to kiss statues of Jesus and Mary en masse all around the country. The *umrah* to Mecca was halted, keeping throngs of Muslims from kissing the Black Stone of the Kaaba. And not unlike the seventeenth-century *untori*, Iranian gate-lickers at the Masumeh shrine in Qom faced prison.[17]

The list continues, echoing numerous episodes in the past concerning the far-flung histories of liturgical kissing, touching, and their medical repercussions. Fear of plague contagion was one of the reasons it became the custom, in many places in the late Middle Ages, to kiss a pax with a devotional image during mass in lieu of direct kissing among the celebrants and congregation, furthering a practice in which the manuscripts of missals would be vigorously kissed, and sometimes even nibbled.[18] One may also revisit the 1656 plague of Rome, when Pope Alexander VII commissioned his artistic impresario Gian Lorenzo Bernini to cast a new series of bronze crucifixes—that is, crucifixes free of any trace of pestilence—for St. Peter's Basilica, as the old ones were granted to the city's lazarettos (or "quarantine stations") to confer plenary indulgences upon moribund individuals who repented, confessed, took communion, and kissed the crucifixes carried by clerics.[19] Bernini's project was literally born out of the tension between the tactile desire for the devotional objects' emanating healing power and the tactile avoidance of the "anti-relics"—the bodies of plague victims—that radiated disease and contamination (just like how medieval Venetian

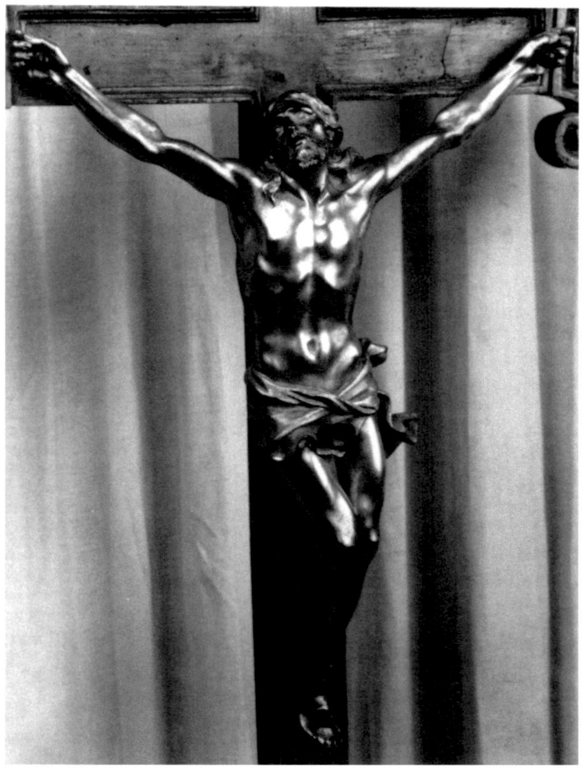

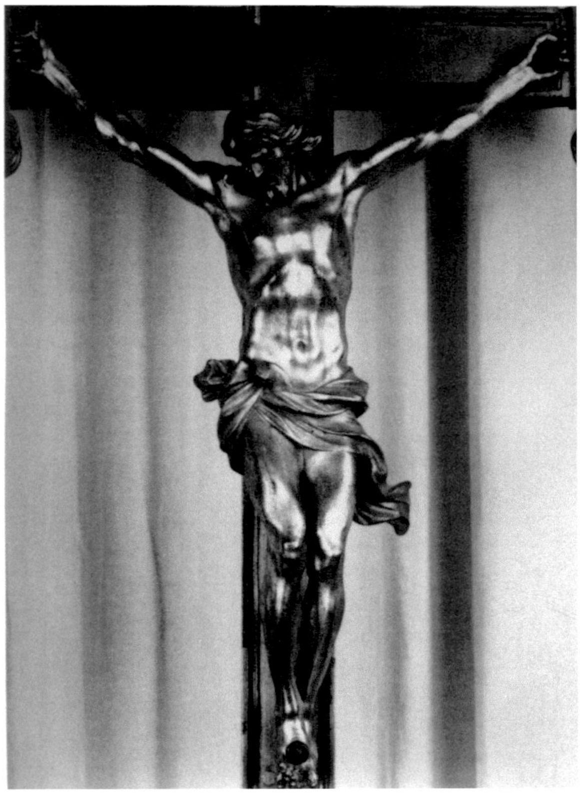

↑ Gian Lorenzo Bernini, modeled by Ercole Ferrata, *Cristo vivo*, 1659, made for the altar of St. Peter's Basilica, Rome. The Basilica of Saint Peter in the Vatican.

↓ Gian Lorenzo Bernini, modeled by Ercole Ferrata, *Cristo morto*, 1659, made for the altar of St. Peter's Basilica, Rome. The Basilica of Saint Peter in the Vatican.

Christians feared touching Jews, since they identified the Jews with corruptive bodily vices, in addition to blaming them for spreading the plague).[20] In the Christian tradition since the early Middle Ages, religious objects have long been associated with the "clean power" of God that could be played out in acts of faith healing.[21] Pope Alexander VII's evasion of touching the crucifixes due to sanitary concerns was therefore particularly anomalous.

One could further claim that the infiltration of a hygienic discourse into sacred space was a sign of religious disbelief. It is no coincidence that during the Protestant Reformation, the cleanliness of the touchable relics became an increasingly palpable issue. In one of his colloquies, the humanist scholar Erasmus offered a curious and most telling instance: on a day in the year 1514, at the dawn of the English Reformation, he set out for a pilgrimage to the Canterbury shrine of Saint Thomas, in company with his friend, Dean John Colet. In the cathedral, they were shown multiple saintly relics that the pilgrims were expected to kiss: the rusty dagger that supposedly pierced the brain of Thomas, the martyr's hair shirt, skull, bones, teeth, the holy rag with which the saint wiped sweat, etc. On their way back to London, an old mendicant offered him a piece of Saint Thomas's shoe to kiss. On this occasion, when Erasmus, to pacify the mendicant, gave him a coin, Colet exclaimed to his friend, "Do these fools wish us to kiss the shoes of every good man? They pick out the filthiest things they can find, and ask us to kiss them!"[22] Colet's hygienic concern surfaced as the fissure between the two tactile attitudes grew deep.

IV With the Protestant Reformation, not only the validity and authenticity of many relics but the efficacy of any relic was put into question.[23] It is no coincidence that doubts toward spurious relics became increasingly widespread in late medieval and Renaissance Europe as the bubonic plague peaked. The saintly power of encounter was on the wane as suspicions of touchable relics abounded. When the sixteenth-century Franciscan François du Moulin made his pilgrimage to the crypt of Basilique Sainte-Marie-Madeleine de Vézelay and was shown Mary Magdalene's skull in reliquary with the supposed impression of Jesus's fingers, he taunted that while the friars called the relic *Noli me tangere* (Touch me not, in reference to Jesus's injunction to Mary Magdalene), it might better be called *Noli me credere*—Believe me not.[24] Touching as anachronistic conversation with invisible divinity was displaced by incredulity, cruelly unmasking the time-bending holy encounter as hoax. Occasions like this, in the words of art historian Christopher S. Wood, are "moments where the deep structure of thinking about artifacts and time are revealed."[25]

Josipovici's two attitudes toward touching correspond to two modes of the sacred artifact's temporality. In the attitude of the devout pilgrim, the artifact she ardently contacts not only constitutes a typological and topological token to the sacred but also always inhabits a destabilized temporal life.[26] It is not so much that the pilgrim travels in space to touch the artifact as that the artifact travels in time to touch the pilgrim, mediating an unbridgeable distance between a tangible now and an invisible past.[27] In the attitude of the skeptic, on the other hand, the artifact's mediation device collapses, mooring the outstretched hand, as it were, onto a precise moment along the chronological line as time's inerrant witness and collator.

These two temporal modes coexist in all sacred artifacts. They are always in play, competing with one another, inducing a constant oscillation between temporal instability and chronology, encounter and verification, gullibility and incredulity, the idea of the relic and the idea of artistic authenticity, Ripamonti's *delibare* and Manzoni's *toccare*.[28] In articulating a relationship to the sacred, the temporal mode of encounter tends to shroud that of suspicion. However, an anomalous situation—such as an epidemic—radically exacerbates their clash, ruthlessly suspending the time-travel license of both the sacred artifact itself and the pilgrims from afar. Yet in situations where sickness threatens to abrogate the anachronistic touch, it also rekindles enchantments in unexpected corners. The mutual redesign of sickness and architecture uncovers the enduring life force of things, their ability to cling to a distant past, and their affect over time.

An earlier version of this essay was originally published by e-flux Architecture in 2020.

1. Giuseppe Ripamonti, *De peste quae fuit anno MDCXXX libri V* (Milan, 1640), 93–95. Alessandro Manzoni could only have read the Latin version, as the book was not translated into Italian until 1841, by Francesco Cusani: Giuseppe Ripamonti, *La peste di Milano del 1630. Libri cinque*, trans. Francesco Cusani (Milan, 1841). For a general history of the *untori* accusations during the 1630 plague of Milan, see Romano Canoso, *Tempo di peste: magistrati ed untori nel 1630 a Milano* (Rome: Angelo Ruggieri, 1985); Samuel K. Cohn Jr., "Plague Spreaders," in *Epidemics: Hate and Compassion from the Plague of Athens to AIDS* (Oxford: Oxford University Press, 2018), 127–160.
2. Alessandro Manzoni, *I promessi sposi* (Milan: Mondadori, 1990), 525. The original text reads, "Come per accertarsi ch'era marmo, stesero essi la mano a toccare. Bastò." English translation by Bruce Penman.
3. Again, Ripamonti was his principal source. For a discussion on Manzoni's *Storia* as a notable historical addendum to the fictional *I promessi sposi*, see Hal Gladfelder's article, "Seeing Black: Alessandro Manzoni between Fiction and History," *MLN* 108, no. 1 (January 1993): 59–86. See also Claudio Povolo, *The Novelist and the Archivist: Fiction and History in Alessandro Manzoni's The Betrothed*, trans. Peter Mazur (New York: Springer, 2014); Marco Codebò, "Records, Fiction, and Power in Alessandro Manzoni's *I promessi sposi* and *Storia della Colonna infame*," *MLN* 121, no. 1 (2006): 187–206.
4. Ripamonti, *De peste*, 94. The English translation is mine; I am grateful to Dong Hao and Zhang Xiaoxi of Princeton University for their help with the Latin.
5. Manzoni's purification and abstraction from *delibare* to *toccare* was not unique: in Francesco Cusani's 1841 Italian translation of Ripamonti's book, which postdated Manzoni's novel by only a few years, the translator similarly reduced, if not utterly converted, the same Latin word to *tasteggiare*, or "to gently touch." Ripamonti, *La peste di Milano*, 85. Cusani translated this sentence as "... e li vide tasteggiare quanto a loro sguardi sembrava pregevole in que' marmi."
6. According to the definition of "architecture"—as opposed to mere "buildings"—of seventeenth-century Europe, the design of churches and other religious spaces assumed the most prominence. Hence religion's supreme pertinence to the discipline of architecture at that time.
7. On blame, hatred, and persecution incurred by past epidemics, see Cohn, *Epidemics*. It may also be mentioned here that there exists a profound and exceedingly old connection between touching and epidemics. In Akkadian (the earliest attested Semitic language), the word for plague literally means "the touch or the blow of god." In the Hebrew Bible, plagues are repeatedly referred to as "the touch," not to mention the Greek and Latin origins of the English word itself, meaning "to strike, to beat."
8. Rudolf Otto, *The Idea of the Holy* (Oxford: Oxford University Press, 1957). See also Douglas A. Marshall, "Temptation, Tradition, and Taboo: A Theory of Sacralization," *Sociological Theory* 28, no. 1 (2010): 64–90; Giorgio Agamben, "The Ambivalence of the Sacred," in *Homo Sacer: Sovereign Power and Bare Life*, trans. Daniel Heller-Roazen (Stanford: Stanford University Press, 1998), 75–81.
9. Carl Abel, *Über den Gegensinn der Urworte* (Leipzig: W. Friedrich, 1884); Sigmund Freud, "The Antithetical Meaning of Primal Words, 1910," in *The Standard Edition of the Complete Psychological Works of Sigmund Freud*, vol. 2 (London: Hogarth, 1957), 153–161. Originally published as Sigmund Freud, "Über den Gegensinn der Urworte," *Gesammelte Werke*, vol. 8 (1910), 213–221.
10. See Gabriel Josipovici, *Touch* (New Haven: Yale University Press, 1996), 58–61.
11. John 20:25, New Revised Standard Version.
12. See Peter Brown, *The Cult of the Saints: Its Rise and Function in Latin Christianity* (Chicago: University of Chicago Press, 1981), 88. Brown's book is one of Josipovici's major references.
13. Josipovici, *Touch*, 61.
14. Josipovici, *Touch*, 62–64. A famous study on the royal touch is Marc Bloch, *The Royal Touch: Sacred Monarchy and Scrofula in England and France*, trans. J. E. Anderson (London: Routledge & Kegan Paul, 1973). The healing touch is incorporated into spiritual rituals in multiple religious traditions. Touching consecrated objects in Buddhism, Hinduism, Sikhism, etc., or drinking (the *Amrita*, for instance), as healing rituals was an ancient practice; in the Gospels one finds numerous accounts of Jesus touching the affected parts of the blind, the lame, or the leprous; the Islamic prophet Muhammad was reported to have performed healing miracles by touching the sick; consuming the Taoist talismanic water (符水 *fu shui*, ashes from burnt talismans dissolved in water) was believed to cure diseases (I am grateful to Du Yalin of Princeton University for this reference); one could continue.
15. See Jacob Magid, "To Kiss or Not to Kiss: The Question for Old City Pilgrims amid Virus Outbreak," *Times of Israel*, March 12, 2020.
16. See Celia Jean, "Western Wall Notes Removed for Passover, Stones Sanitized for Coronavirus," *Jerusalem Post*, March 31, 2020.
17. See Jon Nazca and Silvio Castellanos, "Another Victim of Coronavirus: Spain's Religious Statue-kissing," Reuters, March 6, 2020; Rozina Sini and Armen Shahbazian, "Coronavirus: Iran holy-shrine-lickers face prison," BBC, March 3, 2020; Vivian Yee, "In a Pandemic, Religion Can Be a Balm and a Risk," *New York Times*, March 22, 2020.
18. See Kathryn M. Rudy, "Kissing Images, Unfurling Rolls, Measuring Wounds, Sewing Badges and Carrying Talismans: Considering Some Harley Manuscripts through the Physical Rituals They Reveal," *Electronic British Library Journal* (2011), art. 5; Constance Classen, *The Deepest Sense: A Cultural History of Touch* (Champaign: University of Illinois Press, 2012), 150.
19. See Sheila Barker, "Art, Architecture, and the Roman Plague of 1656," in *La Peste a Roma (1656–1657)*, ed. Irene Fosi (Rome: Università degli Studi Roma Tre—CROMA, 2006), 243–262; Roberto Battaglia, "Crocifissi del Bernini in S. Pietro," *Quaderni di studi romani* 11 (1942): 3–21; and Ursula Schlegel, "I crocifissi degli altari in San Pietro in Vaticano," *Antichità viva* 20 (1981): vi, 37–42.
20. I took the expression "anti-relic" from Constance Classen's discussion on the fear of touching the bodies of plague victims. See Classen, *The Deepest Sense*, 150. For the medieval Venetian Christians' fear and isolation of Jews, see Richard Sennett, "Fear of Touching," in *Flesh and Stone: The Body and the City in Western Civilization* (New York W. W. Norton, 1994), 212–254.
21. On the "clean power" in association with holy sites and sacred artifacts, see Peter Brown, *The Cult of the Saints: Its Rise and Function in Latin Christianity* (Chicago: University of Chicago Press, 1981), 100–105.
22. See Henry Donald Maurice Spence-Jones, *The Church of England: A History for the People*, vol. 2: *The Medieval Church* (London, 1897), 424–427.
23. On the decline of the sacred touch in relation to the Reformation, see Craig Koslofsky, "The Kiss of Peace in the German Reformation," in *The Kiss in History*, ed. Karen Harvey (Manchester: Manchester University Press, 2005), 18–35.
24. See Marjorie O'Rourke Boyle, *Senses of Touch: Human Dignity and Deformity from Michelangelo to Calvin* (Leiden: Brill, 1998), 122. François du Moulin called the skull into doubt because he believed that the evangelists never wrote Jesus touched her forehead.
25. Christopher S. Wood, *Forgery, Replica, Fiction: Temporalities of German Renaissance Art* (Chicago: University of Chicago Press, 2008), 12.
26. Here I am inspired by Alexander Nagel's discussion on the topographical instability of medieval churches (his cases are Giotto's Arena chapel and the Holy Sepulcher of Jerusalem). See Alexander Nagel, *Medieval Modern: Art Out of Time* (London: Thames & Hudson, 2012), 97–115.
27. On the idea of vital/vibrant artifacts, which would not only, as in our context, challenge a traditionally anthropocentric architectural/art historical discourse, but also problematize certain notions of materiality at large, see Jane Bennett's influential book *Vibrant Matter: A Political Ecology of Things* (Durham: Duke University Press, 2009).
28. My claim here on the two temporal modes of the sacred artifact is indebted to Alexander Nagel and Christopher S. Wood's perceptive theoretical construction in their *Anachronic Renaissance*. See Alexander Nagel and Christopher S. Wood, "Plural Temporality of the Work of Art," in *Anachronic Renaissance* (New York: Zone Books, 2010), 7–20.

p175 Courtesy of the Wellcome Collection
p176 Courtesy of The Western Wall Heritage Foundation, September 16, 2020.
p177 Courtesy of the Reverenda Fabbrica of Saint Peter in the Vatican.

ATMO
PHER

S-

ES

HYSTERIA AS SCENOGRAPHY

MARIE DE TESTA

Up until 1968, the Salpêtrière Hospital in Paris exclusively treated women. Between 1872 and 1892, when doctor Jean-Martin Charcot famously endeavored to visually typify hysteria, the medical complex comprised forty-five buildings and approximately five thousand women inmates. Founded by King Louis XIV in 1656 as an institution for the confinement of the poor and their concealment from public view, La Salpêtrière was originally built on the site of a former gunpowder (or *salpêtre*) factory. During the French Revolution, it was the site of an infamous massacre of vulnerable women, which tainted the reputation of its walls as enclosing a "feminine inferno."[1] This historical event only amplified the stigma that came to be associated with its inmates.

During the times of Charcot, women were confined to La Salpêtrière either "voluntarily" or *par office*. The denomination of the former, however, is misleading, for women would often be institutionalized not by their own will but at the request of family members who disproportionately tended to be men—husbands, brothers, sons.[2] The newly created Department of Public Assistance, in association with the police, would also detain *par office*, in the name of public order and safety of the larger population, women who were judged in terms of their "dangerosity"—a conveniently flexible criterion open to the interpretation of the accuser, the judge, or the discriminating medical physician.[3] Women targeted by the police also included those deemed undesirable or in marginal social positions, such as *vagabondes*, *idiotes*, *imbéciles*, children with developmental disabilities (*les arriérées*), and *personnes agés*; women who profited from or asserted their sexuality, such as prostitutes, "seductresses," *débauchés*, and

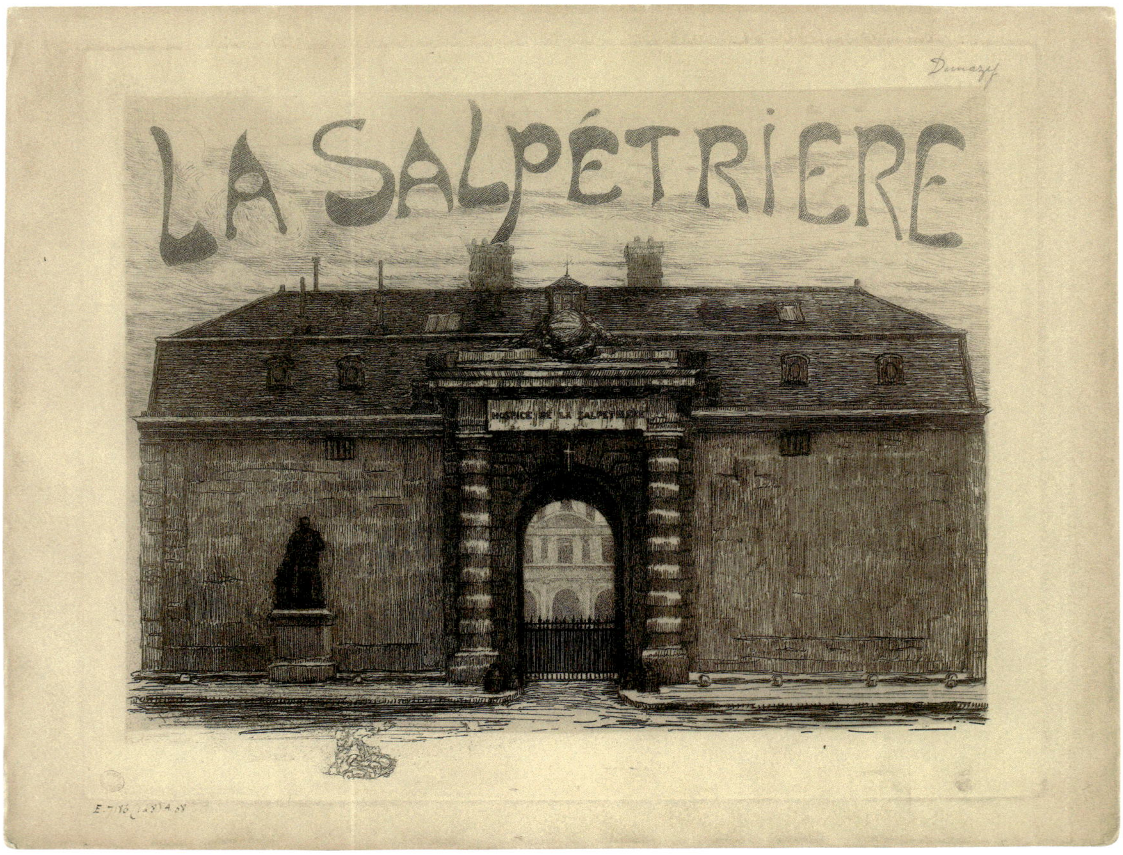

→ J. E. Thierry (engraver), E. Poulet Gallimard (designer), *Plan de L'Hospice de la Salpêtrière*, 1812. Print, 62.8 × 50.1 cm.

↙ Gaston J. C. Demazy, engraving, 1872. Print, 28 × 37 cm.

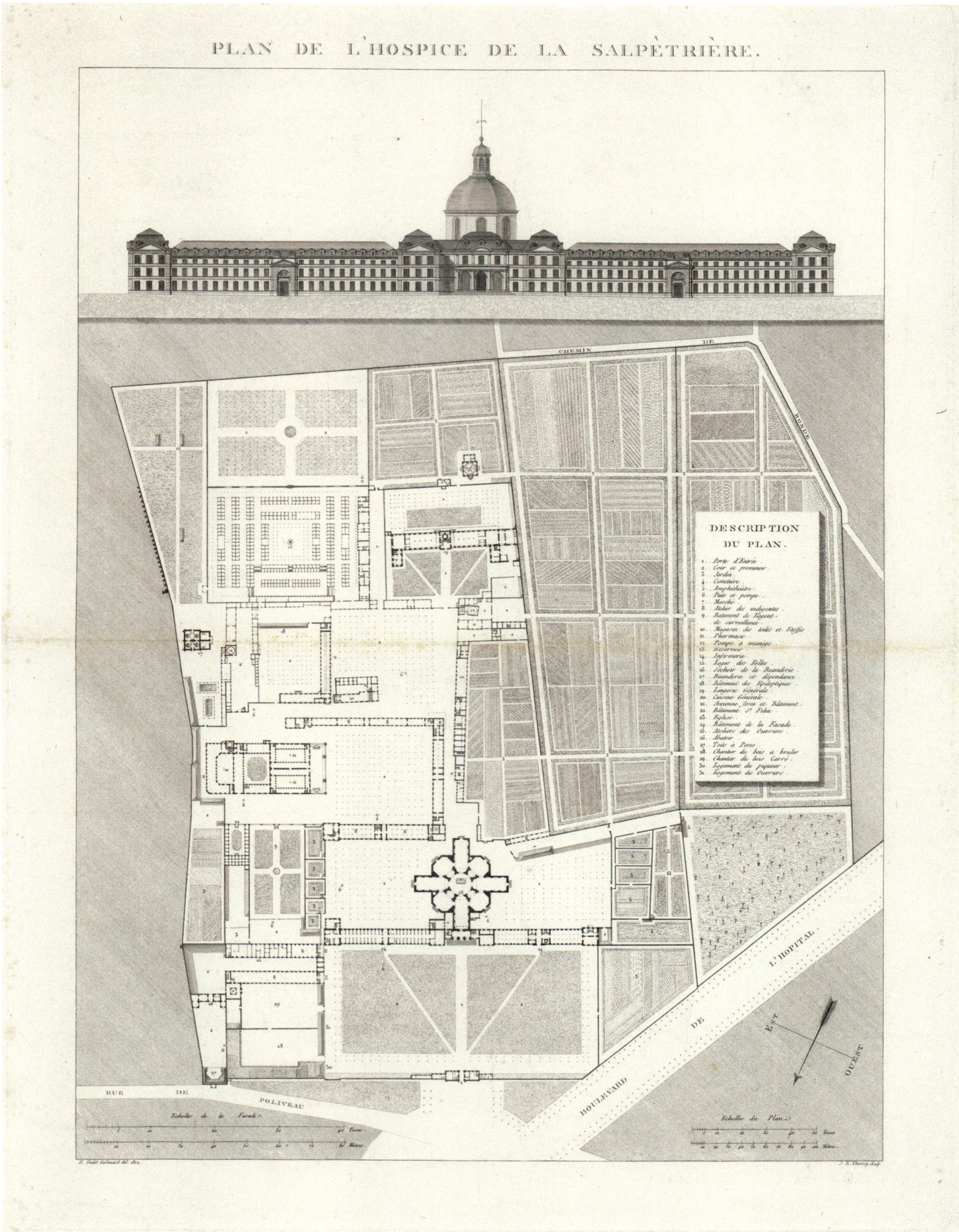

érotomanes; as well as those considered aggressive, such as women who swore, yelled, or could otherwise be considered indomitable (*insoumises*, *agitées*, *indisciplinées*).[4] Women would enter as medical patients, but often become *filles de salle*—permanent residents at the hospital from which they would never be released.

La Salpêtrière existed as a permanent threat for women inclined to what society proscribed as undesirable behavior. At the time of Charcot, the display of a certain type of female subjectivity in private, public, or political domains was deemed not only transgressive but pathological, and therefore to be repressed and treated.[5] Displays of transgressive femininity were perceived as menacing and could only be permitted at the margins, made invisible, or shown in a highly controlled light. The walls of La Salpêtrière defined a place of stigma, one that identified, enclosed, and visibly excluded unsanctioned difference.

Architecture staged hysteria at La Salpêtrière, both its marginalization and its spectacularization. Relays of visual barriers blocked views from the city into the precinct. Successive walls constructed the symbolic demarcation and built up the effective seclusion of female inmates. Symmetrical wings acted as framing devices around a central opening,

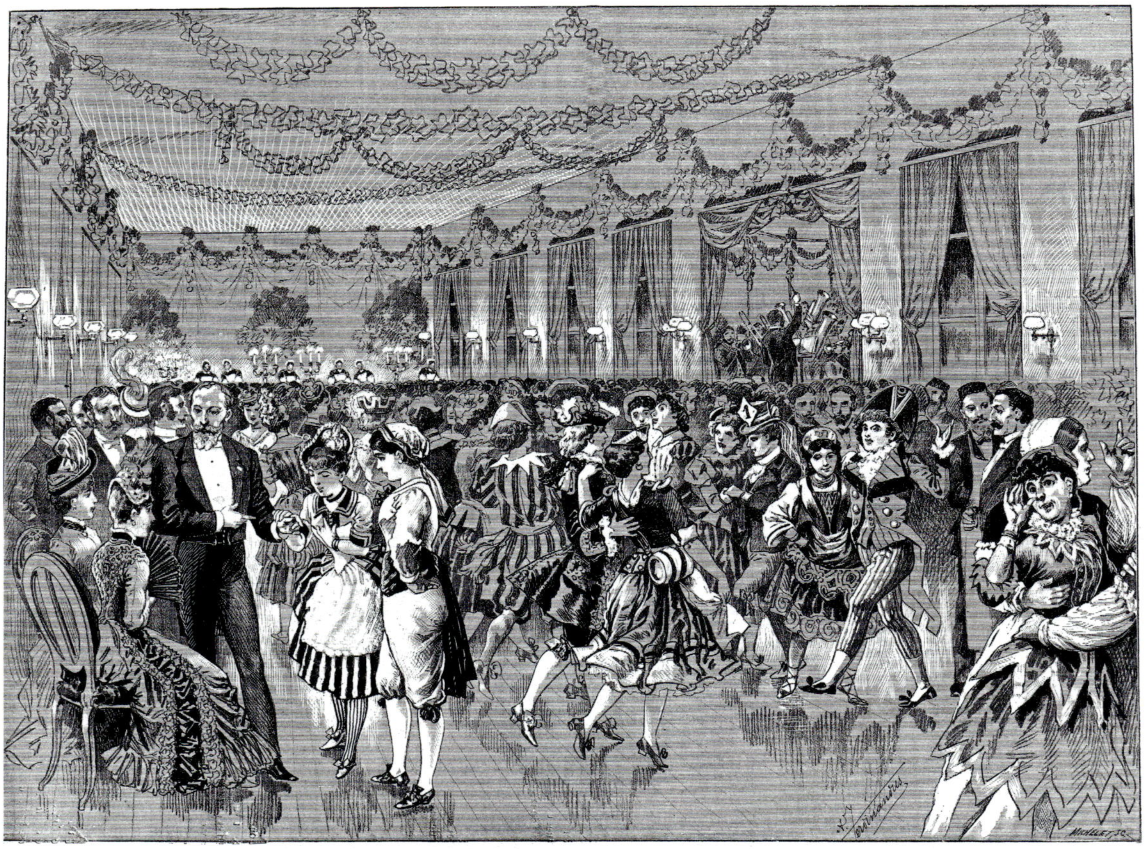

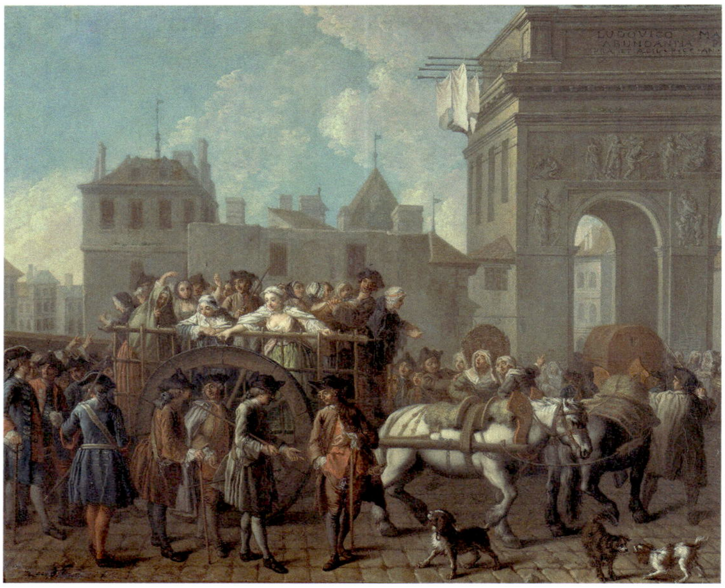

which was immediately blocked by the Saint Louis Chapel.[6] Beyond the prominent volume of the chapel, the sightline of an outsider was tunneled through an old prison and surveillance pavilion. Walls perpendicular to the observer's point of view further restricted their line of sight toward the patients' wards, hidden at the back of the complex. These, in turn, were flanked by gardens, serving as visual and potentially acoustic buffers to adorn and distract from a presumably terrifying sight, or at least a nuisance for city dwellers deemed sane.

While what happened inside its walls remained largely concealed from public view, the detainment of women was highly public and publicized. The transport of new inmates to La Salpêtrière was purposefully designed as a procession of shame. The tension between concealment and exposure produced by the architecture of La Salpêtrière at the scale of the city was reproduced in its interior furnishings. Patient quarters were also referred to as "display pavilions," with "several dozen beds lined up," some closed by curtains, veiling the "relaxing, often incurable, bedridden."[7]

Visibility as Occlusion

From as early as 1835, a yearly public event was organized by the Department of Public Assistance and hosted at La Salpêtrière as part of the Carnival of Paris, the so-called Ball of the Mad (*Bal des Folles*), during which an audience of outside guests and the public at large was invited to spend an evening dancing to

↑ "Le Bal des Folles à l'Hôpital de la Salpêtrière," originally published in *L'Univers illustré*, Paris, March 17, 1888, p. 473.

↓ Étienne Jeurat, *La Conduite des filles de joie à la Salpêtrière: le passage près de la porte Saint-Bernard*, 1757. Oil on canvas, 65 × 82 cm.

orchestral music alongside interned women called upon to perform their illness. The event was considered therapeutic treatment for the inmates and "joyous entertainment" for those in attendance.[8] Charcot himself would select the guests to invite, which served as an opportunity to showcase the claimed modernity of his experimental methods to a target audience.[9]

The ball was a public showcase of the theatricalization of madness. According to Maxime Du Camp, a journalist who reported on the 1893 ball, "the [hysteric] woman ... exaggerates her role, speaks, gesticulates, tells and initiates, at first sight, to all the mysteries of her aberration."[10] Inmates were offered the exceptional opportunity to participate in a social event, even if the pathological judgment of women's behavior ultimately remained in place. In the words of a reporter who attended the 1884 ball: "What do you want, women remain women everywhere and always, at La Salpêtrière as elsewhere."[11]

Other than the desire to please, and to be applauded by the same society which had marginalized, judged, incriminated, excluded, and incarcerated them, inmates were given the pleasure of performance, as well as, and perhaps more importantly, the pleasure of asserting themselves and their desires. The hysteric woman embodied her desire by performing herself, or the woman she wished she could be, in the form of her "hyperbolic incarnation."[12] Through the "considerable magnification" of *pathos*, the symptomatology of the hysteric became akin to the art of the histrionic.[13]

Inmates spent months anticipating the festivity and preparing their costumes ("the most varied, the most picturesque, the freshest").[14] In his recount of the ball of 1889, psychiatrist and invitee Dr. Frédet noted that the hysteric women presented themselves in such a manner that "one would believe oneself to be within one of the most elegant societies."[15] Conversely, he noted that it was the guests, rather than the hosts, who "were the less tranquil, who made the most noise, who were the most agitated, and those whom an impartial spectator would think at first sight are the inhabitants of the house."[16]

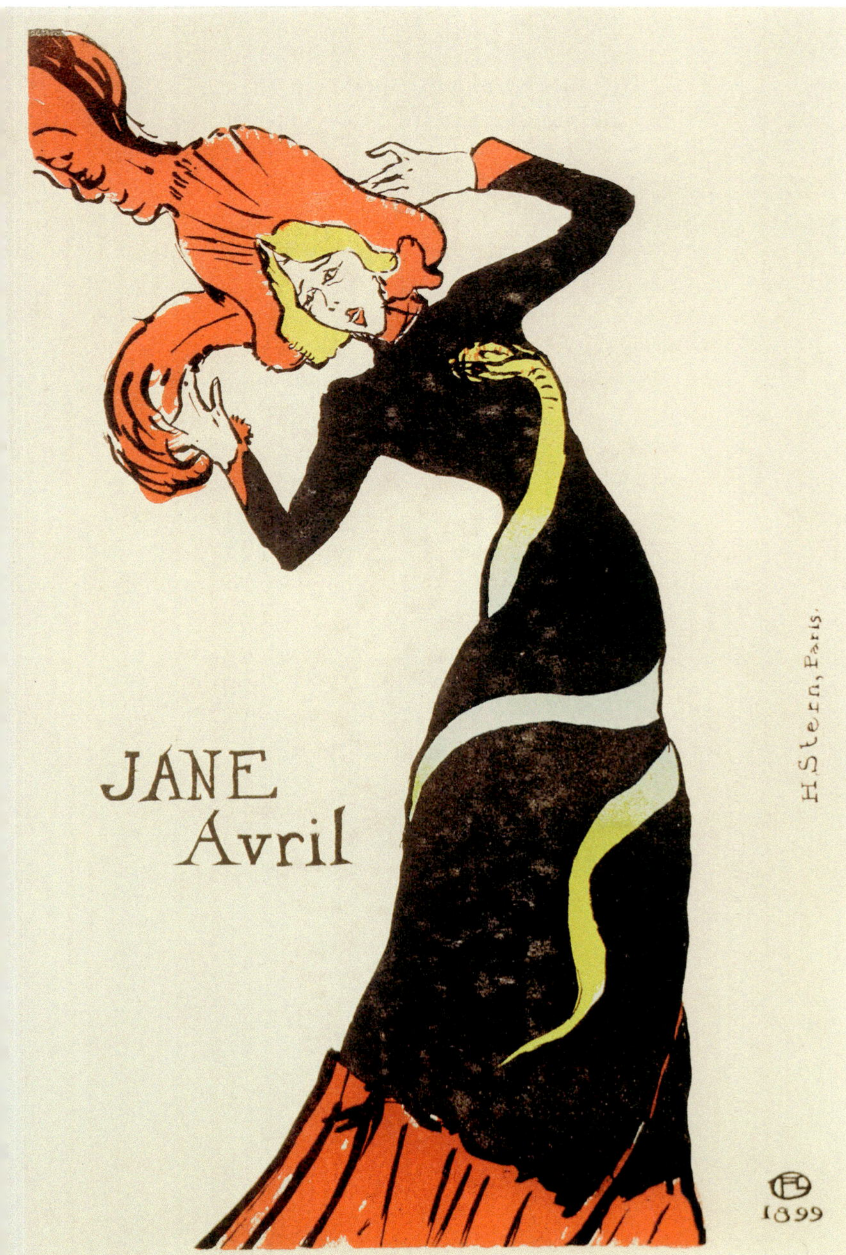

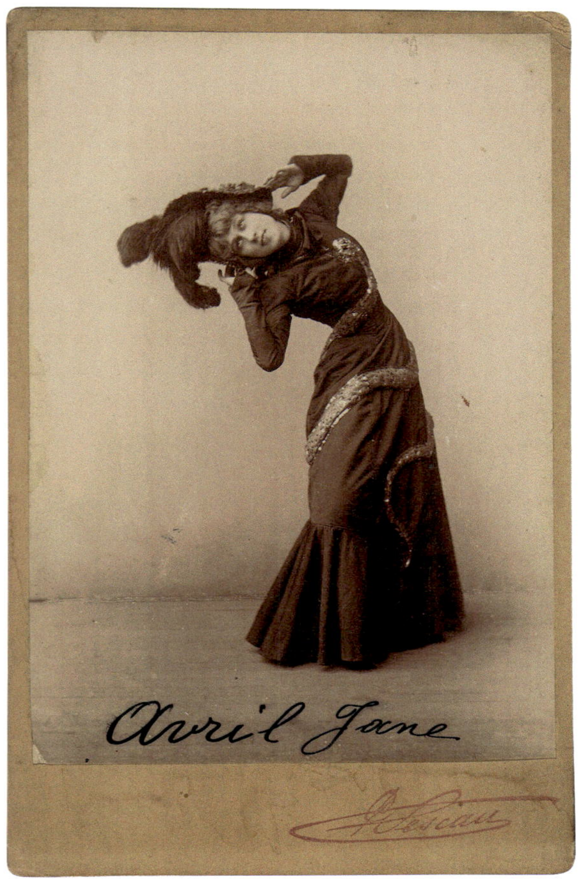

↑ Paul Sescau, *Jane Avril*, dancer of the Moulin Rouge (and patient at La Salpêtrière), ca. 1890.

← Henri de Toulouse-Lautrec, *Jane Avril*, 1899. Color lithograph on tan wove paper, 55.6 × 37.6 cm.

Not only did the occasion facilitate the exceptional reversal of order and societal values allowed by the days of carnival, it may also have provided space for the showcase and rehearsal of new attitudes and modes of behavior. The hosts imitated reason and the guests imitated madness, thus rendering hysteria potentially contagious beyond the psychiatric walls.

The Clinical Stage

Other than the yearly ball, Charcot hosted his famous weekly Tuesday lessons, which became well-attended events by a large spectrum of Parisian society including Sigmund Freud, the Goncourt brothers, Guy de Maupassant, Octave Mirbeau, Alphonse Daudet, Jane Avril, and Rachel and Sarah Bernhardt. During these "lessons," Charcot would publicly perform a real-time consultation and diagnosis of new incoming patients.[17] These were highly produced multimedia events which included the use of printed photographs, photographic projections, drawings quickly executed in chalk, live hysteric bodies performing movement and speech, mimes enacted by Charcot himself, picturesque narratives, dramatic interrogations, and more. The repertory scenes of hysteria that Charcot offered to his audience were scripted in real time, directed live, and supertitled. He would enunciate descriptions that would serve at once as stage directions for the women and as a synopsis guiding the audience in the unfolding of the hysteric plot: "The patient who has just been placed under your eyes is ..."[18]

Charcot simultaneously performed the role of the medical authority, master of ceremonies, and omniscient live narrator. The "leading ladies of hysteria"—Louise Glaiz, Alphonsine Bar, Blanche Wittman—would strike poses, articulate gestures, and enact didascalies to compose the unfolding image of hysteria the physician was trying to recreate.[19] Charcot used their bodies to direct an indexical form of hysteria as visually described in the manuals of neurology he himself had produced in order to typify it. Reenacting a constructed archetype, women became effigies of the illness they were directed to portray and embody. The women's diligence in following directions was such that they were compared to "puppets," "mannequins," and "automata."[20]

During the lessons, women were manipulated and penetrated with medical props.[21] Allegedly, the hysteric woman would relentlessly recreate the symptoms that could only be alleviated, through transference, by degrees of sexual interaction or outright intercourse with the medical doctor or intern most readily available, which she would herself vocally solicit. Reciprocally, the physician would be enamored by the living proof of his scientific research: she who would guarantee his professional success, consent to enact his medical fantasies word by word, and provide sexual satisfaction.[22] The almost compulsive acting-out of roles by the women must have proven highly erotic to the audience.[23]

Emergence of a New Femininity

The amphitheater in which Charcot's famous lessons took place no longer exists, and no photographic documentation survives of his public demonstrations of hysteria. However, the painting *Une leçon de clinique à la Salpêtrière* (1887) by André Brouillet has filled the collective imagination with spatial evidence of these events. The *tableau* presents a central male figure, standing, dressed in a black suit, white shirt, and black bowtie, with his finger pointing toward the viewer. The gesture may be one of instruction, or direction, but also a silent warning. The twenty-four other men gathered around him are dressed alike and pay close attention to him. Most sit on wooden ladder-back chairs, while a few stand at the back of the room. Some seem perplexed, others take notes. All await what Charcot has to say.

At the center of the painting is an armchair with leather upholstery next to a simple table exhibiting medical props. The leading lady of the scene is in *arc-en-cercle*—an iconic posture associated with a woman performing hysteria, which is also popularly

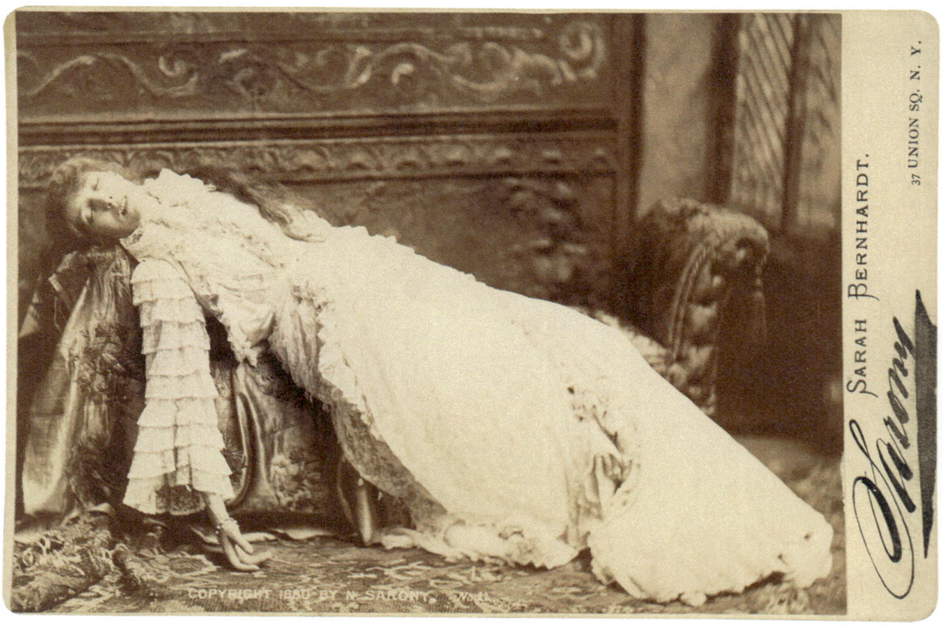

→ Napoleon Sarony, *Sarah Bernhardt*, ca. 1880.

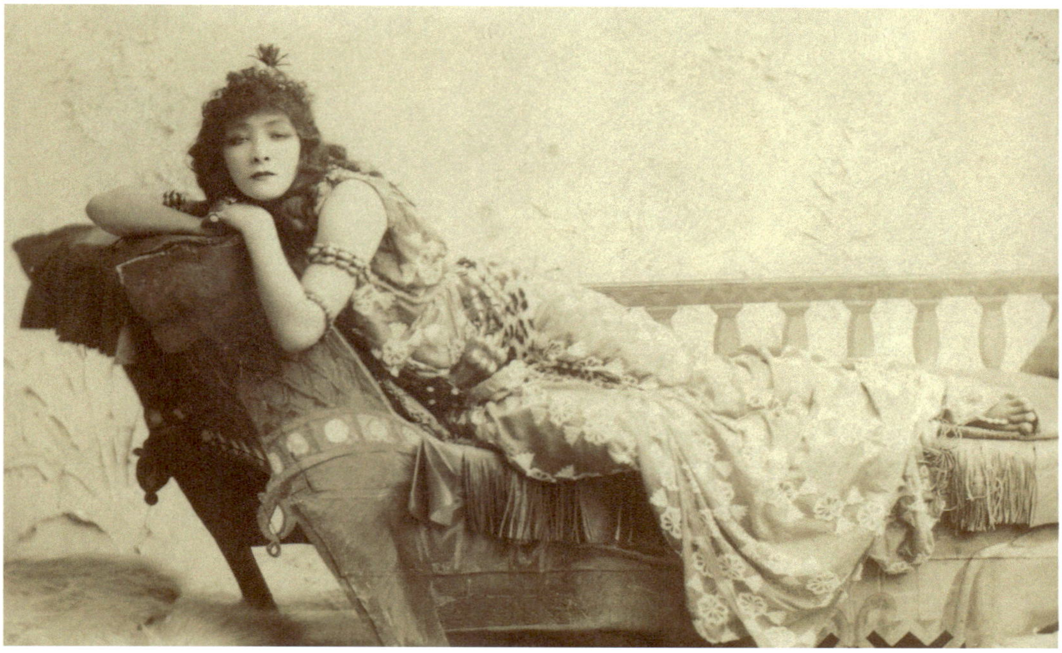

→ Cabinet card image of Sarah Bernhardt, dressed as Cleopatra, photographed by Napoleon Sarony, 1891.

considered, to this day, a highly erotic posture. She is held from behind by a man whose gaze is focused on her neck. Her costume consists of a white off-the-shoulder blouse with a revealing *décolleté*; her corset seems to be untightened. She might be in the process of being unclothed, before the eyes of all attendees, for the upper part of her dress has been unbuttoned and hangs down her waist. The lighting of the scene makes her chest the focal point, which is precisely where the sightlines of most of the depicted men converge. The brightest whites in the picture take the viewer's eye from her body to the adjoining bedsheets, untidy on the stretcher, one of the few other explicit props on stage. On the back wall, two large windows allow daylight to come in but screen the view toward the outside.

The colors of the set are warm, while the gaze of the men is not: they seem interested, but not concerned; certainly not worried or alarmed. The scene is repetitive and has become routine; it appears normal. Another attendant, an older woman, highly covered in her attire, extends her hands toward the fainting woman, as if anticipating what comes next. Her skirt is white, pleated, and clean. Two of the seated men wear dirty aprons. A third woman's face barely makes it into the frame. Suspended on the left wall is a chalk drawing of a woman in the *arc-en-cercle* posture; arching her back on a bed, her left breast again highlighted, her clothing thin enough that it allows the contours of her figure to be seen.

The group portrait of the ensemble whose performance defined modern hysteria was first shown at the Paris Salon of May 1887.[24] Charcot himself kept a reproduction of Brouillet's painting in his living room all of his life, and Freud displayed one in both his Vienna and London medical cabinets. The original painting is now exhibited at the Paris Descartes University, near the entrance of the Museum of Medical History. The variation of institutional contexts wherein the painting has been displayed mirrors the ambiguous position of Charcot's lessons, between the realm of art and representation and that of modern science.

Other descriptions of Charcot's amphitheater were published in writing at the time. In an article for *L'Événement* in 1885, Octave Mirbeau writes of a long hall half-occupied by rows of seating; a space where all windows were "hermetically closed and obstructed" and where no daylight could "pierce through the obscured light produced by the gas lamps."[25] He reports empty seats due to an avid audience gathered around the professor, the patients and the medical aids. He describes two small tables with a "few electrical instruments, demonstration boards and a large chalkboard." He ends his article with the words "Voilà la mise en scène [This is the staging]."[26]

The women of La Salpêtrière redefined femininity in the public eye. They were displayed on Charcot's stages—the architectural complex of La Salpêtrière itself, the yearly showcases held within its premises, and the weekly public lessons in its amphitheater. They were mediatized by photography in Charcot's compendia of neurology, and popularized and catapulted to fame by word of mouth. Yet Charcot's media machine inadvertently advanced the plight of women by amplifying and distributing their image as an overtly sexual subject whose sexuality was transgressive of preestablished limits of normalcy. Indeed, there were other women in the audience—both those directly witnessing the medical performances and those who accessed it through the media and culture of fame—who might have felt liberated seeing these images.

The spectacle of hysteria sublimated the collective oppression of women and emerged as a

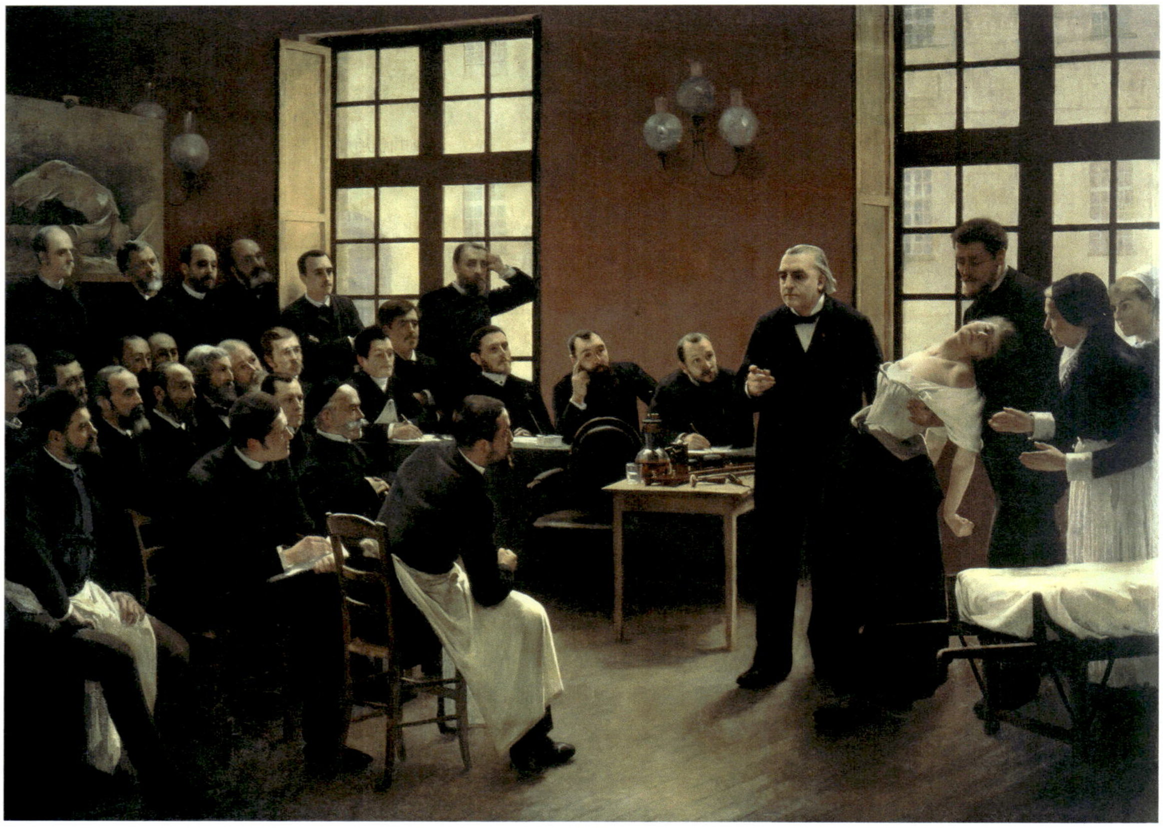

scandalous, shockingly visual manifestation of transgression. In a hysteric attack, the patient performs a highly active and visible dispossession of her inhibited self; a body violently reclaiming its sexuality, unapologetically exhibiting its desire and assertively enacting its satisfaction in public. The effect on (presumably oppressed) women who witnessed other (allegedly ill) women reclaiming their subjectivity and sexual expression must have been inspiring and contagious.

Charcot himself played with the fact that hysteria was perceived as highly transmissible, and addressed his audience with the following warning: "look at it [hysteria] and try not to be influenced, suggested, or intoxicated by what you will see and hear."[27] His warning may have worked as a threat, a demonstration of what could happen to any woman who behaved deviantly. But it also might have served as a covert invitation to perform. Women joining the ranks of hysteria might have proven that they were better off confined than outside the psychiatric wards. By mutual identification—and in solidarity with each other—hysterics proclaimed a new form of femininity. The expansive character of hysteria led it to be considered *the* epidemic of the *fin de siècle* and a public health concern, while the term "collective hysteria" has come to signify the susceptibility of the masses to suggestion.[28] Hysteria, then, took place collectively as an event, while advancing the cause of another, subsequent epidemic in gestation: a femininity publicly assertive of its sexuality.

↑ André Brouillet, *Une leçon de vlinique à la Salpêtrière*, 1887. Oil on canvas, 290 × 430 cm.

An earlier version of this essay was originally published by e-flux Architecture in 2022.

1. "On September 3, 1792, men drunk on the blood spilled in all the prisons of Paris went to La Salpêtrière Hospital and asked to be presented with the forty-five [female] prisoners. ... They decimated them in place, the Desrues woman was one of the first victims. [Le 3 septembre 1792 des hommes ivres du Sang versé dans toutes les Prisons de Paris, allèrent à l'Hôpital de la Salpêtrière, se firent représenter les prisonnières au nombre de quarante-cinq et ... les assommèrent sur la place, la femme Desrues fut une des premières victimes.]" This and all subsequent translations are mine. See inscription on the back of "Massacre of Prostitutes at the Salpêtrière Hospital on September 3, 1792, current 13th arrondissement," print no. 165, *Journal des Révolutions de Paris*, September 1–8, 1792, 430.

"Feminine inferno" is one of the expressions employed by Georges Didi-Huberman to describe La Salpêtrière. See Georges Didi-Huberman, *Invention of Hysteria: Charcot and the Photographic Iconography of the Salpêtrière* (Cambridge, MA: MIT Press, 2003), xi. Octave Mirbeau called it "città dolorosa," and Jean-Martin Charcot referred to it as "The Versailles of Pain [Le Versailles de la Douleur]."

2. See Yanick Rippa, *La Ronde des folles: Femme, folie et enfermement au XIXe siècle (1838–1870)* (Paris: Aubier, 1986), 30–32.

3. "You are this, you are that, you are at last what all women are from the beginning of time Hysteric! [Vous êtes ceci, vous êtes cela, vous êtes enfin ce que sont toutes les femmes depuis le commencement du temps. Hystérique!]" See Guy de Maupassant, "Une femme," *Gil Blas,* August 16, 1882.

4. Rippa, *La Ronde des folles*, 27–33.

5. If La Salpêtrière as an institution targeted certain expressions of feminine sexuality, it paradoxically served, this chapter argues, as a platform for women to publicly enact their liberation.

6. The neoclassical, rational, and symmetric facade of La Salpêtrière was the face it gave to the city. Its defining architectural element, the perimeter wall, an enclosure

denoting confinement, was demolished before the time of Charcot. But the imposing entrance, the threshold marking the limits between normalcy and deviance and innocence and guilt—under the guise of sickness and health—still stood. The vestibule to the modern hospital complex remained as a perspectival court garden stressing the magnificence of the charity that had given rise to it and its royal origins, while the prominent chapel granted further grandeur to the pious who had commissioned it, as it symbolically maintained its pledged allegiance to the Catholic Church.

7. I here reprise the term *Pavillion Vitrine* and description offered by Yann Diener, psychoanalyst, in an interview for *France Culture*, February 15, 2020. At the time of the founding of La Salpêtrière, allegedly "mad" women assigned to confinement were considered "ferocious beasts" ("La folle furieuse était considérée comme une bête féroce"). Inmates lived in underground quarters behind bars and were often chained. They slept on a floor covered with straw which was changed monthly. Daily provisions consisted of bread and water. It was not until 1792, when Dr. Pinel revolutionized the status of madness by claiming "the mad are ill [Les fous sont des malades]," that these women were considered patients, released from their chains, and offered medical treatment. See Alfred Edwards, "Le bal des folles, une grande fête à la Salpêtriere," *Le Matin Derniers Télégrammes de la Nuit*, March 21, 1884.

8. "Un joyeux divertissement pour le public parisien." Edwards, "Le bal des folles."

9. Not all attendees were persuaded. Consider the following words by another journalist who attended the *bal*: "upon leaving, while traversing the precinct, the immense courtyards of this city called La Salpêtriere ... my thoughts go back despite myself to the Salpêtrière of other times, the Salpêtrière before the revolution, such as it was from Louis XIV until Pinel. ... It would seem a novel. It is history, *hélas*. [En traversant, pour m'en aller, les préaux, les cours immenses de cette ville qui s'appelle la Salpêtrière, qui compte quarante-cinq corps de bâtiments, cinq mille fenêtres environ, cinq mille malades, ma pensée se reportait malgré moi sur la Salpêtrière de jadis, la Salpêtrière d'avant la Révolution, telle qu'elle fût depuis Louis XIV jusqu'à Pinel. ... Cela a l'air d'un roman. C'est de l'histoire, hélas.]" See Edwards, "Le bal des folles."

10. Maxime Du Camp, *Paris, ses organes, ses fonctions et sa vie dans la seconde moitié du XIXème siècle*, vol. 4 (Paris: Hachette, 1893–1894).

11. "But this ball of mid-Lent is like a break, a pause for all those victims of neurosis, the great disease of the century, for all those heads devoid of reason or peopled with incoherent thoughts, called the crazy. The ball is everything, a fortnight before and fifteen days after. ... More than one agitated madwoman calms down. More than one atrophied or softened brain seems to regain a flash of thought. What do you want, women remain women everywhere and always, at the Salpêtrière as elsewhere. You have to look pretty for the ball. [Mais ce bal de la Mi-Carême, c'est comme une halte, c'est comme un repos pour toutes ces victimes de la grande maladie du siècle la névrose, pour toutes ces têtes vides de raison ou peuplées de pensées sans suite, qu'on appelle des folles. Le bal est tout, quinze jours avant et quinze jours après. ... Plus d'une folle agitée se calme. Plus d'un cerveau atrophié ou ramolli semble retrouver un éclair de pensée. Que voulez-vous la femme reste femme partout et toujours, à la Salpêtrière comme ailleurs. Il faut se faire belle pour le bal.]" Edwards, "Le bal des folles."

12. Charles Féré, "Sensation and Mouvement," *Revue Philosophique* 20 (1885): 364–365. Cited in Bertrand Marquer, *Les Romans de la Salpêtrière: Réception d'une scénographie clinique: Jean-Martin Charcot dans l'imaginaire fin-de-siècle* (Geneva: Droz, 2008), 130.

13. Charcot explained, "it is a characteristic of hysterical patients to exaggerate their phenomena and they are more prone to do so when observed or admired." See Christopher G. Goetz et al., *Charcot: Constructing Neurology* (Oxford: Oxford University Press, 1995), 173. A former patient turned can-can dancer recalled: "There were crazy girls, whose disease, called 'hysteria' consisted above all in simulating it. [Il y avait ces folles filles, don la maladie, denominée 'hysterie' consistait surtout à la simuler.]" See Jeanne Avril, J. P. Morel, and C. Brécourt-Villars, *Mes Mémoires* (Paris: Phébus, 2005), 437.

14. Docteur Frédet, "Un bal à la Salpêtrière," *Mélanges nouvelles historiques et scientifiques, Bulletin historique et scientifique de l'Auvergne* (1889). Cited in Julie Froudière, "Littérature et aliénisme: Poétique romanesque de l'Asile (1870–1914)," *Littératures* (Dissertation Université Nancy 2, 2010) 142.

15. "There are about 150 women there, young for the most part and some of whom are very beautiful, who walk around, waiting for the call of the orchestra, dressed in the most varied, the most picturesque, the freshest costumes, and some of which, I must say, are worn with arrogance, a totally aristocratic ease. It really feels like being in the world and in a most elegant society. [Il y a là environ cent cinquante femmes, jeunes pour la plupart et dont quelques-unes sont fort belles, qui se promènent, en attendant l'appel de l'orchestre, revêtues des costumes les plus variés, les plus pittoresques, les plus frais, et dont quelques-uns, je dois le dire, sont portés avec une crânerie, une aisance tout aristocratique. On se croirait vraiment dans le monde et dans une société des plus élégantes.]" Frédet, "Un bal à la Salpêtrière."

16. "Ce sont ceux-là, je dois le dire, qui sont les moins tranquilles, qui font le plus de bruit, qui s'agitent le plus, et qu'un spectateur impartial prendrait peut-être, à première vue, pour les habitants de la maison." Frédet, "Un bal à la Salpêtrière."

17. He spoke slowly with impeccable diction; he did not gesture; sometimes he sat and sometimes he stood. His presentation was always remarkably clear. He gave the impression of wanting to instruct and convince." Didi-Huberman, *Invention of Hysteria*, 281, quoting J. M. Guillain, *Charcot, sa vie, son œuvre* (Paris: Maison et Cie, 1955), 53–54.

18. Charcot cited in Didi-Huberman, *Invention of Hysteria*, 183.

19. Expression borrowed from Didi-Huberman.

20. Joseph Delboeuf, "Une visite à la Salpêtrière," *Revue de Belgique* 54 (October 15, 1886): 49. Cited in Andreas Mayer, *Sites of the Unconscious: Hypnosis and the Emergence of the Psychoanalytic Setting* (Chicago: University of Chicago Press, 2013), 99.

21. Such as the "ovarian compressor."

22. This deceptively win-win situation would have indefinitely perpetuated the dynamic named hysteria. Didi-Huberman, *Invention of Hysteria*, 171–174.

23. Mirbeau considered the spectacle offered by the lessons a "dream" from "troubled sleep." He wrote: "Here enters a woman. This is where the dream starts." See Octave Mirbeau, "Le siècle de Charcot," *L'Événement*, May 29, 1885, in *Chroniques du diable, Annales littéraires de l'Université de Besançon*, no. 555 (1995): 121–122. My translation. In Marquer's words, the phantasy was indeed "the erotic dream of male omnipotence." Marquer, *Les Romans de la Salpêtrière*, 7.

24. Brouillet's painting features Dr. Jean Martin Charcot, medical artist Paul Richer, chrono-photographer Albert Londe, Jules Clarétie, journalist and author of *Les amours d'un interne* (1881) and who interestingly was to become the administrator of the Comédie-Française, and Blanche Wittman—one of Charcot's most famous patients. Brouillet is not known to have sat in the room to portray the event while it unfolded. We do not know whether he composed the group portrait from individual studies of each person represented; we do not know either if Wittman posed for him or if her portrait was painted based on the abundant photographic documentation which was being produced and circulated in the publications of La Salpêtrière.

25. Octave Mirbeau, "La Névrose au village," *L'Événement*, March 29, 1885.

26. Mirbeau's description closely resembles Brouillet's painting except, and tellingly, for the lighting of the space and its windows. Mirbeau underlines the controlled low light that Charcot preferred to submerge his audience in. Starting from a dark space, Charcot chose which effects to deploy.

27. "Leçons du mardi à la Salpêtrière," in *Policlinique 1887–1888. Notes de Cours de M. M. Blin, J. M. Charcot, et H. Colin* (Paris: Babé et Cie, 1892), 6.

28. Jules Clarétie named hysteria "the illness of the century [le mal du siècle]." Bertrand Marquer attributes its seemingly contagious character to its seductive power: "The epidemic character of hysteria is a metaphor of its power of seduction." See Marquer, *Les Romans de la Salpêtrière*, 232.

p182, 183 CCØ Paris Musées / Musée Carnavalet—Histoire de Paris.
p184 Bibliothèque nationale de France, département Philosophie, histoire, sciences de l'homme.
p185 The Art Institute of Chicago. Mr. and Mrs. Carter H. Harrison Collection.
p186 Library of Congress Prints and Photographs Division. Control Number: 2004679983.
p187 Harvard Theater Collection, Houghton Library, Cambridge, MA.
p188 FNAC 1133. Centre national des arts plastiques. Domaine public / Cnap. Photo: Musée d'histoire de la médecine—Ministère de la jeunesse, de l'éducation nationale et de la recherche.

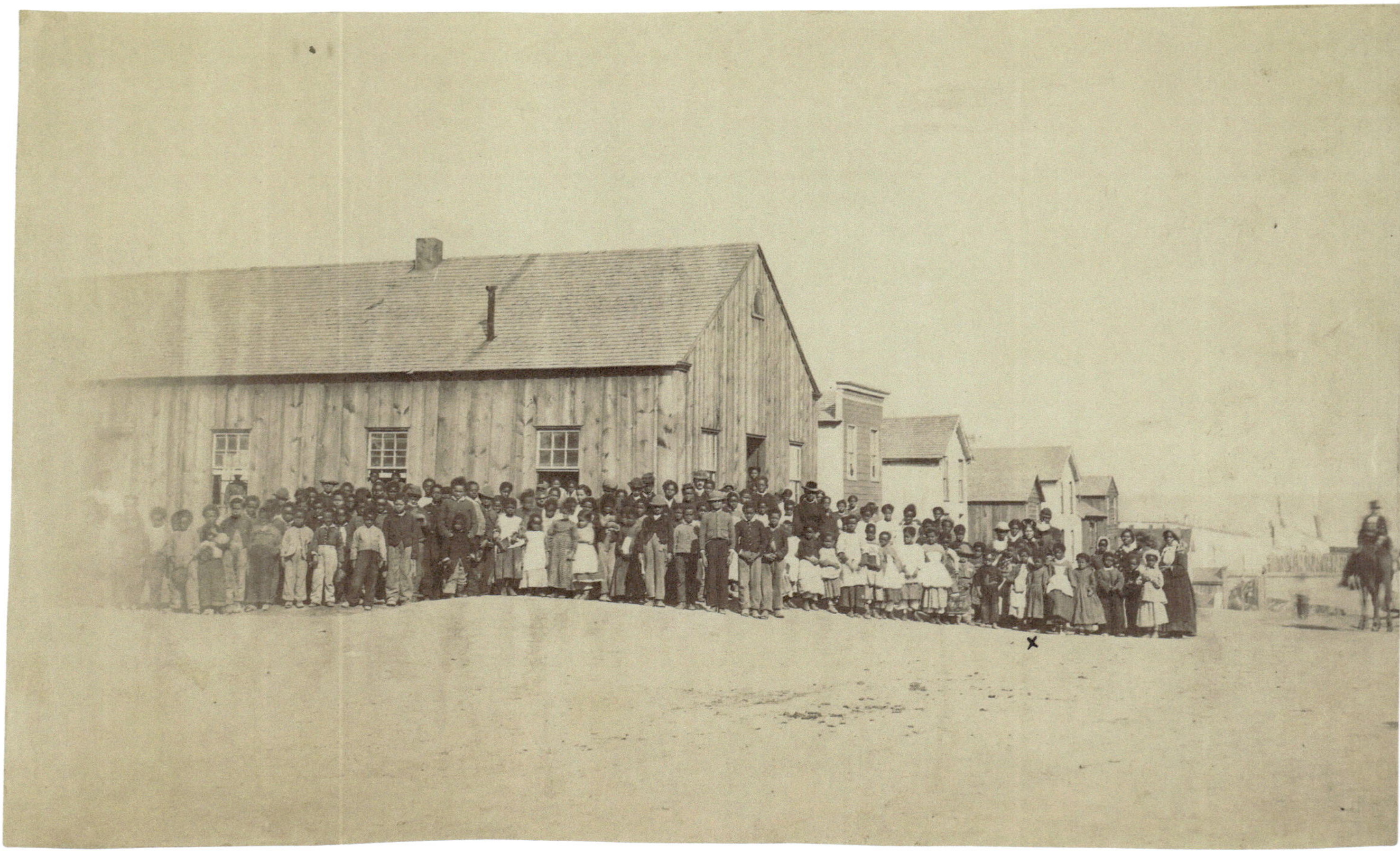

↑ "Coloured school at Alexandria, Va, 1864, taught by Harriet Jacobs & daughter agents of New York Friends."

CONTAGION ON THE PLANTATION

EDNA BONHOMME

As far as Harriet Ann Brent Jacobs knew, life for an enslaved person was ghastly, and like many enslaved people, she had learned to navigate the thin line between survival and death. When she fell ill, she recalled a "chilliness and deadly sickness" that came over her. Although she never received a diagnosis, one thing she elucidated was that during this period of being both enslaved and sick, she "prayed to die, but the prayer was not answered." Her sickness had become part of her way of life, and for an entire year, she rarely had a day without a deluge of chills or fever. For Harriet Jacobs, death was on the precipice of life.

This reflection on the interlacing of confinement, sickness, and mortality was documented in her autobiography, *Incidents in the Life of a Slave Girl*, written between 1853 and 1858.[1] In this memoir, Jacobs moves from captivity to freedom through a series of harrowing trials not uncommon for enslaved Black women during the mid-nineteenth century. Jacobs's memoir summons tragic watersheds from her life during her enslavement and after her manumission, the everyday anxieties on the plantation, and the plausibility of having her newfound freedom taken away.

Rapidly we retraced our steps back to the plantation. About halfway we were met by a company of four patrols. Luckily we heard their horse's hoofs before they came in sight, and we had time to hide behind a large tree. They passed, hallooing and shouting in a manner that indicated a recent carousal. How thankful we were that they had not their dogs with them! We hastened our footsteps, and when we arrived on the plantation we heard the sound of the hand-mill. The slaves were grinding their corn.[2]

The thrust of what Jacobs describes from her life during enslavement and after her manumission exists beyond the lexicon of captivity; a state of unrest that inculcates how labor was toiled within a carceral landscape, where watchmen dictated and limited the movement of the enslaved. As she wryly notes, the plantation not only created the conditions that fueled psychological, physical, and sexual assault but also incited a modicum of resistance. Throughout the text, Jacobs weaves together her desire to escape and her physical breaking points. One of these moments of entanglement came when, at the age of thirteen, Dr. James Norcom, who was her de facto enslaver, tried to assault Jacobs sexually. As a plantation owner, Dr. Norcom's actions were hewing to the tenets of slavery's evils—transgression, assault, and abuse. But Harriet came to realize something even more difficult, that some doctors, who were meant to provide care, were not only complicit within the plantation system; they were also meant to ensure that the breathing and thinking "property" could live under one condition: dejection.

When I first read Jacobs's testimony, I was flooded with a range of emotions, including the heavy weight of knowing that her enslaver, by design, did not have her physical well-being in mind and that the infractions imposed planted the seeds of her suicidal ideation. Jacobs shows how the relationship between slavery's surveillance system and illness can bring the enslaved to wish for death. So many autobiographies of the formerly enslaved during this period—from Solomon Northup's *Twelve Years a Slave* to Frederick Douglass's *Narrative of the Life of Frederick Douglass, an America Slave*—open up about the brutality of the plantation as the site of social death. But in contrast to her male counterparts, Jacobs's narrative is a nuanced exploration of a Black enslaved woman's journey to freedom, her family history, and how the racial logic post-emancipation left many Black people in America neglected, tired, and broken. Her memoir is a cipher into malady's journey into the plantation, and how the environment caused harm, but also how the enslaved did their best to aid each other to full recovery.

Jacobs's book bears affinity to the other markers of the freed who narrated confinement, sickness, and death on the plantation. For instance, in his autobiography *From Slave Cabin to the Pulpit* (1893), Rev. Peter Randolph sketches plantation life and malaise.[3] The text is a conventional slave narrative of the time, highlighting his early childhood memories, his kin, and his path to freedom. In the text's fourteenth chapter, he lists his friends' full names, carefully marking their initials when known. He justifies this chapter, stating that these are the friends who have been part of "the changing scenes of my life."[4] This follows from an earlier point he makes in the text that "he who has friends must show himself friendly."[5] Randolph was enslaved with eighty-one other Black people by Carter H. Edloe on Brandon Plantation in Prince George County, Virginia. Unlike most of the enslaved on the plantation, Randolph learned to read and write. After lamenting the perils of slavery, he noted: "The cholera came among the slaves and carried many to their rest. The very atmosphere, at this time, seemed to burn with evil and wrong for the poor Negroes, so that death was their best friend."[6] Randolph suggests that death was more appealing than a life of enslavement. But underlying his testimony is a disquieting reality: enslavement provokes outbreaks.

Slavery is often a condition that is remembered without giving voice to the enslaved. But as Yogita Goyal has noted, slave narratives were a tool for the formerly enslaved to provide heartbreaking and sentimental appeals for abolition. Indeed, they do more than just that: they narrate how the enslaved were actively battling the menace of captivity, which reduced their lives, their labor, and the scope of their humanity to their skin color. For the formerly enslaved, these narratives were not merely literary devices or memoir. They provide glimpses into the architecture of the plantation: a colonial concentration camp, the origins of modern policing, the site of medical racism, and a reminder of America's hypocrisy. For Jacobs and Randolph, writing was their method for signaling how the plantation was the site of contagion and morbidity.

Cholera marked life and death in mid-nineteenth-century America, but how it was documented was predicated on one's proximity to freedom. With nearly 40,000 reported cholera deaths as of June 1850, the pandemic hit every layer of society.[7] In the pandemic's third outbreak in the nineteenth century (1846–1860), two US presidents perished from the disease: James K. Polk died of cholera morbus in 1849 and his successor, Zachary Taylor passed away from cholera one year later. While elite and free persons had their deaths recorded in state mortality records, enslaved people were listed in the census by their enslaver, not as individuals.[8] At the time cholera was a ubiquitous and mysterious force. In hindsight, the source of this plague was dirty water, but cholera can also be contracted by ingesting food contaminated by excrement that harbors the bacteria. It is the microbe that causes diarrhea, vomiting, muscle cramps, sunken eyes, wrinkled skin, ruptured capillaries, and, if left untreated, death.

Before Filippo Pacini and Robert Koch's independent discoveries of the bacteria *Vibrio cholerae* as the cause of cholera were widely accepted, during the mid- and late nineteenth century, everyone had an opinion about how and why the malady spread. In *Die Cholera Morbus* (1831), Friedrich Schnurrer theorized about the pathology and produced a map of cholera, arguing that there was a relationship between human settlement and cholera prevalence.[9] He believed the built environment was strongly connected to the spread of disease and opined that epidemics are connected to geography. In 1854, John Snow famously traced the source of the cholera outbreak in London to a water pump, eventually persuading public health authorities to remove the contaminated pipe.[10] Amidst Snow's great experiment was a period of reprieve for people in cities who benefited from public health departments and structural programs to stave off cholera. However, these gains were not experienced by everyone. For the enslaved, there was a different rubric for public health. In some cases, it led enslavers and their doctors to theorize about plantation medicine, while in others, an outbreak contributed to revolt. The social and political course of contagion on a plantation created unseen forces—some infectious, others latent.

Enslaved Community and the Intimate Horrors of Contagion

In the United States, cholera was perceived as an urban problem, especially given cities' more substantial and direct links to the broader world. As the historian of medicine Charles Rosenberg noted: "Cholera could not have thrived where filth and want did not already exist; nor could it have traveled so widely without an unprecedented development of trade and transportation."[11] Cholera had a different life in plantations than in free society. As historian Diedre Cooper Owens has noted, the value of Black life shifted during slavery, leading to an investment in plantation medical science and a constellation of ad hoc medical practices.[12] Plantation medicine was not only used to manage endemic diseases; during the height of epidemics, enslavers also sought advice from doctors and consulted medical pamphlets that specifically focused on the plantation, such as *Practical Rules for the Management and Medical Treatment of Negro Slaves, in the Sugar Colonies* (1803).[13] While much can be said about the cholera outbreaks in nineteenth-century cities such as New York City, the plantation was a glaring example of the effects of captivity on disease. Health's iteration—in the age of cholera (1832–1866)—was filtered through a patchwork, racialized medical geography, and fueled by pamphlets. The social-medical contract was based on the will of an enslaver and his network, not the greater goal of the public's health.

The story of cholera on the plantation is not only about the nature of the disease but also about how Southern and Caribbean slavery lacked the capacity and will to undo harm for the enslaved. The network of medical pamphlets that sustained the architecture of the plantations also upheld medical racism. According to a report in Dr. James Ewell's *The Planter's and Mariner's Medical Companion*, cholera was one of the most common diseases on plantations.[14] Published in 1807 at $50—equivalent to $1,500 today—and dedicated to Thomas Jefferson, the text was used as a medical "advice book" for plantation owners to treat the enslaved directly.

On May 1, 1850, R. N. Featherston, a plantation owner, wrote to Dr. New, a physician who specialized in plantation medicine, asking for advice on how to treat an outbreak of cholera on his plantation. Dr. New responded to the letter, which he later published as a modest pamphlet, indicating: "When a well-marked case of Cholera, fully developed in all the characteristics of the disease, appears on a plantation, I would advise the removal of all the well negroes to some remote, comfortable buildings."[15] New advocated for a strict quarantine, like the recommendations of the International Sanitary Commission, which was established by the French government in 1861. Based in Rodney, Mississippi, Featherston used New's pamphlet as a guide to isolate contagion. This correspondence was not unique. Various plantation medicine manuals were published to account for modifying and thereby designing the health of enslaved Black people during the nineteenth century. While the ceaseless war on Black life was carried out in the United States, both plantation owners and the vast regional, national, and global networks sustaining and benefiting from enslavement depended on sufficiently healthy labor for plantations.

That same year, Jamaica, then a British territory, experienced a cholera outbreak, killing 30,000 people out of a population of 400,000. Although this was a period of post-emancipation, many of the newly "freed" Black people still labored in a brutal plantation economy that supplied cotton, sugar, and tobacco to the British Empire. The Scottish physician Gavin Milroy was called to provide treatment to the Black people working in and around horrifically afflicted plantations. He researched fervently, hoping to understand how the cholera epidemic progressed. After months of traveling throughout the island and seeing firsthand what was happening, he became convinced that complete emancipation would be the only way to mitigate disease, arguing that it was the only way to adopt sufficient sanitary reform to improve the health of everyone in Jamaica.

For enslavers like Featherston, slave mortality was principally tied to the profitability of plantation investments, while for physicians like New, Milroy, and Ewell, the practice of caring for the most vulnerable opened broader conversations about contagion and enslavement. Plantation medicine was an uncomfortable space where doctors sought to treat the diseases of those they did not fully deem human.

During slavery, enslavers also employed white physicians or Black midwives on an annual-salary basis to treat the enslaved. One enslaver, John Pope, who owned a plantation near Memphis, Tennessee, had land that was valued at $100,000, with seventy-five enslaved Black people.[16] Given that the 1833 cholera epidemic had ravaged most of the eastern coast of the United States, he decided to concoct a "remedy," which included "a spoonful of spirits of camphor with two of the essence of peppermint and 25 drops of Laudanum," and give it to the slaves who contracted cholera on his plantation. He claimed that using this remedy, he "never lost a patient." John Pope was not unique. Many apothecaries, doctors,

↙ Title pages of medical guidebooks that were used to regulate the health of slaves, late eighteenth to early nineteenth century: Dr. Collins, *Practical Rules for the Management and Medical Treatment of Negro Slaves, in the Sugar Colonies*, 1803.

↓ Title pages of medical guidebooks that were used to regulate the health of slaves, late eighteenth to early nineteenth century: James Ewell, *The Planter's and Mariner's Medical Companion*, 1807.

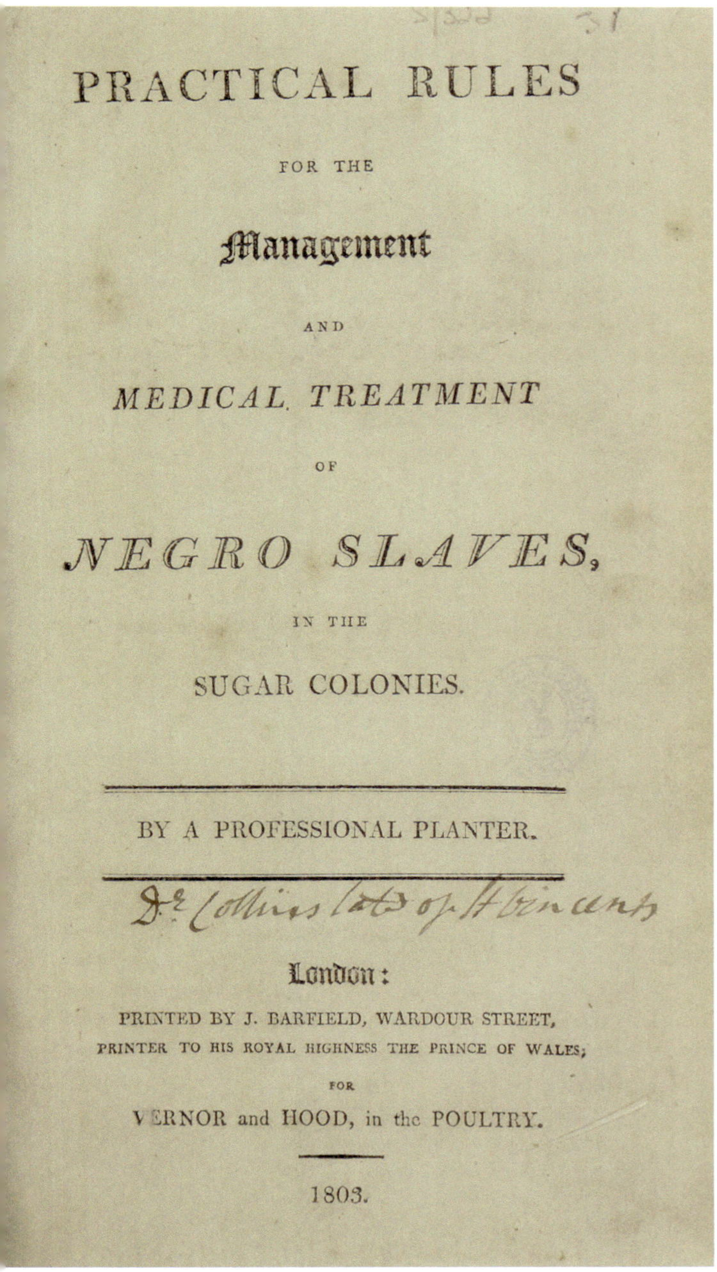

PRACTICAL RULES

FOR THE

Management

AND

MEDICAL TREATMENT

OF

NEGRO SLAVES,

IN THE

SUGAR COLONIES.

BY A PROFESSIONAL PLANTER.

Dr Collins late of St Vincents

London:

PRINTED BY J. BARFIELD, WARDOUR STREET,

PRINTER TO HIS ROYAL HIGHNESS THE PRINCE OF WALES;

FOR

VERNOR and HOOD, in the POULTRY.

1803.

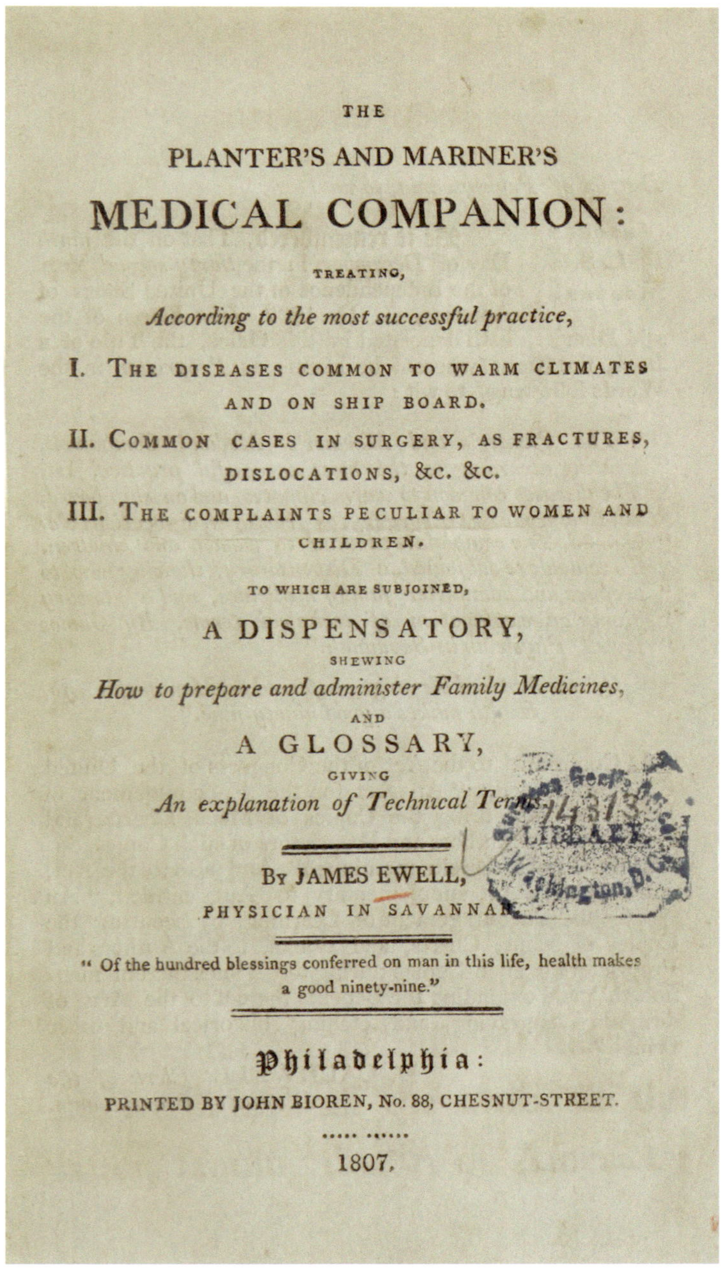

THE

PLANTER'S AND MARINER'S

MEDICAL COMPANION:

TREATING,

According to the most successful practice,

I. THE DISEASES COMMON TO WARM CLIMATES AND ON SHIP BOARD.

II. COMMON CASES IN SURGERY, AS FRACTURES, DISLOCATIONS, &c. &c.

III. THE COMPLAINTS PECULIAR TO WOMEN AND CHILDREN.

TO WHICH ARE SUBJOINED,

A DISPENSATORY,

SHEWING

How to prepare and administer Family Medicines,

AND

A GLOSSARY,

GIVING

An explanation of Technical Terms.

BY JAMES EWELL,

PHYSICIAN IN SAVANNAH.

" Of the hundred blessings conferred on man in this life, health makes a good ninety-nine."

Philadelphia:

PRINTED BY JOHN BIOREN, No. 88, CHESNUT-STREET.

1807.

and enslavers used a panoply of home-based reagents, hoping to prevent or treat cholera. In the preface of one popularly circulated text, *Gunn's Domestic Medicine* (1838), the author, John Gunn, provides medicinal plants "for healing our diseases."[17] The manual provided a quick fix for enslavers seeking homegrown antidotes.

Even after slavery officially ended, plantations in the Caribbean were still, as in Jamaica, spaces where Black people were made to till the land, even as cholera continued to mushroom on the earth. On August 2, 1854, four years after devastating epidemics in Mississippi and Jamaica, the *New York Times* reported that a cholera epidemic "swept over the plantations with a deadly effect" in Barbados, then a British colony.[18] After six weeks of ravaging the island, 34,000 had died. According to the report, more than a dozen doctors were integrating a mixture of homeopathic methods while attending to the sick. In other cases, ersatz doctors used prescriptions such as camphor, one of the early homemade remedies that cholera victims had used in Italy. One enslaver on the St. Philip plantation allegedly "cured" twenty-nine people by administering a spoonful of camphorated spirits and brandy to the patients. For him, the treatment was not just about providing the reagent; it also entailed giving the patients a clean, dry room and covering them with a blanket, which was considered a privilege compared to "normal" conditions. The report does not mention "slave," "slavery," or the names of the people who died, but given that Barbados was one of Britain's many slave economies, the majority of the infected were descendants of the formerly enslaved.

Part of the reason that these medicinal practices were homegrown is because the plantations experiencing such substantial mortality were almost uniformly located in regions that completely lacked public health facilities. Medical pamphlets for enslavers reveal the complicated reality of who was responsible for health, even during a pandemic. The failure of the slave economy to build a robust infrastructure, such as regional health boards, meant that the captive and unpaid labor systems were contained in a sphere that did not think it necessary to procure everyone's salubrity.

Escaping Captivity

While much can be said about how epidemics affect public health measures, more can be done to understand how space, movement, and socially constructed internment contribute to infection. How do we make sense of plantation medicine in times of an epidemic? Achille Mbembe evinces that the plantation economy was one of many technologies of colonialism that denigrated the body through total brutality, a mortifying reality wherein the everyday violence of the plantation created the conditions that made the enslaved more susceptible to illness.[19] Clifton Ellis and Rebecca Ginsburg examine the architecture and landscape of plantation towns in the United States, highlighting how plantations adapted to control the movement and mentally and physically compromise enslaved people.[20] Meanwhile, (formerly) enslaved people, mortified by the trauma of every day, saw in cholera the potential to escape enslavement or even the never-ending trauma of life itself.

Approximately one thousand miles apart, the slave economies of both Mississippi and Jamaica experienced simultaneous outbreaks. With the enslaved and formerly enslaved the most susceptible to infection, that very susceptibility turned illness into resistance. Enslaved people in the American South and the Caribbean were also challenging their vulnerability to contagion by utilizing their own herbal remedies or escaping bondage. With little to no access to medical care and acute susceptibility to ailments such as scurvy and measles, enslaved Africans were able to exercise agency over their bodies, implementing medical care for their own needs. African slaves used ginger to protect their immune systems and castor oil to treat inflammation. Their use of plants and plant parts, from pine to turpentine, also offered them control of how to oversee their own bodies. Coercive forms of medical intervention through confinement in the plantation economy were conspicuous. The parable at the heart

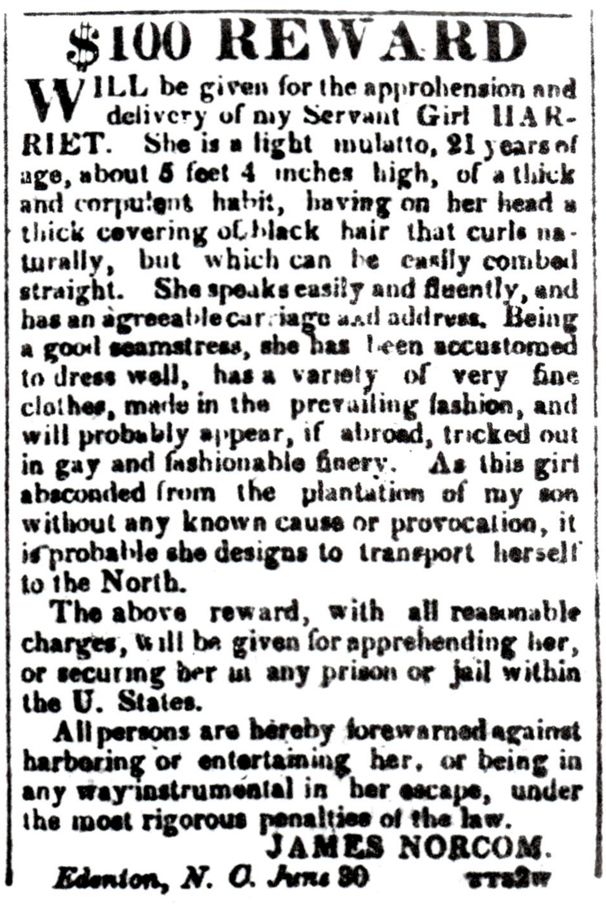
$100 REWARD

WILL be given for the approhension and delivery of my Servant Girl HARRIET. She is a light mulatto, 21 years of age, about 5 feet 4 inches high, of a thick and corpulent habit, having on her head a thick covering of black hair that curls naturally, but which can be easily combed straight. She speaks easily and fluently, and has an agreeable carriage and address. Being a good seamstress, she has been accustomed to dress well, has a variety of very fine clothes, made in the prevailing fashion, and will probably appear, if abroad, tricked out in gay and fashionable finery. As this girl absconded from the plantation of my son without any known cause or provocation, it is probable she designs to transport herself to the North.

The above reward, with all reasonable charges, will be given for apprehending her, or securing her in any prison or jail within the U. States.

All persons are hereby forewarned against harboring or entertaining her, or being in any way instrumental in her escape, under the most rigorous penalties of the law.

JAMES NORCOM.

Edenton, N. C. June 30

↑ Reward notice for the return of Harriet Jacobs by James Norcome (Dr. Flint).

of the plantation system was bound to a new form of medicine, predicated on experimenting on the Black body. But this was not the only outcome.

Enslaved Black people understood themselves apart from confinement and, given the brutality of plantation life, could see an epidemic as an escape. In 1869, when cholera ravaged the eastern portion of Cuba, a group of formerly enslaved insurgent maroons took the opportunity to burn down eighteen plantations.[21] The insurgents targeted Spanish troops and wealthy families from the eastern part of the island by setting fire to the plantations of Corestina, Resolución, Santa María, and Doloritas. At the time, plantation owners believed some insurgents came from Trinidad. By the end of the pandemic, ten Cuban plantations ceased to exist. The uprisings on these plantations were not only fueled by the conditions of confinement, but also by a cholera outbreak. Spatial arrangements can be conducive for pandemics to emerge, reemerge, or even wither. These slave revolts demonstrate that illness is itself a symptom of violent confinement. Yet it also incubates the seed to escape—a liberation that is not just spatial but manifests through text.

The testimony of the enslaved shows how they endured the violence of their enslavement on the one side and illness on the other, culminating in the idea of the plantation as an incubator of resistance and liberation. By the end of her life, Harriet Jacobs paid little mind to the limits of her gender or race. To her, abolition was the only answer to a brutal system, while the other solution was death. In her autobiography, she notes, “At least death frees the slave from his chain.”[22] The back and forth between revolt and death was part of the logic of escaping contagion and confinement. While the plantation might be considered a planet without a suitable life support system, hardened by the abject condemnation of enslaved humans, the plantation is a site of both designed terror and resistance, the very kernel of liberation.

An earlier version of this essay was originally published by e-flux Architecture in 2022.

1. Harriet Jacobs, *Incidents in the Life of a Slave Girl* (Boston: Penguin Books, 2000). First published 1861.
2. Jacobs, *Incidents in the Life of a Slave Girl*, 98.
3. Peter Randolph, *From Slave Cabin to the Pulpit. The Autobiography of Rev. Peter Randolph: The Southern Question Illustrated and Sketches of Slave Life* (Boston: James H. Earle, 1893).
4. Randolph, *From Slave Cabin to the Pulpit*, 141.
5. Randolph, *From Slave Cabin to the Pulpit*, 141.
6. Randolph, *From Slave Cabin to the Pulpit*, 170.
7. US Census Tables, June 1, 1850, https://www2.census.gov/library/publications/decennial/1850/1850b/1850b-03.pdf.
8. US Census, https://www.census.gov/history/www/through_the_decades/index_of_questions/1850_1.html. For a list of Slave schedules in 1850, see https://www.archives.gov/research/census/microfilm-catalog/1790-1890/part-03#virginia.
9. *Die Cholera morbus, ihre Verbreitung und ihre Zufälle etc* (Stuttgart: Universität Tübingen, 1831). Schnurrer also wrote another opus, *Chronik der Seuchen* (1825), which documents the rise of epidemics more broadly. For more information about Friedrich Schnurrer refer to Dietlinde Goltz, “‘Das ist eine fatale Geschichte für unsern medizinischen Verstand’: Pathogenese und Therapie der Cholera um 1830,” *Medizinhistorisches Journal* 33, no. 3/4 (1998): 211–244.
10. Sandra Hempel, “John Snow,” *The Lancet* 381 (2013): 1269–1270.
11. Charles E. Rosenberg, *The Cholera Years: The United States in 1832, 1849, and 1866* (Chicago: University of Chicago Press, 1987), 2.
12. Deirdre Cooper Owens, *Medical Bondage: Race, Gender, and the Origins of American Gynecology* (Athens: University of Georgia Press, 2017).
13. Dr. Collins, *Practical Rules for the Management and Medical Treatment of Negro Slaves, in the Sugar Colonies* (London: Vernor and Hood, 1803).
14. James Ewell, *The Planter's and Mariner's Medical Companion: Treating, According to the Most Successful Practice, I. The Diseases Common to Warm Climates and on Ship Board. II. Common Cases in Surgery, as Fractures, Dislocations, &c. &c. III. The Complaints Peculiar to Women and Children. To Which Are Subjoined, a Dispensatory, Shewing How to Prepare and Administer Family Medicines, and a Glossary, Giving an Explanation of Technical Terms* (Philadelphia: John Bioren, 1807).
15. Dr. New, May 7, 1850.
16. Virginia Jayne Lacy and David Edwin Harrell, “Plantation Home Remedies: Medicinal Recipes from the Diaries of Jonn Pope,” *Tennessee Historical Quarterly* 22, no. 3 (1963): 259–265.
17. John C. Gunn, *Gunn's Domestic Medicine, or, Poor Man's Friend, in the Hours of Affliction, Pain and Sickness* (Louisville: Charles Pool, 1838).
18. “The Cholera at Barbados—Terrible Condition of Affairs,” *New York Times*, August 2, 1854.
19. Achille Mbembe, *Necropolitics* (Durham: Duke University Press, 2019).
20. Clifton Ellis and Rebecca Ginsburg, eds., *Cabin, Quarter, Plantation: Architecture and Landscapes of North American Slavery* (New Haven: Yale University Press 2010).
21. “Eighteen Plantations Earned by the Insurgents—Flight of Cuban Bandits,” *New York Times,* February 6, 1869.
22. Jacobs, *Incidents in the Life of a Slave Girl,* 258.

p190 Courtesy of Emory Libraries.
p193 Courtesy of the Wellcome Collection, London, UK.
p194 Reproduced from *Incidents in the Life of a Slave Girl*, which states that the ad ran in the Norfolk, Virginia newspaper *American Beacon* on July 4, 1835.

↓ Johannes van Doetecum I and Lucas van Doetecum, after Gerard van Groeningen, *Episodes from Ovid's Metamorphoses [Erysichthon and Demeter]*, published by Gerard de Jode, ca. 1572. Engraving, 205 × 293 mm

HUNGER ARCHITECTURE

IASON STATHATOS

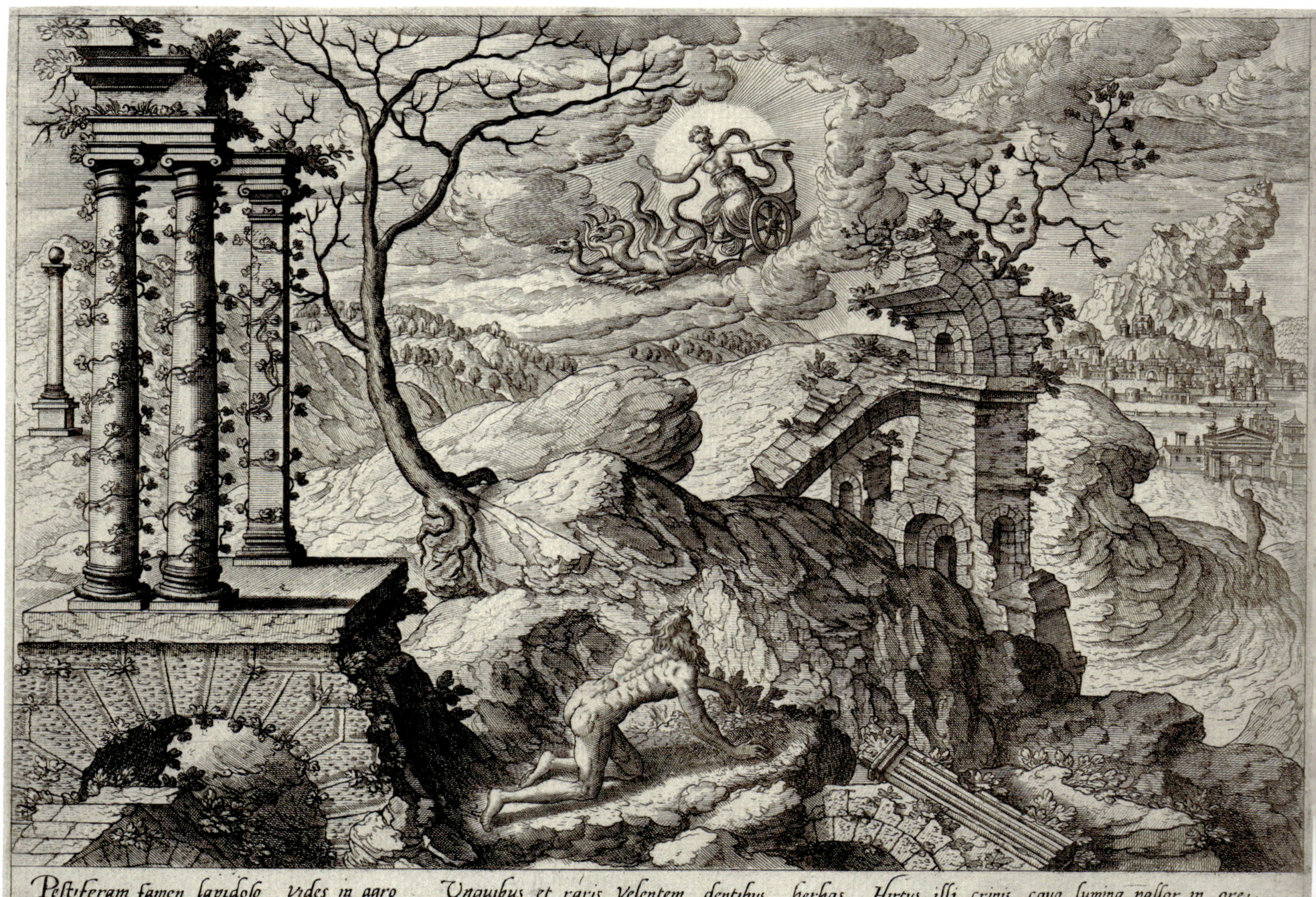
Pestiferam famen lapidoso vides in agro Unguibus et raris velentem dentibus herbas. Hirtus illi crinis, caua lumina, pallor in ore.

Of the many notorious origin myths of architecture, the story that directly relates to the insatiable, primordial human desire to eat is one of the least known. As the story goes, Erysichthon, a legendary king of Thessaly, wished to design and construct an imposing palace.[1] The building was supposed to feature a large feasting hall whose beam construction required substantial quantities of timber. Erysichthon decided that the nearby sacred oak forest dedicated to Demeter would deliver the necessary wood. Unsurprisingly, this was not welcomed by the goddess of the Earth, fertility, and grain. To punish the ambitious king-builder, she sent the personification of hunger, who like a disease invaded the body of Erysichthon through his airways and made it so that the more he ate, the hungrier he became. Erysichthon consumed all the provisions of the palace and then the city before turning to his own body. From its origins, architecture was placed at the intersection of environmental crisis, disease, and hunger.

The fear of hunger haunted Europe for centuries, well beyond the continent's ancient mythologies. Accounts of anthropophagy accompanying famine were seen as late as the seventeenth century. During the civil wars under the reign of Louis XIV, for instance, reports from Picardy claimed that "men eat earth and bark 'and what we would not dare to say if we had not seen it, and which is horrifying, they eat their own arms and hands and die in despair.'"[2] Similarly, in Burgundy, "the carrion of dead animals was sought after. ... Finally, it came to human flesh."[3] When famine occurs it is never just the human stomach that is impacted: "Day by day, the houses were emptied of household goods ... and the hearth became ever darker until it went out completely, the cold penetrating piercingly into the empty and desolate interiors."[4] But even in "normal" times of less acute food shortages, the masses of early modern Europe were largely fed with plant protein and carbohydrates, and were almost entirely deprived of animal protein, vitamins, and fat. This nutritional regime, a structural feature of daily life in the countryside and cities alike, made the majority vulnerable to infectious diseases.

The boundary between famine and epidemics in early modern France was blurry. They were both practically endemic and killed independently, but hunger accelerated the work of disease, which developed more brutally on weakened organisms. When pandemics did occur, however, architecture was used to keep famine at bay. For example, until the end of the seventeenth century, when the plague broke out, concrete architectural apparatuses such as "small wooden canals" were carefully instrumentalized to deliver individual rations of food and wine to the quarantining urban population.[5] Over the course of the eighteenth century, however, architecture went beyond practically ensuring survival to positioning the space of hunger relief as an artificial paradise.

The Mise-en-scène of Hunger

The initial cause of the 1709 famine was the worst winter of Europe's "Little Ice Age." This naturally led to a terrible harvest, whose first victims were those who died from low temperatures. During the month of January alone, Princess Palatine claimed that 24,000 Parisians died, concluding that "the plague is not worse." In spring, grain became increasingly scarce, and by summer, prices even of the old, bad, or imported types rose sharply.[6] Contaminated and spoiled breads were made with ingredients of unusual provenance, such as strange herbs, roots, ferns, nutshells, and clay.[7] But resorting to surrogates for flour came at a cost. Unconventional types of bread were known to alter mental states and cause delirious visions just like hunger itself, which "like mescaline produces hallucinations and the tremors of dementia."[8]

By September, the famine laid the groundwork for dysentery, typhoid fever, and scurvy to spread throughout the city. "It was," as Marcel Lachiver put it, "difficult to tell the difference between an empty stomach and a sick body."[9] In total, in less than two years, 800,000 people died, or about 3.5 percent of the French population. But for many who remained, survival depended on the consumption of these strange breads. A huge stratum of the population now "lived in a world ... altered in the relations of time and space: a universe of completely unreal extrasensory perceptions."[10]

As much as the famine might have derived from natural causes, the image of hunger and its relief was constructed. An anonymous etching of the 1709 famine held at the National Library of France depicts an operation where bread is being distributed by King Louis XIV to a desperate crowd in front of the Tuileries Palace. Jean Delumeau described a similar event as follows: "thousands of poor people, along the hedges, with blackened and bruised faces, subdued like skeletons, most of them leaning on sticks and dragging themselves along as best they could to ask for a piece of bread."[11] In the lower left corner of the etching, a seemingly incalculable mass of hungry—and intoxicated—Parisians stands on the gridded pattern of the palace courtyard and outer fence. A glimpse into an undisturbed world of plenty is offered to the crowd through the windows of a temporary bakery constructed on the axis of symmetry of the palace's *Pavillon de l'Horloge*, or Clock Pavilion. To relieve the king's delirious subjects from the famine, the operation of ensuring urban food security came to project its own "relations of time and space."[12] The hungry Parisians needed non-narcotic bread, but they were also fed with architecture.

Franz Kafka's *Ein Hungerkünstler* (*A Hunger Artist*), a novel published in 1922, shortly before his death from tuberculosis, also constructs the tension between starvation and abundance as a spectacle.

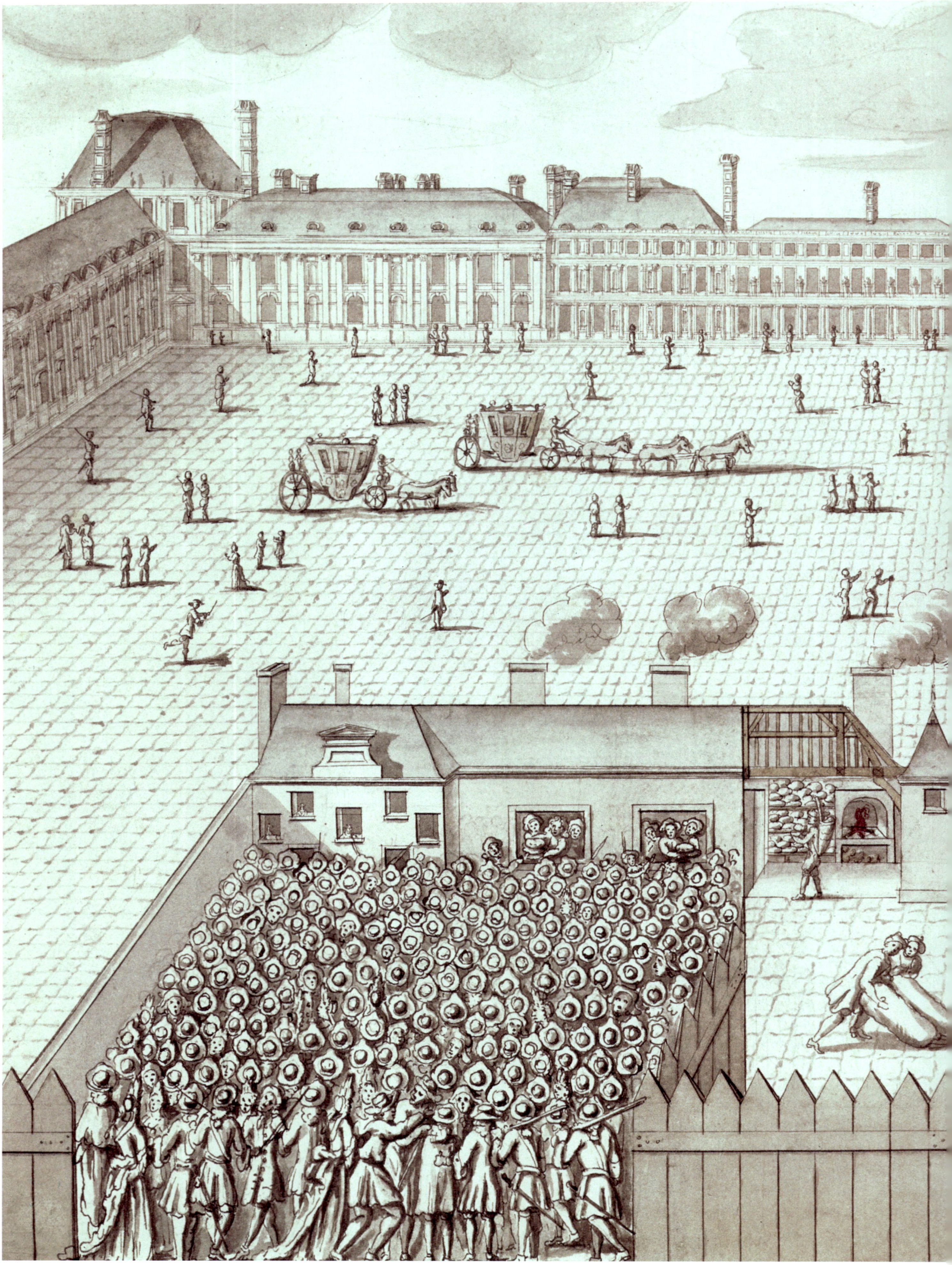

↑ Distribution of bread at the Tuileries, Paris, 1709.

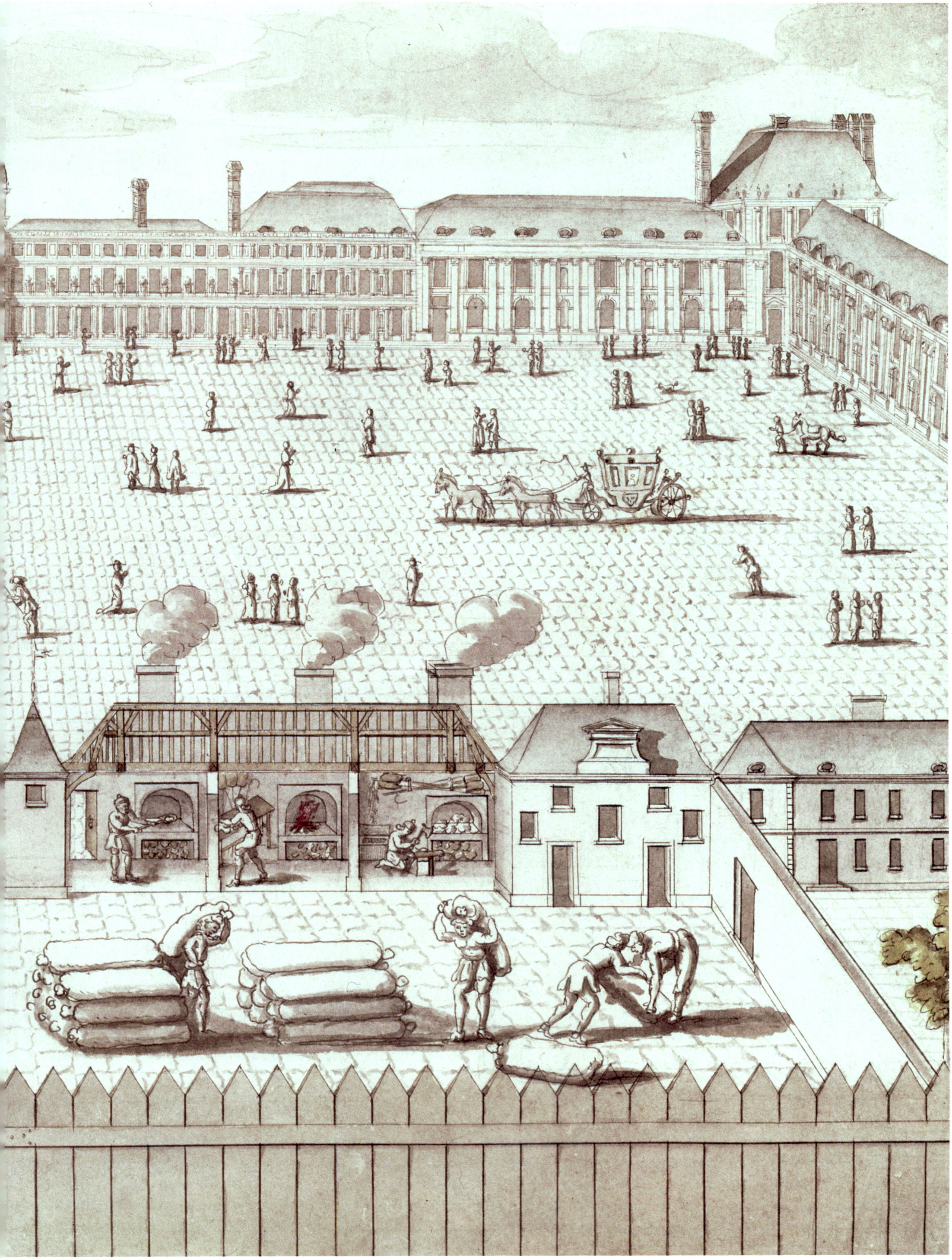

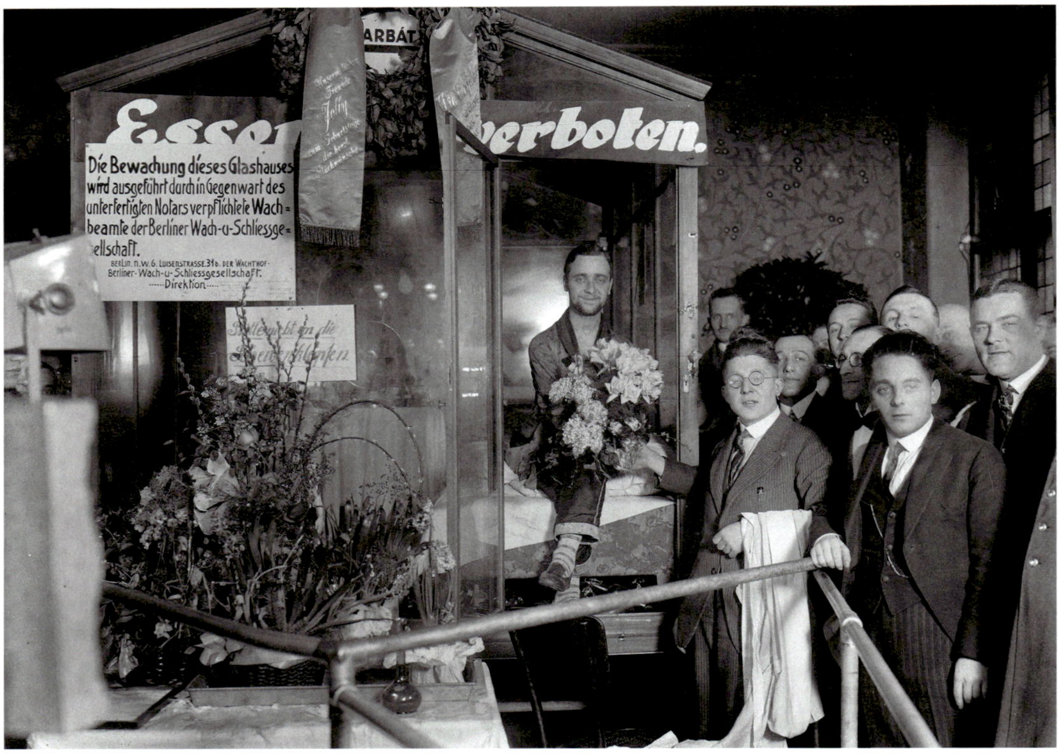
verboten.
Die Bewachung dieses Glashauses wird ausgeführt durch in Gegenwart des unterfertigten Notars verpflichtete Wach=beamte der Berliner Wach-u-Schliessge=sellschaft.

← Starving record: hunger artist "Jolly" reached the new hunger record with 44 days, March 29, 1926 (in a glass cage, guarded by the Berlin Wach-u-Locking company). Photograph, 13 × 18 cm, Willy Römer.

→ Les Halles de Paris on June 18, 1927. Photograph, 13 × 18 cm.

↘ Les Halles, 1916. Photograph, 13 × 18 cm.

Kafka describes a barred cage containing the body of the artist who deprives himself of nourishment in the center of a heavily decorated hall. The cage, an architecture of hedonistic voyeurism, allows the examination of every sign of malnutrition, and attracts hundreds of excited spectators. The most determining feature of the story, however, is the clock, which counts down the forty-day duration of the quarantine-like performance. Kafka's clock validated and made the accumulated time spent under the regime of starvation visible, gradually building suspense. And in the last day, in a perverse recognition of the artist's extreme malnutrition, the room was turned into a huge feasting hall. In Kafka, as in the Tuileries, the satiation of hunger can occur by simply crossing a spatial or temporal boundary. The threshold between life and death becomes uncomplicated, medicalized, and modern, describable in mere calorific terms.[13]

The Ground of Paris

The Tuileries etching is not a depiction of a historical event but rather a fictional architectural project.[14] Indeed, these large, white, clean gridded surfaces where Parisian bodies are controlled and fed was certainly not the ground of Paris of the early eighteenth century. The etching might be better understood as an illustration of the proto-science fiction novel by Louis-Sébastien Mercier, *The Year 2440: A Dream If Ever There Was One* (1771). Mercier's novel is organized around an imaginary walk through Paris in the twenty-fifth century. The city is an idealized, hygienic city that provides two fundamentals for its people: medical treatment and proper nourishment. In case of famine, large public granaries open to provide necessary food to citizens, while sick patients are properly treated in twenty small peripheral clinics (but which are hardly needed, since citizens rigorously follow hygiene protocols).[15]

The reality of Paris in the eighteenth century was far from Mercier's vision. Its air was seen as stagnated and immovable, which was believed to derive from specific architectural forms. Houses on top of the city's bridges, for instance, were thought to act as screens blocking the air from circulating freely, while other structures, like the hospital of Hôtel-Dieu, were alleged to perpetually emanate miasmatic air.[16] This was not just the period that saw the emergence of hygienist literature that obsessively focused on doctrines of ventilation and the free circulation of air within the city. It also gave rise to the theory that the urban ground itself can be a source of the "toxic" vapors thought to be responsible for multiple diseases and even death.[17] For example, in 1786, Pierre Bertholon published a book whose title was *On the Insalubrity of the Air in the Cities*, but whose stated intention was to "cast light on the tenebrous art of paving."

Examining the city's surfaces as sources of contagion offers a renewed understanding of how certain architectural forms emerged and worked within the larger framework of the medicalization of the urban space in eighteenth-century Paris. The ground of Les Halles, for instance, the central market where both healthy and sick bodies were fed, was described by Fernand Braudel as "pestilential mud," while others preferred words such as "disgusting" or "infectious."[18] Françoise Boudon wrote about "a thick mud which was mixed with rubbish and urine." It was

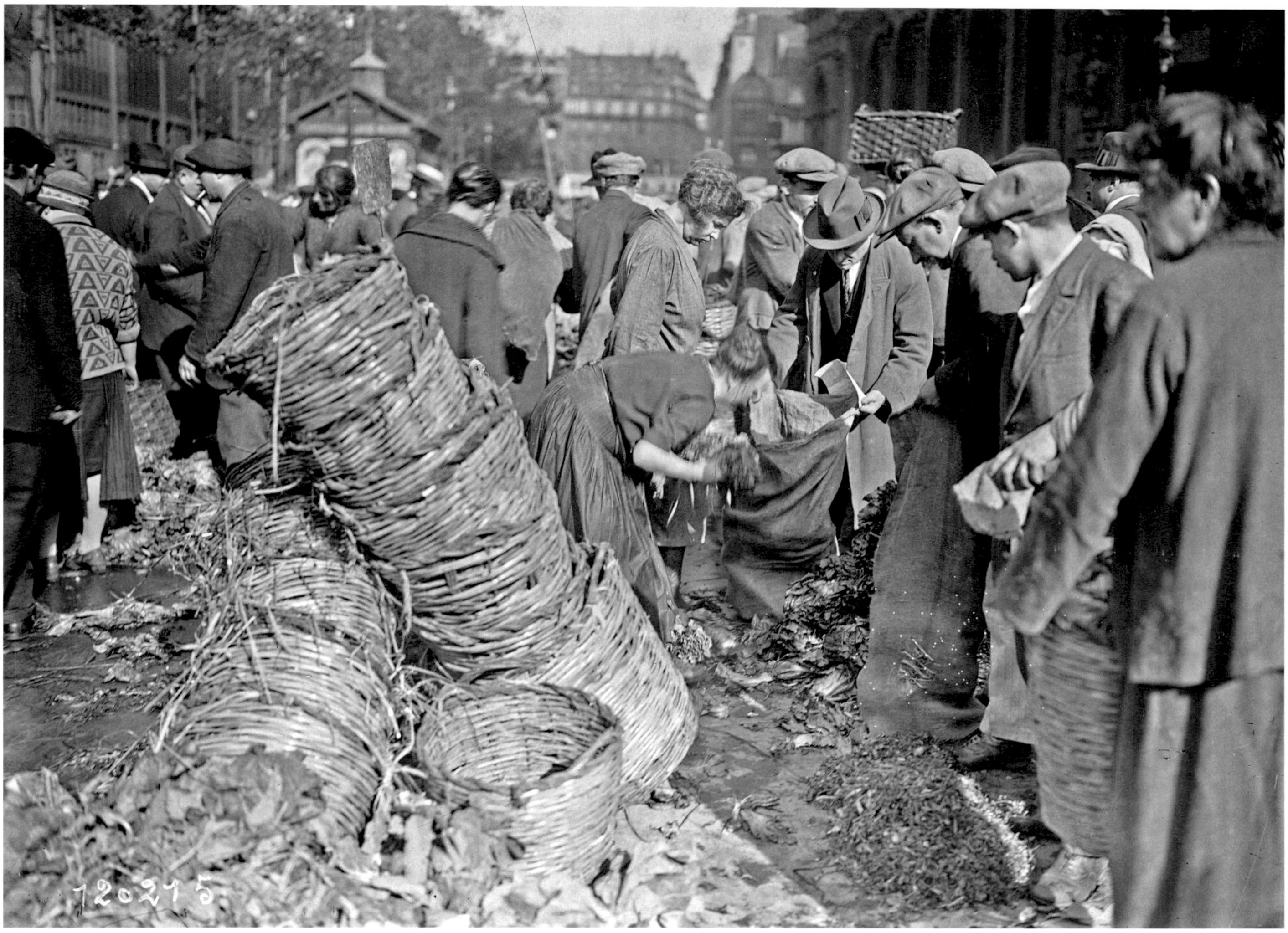
120275

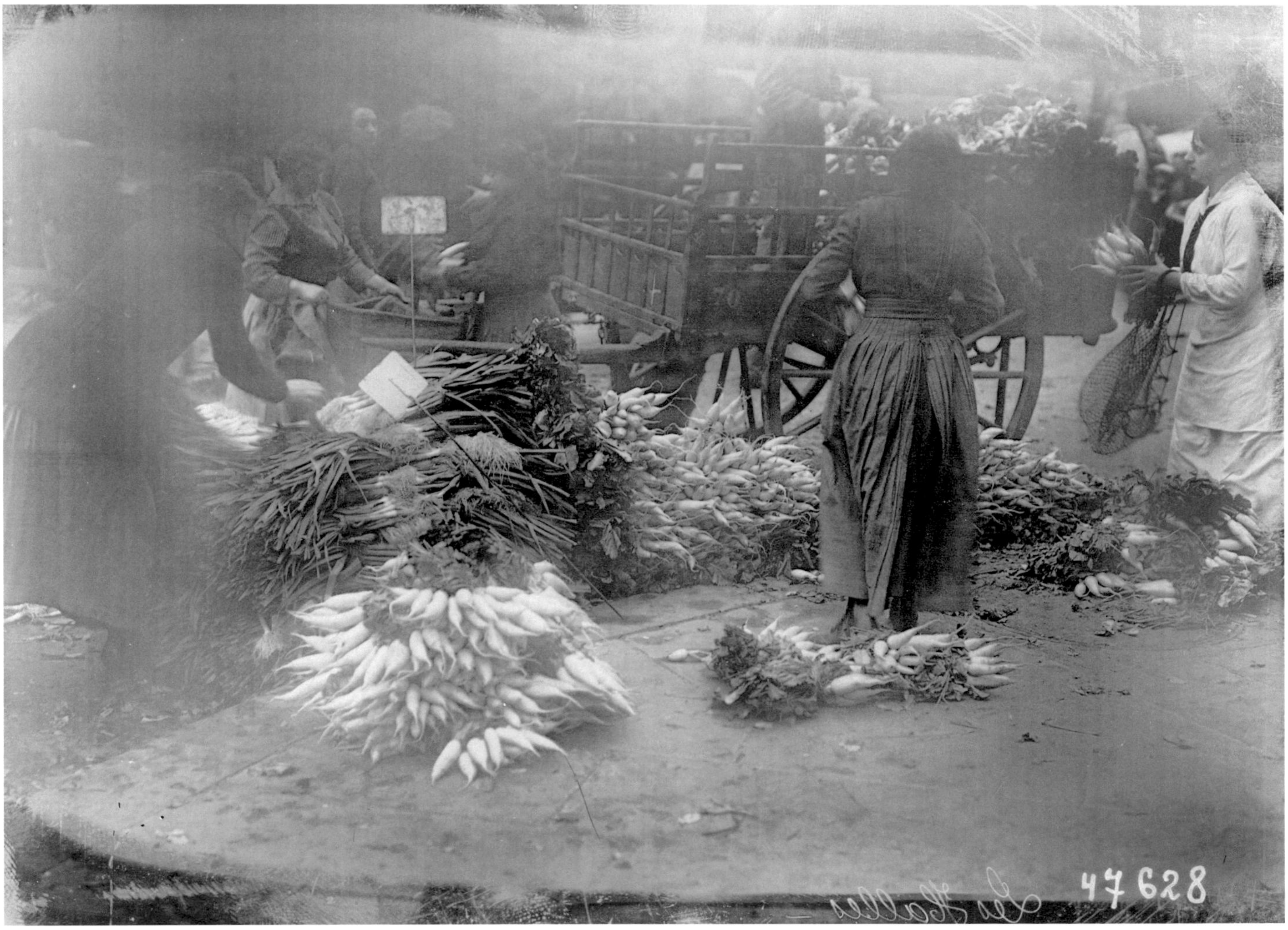
47628

a place where “the dirt appeared in its real terms: monstrous, invasive, always present.”[19] At Les Halles, the excrement of animals that pulled carriages would be added to the chamber pots of nearby inhabitants, who did not hesitate to evacuate them directly onto ground—the same ground where bags of grain were sold.[20] Both the ground and the bread distributed to the working classes in eighteenth-century Paris was not white but black.

The Granary and the Hospital

During this time, grain was seen to be like air in that it should never be stagnant. In Les Halles, one important principle that governed trade was that storage was not allowed. The absence of a market canopy was, above all, an issue of public health: it ensured the continuous replacement and ample ventilation of the grain that was sold.[21] It was also thought to accelerate the sale of bread while keeping the prices low.[22] The open-air market was the architectural apparatus designed to secure the constant flow of calories from the countryside to the stomachs of citizens. But without the possibility of storage, food security had very thin lines of defense. Les Halles’s primordial role in Parisian homeostasis became evident with only the slightest disruption in the grain market or supply chain.

Les Halles soon became the laboratory for the modern healthy, hygienic, and safe city. Within fifty years after the 1709 famine, its architecture of the flow, consumption, and storage of calories had undergone dramatic evolution. In 1763, the Halle au Blé, a new public granary at the heart of the market, designed by Le Camus de Mézières, was devised to separate the food from its ground, sterilizing Parisians’ nourishment by insulating it from any “toxic” exhalations. However, this design did not just attempt to remove the fear of disease; it also aspired to control the fear of hunger. By lifting the grain approximately nine meters overhead, above the market floor, the public was now able to hedonistically inspect whether enough provisions were available and if famines were anywhere to be seen. This form of transparency was welcomed by police officers who manipulated the stocks, intoxicating Parisians’ fear of hunger whenever necessary.[23] Conversely, an image of abundance was often put on display, regardless of whether it was real or not.

The typological development of the public granary ran in parallel with that of another new typology, the public hospital.[24] In fact, much of the “machine to heal” could also be found in the “machine to feed.” The functional and compositional parallels between the two were expressed most succinctly by the architect Charles de Wailly in 1785, who appropriated

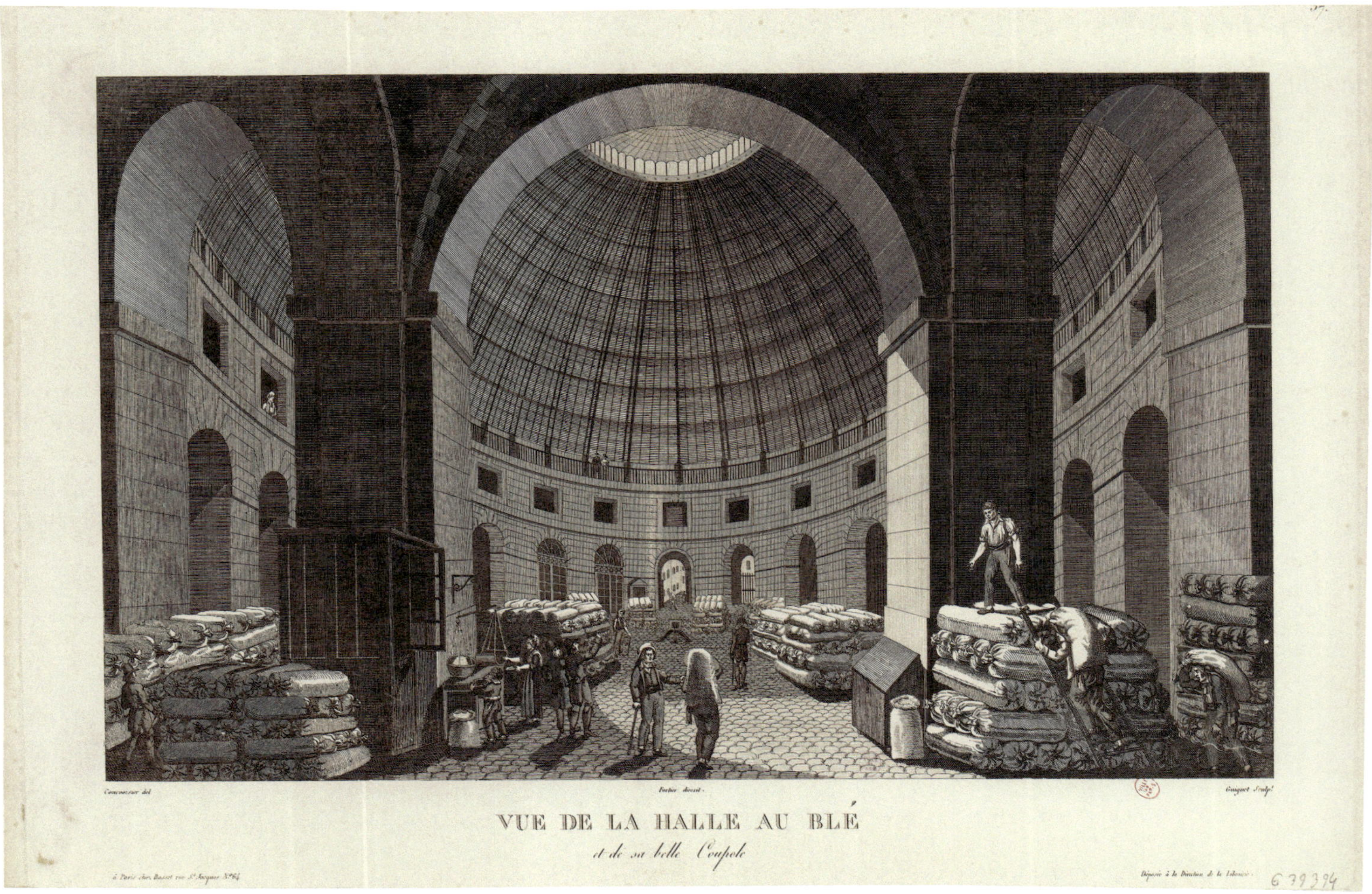
VUE DE LA HALLE AU BLÉ
et de sa belle Coupole

↑ Henri Courvoisier-Voisin, *Interior of the Halle au Blé*, in *Vues de Paris*, ca. 1850. Etching, 31 × 48 cm.

↗ Charles de Wailly, *Plan général du projet des embellissements de Paris* (detail), 1785.

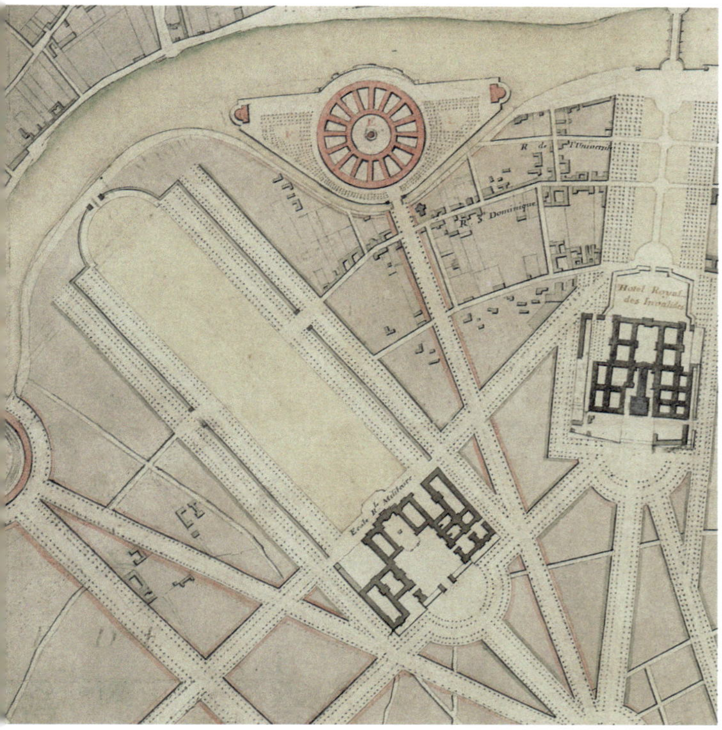

Bernard Poyet's project for a new Hôtel-Dieu and coupled it with a new Halle au Blé when proposing a new configuration for the Champ-de-Mars area. Here, the granary and hospital were not simply juxtaposed but appeared as complementary, two poles that treated the sick and healthy bodies of the Parisians in two different ways. The public granary was, according to de Wailly, more than a place for supplying grain and bread; it had become a place of well-being. His project offered the possibility of using the granary's water basin during summer months for recreational swimming and even water sports.

In only a few decades, then, the distribution of bread was transformed from a space of necessity, disease, scarcity, and anxiety to a space of commodity, hygiene, pleasure, and spectacle. The architecture of hunger transformed necessities into commodities by creating new artificial paradises, microcosms of ideal cities and model apparatuses through which the promise of a hygienic, abundant modernity projected itself onto those experiencing its unbearable realities.

An earlier version of this essay was originally published by e-flux Architecture in 2022.

1. Callimachus (*Sixth Hymn to Demeter*, third century BCE) and Ovid (*Metamorphoses* 8, first century BCE and first CE) are the primary ancient sources for this myth.
2. Jean Delumeau, *La peur en Occident (XIVe–XVIIe siècles): Une cité assiégée* (Paris: Fayard, 1978), 164.
3. Delumeau, *La peur en Occident*, 164.
4. Piero Camporesi, *Bread of Dreams: Food and Fantasy in Early Modern Europe*, trans. David Gentilcore (Cambridge: Polity Press, 1989), 56. For an excellent, more recent study of how famines intersect with architecture, see Ateya A. Khorakiwala, "The Well-Fed Subject: Modern Architecture in the Quantitative State, India (1943–1984)" (PhD diss., Harvard University, Graduate School of Arts and Sciences, 2017).
5. Michel Foucault, *Discipline and Punish: The Birth of the Prison*, trans. Alan Sheridan (New York: Vintage, 2012), 195.
6. Pierre Goubert, *Louis XIV et vingt millions de Français* (Paris: Fayard, 1991), 272.
7. Marcel Lachiver, *Les Années de misère: La famine au temps du Grand Roi, 1680–1720* (Paris: Fayard, 1991), 356.
8. Camporesi, *Bread of Dreams*, 127.
9. Lachiver, *Les Années de misère*, 354.
10. Camporesi, *Bread of Dreams*, 127.
11. Delumeau, *La peur en Occident*, 163.
12. Camporesi, *Bread of Dreams*, 127.
13. See Agustí Nieto-Galan, "Mr. Giovanni Succi Meets Dr. Luigi Luciani in Florence: Hunger Artists and Experimental Physiology in the Late Nineteenth Century," *Social History of Medicine* 28, no. 1 (February 2015): 64–81; also Jenny Edkins, *Whose Hunger? Concepts of Famine, Practices of Aid* (Minneapolis: University of Minnesota Press, 2000), 15–41.
14. The north wing of the palace is entirely fictional, while the open square in front of the building is devoid of all the constructions built at the time.
15. Louis-Sébastien Mercier, *L'An deux mille quatre cent quarante: Rêve s'il en fût jamais* (London, 1771), chapters 8, 14, 23.
16. See Richard Etlin, "L'air dans l'urbanisme des Lumières," *Dix-huitième Siècle, Le sain et le malsain,* 9 (1977): 124. Also Nikolaus Pevsner, *A History of Building Types* (London: Thames & Hudson,1976), 146.
17. See Sabine Barles, "La pédosphère urbaine: Le sol de Paris XVIIIe–XXe siècles" (PhD diss., École Nationale des Ponts et Chaussées, 1993), 91–123.
18. Fernand Braudel, *Capitalism and Material Life, 1400–1800*, trans. Miriam Kochan (London: Weidenfeld & Nicolson, 1973), 437.
19. Françoise Boudon, "La salubrité du Grenier de l'abondance à la fin du 18e siècle," *Dix-huitième Siècle, Le sain et le malsain,* 9 (1977): 171–180.
20. Also see Steven Laurence Kaplan, *Les ventres de Paris: Pouvoir et approvisionnement dans la France d'Ancien Régime,* trans. Sabine Boulonge (Paris: Fayard, 1988), 92–93.
21. Mark K. Deming, *La Halle au Blé de Paris, 1762–1813: "Cheval de Troie" de l'abondance dans la capitale des Lumières* (Brussels: Archives d'architecture moderne, 1984), 58.
22. At least, this was La Reynie's argument when he opposed the grain merchants' request for the construction of a roof, claiming that if the merchants did not have to fear the rain, they would be in no hurry to sell, and prices would inevitably rise. See Léon Bernard, *The Emerging City: Paris in the Age of Louis XIV* (Durham: Duke University Press, 1970), 253.
23. Deming, *La Halle au Blé*, 116.
24. About the Halle au Blé, its role in relation to hospitals, grain circulation, and hygiene, see Meredith TenHoor, "Architecture and Biopolitics at Les Halles," *French Politics, Culture and Society* 25, no. 2 (2007): 73–92; Meredith TenHoor, "Markets and the Food Landscape in France, 1940–72," *Dumbarton Oaks Colloquium on the History of Landscape Architecture* 36 (2015): 333–351.

CORPORATE CAPTURE: DESIGNING TOXICITY'S ABSENCE IN THE DEUTSCHER WERKBUND

JESSICA VARNER

On October 6, 1907, the Deutscher Werkbund (German Work Federation) was established by twelve prominent men, including Peter Behrens, Theodor Fischer, Hermann Muthesius, Friedrich Naumann, Josef Olbrich, Bruno Paul, and Richard Riemerschmid, together with twelve notable companies, including Allgemeine Elektricitäts-Gesellschaft AG (AEG), Badische Anilin und Soda Fabrik (BASF), Bayer, Benz, Bosch, Daimler, Siemens, Krupp, and Leverkusen. The group, which comprised architects, artisans, politicians, scientists, industrialists, and corporate firms, allied to form an applied arts association, forging ties between tradespeople, art professionals, and industrial businesses. With ambitious goals, the Werkbund proposed a synthesis between the arts and industry—from "the sofa cushion to urban planning."[1] One of twentieth-century Germany's most prominent artistic movements, the organization would go on to sponsor lectures, organize conferences, assemble exhibitions, start a museum of applied arts (the Deutsches Museum für Kunst in Handel und Gewerbe, or German Museum for Art in Trade and Industry), and establish a publication (the *Werkbund Jahrbücher*).

From the group's founding in 1907 to its dissolution in 1933 (not including post-World War II iterations that would reignite the Werkbund), the Werkbund focused on "coming to terms with the modern age" and the "forces that shaped twentieth-century Germany."[2] Yet the Werkbund selectively confronted certain aspects of the modern age and omitted others, focusing on artisanal work and building industrial relationships while disregarding the growing industrial laborers and *Arbeiterklasse* almost wholesale. The Werkbund held no meetings on emerging industrial hygiene topics during the organization's founding, and industrial toxicology or worker safety never registered in the *Werkbund Jahrbücher*. This is surprising, given that the foundation of industrial hygiene was forged in the same factories with which the Werkbund was allied. Already at the end of the nineteenth century, BASF, Bayer, and Leverkusen—all growing, profitable dye corporations—drew scrutiny over their labor practices, polluting practices, and lack of industrial hygiene safeguards.[3] Despite growing public awareness about the harms of the chemical dye industry, the Werkbund mainly remained disengaged from the broader German industrial hygiene movement taking place in factories, health clinics, and labor protests at the time.[4]

In 1883, Chancellor Bismarck had enacted sickness insurance, a prototype for contemporary worker's compensation meant to appease the growing socialist revolution aimed at worker conditions in Germany (amidst a transition from Prussian rule).[5] And the 1906 Berne Convention prohibited the manufacture or import of white-phosphorus matches

→ Linoleum and dye advertisements in Deutscher Werkbund, *Jahrbuch des Deutschen Werkbundes* (Jena: Eugen Diederichs, 1912).

and recommended the substitute of nonpoisonous sesquisulfide after rising public protests and phossy jaw cases resulting from match factories' dangerous exposure levels.[6] German exposure science and industrial hygiene practices also guided their development in other countries, such as the United States, throughout the twentieth century.[7]

While the factory has been a historical site of labor reform and a target for industrial hygiene improvements in Germany, it has also been a site of corporate pushback. The German dye industry experienced rapid growth in the early twentieth century thanks to public- and private-sector investments in organic chemistry and the science of synthetic chemical production. With this growth came increasing industrial disease occurrences among the industry's workers. As a result, German scientists looked to reform the synthetic dye industry.[8] Yet the industry was quick to refute claims that their factories were the cause of their workers' ailments. This rebuttal initially emerged in 1880, when the first book on the health of dye workers was published by an in-house physician at Höchst (a dye company later associated with BASF), which claimed that the problems reported were not work-related.[9] Höchst physicians repeated this denial when Ludwig Rehn, a surgeon in Frankfurt-am-Main, found the first cases of bladder cancer in 1895 in dye laborers from Leverkusen. Of the forty-five cases of workers who developed cancer, three were laborers who toiled in the production of fuchsine, an early aniline dye. Others developed nonmalignant bladder diseases.[10] Debates followed, with decades-long pushback from the industry that the disease was not linked to exposures in the factory doing dye work.

These debates about industrial labor and its sicknesses were, therefore, a crucial part of the context in which the Deutscher Werkbund emerged, yet at the same time they were systematically occluded by it. Lecturing in 1907 on the occasion of his inaugural chair appointment at the Berlin Handelshochschule, Hermann Muthesius—architect, trained mason, once Prussian Ministry of Trade bureaucrat, and soon-to-be Deutscher Werkbund founder—voiced his objections about recent developments in German object design and industry. Muthesius's points spanned cheap production, misuse of raw materials, and labor problems. The controversial address catalyzed the alliance between workers, companies, industrialists, and political figures that became the Werkbund. He foretold issues with the industry's growing political and economic emphasis and the resultant externalities, including troubles in the division of labor. "In a field of activity that is a business as well as an art, the new movement [in design] has to find its feet in economic terms."[11] For Muthesius, artists needed to heed economic factors and understand they were part of the broadening labor workforce tied to capitalist ethos: profit and more work.

One of the most influential pro-labor ideas at the end of the nineteenth century came from Werkbund founder and political figure Friedrich Naumann, whose unique personal experience in working-class misery and the slow degradation of working people sparked a search for better solutions as early as the 1890s.[12] In *Deutsche Gewerbekunst*, a pamphlet produced for the association's first annual meeting in 1908, Naumann tied the economics of labor to the growing divides in upper- and lower-class work, calling for a return to labor's joy.[13] The Werkbund could, Naumann argued, "raise the value of labor, improve the worker's status, increase his joy in work, and thus reverse the trend to proletarianization hitherto associated with the advance of capitalism."[14] He believed the working class should not be dismissed as "the dregs" of society. Instead, this demographic was an important consideration and formed the foundation of a stable work force, growing rapidly as the most significant population for modern development.[15]

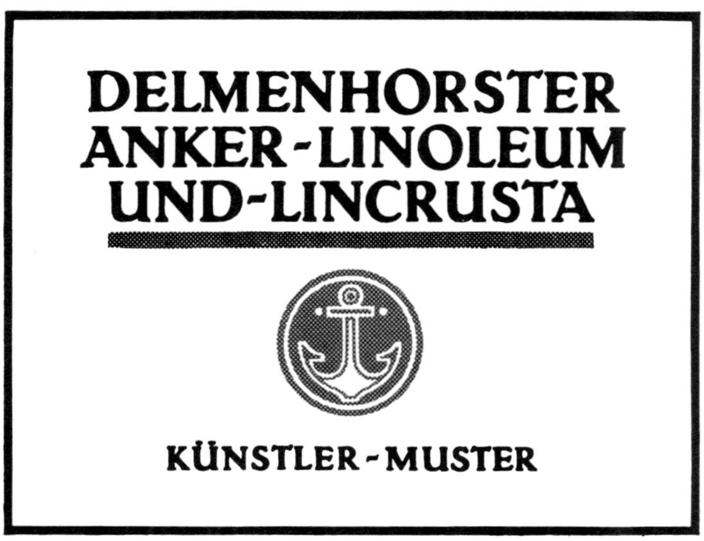

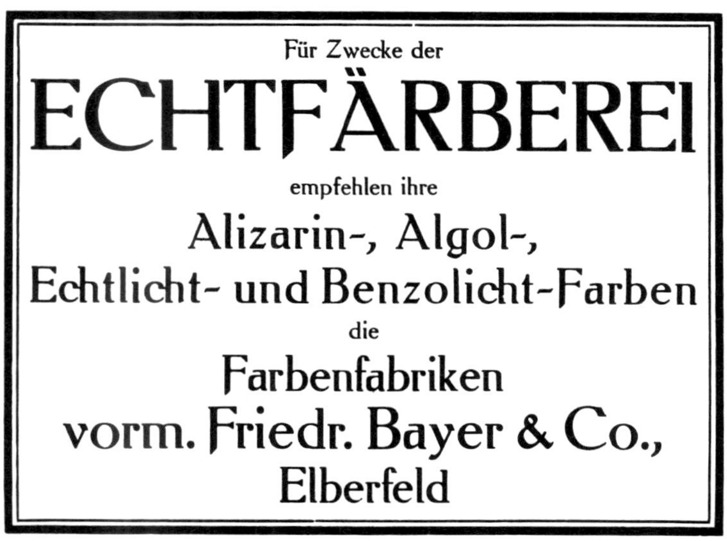

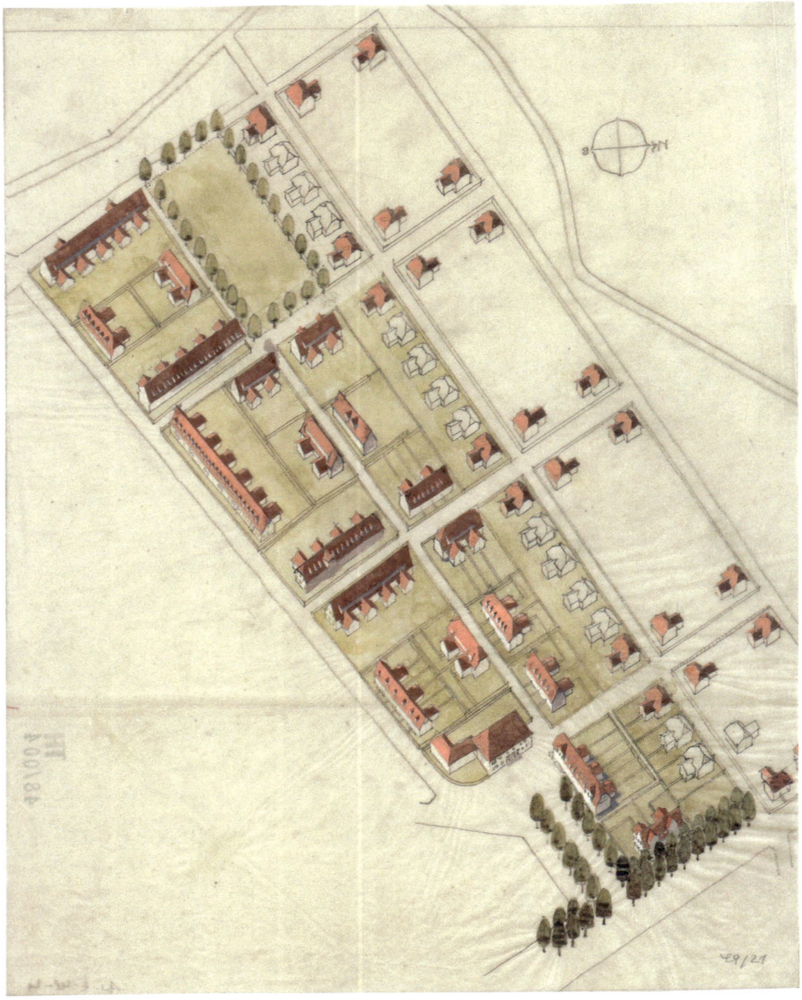

← Theodor Fischer, Badische Anilin- und Soda-Fabrik, Arbeiterkolonie Limburgerhof (1911).

↓ Theodor Fischer, Badische Anilin- und Soda-Fabrik, Arbeiterkolonie Limburgerhof (1911).

→ Deutscher Werkbund Ausstellung, Cologne, 1914, *Offizieller Katalog* (Cologne: Verlag von Rudolf Moose, 1914), 201.

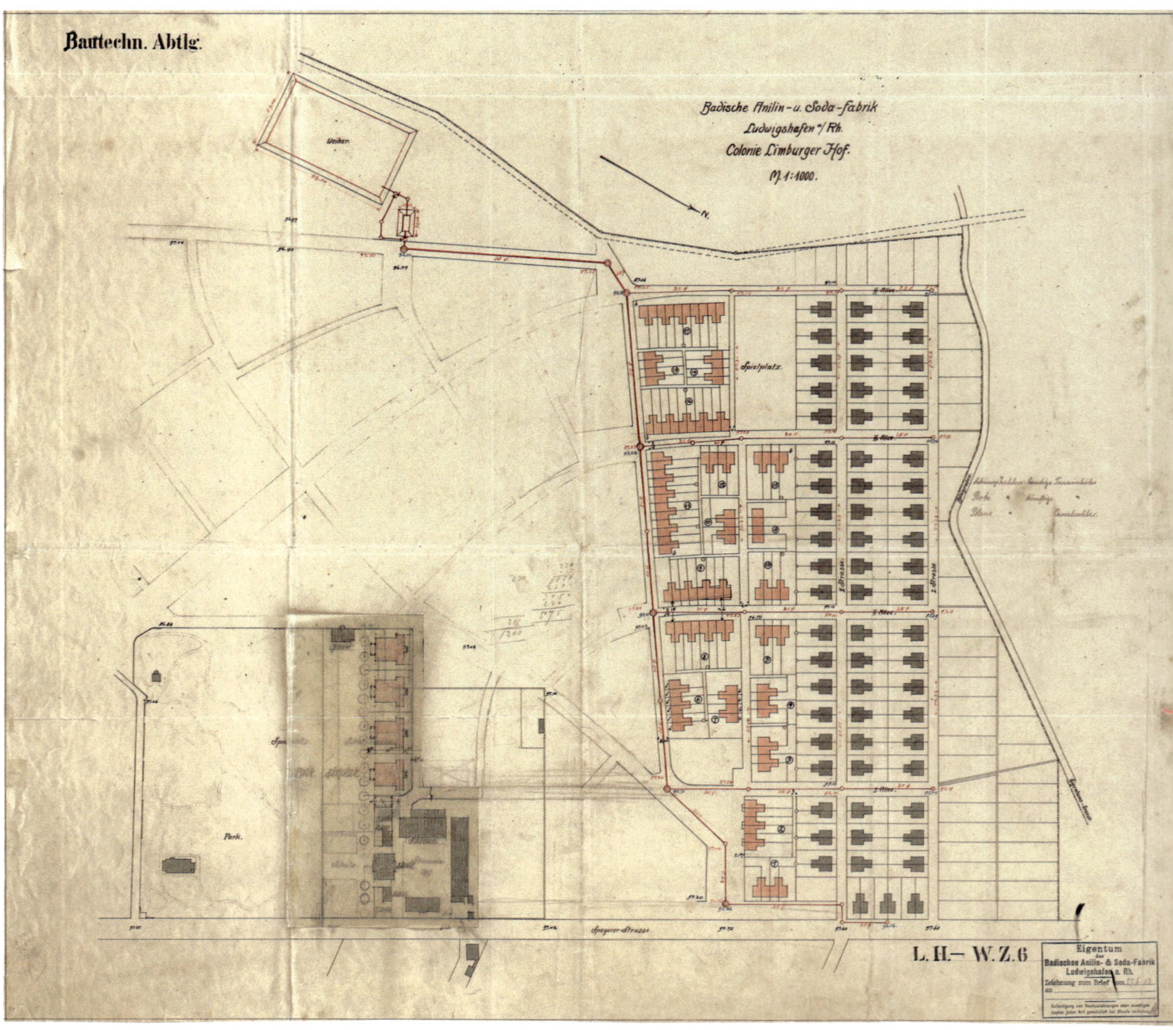

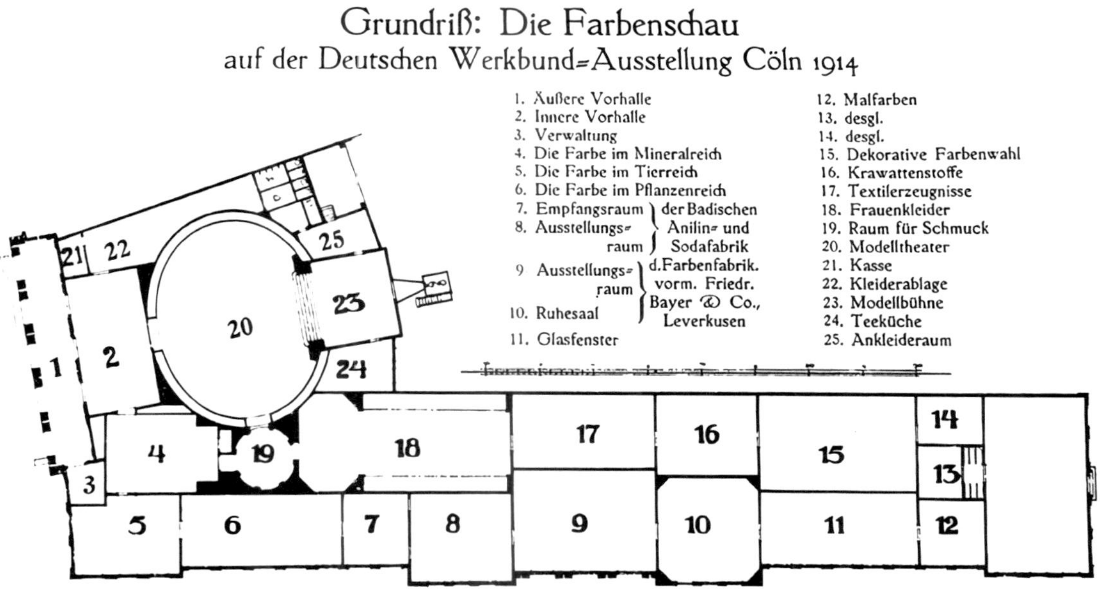

Naumann proclaimed "organization," or the idea that business, economies, and German bureaucracy needed to harness the growing labor force and bend to the rise of the corporation, as critical to growth:

> All relations are pervaded by the thought of organization, that is, the regulation of the masses. It will be a man's pride to belong to great associations, societies, unions, syndicates, to serve in great enterprises, to be drawn into extended ties. Often this pride is mixed with a painful look back to past times, when the individual by himself meant something. But what's the use?[16]

Naumann believed that strong unions could fight against corporate employers for things like improved health conditions, better compensation, medical treatment, etc.[17] As a result, he did not believe that state or governmental intervention in industrial affairs was necessary, as internal organizational issues could be handled locally. Naumann's stance as an economic liberal went as far as insisting that the Werkbund remain independent from state guidance or subsidies.[18]

Of all the Werkbund members, Naumann's concerns remained closest to the interests of the laboring class, even if those ideals did not enter into the Werkbund's overall agenda due to disagreement or differing aims. Historian John Maciuika asserts that key Werkbund members such as Muthesius and Naumann could not agree on a common *Sozialpolitik* (social policy) around the treatment of German workers.[19] Instead, and more commonplace in the groups' publications, the Werkbund's views reflected industrial agendas and followed corporate commissions.[20]

The early Werkbund years saw relationships flourish with chemical dye corporations. BASF's Carl Immerheiser, a leading chemist and research scientist, became an elected member of the Werkbund during the 1909/1910 annual meeting program.[21] Starting in 1911, the architect and Werkbund founder Theodor Fischer constructed worker housing for BASF, extending his growing industrial project portfolio. Named the Arbeiterkolonie Limburgerhof, the sizable, planned subdivision in Ludwigshafen accommodated all ranks of the *Chemie-Proletariat*, including supervisors, with single-bed barracks for lower-ranked chemical laborers.[22] Fischer's connection to BASF reinforced the Werkbund's role in the division of labor, product innovation, and cheap chemicals. Housing created a stable workforce for the growing chemical corporation. Fischer, the Werkbund, and BASF were tied together through dependent economic and aesthetic means.

The 1914 *Cöln Deutsche Werkbund Ausstellung* (Cologne Werkbund Exhibition) demonstrates the strong relationship between the Werkbund and the synthetic chemical dye industry.[23] The design and interior of the *Farbenschau* (Color Show)—a central building on the axis with the main promenade, which presented "technical" colors (those derived from synthetic chemicals) sweeping German and international markets at the time—is credited to Werkbund founder Hermann Muthesius. However, the final displays and presentations were decided upon by an exhibition team that also included chemists Hess and Walter from Bayer, Innenheisse from BASF, and the director of the Krefelder Dyeing School, Heinrich Lange. Chemist Friedrich Carl Duisberg, from Friedr. Bayer & Co., was appointed the exhibition's honorary president to secure Bayer's participation.[24]

Growing a consumer audience for dyes in Germany largely depended upon the development of new applications for the home. As part of the color show pavilion, Bayer, Leverkusen, and BASF presented large displays and entire rooms. Bayer focused on new developments in lacquer house paints in an austere and refined lounge featuring polished

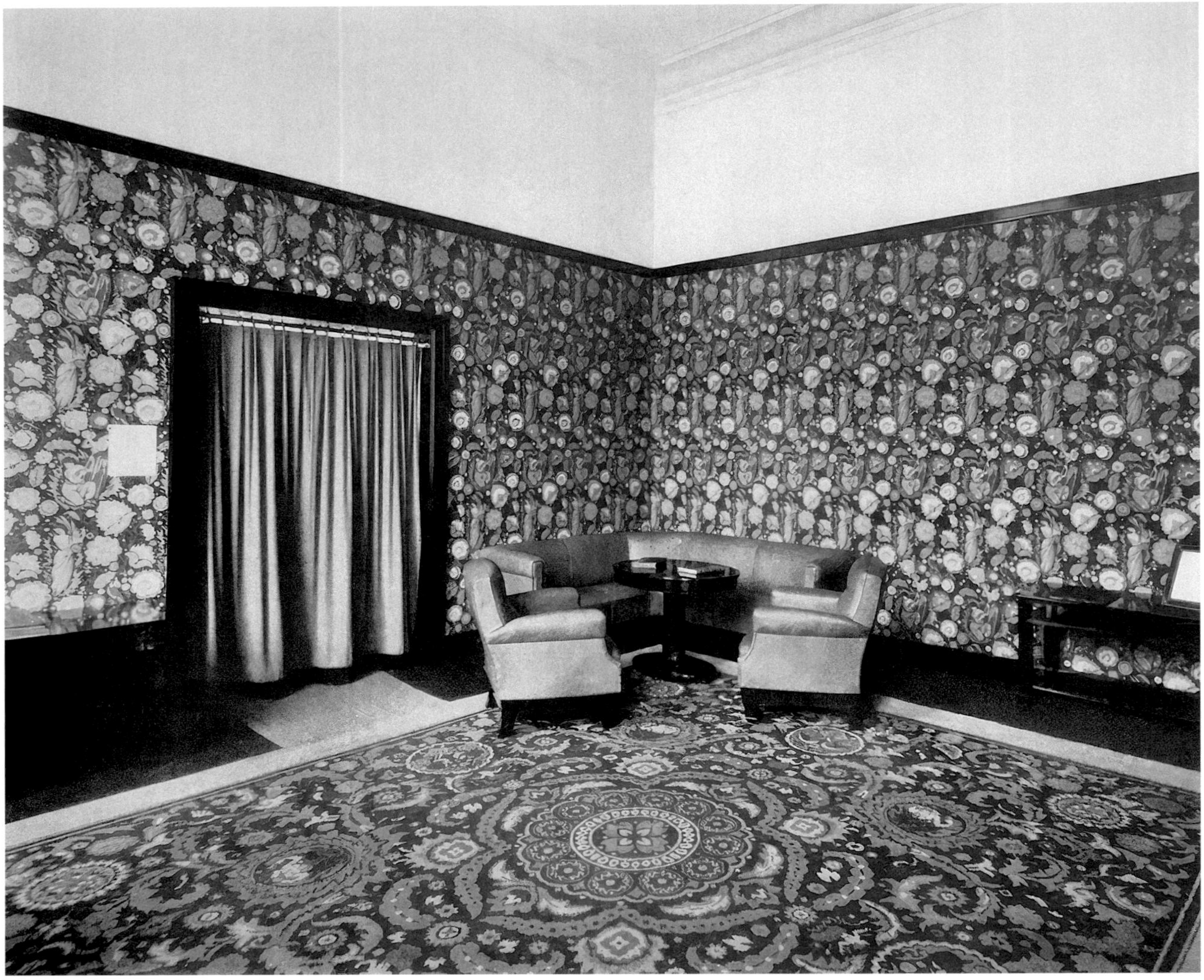

cherry wood paneling, painted surfaces, and glass vitrine display cases. Bayer's contribution not only represented the company's desire "to present our real colors in an appropriate way" but also the "conservative ideas of the Bayer management."[25] BASF, conversely, presented its newest dye class, Indanthren dyes—a colorfast, durable formula invented to replace natural dyes used for carpets, upholstery, wallpaper, and other home goods for the growing consumer classes—in a "restless" reception room containing carpets impregnated with synthetic dyes, pilasters coated with synthetic paints, and wallpapers in florid reds, blues, and greens.[26] Despite their aesthetic differences, both rooms presented a compromise: modernity was used as a vehicle for corporate product placement, the industrial chemists' view of progress, and corporate management-imposed aesthetics.

As historian Joan Campbell contends, the Werkbund founders forged industrial ties by creating an organization composed of Germany's most significant corporate members, who believed that quality design would result in higher profits.[27] The 1914 Cologne exhibition provides one concrete example of the aesthetics of corporate influence in the Werkbund, in which "aesthetics" were "subordinate[d] ... to commercial considerations."[28] The early alliance and exhibition with the dye industries proffered a promotional and pro-innovation stance for new products and production methods. Modern aesthetics propelled by the Werkbund movement were ultimately subordinate to consumer taste and the vivid modernity sold by dye companies.

As evidence of the harms of dye work continued to mount, the minds of designers started aligning with those of industrialists to sell dyes despite health concerns. The Werkbund as well as its exhibition program and promotion of dyes were instrumental in the promotion of an aesthetic regime that was seen to sustain workers' health—even if that work was toxic and often lethal. Werkbund founder Peter Behrens was the artistic consultant for the Allgemeine Elektricitäts-Gesellschaft (AEG) and controlled the corporation's visual identity, from product designs and posters to exhibitions and factories.[29] For Behrens, company buildings presented an impression of the corporation to the world and reflected directly back on it. He also believed factory design could ameliorate working conditions: "Better work is performed in well-lit and friendly factory halls

← Hermann Muthesius, BASF Room at the Cologne Werkbund Exhibition, 1914. 'Ausführung von Hermann Gerson, Berlin, Teppich und Tapete von H. Bengen Charlottenburg, Lichtecht gefarbt von der Badischen Anilin- und Soda-Fabrik, Ludwigshafen A. Rh." (1914, Köln Ausstellung, BASF, 123.)

impeccably designed according to the basic laws of health than in constricted and smoky sheds."[30]

The Werkbund's 1916 *Ausstellung für soziale Fürsorge* (Social Welfare Exhibition) in Brussels hosted a side display on accident prevention, including safety devices, models, and diagrams. A central Hugo Kaufmann sculpture titled *Betriebssicherheit* (*Operational Safety*) played against models of factories that Behrens designed for AEG presenting workplaces "incorporating wide-ranging health precautions against all types of harmful influences in factory work."[31] The models reflected a basic level of improved light conditions and ventilation. However, these narrow engagements in health hygiene do not compare to what was being recommended by the sophisticated occupational disease research developed by physicians and health officials in nearby factories at the time.

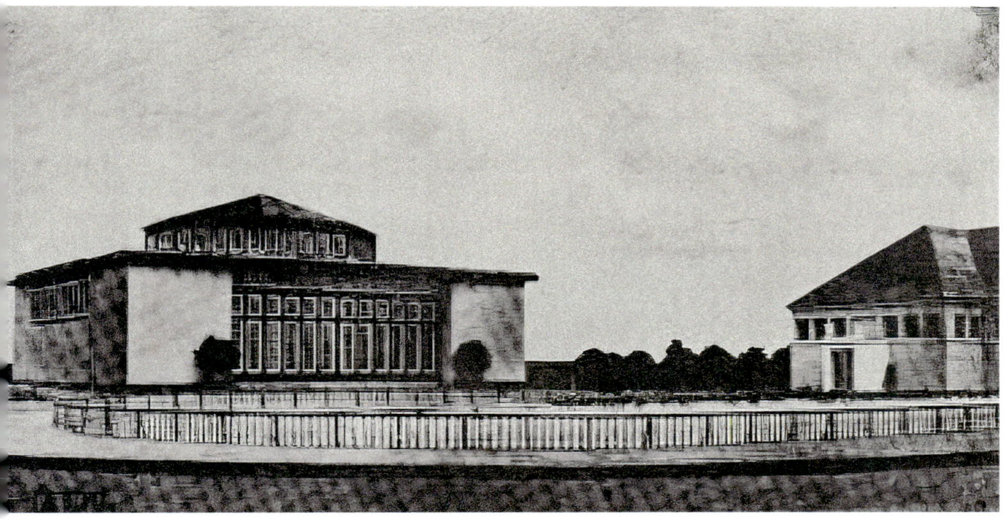

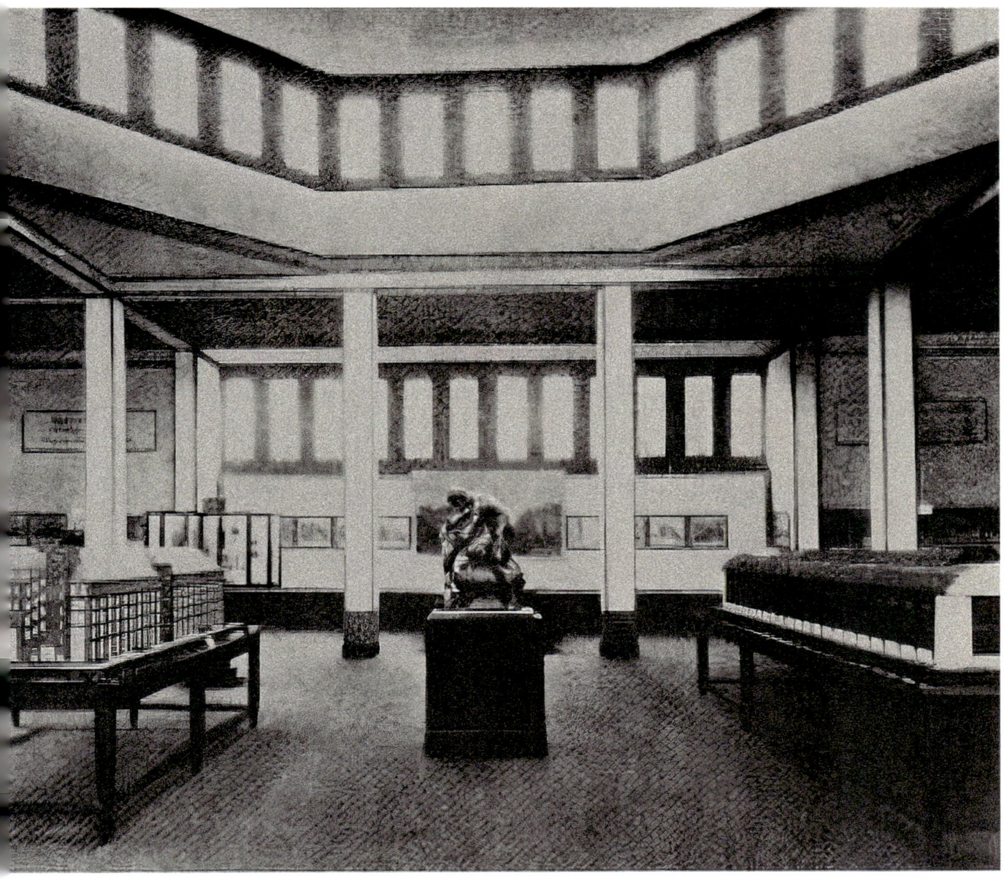

↖ Peter Behrens, 1916 Ausstellung für soziale Fürsorge, *MdBEW* 12, no. 10 (October 1916): 157.

← Peter Behrens, 1916 Ausstellung für soziale Fürsorge, *MdBEW* 12, no. 10 (October 1916): 157.

As the Werkbund focused on design and dye sales, it avoided contemporaneous developments regulating growing industrial harm, specifically within the chemical dye industry. The concept of regulatory capture describes how regulatory entities and state governance are dominated by the interests they regulate and are skewed to favor corporate growth.[32] Regulatory capture occurs in various ways—from direct political influence to cultural ties and social capture.[33] By practicing industrial allegiance, strategic ignorance around growing industrial reforms, and unknowing industrial hygiene developments (many related to building construction, spatial configurations, and ventilation design), the Werkbund was part of an emerging era of regulatory capture.[34]

Suggesting that corporate coalition members influenced the Werkbund goes against the common historiographies that focus on the group's artistic motivations and treat its pursuit of modern style as the primary objective.[35] The Western canon of modern architecture is commonly tied to the Werkbund's origins. Given the Werkbund's intimate ties to the chemical industry, however, this canon is grounded in chemical capitalism's expansion and its associated toxicities. The greatest legacy of the Werkbund might therefore ultimately be that of corporate influence and cultural capture. Questioning its silence on matters of industrial labor and occupational health reveals the role the Werkbund played in increasing corporate chemical profits and early forms of regulatory capture while shifting the focus of design away from health concerns during a period of vast expansion and industrial growth. In this light, the Werkbund can be understood to have designed ignorance to toxicity, from the architect's office to the factory floor.

1. Joan Campbell, *The German Werkbund: The Politics of Reform in the Applied Arts* (Princeton: Princeton University Press, 1978), 16. Campbell likely attributes this phrase to Hermann Muthesius from "Wo stehen wir?" *Jahrbuch des Deutschen Werkbundes* (1912): 16.
2. Campbell, *The German Werkbund*, 6.
3. For longer debates around BASF and the synthetic chemical development of Indanthren, Jessica Varner, *Chemical Desires: When the Chemical Industry Met Modern Design (1870–1970)* (forthcoming). See also Jessica Varner, "Chemical Desires: Dyes, Additives, and Foams; Making the Architectural Materials of Modernity (1870–1970)" (PhD diss., Massachusetts Institute of Technology, 2020).
4. Frederic J. Schwartz, "Commodity Signs: Peter Behrens, the AEG, and the Trademark," *Journal of Design History* 9, no. 3 (1996): 153–184; John V. Maciuika, "Art in the Age of Government Intervention: Hermann Muthesius, Sachlichkeit, and the State, 1897–1907," *German Studies Review* 21, no. 2 (1998): 285–308; Robin Schuldenfrei, "Objectivity: The Werkbund Display Window and Architecture's Object," in *Luxury and Modernism: Architecture and the Object in Germany 1900–1933* (Princeton: Princeton University Press, 2018), 59–115.
5. Herbert K. Abrams, "A Short History of Occupational Health," *Journal of Public Health Policy* 22, no. 1 (2001): 47.
6. Alice Hamilton, "Nineteen Years in the Dangerous Trades," *Harper's*, October 1929, 580.
7. Physician, industrial hygiene stalwart, and Hull House reformer Alice Hamilton looked to German dye factories in the 1910s while working for the state of Illinois for evidence and reform.
8. The modern industrial hygiene movement and government chemical regulations began in Werkbund Alliance dye factories. John Joseph Beer, *The Emergence of the German Dye Industry* (New York: Arno Press, 1981). See also Carsten Reinhardt and Anthony S. Travis, *Heinrich*

Caro and the Creation of Modern Chemical Industry (Dordrecht: Springer, 2010); and Frank Uekötter, *The Greenest Nation? A New History of German Environmentalism* (Cambridge, MA: MIT Press, 2014).

9. In 1880, Wilhelm Grandhomme, a physician at Höchst, published the first book on the health problems of tar and aniline dye workers. Grandhomme quickly took the stance that occupational and "social" conditions of workers were to blame. Fritz Schuckmann, "The History and Practice of Occupational Medicine in the Federal Republic of Germany," *Journal of Occupational Medicine* 28, no. 3 (March 1986): 212.

10. By 1906, just one year before the Werkbund's founding, Rehn identified thirty-eight additional cases of bladder cancer linked to the German dye industry. Later, in 1913, another physician, David Michaels, found over 100 more cases of dye-related bladder cancers in Germany. David Michaels, "Waiting for the Body Count: Corporate Decision Making and Bladder Cancer in the US Dye Industry," *Medical Anthropology Quarterly* 2, no. 3 (October 2009): 217.

11. Hermann Muthesius, "The Significance of Applied Art," in *The Theory of Decorative Art: An Anthology of European and American Writings, 1750–1940*, ed. Isabelle Frank, trans. David Britt (New Haven: Yale University Press, 2000), 79.

12. Conze, "Friedrich Naumann: Grundlagen und Ansatz seiner Politik in der nationalsozialen Zeit," in *Schicksalswege deutscher Vergangenheit: Beiträge zur geschichtlichen Deutung der letzten hundertfünfzig Jahre*, ed. Walther Hubatsch (Düsseldorf, 1950), 357–358.

13. Friedrich Naumann, "Deutsche Gewerbekunst," *Werke* 6 (1908): 254–289.

14. Campbell, *The German Werkbund*, 17.

15. Friedrich Naumann, *Neudeutsche Wirtschaftspolitik* (Berlin, 1911), 19. Quoted in Kevin Repp, "'More Corporeal, More Concrete': Liberal Humanism, Eugenics, and German Progressives at the Last Fin de Siècle," *Journal of Modern History* 72, no. 3 (2000): 683–730.

16. Friedrich Naumann, *Neudeutsche Wirtschaftspolitik* (Berlin, 1906), 26–27. Quoted in David Meskill, *Optimizing the German Workforce: Labor Administration from Bismarck to the Economic Miracle* (New York: Berghahn Books, 2019).

17. Throughout the history of labor movements and industrial health reform, the workers themselves (and their actions and advocacies) remained crucial to each advancement in legislation, compensation, correction, or even attempts at prevention. The reforms occurred through labor unrest, protests, strikes, lawsuits, and media attention in catastrophic emergencies. Workers and their actions were vital catalysts for change. Meskill, *Optimizing the German Workforce*, 23.

18. Joan Campbell points to how Naumann wanted to stay independent of the state to remain an effective organization; however, the corporation posited influential views internally via sponsorship that remain underexplored. Campbell, *The German Werkbund*, 18. Schwartz comes the closest to this analysis but remains on the theoretical level of capitalism and does not deepen his analysis of the corporation's role within the Werkbund ideals. Frederic J. Schwartz, *The Werkbund: Design Theory and Mass Culture before the First World War* (New Haven: Yale University Press, 1996).

19. Schwartz, *The Werkbund*, 251. Maciuika also gives the example of "types" in Werkbund debates occurring in 1914. For Maciuika, the "types"—or *Typisierung*, a heavily debated concept in the Werkbund's history—were less about aesthetic aims and more about trade acceleration, production ease, and Germany's colonial and global goals at the time. John Maciuika, "*Werkbundpolitik* and *Weltpolitik*: The German State's Interest in Global Commerce and 'Good Design,' 1912–1914," *German Politics and Society* 23, no. 1 (Spring 2005): 102–127, see 108.

20. Maciuika "*Werkbundpolitik* and *Weltpolitik*," 108.

21. Deutcher Werkbund EV, "Gründung und Programm (1909/1910)," Museum der Dinge, Werkbund Archiv.

22. *Chemie-proletariat* was used to describe chemical workers as labor resistance rose at the BASF factory in the 1910s. See the newspaper of the Communist Party of Germany cell at BASF, Ludwigshafen, *Der Aniliner*.

23. Museum der Dinge, Werkbund Archiv.

24. *Die Deutsche Werkbund-Ausstellung Cöln 1914* (Kölnischer Kunstverein), 209. Museum der Dinge, Werkbund Archiv.

25. *Die Deutsche Werkbund-Ausstellung Cöln 1914*, 209.

26. *Die Deutsche Werkbund-Ausstellung Cöln 1914*, 210.

27. Campbell, *The German Werkbund*, 49.

28. Campbell, *The German Werkbund*, 70.

29. Stanford Anderson, "Modern Architecture and Industry: Peter Behrens and the Cultural Policy of Historical Determinism," *Oppositions* 11 (Winter 1977): 69; Stanford Anderson, *Peter Behrens and a New Architecture for the Twentieth Century* (Cambridge, MA: MIT Press, 2002).

30. "Artistic Values in Factory Building and Their Effect as Publicity," *Das Plakat* 11, no. 6 (June 1920): 269–273.

31. *MdBEW* 12, no. 10 (October 1916): 157. Quoted in Tilmann Buddensieg and Henning Rogge, *Industriekultur: Peter Behrens and the AEG, 1907–1914* (Cambridge, MA: MIT Press, 1984), 269.

32. George J. Stigler, "The Theory of Economic Regulation," *Bell Journal of Economics and Management Science* 2, no. 1 (1971): 3–21; and Michael E. Levine and Jennifer L. Forrence, "Regulatory Capture, Public Interest, and the Public Agenda: Toward a Synthesis," *Journal of Law, Economics, and Organization* 6 (1990): 169–170.

33. Legal scholar James Kwak offers the concept of "cultural capture" as an expanded effect of regulatory capture to explain the indirect ways that regulatory bodies can be influenced to create or enforce pollution laws, reduce worker harm, and more—through cultural norms, relationships in the world, or social associations or consumer trends and knowledge. For Carpenter and Moss, cultural capture occurs more in a system of regulators tied to industry directly. "Cultural Capture and the Financial Crisis," in Daniel Carpenter and David A. Moss, *Preventing Regulatory Capture: Special Interest Influence and How to Limit It* (Cambridge: Cambridge University Press, 2013). Similarly, legal historian Davidoff discusses "social capture," where social network composition influences regulators' decisions: "These men and women may believe they are doing their best, but their worldview is affected by the people they interact with." Steven M. Davidoff, "The Government's Elite and Regulatory Capture," *New York Times,* June 11, 2010, 39.

34. This conceptual reframing builds on McGoey's concepts of strategic ignorance and Proctor's work on corporate unknowing. Linsey McGoey, *The Unknowers: How Strategic Ignorance Rules the World* (New York: Zed Books, 2019); and Robert Proctor and Londa L. Schiebinger, eds., *Agnotology: The Making and Unmaking of Ignorance* (Stanford: Stanford University Press, 2008).

35. There are three main historiographical narratives about the Werkbund's role in the twentieth century. One focuses on the origins of modern design, whether in artisanal revival, aesthetic dogma toward clean factory lines or modern materials, and its later connections to German modern design tradition and education, including the Bauhaus. Campbell's work remains a lasting reference for the history of the Werkbund (Campbell, *The German Werkbund*). The second focuses on the Werkbund's political or antipolitical role, coinciding with the timing before World War I and World War II, as avant-garde modern design came under attack from the state. Maciuika's work best contextualizes the Werkbund's role in larger political and social movements, including in "modernity" and "anti-modernity" debates, and the agency the artists maintained with and against growing government influence. John V. Maciuika, *Before the Bauhaus: Architecture, Politics, and the German State, 1890–1920* (Cambridge: Cambridge University Press, 2005). Jarzombek recuperates Joseph August Lux to outline the Werkbund's political issues in an emerging rationalist worldview. Mark Jarzombek, "Joseph August Lux: Werkbund Promoter, Historian of a Lost Modernity," *Journal of the Society of Architectural Historians* 63, no. 2 (2004): 202–219. The third focuses on the outsized role industry had in design in the twentieth century. Schwartz, Maciuika, and Schuldenfrei partially address industry's influence within the Werkbund. Schwartz uses the term "capitalese" to suggest the Werkbund's tight relationship with industrial capitalism in trademark and logo design. Frederic J. Schwartz, "Commodity Signs: Peter Behrens, the AEG, and the Trademark," *Journal of Design History* 9, no. 3 (1996): 153–184. Maciuika outlines the vast state and industry relationships forged in early twentieth-century Germany. John V. Maciuika, "Art in the Age of Government Intervention: Hermann Muthesius, Sachlichkeit, and the State, 1897–1907," *German Studies Review* 21, no. 2 (1998): 285–308. Schuldenfrei finds evidence deep in object history, extending industrial capitalism's influence into the Werkbund's window displays. Robin Schuldenfrei, "Objectivity: The Werkbund Display Window and Architecture's Object," in *Luxury and Modernism: Architecture and the Object in Germany 1900–1933* (Princeton: Princeton University Press, 2018), 59–115.

p206 TUMunich Archiv.
p207 Deutscher Werkbund Archiv (Berlin).

VITAMIN D ARCHITECTURE

XHULIO BINJAKU

Plague Clouds On August 27, 1883, the volcano of Krakatoa in the Indonesian islands erupted. Ashes and rocks flew miles high. Barometers wobbled three and a half times as they recorded the atmospheric pressure wave circumnavigating the globe. The noise was heard across the Indian Ocean and Australia. For years, small ash particles floated in the atmosphere, diffusing the sun's light and scattering colors around the world.

The sublime event was an immense creative influence for artist and writers. Edvard Munch's iconic painting *The Scream* (1893) was a response to the swirling red-orange skies he saw in Oslo that resulted from the eruption. In the chthonic shockwaves, Munch said he felt "a great unending scream piercing through nature."[1] John Ruskin discussed the eruption in his 1884 lecture *The Storm-Cloud of the Nineteenth Century*, in which he told his audience, in "the plague-wind, every breath of air you draw is polluted, half-round the world," and that the sun itself is "choked out of the whole heaven."[2]

To Ruskin, these volcanic repercussions were not just an environmental disaster, but a medical and moral one too. The skies, to him, were a "plague cloud," an outcome of both bad climate and polluted industrialization that produced sickened citizens and instilled moral failings.[3] For Ruskin, the plumes of Krakatoa were an allegory for Manchester's chimney stacks: dark burdens on the metaphorical English body, fumes that destroyed it from within.

By the end of the nineteenth century, the scant amounts of sunlight in the English climate had produced artistic, literary, and medical responses. Sunlight's absence led to intense research into two endemic diseases at the time: tuberculosis, whose impact on modern life, urban space, and architecture has been extensively studied;[4] and the lesser-known rickets, a disease caused by vitamin D deficiency, which at the time affected sixty to ninety percent of children living in urban areas of northern Europe, deforming their bones and musculoskeletal systems.[5]

Rickets was labeled an "urban disease," as well as "the English disease" because it was especially widespread the British Isles, where manufacturing cities like London and Manchester had large populations

→ Explosion of Krakatoa, August 27, 1883, engraved by Parker & Coward from a photograph.

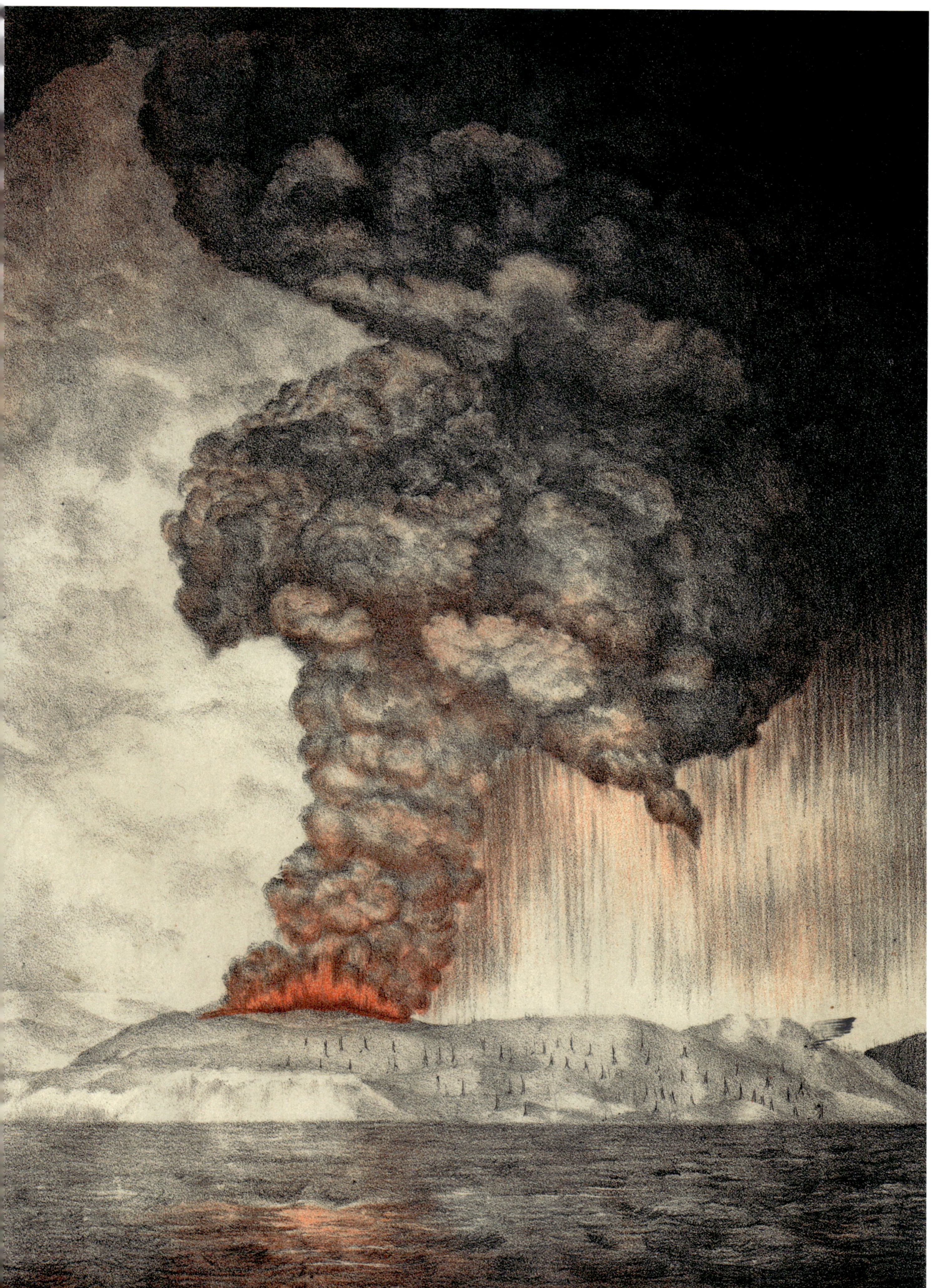

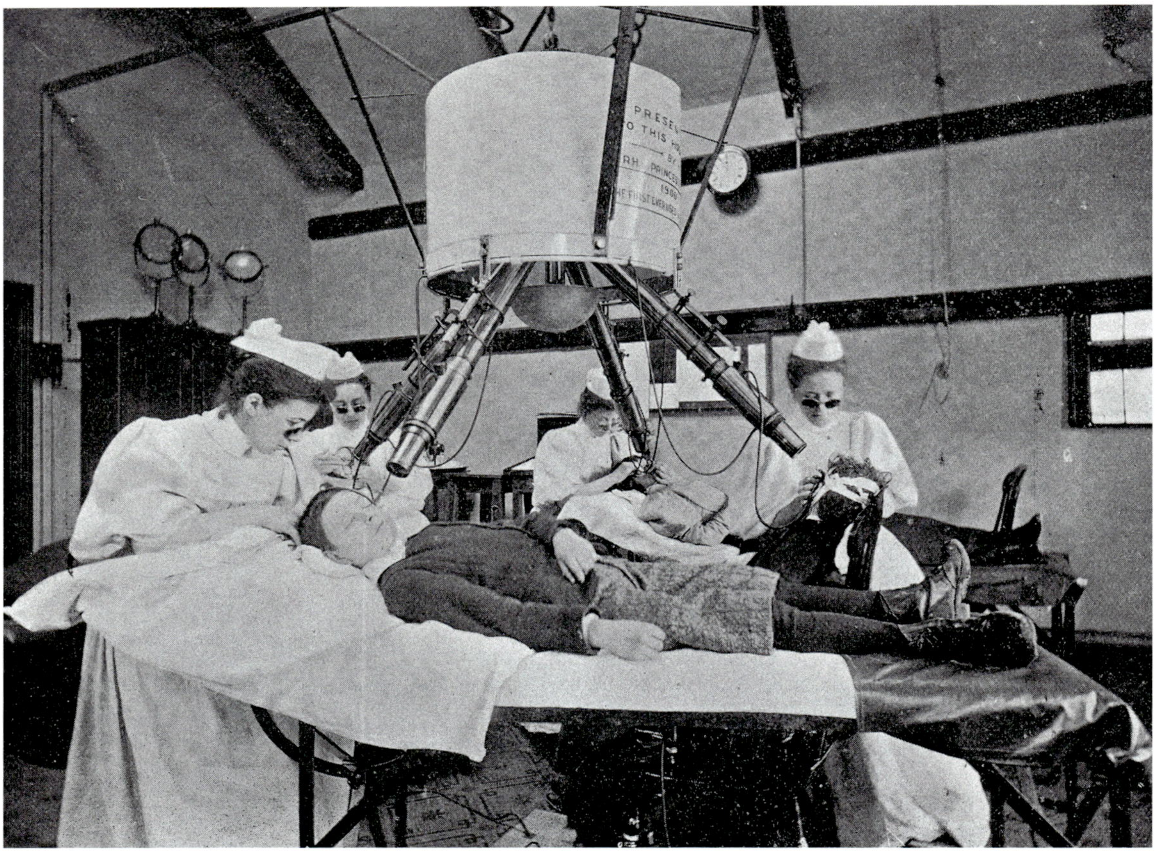

← Finsen lamps used to treat young patients with ultraviolet rays at the Finsen Institute in Copenhagen, Denmark, ca. 1901.

living with poor nutrition, hygiene, and little access to direct sunlight. Unlike tuberculosis, which was an “ancient disease,” rickets was a “modern disease,” first being diagnosed only in 1645, with recorded cases increasing during the Industrial Revolution.[6]

If, as Beatriz Colomina states, “a map showing the distribution of modern architecture would echo a map of the distribution of [tuberculosis],” that map would also neatly overlap with rickets.[7] Indeed, many of the same techniques that were applied to patients with tuberculosis, like light therapy and long stays in open-air sanatoria, were also used on those with rickets. Both diseases produced the same languid patient and new types of modern architecture. Although rickets was caused by a lack of sunlight, and tuberculosis by bacteria, both diseases were symptoms of profound changes in urban life at the turn of the twentieth century. During this period, medicine and modern architecture became entangled in the study of sunlight and its effects on the human body. Architecture was paradoxically seen as both cause and cure.

Chemistry of Light: Phototherapy and Heliotherapy

The science of light therapy quickly developed between 1890 and 1920 in order to deal with both rickets and tuberculosis. Theobald A. Palm, a British medical missionary researching rickets in impoverished children in Japan, was witness to drastic outcomes of the Krakatoa eruption: for six years, suspended ash particulates occluded sunlight, average temperatures dipped by more than two degrees, and weather patterns became extremely erratic.[8] In a report compiled in 1890, he was “struck by the fact that children in tropical zones were exposed to filth, inadequate sanitation, unsafe water, and dysentery, yet they were free of rickets.”[9] Like Ruskin, he blamed the British atmosphere and urban planning, where citizens are “under a perennial pall of smoke, and where high-houses cut off from narrow streets a large proportion of the rays which struggle through the gloom.”[10]

Palm was one of the first to collate global data on rickets and tuberculosis. Utilizing the British Empire’s vast medical missionary network, he came to “the theory that sunlight is essential to the healthy nutrition” and that a deficiency of sunlight characterizes the conditions of those with rickets.[11] In the same research, Palm called for a new study into the “Chemistry of Light” to further deduce the health properties of sun exposure. A few years later, two methods of light therapy were developed: phototherapy (also called actinotherapy), where artificial light is applied to specific areas on the body; and heliotherapy, where natural daylight is applied to the entire body.

In 1893, Danish physician Niels Finsen initiated modern phototherapy by applying limited amounts of light directly onto skin infected with *lupus vulgaris*, a visible form of tuberculosis. Two years later he cooperated with the Copenhagen Electric Light Works to design and produce lamps emitting artificial ultraviolet light that proved to be highly successful medical instruments. Soon after, Finsen established the Medical Light Institute (later named Finsen Institute) to cure patients from lupus and tuberculosis. The main discovery behind Finsen's lamps was the germicidal attributes of ultraviolet rays, which won him a Nobel Prize in 1903. Finsen's scientific achievements with phototherapy were so popular that by around 1910 there were forty Finsen Institutes in Europe and the United States.[12]

Phototherapy's growing demand would quickly move from hospitals into homes. The German electrical company Allgemeine Elektrizitäts-Gesellschaft (AEG) hired artist László Moholy-Nagy and architect Peter Behrens in 1926 and 1927 respectively as design consultants to create ultraviolet lamps based on Finsen's designs. Moholy-Nagy's design for the "Original Hanau" lamp was widely used in private homes until 1973, a testament to both its design and the proven methods of phototherapy.

Meanwhile, in 1903 the Swiss physician Auguste Rollier began applying Finsen's techniques all over patients' bodies in an approach called heliotherapy. His Leysin Sanatorium in the mountains of Switzerland—a Victorian-era hotel converted into a modern building with protruding sun balconies on every facade—was a haven for patients, most of whom were children suffering from tuberculosis, rickets, or sometimes both. Rather than apply light to treat specific areas the body, patients took daily sunbaths, even in the winter months.

Rollier was a masterful promoter of his craft: he employed several photographers to take before-and-after shots of his patients, and made use of recently invented X-rays and even early color photography.[13] His work was influential to the development of modern architecture—Le Corbusier, claimed Rollier, was inspired by the design of Leysin.[14] He also treated Bessie Bruce, the partner of Adolf Loos.[15] By 1933, the Royal Institute of British Architects (RIBA) was promoting his ideas.[16] Rollier's diagrams for a gradual solarization of the body, beginning with the ankles for five minutes and gradually moving to the face, recall the silhouettes and subdivisions of Le Corbusier's Modulor. Le Corbusier even enshrined the principles of light therapy in the 1933 Athens Charter for CIAM:

> Science, in its studies of solar radiations, has disclosed those that are indispensable to human health and those that, in certain cases, could be harmful to it. The sun is the master of life. ... The sun must penetrate every dwelling several hours a day even during the season when sunlight is most scarce. Society will no longer tolerate a situation where entire families are cut off from the sun and thus doomed to declining health. ... To introduce the sun is the new and most imperative duty of the architect.[17]

↓ Original Hanau lamps were designed by László Moholy-Nagy at the AEG in the early twentieth century.

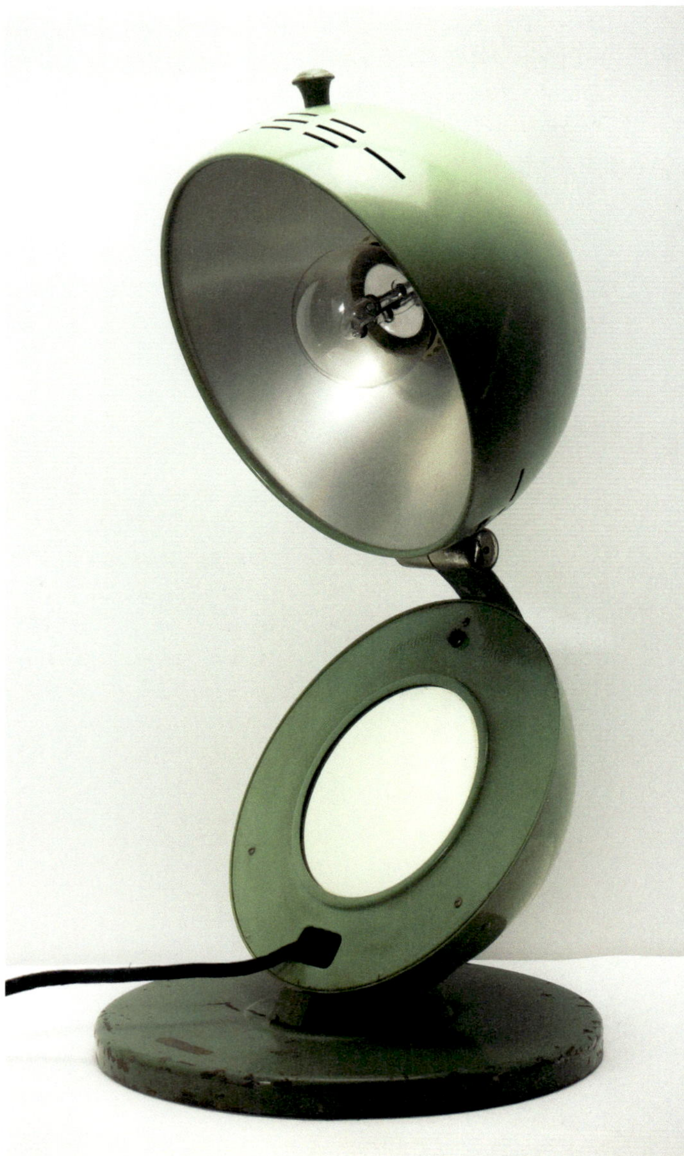

↓ Rollier's sun exposure chart.

→ All activities at Rollier's Alpine sanatorium in Leysin, even skiing in winter, were part of the heliotherapy methods.

The Discovery of Vitamin D

While architects found an ally for modern styles in Rollier's techniques, medical professionals were not impressed. In the early decades of the twentieth century, the medicalization of sunlight moved from the macro to the molecular scale. Advancements in vitamin research rendered Rollier's holistic techniques unreliable and suspicious. When Rollier presented his results to other physicians in Paris, the crowd walked out,[18] and by 1934, the American Medical Association's Council on Physical Therapy noted that "there is hardly a skin disease or condition for which some physician has not failed to claim good results with ultraviolet radiation."[19] Heliotherapy and the sanatoria design it produced were quickly relegated to pseudoscience.

Simultaneous to the development of light therapy, physicians began nutritional experiments on children and animals with rickets. While scientists understood that rickets was prevalent in unsanitary and sun-deprived urban living conditions, they could not isolate its specific causes. Already in 1912, Polish biochemist Casimir Funk hypothesized that some diseases could not be explained by bacteria or environmental influences, but by a lack of "accessory food factors."[20] Funk speculated that specific nutrients in food could cure common deficiency diseases of the time. Some of these, like those in fish oils and lemons, had been known as ancient folk remedies but

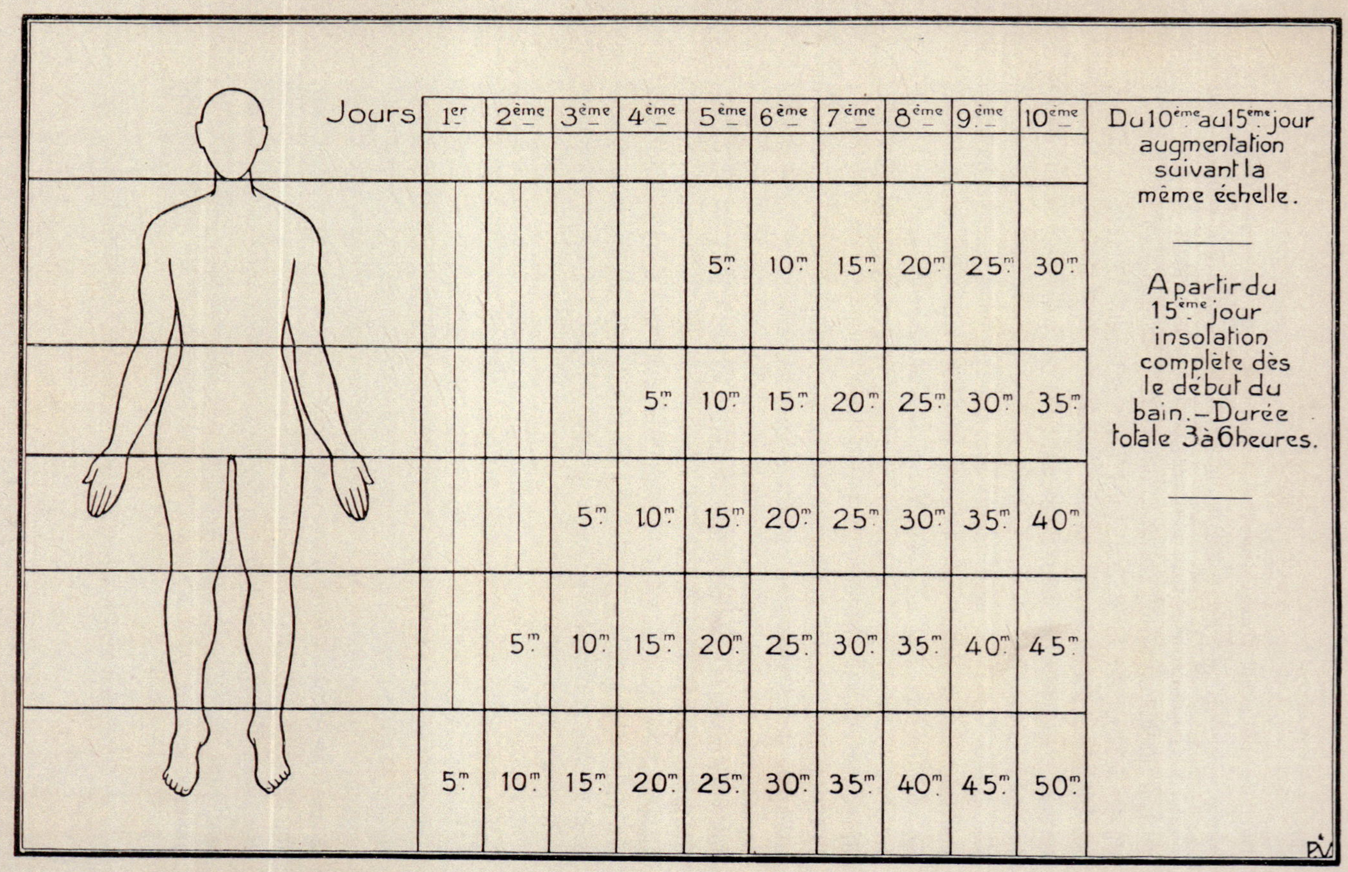

Fig. 8.
Notre schéma d'insolation. — Progression suivant laquelle le malade est exposé au soleil.

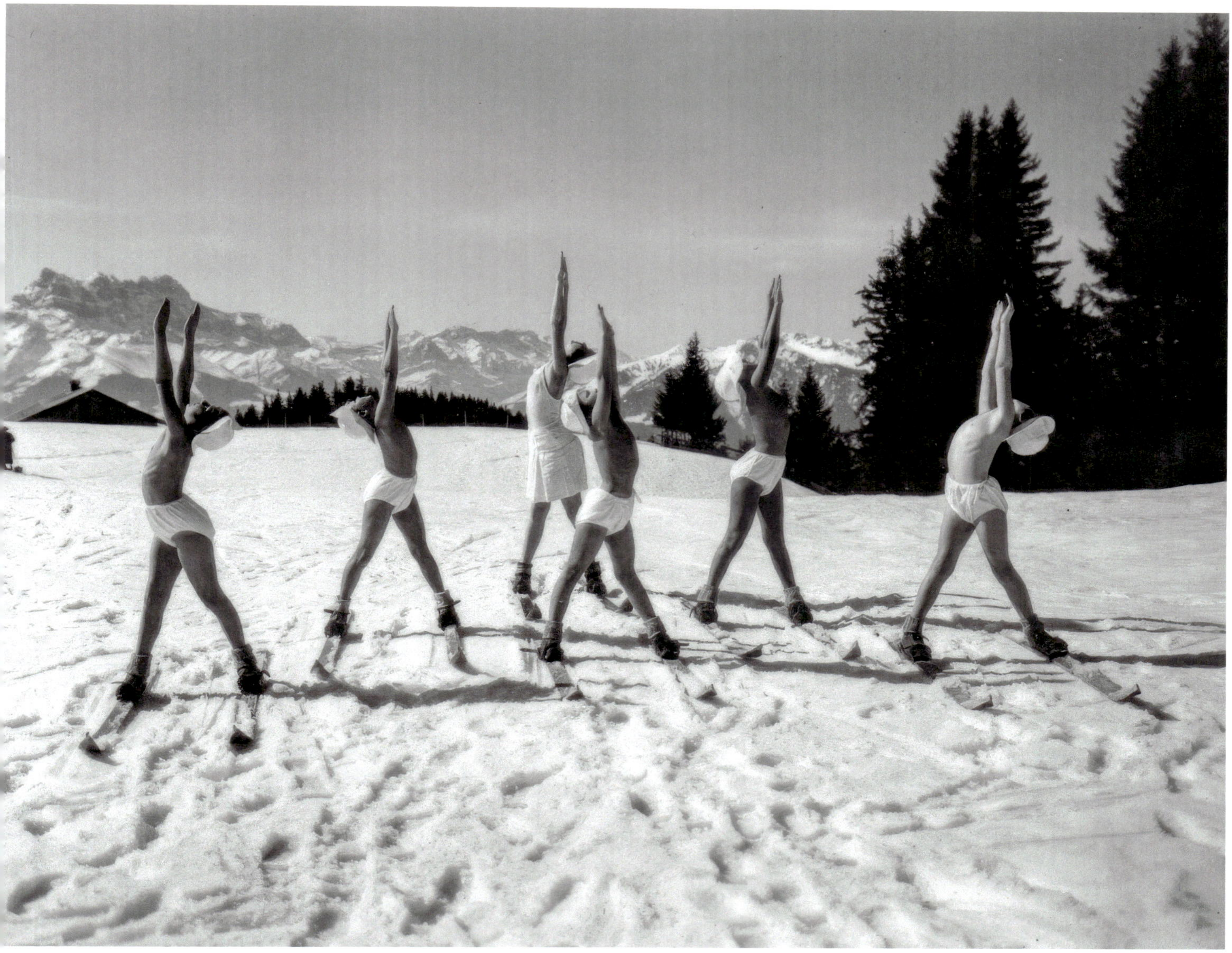

were only just being isolated by scientists. He termed these essential substances "vital amines," later shortened to "vitamines," and finally "vitamins" because not all of the compounds come from the amine group.

Between 1910 and 1920, four vitamins were discovered, named with an alphabetical letter and attributed as a cure for a common deficiency disease: vitamin A, found in fish oils, cured night blindness; vitamin B, found in brown rice, treated beriberi, a cardiovascular disease; vitamin C, found in citrus fruits, cured scurvy; and vitamin D, found in cod liver oil, cured rickets.[21] Concurrently, scientists working with Finsen's lamps specified that ultraviolet light in the B range (between 280 and 315 nanometers) could synthesize vitamin D on the skin.

By the early 1920s, vitamin D had two completely different sources: one from ultraviolet light, and the other from dietary sources. These twin sources were immediately conflated by advertisers sensing an opportunity to profit, claiming that ultraviolet light had become an essential nutrient, and supplement manufacturers declaring "light is food." Citizens were not only malnourished but in fact "sun-starved."[22] One British advertisement went on to clarify, "sunlight has become, for the whole world, a commodity rather than a mere stimulus ... the conception of a 'place in the sun' is giving way to the conception of a 'ration of sunlight,' something to be possessed and consumed."[23]

Architecture as Vitamin

At the turn of the twentieth century, captive animals at the London Zoo also regularly suffered from rickets. Francis Lamplough, a technologist who worked for Chance Bros., the company that provided the sheet glass for Joseph Paxton's Crystal Palace, was urged by the zoo's director to come up with a solution. Finsen had observed that regular sheet glass absorbs ultraviolet radiation, and another scientist found that traces of iron impurities present in glass production was the cause. By 1925, Lamplough had developed a method of sheet glass production that removed these ferrous bits to create a new type of window glass that effectively transmits ultraviolet B

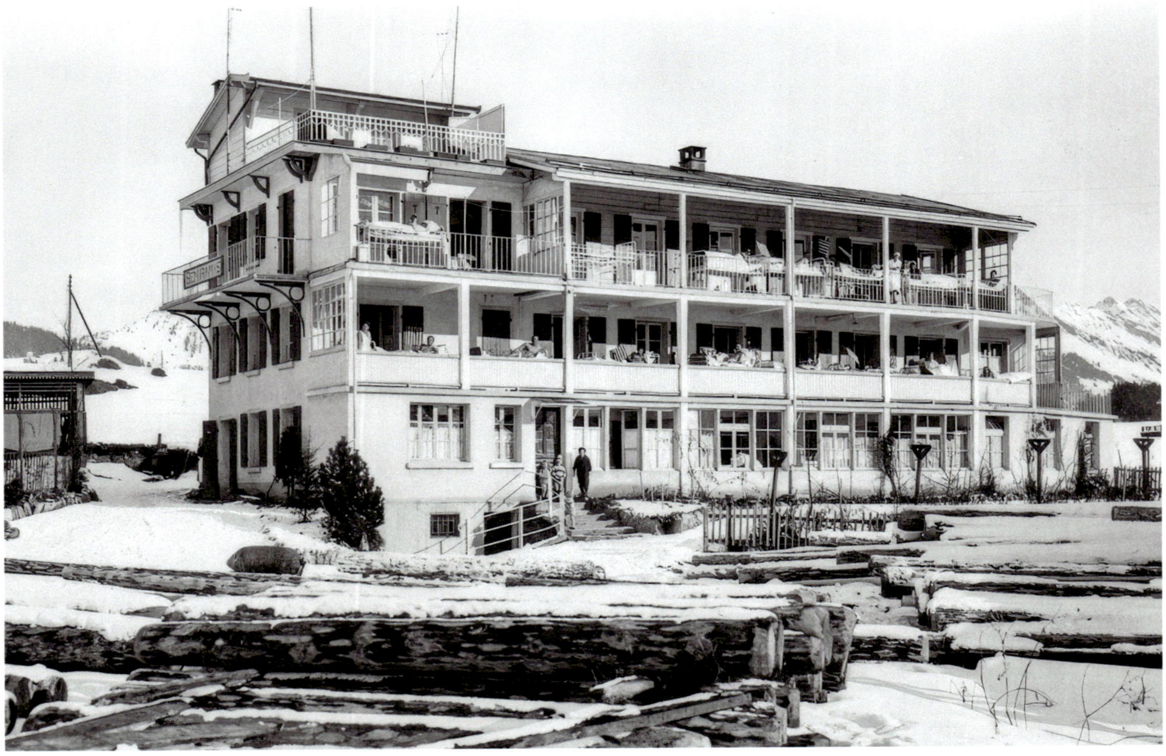

← Rollier's sanatorium, Leysin, Switzerland, ca. 1930. Building designs always called for south-facing balconies in order to maximize sun exposure.

→ Vitaglass advertisement.

rays directly into buildings.[24] The first installation of this experimental glass was at the Monkey House in the London Zoo, to positive effects. Chance Bros. immediately saw an economic opportunity for the glass in private homes, and began advertising their reduced-iron glass as "Vitaglass," short for "vitamin glass."

Beyond the name, Vitaglass was marketed with explicit reference to nutrition and aimed toward health-conscious consumers, Le Corbusier being one of them. In *The Radiant City*, he proposes a "Questionnaire to Doctors," which specifically asked about glass that allows ultraviolet light.[25] Modern architecture with scientific glass turned the space of the home into "an investment for health."[26] Working with the Vitaglass Corporation, the marketing firm F. E. Prichard & Company inflated research on vitamin D, emphatically stating that "the case for Vitaglass is really exactly the same as that used for baby and adult proprietary foods."[27]

Vitaglass was used in hospitals and schools worldwide.[28] It was also used in domestic projects, such as Richard Neutra's Health Demonstration-House (1927–1929) for Philip and Leah Lovell in Southern California. Philip Lovell was a practicing naturopath, an anti-drug physician who advocated for natural methods, and a "radical" in dietary and health matters.[29] The house was a showcase of all the most up-to-date natural healing methods: sunbathing, natural lighting, ventilation, sports facilities, and sleeping balconies. In "Care for the Body," a weekly column that Lovell wrote for the *Los Angeles Times*, he promoted the newly built home and laid out its health benefits:

> There are plenty of opportunities throughout the house for nude sunbaths privately taken for each member. Many of the windows are of the latest invention of glass, admitting ultraviolet light. Sanitation and hygiene are the key note. The ventilation, sunshine, and light ideas are exceedingly modern.[30]

Lovell's modern home was for the whole family, but it would primarily benefit children. The bulk of Rollier's patients were children, and even advertisements for Vitaglass present the body of a child as the primary benefactor. Lovell stated: "This home, in a sense, is being built mainly for the little ones. It is really a social school in which they will learn their life habits. Their customs will be molded and shaped therein."[31]

After the Lovell house, Neutra used ultraviolet glass again in 1935 at the Corona Avenue School. The building's southern-facing glass walls made from Lustraglass, a Vitaglass competitor, opened out directly into the garden.[32] Known as the "Test Tube School," its nickname serves as a metaphor for the extensive use of transparent glass, while also suggesting the growth, development, and care of children in a highly monitored and medicalized environment.[33]

Unlike Le Corbusier's commands to let the sun in, Neutra sought subtler methods, arguing that the modern architect should "digest the complex problems of today's house into a new formal solution."[34] The use of the word "digest" here is striking. Perhaps Neutra was following Lovell's decree that "next to diet ... it is the physical or, in other words, the architectural environment of our nurseries which imprints itself most forcibly on our early physical and mental

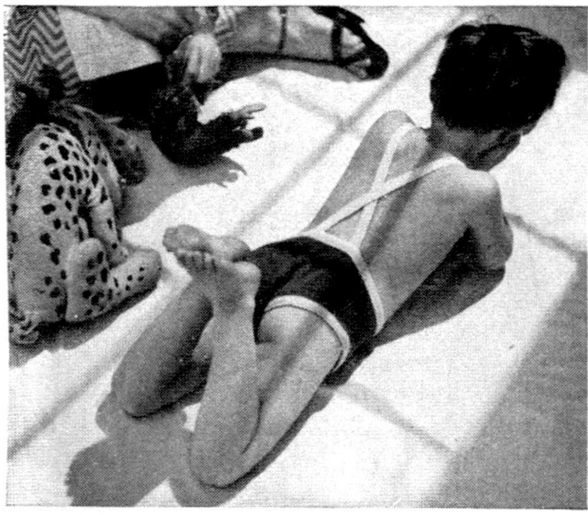
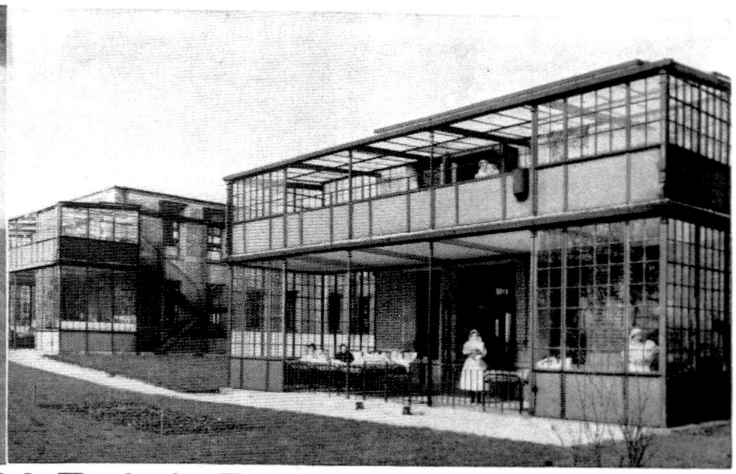

LET IN THE HEALTH RAYS OF

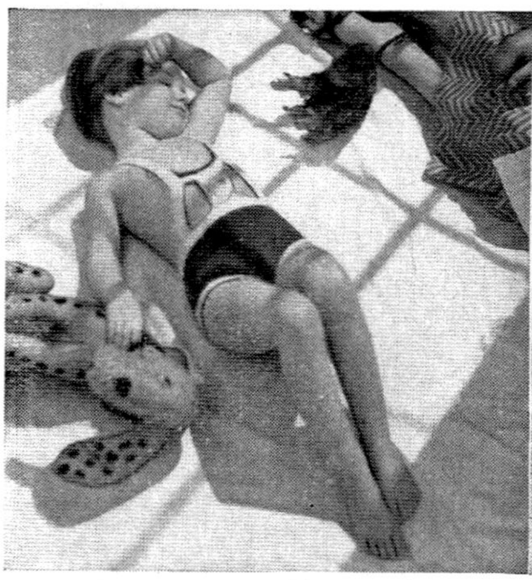
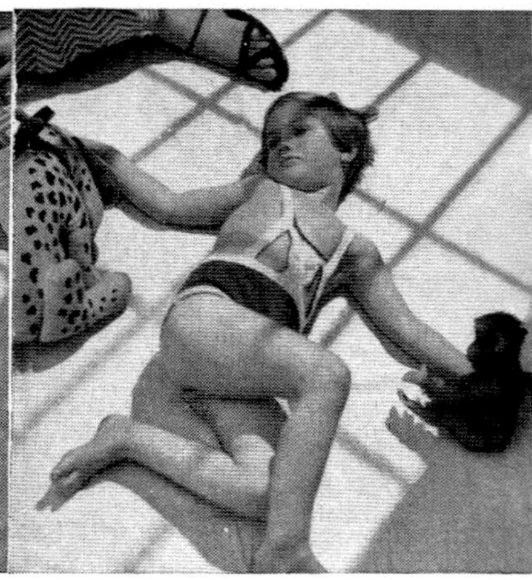
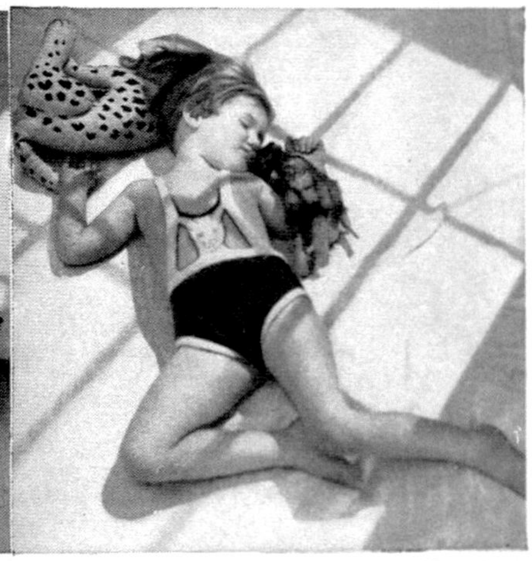

DAYLIGHT PERMANENTLY THROUGH

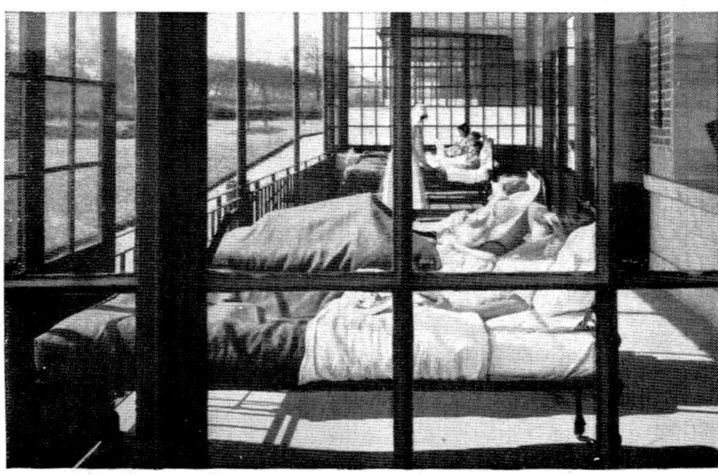
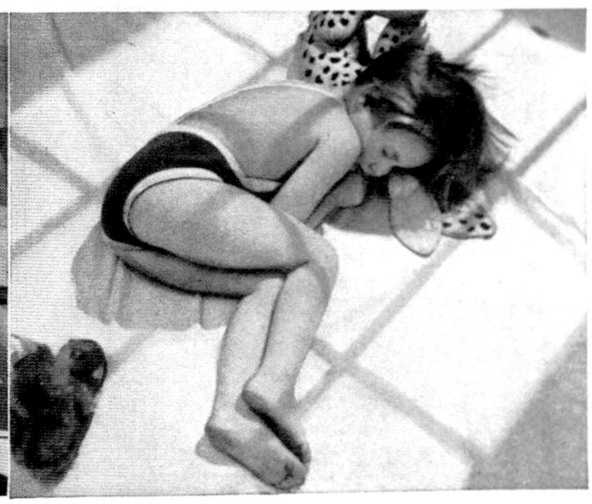

"VITA" GLASS WINDOWS

Ordinary window glass shuts out the ultra-violet health rays of daylight. "Vita" Glass admits them permanently. The properties of "Vita" Glass do not fade away in a year or two; they are guaranteed permanent, and that guarantee has been confirmed by tests made by the Building Research Station. (Write for copy of report 62/B.R.S. 36/12/4—Nov. 1933.) Two views are shown above of the "Vita" Sun Balconies at Harrogate Infirmary. Roof glazing in $\frac{3}{16}$ "Vita" cathedral by Mellowes & Co. Ltd., Sheffield. Side glazing in $\frac{5}{32}$ plate "Vita" Glass. "Vita" Glass is obtainable from local glass merchants, plumbers, glaziers and builders. "Vita" is the registered trade mark of Pilkington Brothers, Limited, St. Helens, Lancs, whose Technical Department is available for consultation regarding properties and uses of glass.

habits."[35] Modern architecture could create a healing environment, but proper nutrition always preceded it.

The Corona Avenue School was possibly the last use of UV glass in Neutra's work. The Great Depression and the looming war made luxury vitamin glass difficult to justify. Architectural historian John Stanislav Sadar explains that as soon as Vitaglass was produced, there was criticism toward its quantitative effects. A hygienist at Johns Hopkins University, for instance, showed that receiving sun through Vitaglass was not as effective as simply going outside for a walk.[36] Furthermore, pollution, grime, and dust accumulates on the outside of the window and reduces rates of transmission, and inside, people often wear clothes, which further reduces the direct transmission of UV radiation onto skin. The skeptical scientist also questioned how many hours a day someone might spend right next to the window.

As the economics and science of ultraviolet glass dwindled, scientists found more cost-effective ways of distributing and ameliorating vitamin D deficiency though food. During World War II, the American Medical Association recommended radiating milk and wheat with ultraviolet light, thereby fortifying it with vitamin D. Quickly administered during and after the war, this practice effectively eradicated rickets together with the architectural market for ultraviolet glass.[37] Still, modern architecture's commitment to sunshine endured. Modern architecture was not so much a response to changes in technology and medicine as medical equipment itself.[38]

↙ Richard Neutra designed the Corona Avenue School in Bell, California, with an ultraviolet glass facade that easily connected the schoolchildren to outdoor garden spaces.

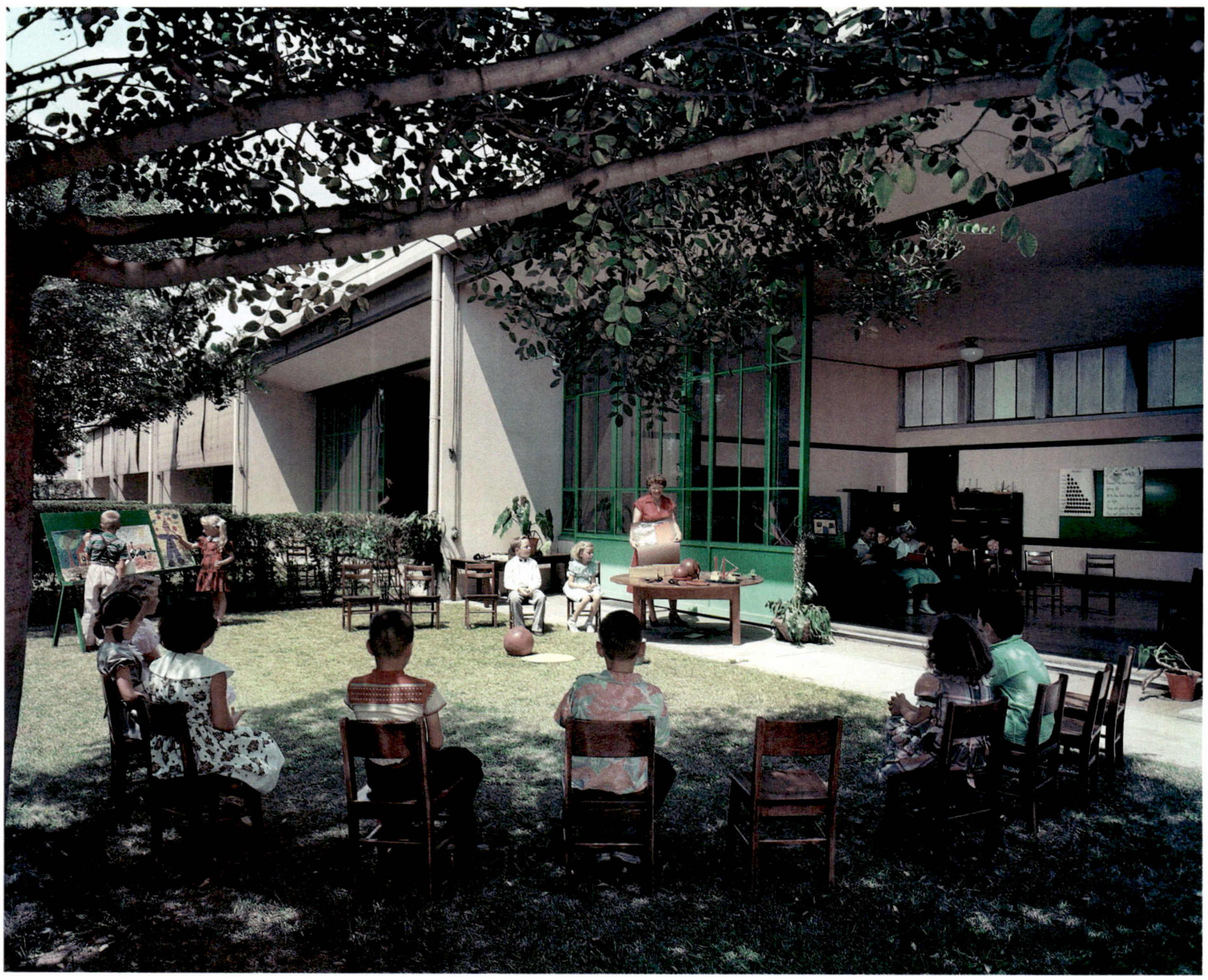

An earlier version of this essay was originally published by e-flux Architecture in 2022.

p213 Reproduced from *The Eruption of Krakatoa and Subsequent Phenomena. Report of the Krakatoa Committee of the Royal Society* (London: Trubner & Co., 1888).
p214, 216 Courtesy of the Wellcome Collection, London, UK.
p215 Courtesy of Bukowskis Auctioneering, Stockholm, Sweden.
p216 Originally published in Auguste Rollier, *La cure de soleil* (Paris: Baillière & fils, 1915).
p217, 218 Multiple photographers.
Reproduced from Auguste Rollier, *Quarante ans d'héliothérapie* (Lausanne: F. Rouge & Cie, 1944).
p219 Reproduced from *Architectural Review*, January 1935.
p220 Photo: Julius Schulman, 1953. © J. Paul Getty Trust. Getty Research Institute, Los Angeles (2004.R.10).

1. Marilynn S. Olson, Donald W. Olson, and Russell L. Doescher, "On the Blood-Red Sky of Munch's *The Scream*," *Environmental History* 12 (January 2007): 131. For more artists influenced by the eruption, see C. S. Zerefos, V. T. Gerogiannis, D. Balis, S. C. Zerefos, and A. Kazantzidis, "Atmospheric Effects of Volcanic Eruptions as Seen by Famous Artists and Depicted in Their Paintings," *Atmospheric Chemistry and Physics, European Geosciences Union* 7 (August 7, 2007).
2. John Ruskin, "The Storm Cloud of the Nineteenth Century," in *The Seven Lamps of Architecture: also, Lectures on Architecture and Painting; The Study of Architecture; Sesame and Lilies; Unto This Last; The Queen of the Air; The Storm-Cloud of the Nineteenth Century* (Boston: Aldine, 1890), 391.
3. Seth T. Reno, *Early Anthropocene Literature in Britain, 1750–1884* (London: Pallgrave Macmillan, 2020), 104–107.
4. See Beatriz Colomina, *X-Ray Architecture* (Zurich: Lars Müller, 2016); Paul Overy, *Air, Light, and Openness* (London: Thames & Hudson, 2007).
5. J. Zappert, "Rickets (rachitis)," in *Diseases of Children*, ed. A. Jacobo (New York: Appleton, 1910), 12.
6. Daniel Whistler, *De moro pueril anglorum, quem idiomate indigenae vocant The Rickets* (Leiden, 1645).
7. Colomina, *X-Ray Architecture*, 10.
8. Russell W. Chesney, "Theobald Palm and His Remarkable Observation: How the Sunshine Vitamin Came to Be Recognized," *Nutrients* 4 (2012): 45.
9. T. A. Palm, "The Geographical Distribution and Ætiology of Rickets," *Practitioner* 45 (1890): 272.
10. Palm, "The Geographical Distribution and Ætiology of Rickets," 335.
11. Palm, "The Geographical Distribution and Ætiology of Rickets," 274; emphasis original.
12. Andrzej Grzybowski and Krzysztof Pietrzak, "From Patient to Discoverer—Niels Ryberg Finsen (1860–1904)—the Founder of Modern Phototherapy in Dermatology," *Clinics in Dermatology* 30, no. 4 (2012): 451–455.
13. See Tania Anne Woloshyn, "Patients Rebuilt: Dr. Auguste Rollier's Heliotherapeutic Portraits, c. 1903–1944," *Medical Humanities* 29 (March 2013): 38.
14. Le Corbusier was familiar with Swiss sanitoria designs and kept current with health issues and design. Coincidentally, Le Corbusier and Rollier were born in small villages near each other in the Neuchâtel canton, Switzerland. See Colomina, *X-Ray Architecture.* Also Margaret Campbell, "What Tuberculosis Did for Modernism," *Medical History* 49 (2005): 469; Lyra Kilston, *Sun Seekers: The Cure of California* (Los Angeles: Atelier Éditions, 2019), 63. For more indirect connections between Rollier and Le Corbusier see Richard A. Hobday, "Sunlight Therapy and Solar Architecture," *Medical History* 42 (1997).
15. Tania Anne Woloshyn, *Soaking Up the Rays: Light Therapy and Visual Culture in Britain, 1890–1940* (Manchester: Manchester University Press, 2017), 45, n76.
16. Royal Institute of British Architects, *The Orientation of Buildings* (London: Royal Institute of British Architects, 1933), 3.
17. Le Corbusier, *The Athens Charter* (New York: Grossman, 1973), article 26.
18. Hobday, "Sunlight Therapy and Solar Architecture," 464.
19. G. M. Mackee, "Ultraviolet Therapy in Dermatology," *Journal of the American Medical Association* 83, no. 18 (1932): 1553–1561.
20. Casimir Funk, *The Vitamines,* trans. Harry E. Durbin (Baltimore: Williams & Wilkins Company, 1922).
21. For more on the development of dietary vitamin D, see Philippe Hernigou, Jean Charles Auregan, and Arnaud Dubory, "Vitamin D: Part II; Cod Liver Oil, Ultraviolet Radiation, and Eradication of Rickets," *International Orthopaedics* 43 (2019): 740–742.
22. Woloshyn, *Soaking Up the Rays*, n.p.
23. Woloshyn, *Soaking Up the Rays*, n.p.
24. John Stanislav Sadar, "The Healthful Ambiance of Vitaglass: Light, Glass and Curative Environment," *Architecture Research Quarterly* 12, no. 3/4 (2008): 272.
25. Le Corbusier, *La Ville Radieuse* (Paris: Vincent, Fréal, 1964), 48. Originally published 1934.
26. John Stanislav Sadar, *Through the Healing Glass: Shaping the Modern Body through Glass Architecture, 1925–35* (London: Routledge, 2017), 11.
27. Sadar, *Through the Healing Glass*, 11.
28. Sadar, *Through the Healing Glass*, 11.
29. Thomas S. Hines, *Richard Neutra and the Search for Modern Architecture: A Biography and History* (Berkeley: University of California Press, 1994), 96.
30. Philip Lovell, "Care for the Body," *Los Angeles Times*, December 15, 1929.
31. Likely from Philip Lovell's "Care for the Body" column in the *Los Angeles Times*; quoted in Hines, *Richard Neutra and the Search for Modern Architecture*, 108.
32. On Lustraglass see Sadar, *Through the Healing Glass*, 168.
33. "'Test Tube' School Open," *Los Angeles Times*, October 14, 1935, 9.
34. Richard J. Neutra, "Contemporary Developments of the Unconventional House," in Greta Grey, *House and Home: A Manual and Textbook of Practical House Planning*, 3rd ed. (Philadelphia: J. B. Lippincott, 1935), 194.
35. Neutra, "Contemporary Developments of the Unconventional House," 194–195.
36. See Sadar, *Through the Healing Glass*, 15.
37. Judith A. Quick and Elizabeth W. Murphy, eds., "The Fortification of Foods: A Review," United States Department of Agriculture, Food Safety and Inspection Service, Agricultural Handbook Number 598 (July 1982), 2.
38. Colomina, *X-Ray Architecture*, 94.

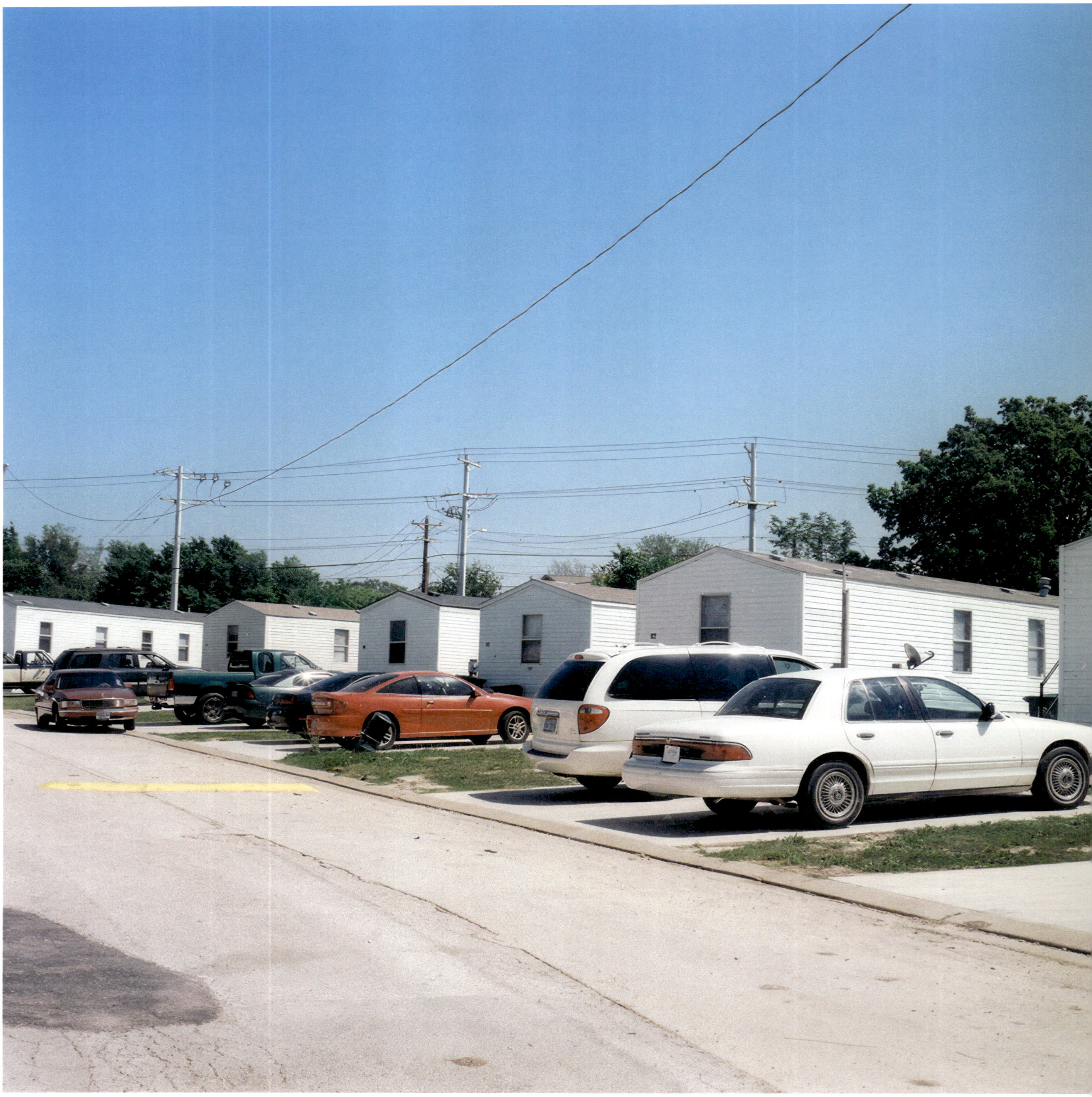

↑ A mobile home park in Oklahoma comprised entirely of former FEMA trailers. Typical rent is $750.00 a month.

→ FEMA trailer with sticker (upside down) in window indicating "Not to be used for housing." The image was created for a video about the potentially hazardous conditions, resale, and use of FEMA trailers, entitled *Where Have All the Trailers Gone?*

MANUFACTURED HOME SYNDROME

NICHOLAS SHAPIRO

> I am convinced that the trailer or an improved version of it is, for better or for worse, the low cost dwelling of the future—lacking in solidity, lacking in charm, but inexpensive, convenient and mobile.
> —J. B. Jackson[1]

In the spring of 2011, on one of my many trips to Texas, I visited a trailer park twenty minutes outside Houston's perimeter highway. I was in my second year of traveling the country to track down the quasi-legal resale of 120,000 emergency housing units that were initially deployed to the Gulf Coast after Hurricanes Katrina and Rita of 2005. These 150-square-foot travel trailers were bought by the Federal Emergency Management Agency (FEMA) and later reclaimed after their interior atmospheres were found to bear elevated levels of the irritant, allergen, neurotoxin, and human carcinogen known as formaldehyde. After the federal government washed its hands of these toxic assets via massive auctions beginning in 2010, they wound their way through gray markets with resellers making a few hundred to a few thousand dollars with each exchange. Before setting out, I had mined a 150,000-line spreadsheet, acquired by way of a Freedom of Information Act request, for resellers along my planned route. From this list, I came to know that this trailer park outside Houston had acquired just under 100 FEMA trailers, a quarter of which were designated as scrap. This represented mid- to small-scale reselling, yet still cost over $215,000.[2]

When I arrived, there was some road work underway on the nearby highway and the air was inked with the smell of asphalt. Most of the trailers in the small, perhaps five-acre trailer park bore deep grime. Dirt mixed with green mildew edged up the sides of the trailers. The park consisted of two lots. One hosted the office, a remodeled modular home fitted with a generous deck out front, and trailers to rent on site. The other lot was dedicated to reselling used mobile homes and trailers. After having heard hundreds of accounts of the warped life-worlds of resold trailer inhabitants, my goal for this trip was to understand how the toxic trailer market understood itself.

As I walked into the office, a white woman in her late thirties with tight blond curls and carefully painted eyebrows asked from across the room, "Can I help you?" I got my voice together and did my spiel. She looked concerned, at first, then pointed me to the faux-wood-paneled back office of the owners, Tina and Darryl.

Behind a large desk Tina sat with the posture of a mom—strong but not wasting energy on elegance—filling out contracts, barking out orders to the front office and a roving handyman. Even while she talked to me, she was listening to the conversations in the front room, and from time to time would intervene with no-nonsense assertiveness.

Darryl came in as we talked over the consent form. They both perked up at my mention of formaldehyde. Darryl dove straight in, "We have always had to deal with formaldehyde issues in the mobile home business. This is nothing new. I always have people sign a formaldehyde release before they buy or move in." Darryl was crouching next to the desk. He kneeled, suspended in pensive thought before continuing, "Everybody knows that they have formaldehyde in 'em. They don't just spray it in there. They put it in as a preservative."

"It isn't the formaldehyde that made them sick," Tina chimes in, "When we drove into Louisiana [after Katrina], we just got stuffed up. It was like a wall of mold and allergens when we drove in. I would be sick too if I lived there. The trailer was protection from that, if anything. They got sick from their environment ... not their home." While formaldehyde is always an issue, always warranting a legal release, they asserted that formaldehyde is never a cause of illness. The paradox hung heavily in the air, one that I encountered time and time again when speaking with resellers or park owners.

After several heated minutes of back and forth that wasn't moving anywhere—fairly standard for my conversations with resellers—I looked for a way out. I asked if residues of the trailers' previous use in catastrophe negatively affected their current value. "Having had those people in Louisiana in there before doesn't matter now. I've had mobile homes that people have died in, ones where some guy blew his brains out. That is just part of the business," Darryl answered frankly, running his hand down his cheek to his chin slow enough that the rasp of each follicle of stubble passing under his hands was almost audibly distinct. "Once he bought one [a mobile home] from a repo auction that ended up having a body in it," Tina goaded. Darryl blushed and turned his eyes toward the carpet, his gaze hovering over a plastic toy stethoscope that had tripped me up earlier as I entered the room.

Tina kept the conversation going, distracting from Darryl's palpable discomfort. "There were some that had voodoo in them. Those Louisiana people had smeared ashes over the door to protect them from evils."[3] Looking back up, Darryl interjected, "There

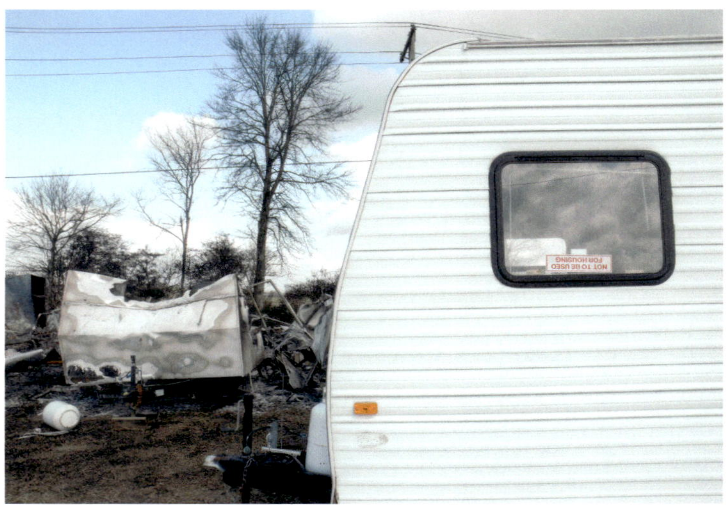

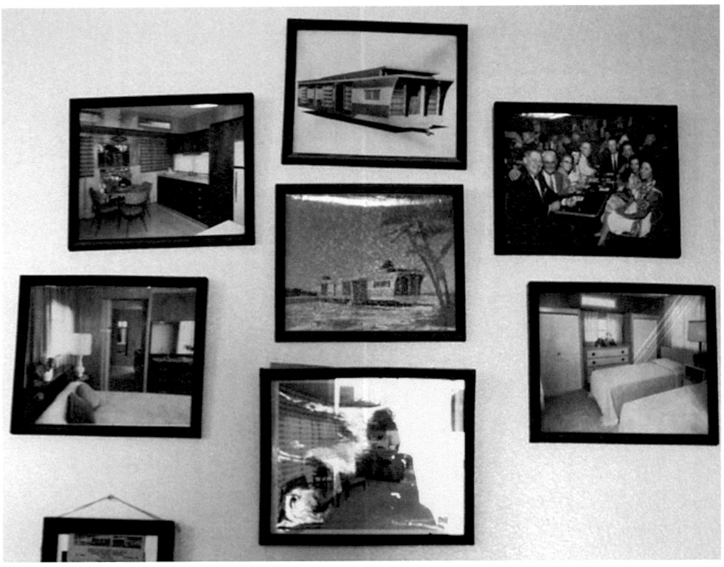

were bamboo crosses and all that. No one would bid on them." One of their sons, in his red and white little league uniform, slinked into the office and climbed into his mother's lap without saying a word. His mouth hung open slightly as he silently stared across the desk at me, unflinching to my playful faces. Darryl looked at his son, then up at the clock, and with a jolt, hopped up from the crouch he had held for nearly an hour. "Okay, we need to head out to his game."

As we walked out together, I asked him how he got started in the trailer business. With a prideful smirk and a mysterious "let me show you something," he led me to the front office and a small collection of black and white photographs from the 1950s featuring a high-end mobile home. "My grandmother was 'Mrs. mobile home' in Florida in 1952," he proudly related, gesturing to a yellowing newspaper clipping. "My grandparents designed the first mobile home in Florida, 'The Futuro.' It was all custom. Here ya got: them, cousins, and the investors. Mobile homes are in my blood." Flush with vigor and pride, he recounted the particulars of each shot, the model's features, and every one of his depicted relations. An antithetical disposition to that of his earlier explanations, full of backpedaling, grimaces, and sighs. Times were no doubt hard. The FEMA trailers sold well, but Darryl and Tina were ensnared in a lawsuit with a former tenant over maintenance issues. He was selling and renting bare-bone homes to desperate folks barely staying afloat, not those playing out their dreams of mobility and luxury. After a wistful pause, he rushed out, playfully pushing his son out the door.

I stood in their front office, staring at the collection of images. Beaming men proudly standing by the first Futuro off the line. Airy shots of the mobile home's interior: ample seating, some fixtures built in for mobile efficiency, convenience, and sturdiness. Freely movable stools, chairs, and end tables lent the feeling of a conventional home. An illustration of the Futuro hovering in a white abstract landscape, replete with design flourishes similar to the more expensive automobiles of the day. A series of gill-like windows encircle the home, lending it resemblance to spacecraft. And finally, the centerpiece of the constellation: the Futuro in situ on a secluded beach, palm fronds leaning into the frame from the right.

As I stood in the reception area, regarding this shrine to the Futuro, I got lost in the expanse between the sixty-year-old dreamworld of mass-produced comfort and escape and the seemingly inescapable hardscrabble realities of the current mobile home business surrounding me. I thought about the long histories of mobile dwellings in North America and how European prefabricated homes entangle with resource extraction and settlement. How the rise of petrochemistry enabled the creation of the midcentury manufactured home, made primarily from engineered woods held together by formaldehyde. How Walter Benjamin concisely summarized the connection between the material constituents of the built environment and dreamworlds: "Construction plays the role of the subconscious."[4] I wondered about how to even begin unpacking the various tributaries that fed into these starkly contrasting realities and how to imagine healthy affordable housing beyond them.

The receptionist punctured my reverie. "Ya know, those Louisiana people bought Cadillacs with their FEMA money," she called out from across the room, with a hint of venom. The phantasmagoria of the Futuro sputtered to a halt. I returned from the nostalgic futurism of the photos to the shag carpet I was standing on that resembled a dog's coat after a day at the beach. To the mildewing shelters of last resort that they rented out to the down-on-their-luck or the newly evicted. To a manufactured interior space where nothing is custom-built like the Futuro. To the news story about Darryl buying a mobile home with a dead body in it, which hung discretely in a back corner. To the grounded dream of the mobile home.

"Cadillacs got formaldehyde in 'em too, why couldn't that be what's making 'em sick?" she continued, pursing her lips and raising her painted eyebrows when I turned to look at her. "Well," I thought out loud, "You don't live in your car—I mean, you don't spend as much time in it. ... It's easier to ventilate ... um, there is probably less formaldehyde in it because there are no engineered woods in 'em ... and how many people really bought new Cadys with their FEMA money?" She waggled her head disapprovingly at my answer and turned to her paperwork. A gust of asphalt-singed air blew into the room as a Latina woman pushed open the front door, a baby slumbering on her breast. "Do you have anything I can move into today?" She asked in a thick accent as I left, pushed out by the receptionist's glare.

During a six-month stay in a travel trailer in rural Oklahoma, a three-year-old developed small red

← Photographs of the Futuro in a trailer park outside Houston.

↑ Manning, Portable Colonial Cottage, ca. 1833. Diagrams after Loudon, *An Encyclopaedia of Architecture;* advertisement: *South Australian Record*, November 27, 1837.

↓ Warehouse prefabricated for the California Gold Rush.

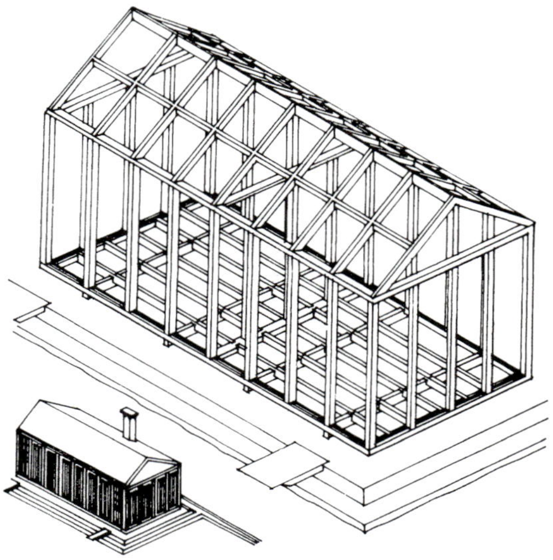

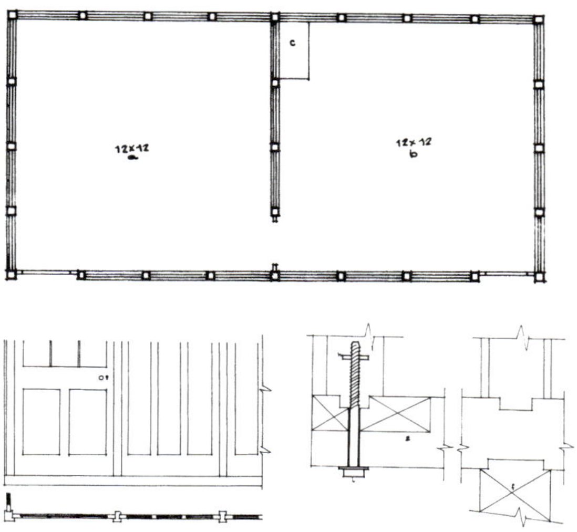

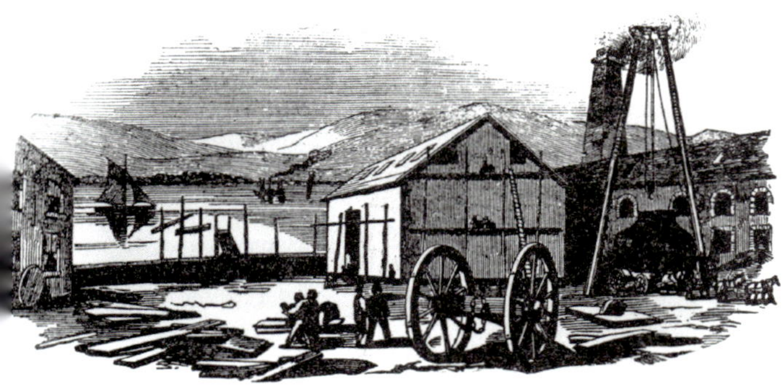

dots on the backs of her ears, began bruising more easily, and walked through the world more clumsily, constantly toppling over. An older Indiana woman descended into a fog of "fuzzy thinking" and felt that her body was deteriorating at a slightly accelerated rate. A middle-aged man in Ohio sustained a "sick stuffy nose" and "throat problems" for a year and a half. Eye and respiratory-tract irritation, headaches, insomnia, and fatigue slowly crept into the body of a single father in rural Florida. His dreams, which became increasingly menacing over a matter of months, abated in intensity only when he slept next door at his grandparents' house. The stool of a nurse in Texas gradually loosened in consistency. A grandfather on a reservation in Washington almost entirely ceased eating as his sense of taste began to dull. His wife, experiencing the same sensorial skewing, doused her food with large quantities of salt and noted the "weird air" in their home. These people, and hundreds of others I've spoken with over the years, all began developing subtle and ongoing alterations to their physical constitution after spending time in a manufactured home that would eventually be suspected of sustaining elevated levels of airborne formaldehyde.

Homesick Beginnings

> We would especially call the attention of emigrants and colonies locating in the West, and also of emigrant and land associations to the advantages of these houses for the use of settlers.
> —*The Clemens' Ready Made Sectional Houses*, 1862

The social projects that give historical form to this quintessentially rural and suburban habitation extend well beyond the techno-utopianism of the 1950s, back to the fledgling days of North American colonization. Settler colonialism can be thought of as a process of manufacturing home on top of and in place of the homes of a land's original human inhabitants. Bringing a diminutive architecture of home along on voyages of conquest, settlement, and extraction was crucial to European colonial expansion. Making the colonist's home mobile and exportable is foundational to the settler colonial project.

Manufactured housing dates back to 1587, when the first prefabricated dwelling in North America failed to be built. The wooden structure had been shipped from England to house a hundred gold miners for the winter in what is now known as Baffin Island, Canada. Two of its walls never arrived. Other parts were lost to the icy sea. The crew ended up sailing back to England as the brutal Arctic winter closed in.[5]

Two centuries later, as the empire prepared to accelerate its colonial emigration efforts, industrial manufacturing techniques of prefabrication and

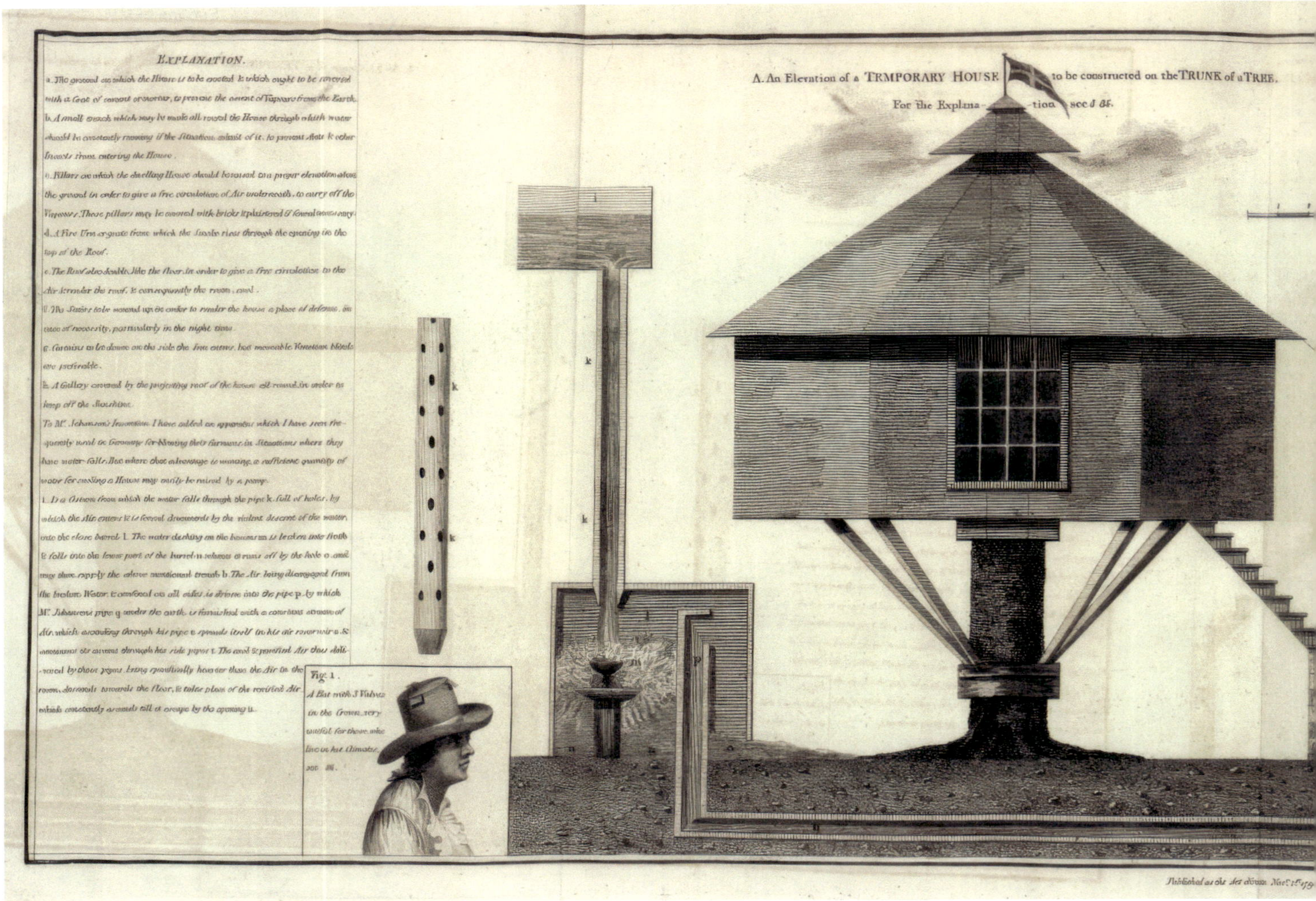

modular paneling began refining English architectures of occupation. In the 1790s, the British dispatched prefabricated houses, shops, a church, and hospitals to Freetown, purchased by the Sierra Leone Company. Simultaneously, flatpack storehouses and cottages sailed toward Sydney, where they met "the first *real* building in Australia ... brought from England by Captain Arthur Phillip in 1788."[6] Despite being ill-adapted to the Australian climate, these premade buildings were, in the eyes of the settlers, physical manifestations of white supremacy, disqualifying Indigenous architecture as inferior and illegitimate. As thousands of Brits were paid to emigrate to South Africa in the 1820s to curtail severe unemployment at home, the Colonial Office shipped demountable housing along with them.

Difficulties with transportation and assembly led to further streamlining and the development in 1833 of the Manning Portable Colonial Cottage, which required no nails to erect and had standardized components that were small enough that "a boy could carry [them] for several miles."[7] These cottages were purchased en masse by Australian settlers and, with their popularity, established a market for settler prefabricated dwellings. Their designs were quickly appropriated by an architect in Baltimore for use by argonauts headed to the California gold rush in 1849, and later by settlers of the North American prairies who had only a few trees for lumber, save for small groves of cottonwoods near streams.[8] Already by the mid-nineteenth century, the center of the prefabricated home market began to shift from Britain to the United States.[9] Like contemporary mobile homes, which 95–97 percent of the time never move from the ground of their initial placement, these US-made structures were not designed for seasonal or occupational migration but for singular, rapid settlement.[10]

Prefab homes enabled the mobility of imperialism. With prefabrication, European colonists were able to instantly reproduce the aesthetics of home, seize territory through European legal doctrines like *terra nullius*, advance ideas of universal white superiority, protect and advance regimes of private property, actively remain ignorant of local materials, local ecologies, and place-based practices of homebuilding, and rapidly scale settlement. The early manufactured houses that proliferated across the globe like imperial flags staked into the ground were not only foundational to the stealing of Indigenous land, but also to the "instant" transition of rural settlements into urban ones. For example, a prefab home was the first settler

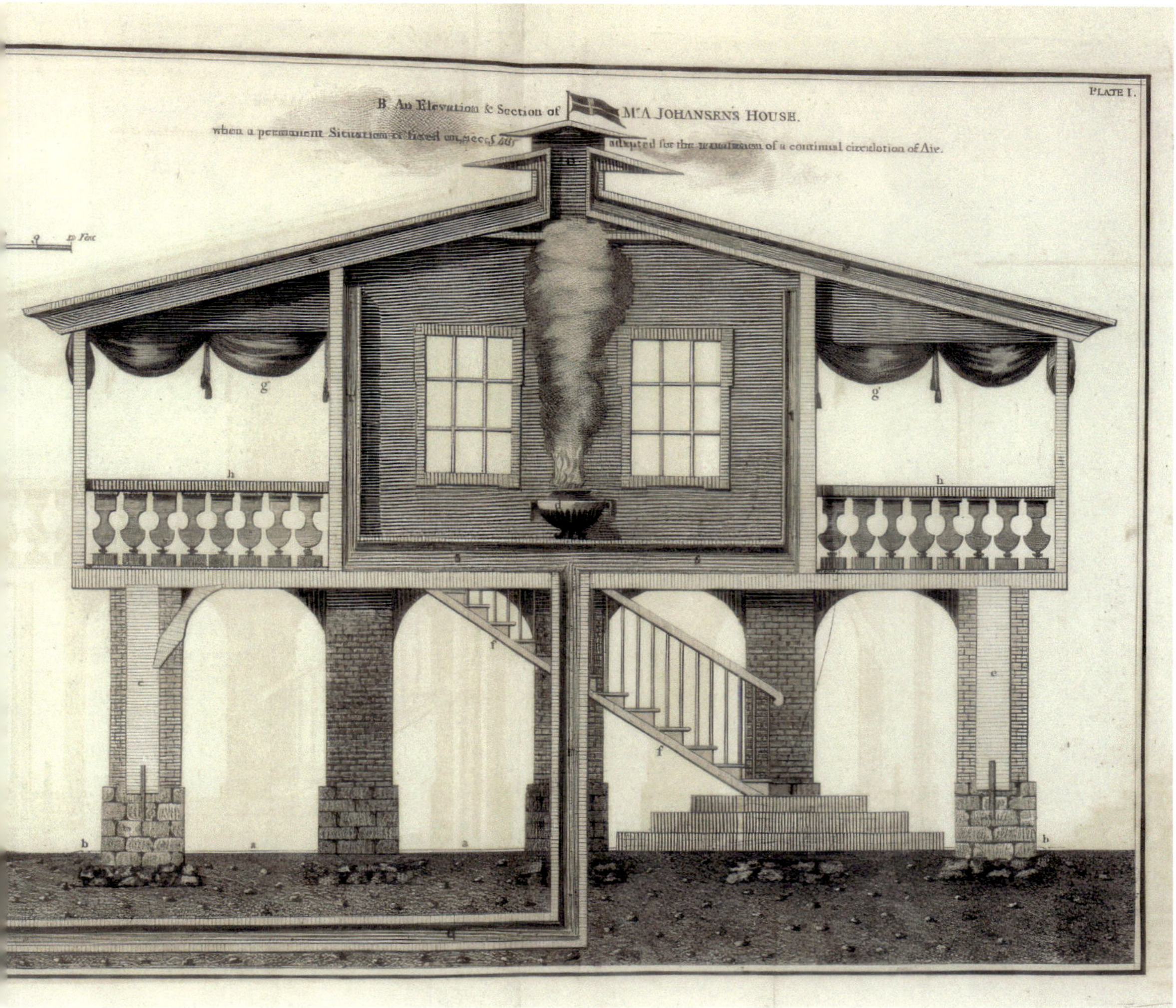

← Section of Major Johansen's House, featuring continual air circulation, a protective trench, and an elevated structure to enhance airflow and prevent insect intrusion.

structure built in what is now San Francisco, and these structures multiplied to become the scaffolding upon which the city was built. Today, nearly one in five homes in the United States is built in a factory. And while more than half are located in rural areas, their influence on urban density and form lingers in the history of colonial cities across the globe.

The mobile home's contemporary relationship to colonialism is not solely that of a vessel for fast, affordable settlement. Native nations are flooded with manufactured housing. Indeed, between 2007 and 2009 1,300 formaldehyde-ridden FEMA mobile homes were given to eighty-eight tribes, of which members from about a dozen have contacted me about formaldehyde testing.[11] The disproportionate use of mobile housing on Native lands is an indicator of the limits to tribal sovereignty under the colonial reservation system, which holds most Native land in federal trust and separates it from homeownership. In 2016, American Indians and Native Alaskans living on reservation land were twenty-one times more likely to finance a mobile home loan versus a conventional home loan than the average American.[12]

Warren Buffett's Berkshire Hathaway owns Clayton Homes, which operates a network of over 1,600 dealerships and sells almost half of all manufactured housing in the United States. The Clayton Homes subsidiary Vanderbilt Mortgage provides the majority of Indigenous, Black, and Latinx mobile home lending, while only servicing thirty-one percent of the white mobile home market. Its interest rates are 0.73 percent higher for minorities than for white customers, which regularly results in default and repossession of mobile homes on reservations or the seizing of land that had been black-owned since Reconstruction and "put up" to secure a predatory loan.[13]

The majority of mobile home purchases are financed via personal property loans like cars (and tend to similarly decrease in value, as opposed to the wealth-building of conventional homes). While quicker to approve, these loans bear higher interest rates than mortgages and fewer consumer protections. Together, these attributes make falling behind on payments easy and repossession swift. Defaulting owners sometimes return home not to foreclosure notices but to the negative space of their home towed away to an impoundment lot. Factory-building as opposed to site-building homes also allows not only for the full confiscation of the home but also the concentration of profits in a small number of firms, which more efficiently systematizes the racialization of predatory lending.

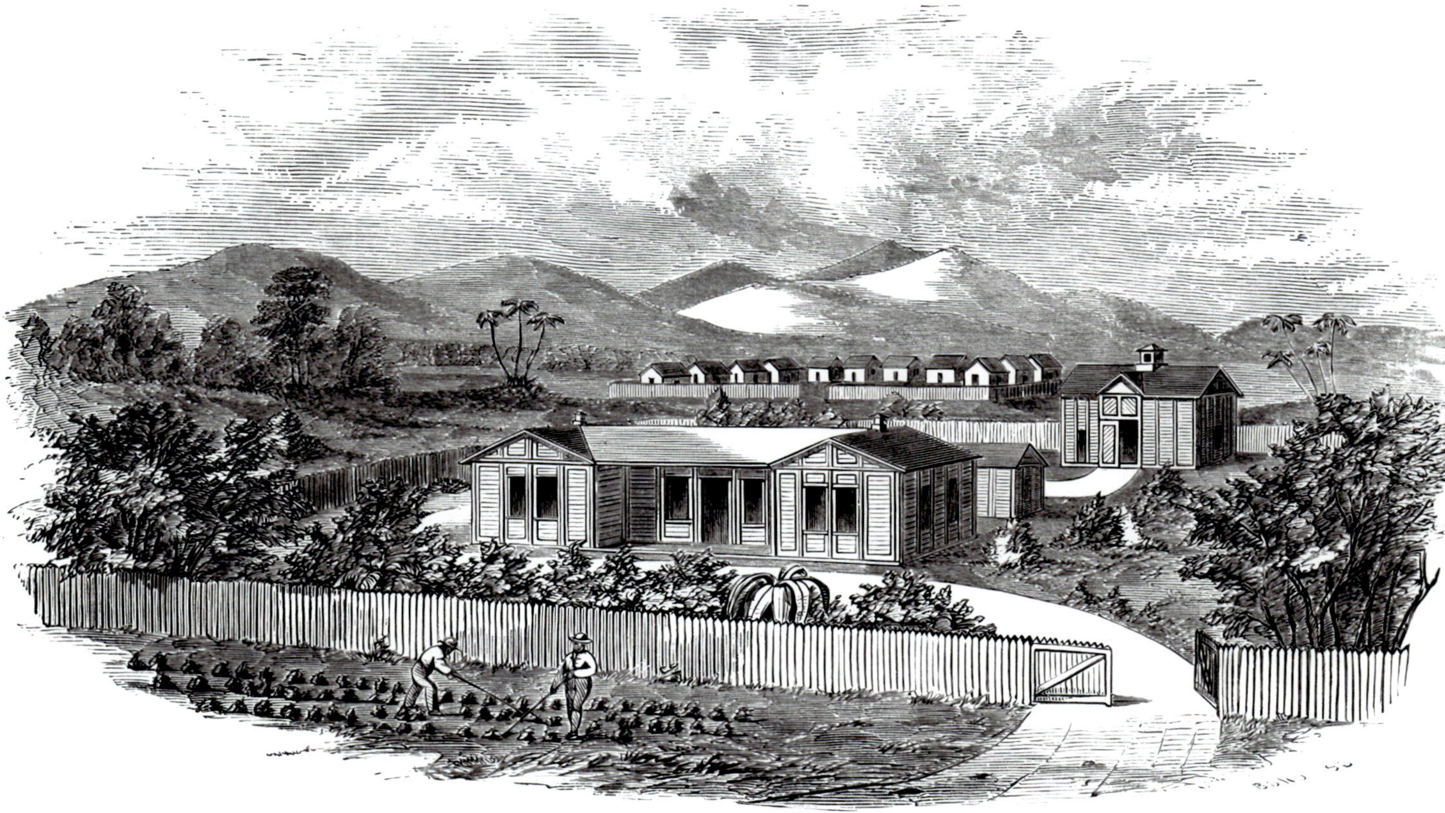

Toxic Loans and Toxic Homes

The domicile that became known as the mobile home, one that was factory-assembled and towable behind a truck rather than assembled onsite like a prefab home, first became a coherent phenomenon in the 1930s during the bleakest days of the Great Depression.[14] As the consequences of loose credit and rampant stock speculation stalled housing construction and drove up unemployment, more and more people were forced into living permanently in trailers.[15] In the US the ever-increasing network of roadways and devotion to the automobile also beckoned new valuations of mobility that made these emergent forms of roving domesticity possible.

War intensified what finance had begun. During World War II, military personnel and other defense industry workers were housed in over 120,000 mobile homes distributed across the US in thousands of trailer villages that supported war efforts like the Manhattan Project. After the war, returning servicemen quickly oversaturated the conventional housing market, and veterans starting new families streamed into mobile homes. The wide variety of Americans who inhabited trailers in the war effort helped to partially transform mobile homes in the national imagination from dwellings on the itinerant fringe into a legitimate residential alternative.

As homebuilders scrambled to keep up with housing demand after the war, the war effort helped a host of new plastic and plastic-infused building materials reach maturity. The chemical reactions that

↑ Illustration of an arrangement of prefabricated houses for slaves in West Indies plantations from the prefabricated houses catalog by Skillings and Flint allowing “a village almost in a day,” 1861.

formed the first plastic—phenol and formaldehyde in Bakelite—were adapted into the adhesives that held together plywood. These standardized sheets of wood-plastic mixtures resisted decay, cut and deskilled installation labor, and reduced the amount of nails used in average home construction by half. Their influence is most concentrated in the mobile home but extends to all housing types. The average square footage of structural plywood incorporated into site-built homes across the country more than quintupled from 1950 (1,707) to 1992 (9,668), and usage of particle board, another plasticized wood, increased by three thousand percent between 1954 and 1992.[16]

Due to their expense, phenol-formaldehyde resins were soon relegated to exterior-grade plywoods only, while cheaper urea-formaldehyde resins took hold of interior spaces through interior-grade plywood, particle board, chipboard, luan, and a host of other engineered woods. The chemical bonds of urea-formaldehyde plywood are more unstable than phenol resins, continuously and quietly sublimating formaldehyde into enclosed indoor atmospheres. Elevated formaldehyde levels are found across all homes that utilize engineered woods, but in mobile homes these materials are so pervasive that they harbor three to four times the chemical load of conventional homes. As these toxic vapors suffuse into the bodies of inhabitants, they have given rise to a novel constellation of chronic, enervating symptoms, dubbed "mobile home syndrome."[17]

Formaldehyde-based resins that held together the postwar home are material co-constituents of the fiscal instrument of the American mortgage. To ensure that the bottom would not drop out of the postwar construction boom, the Federal Housing Administration (FHA) significantly liberalized its mortgage terms, first in 1948 by increasing the maximum payback term from twenty to thirty years (thus reducing monthly payments), and then in 1956, by decreasing the minimum down payment required from twenty to five percent for new construction and to ten percent for existing homes. What could be considered the birth of the contemporary mortgage industry began a year later when the Mortgage Guarantee Insurance Corporation allowed lenders to make even riskier loans than those of the FHA.[18] Down payments decreased by around $15,000 contemporary (2021) dollars in the decade following this change, even as the average home price soared by over fifty percent.[19]

With their vastly reduced labor costs, polymerized wood products subsidized the postwar spike in home construction and ownership, of which the latter grew by nearly seventy percent between 1940 and 1980.[20] This new access to homeownership, facilitated by both cheaper housing and liberalized financing options, ratcheted up the mortgage debt burden relative to total household income shouldered by homeowners. Mortgage debt was twenty percent of household income at midcentury, but over seventy percent of household income by the turn of the millennium.[21] This debt was cast as a social good through the valuation of homeownership, which enhanced the predictability of housing, financial, and labor markets.[22]

In the late 1960s and early 1970s, when inflation was steadily mounting and the price of housing began inching out of reach for almost half of American families, mobile homes again became an increasingly popular fallback means of accessing homeownership. Of all single-family homes sold in 1969, over forty percent were mobile homes.[23] And in a 1970 Housing and Urban Development (HUD) report, the Nixon administration praised the mobile home industry for mitigating the effects of the housing crisis on those with low and moderate incomes. Notably, in this same report, HUD first began counting mobile homes as residences, increasing the likelihood that their statistics would support the administration's home construction goals.

Tantalized by its unique properties, architects and chemists alike had seized upon the possibility of "all-plastic homes" in the postwar period. From rapidly assembled humanitarian huts to UFO-like modernist mansions, plastic home prototypes proliferated from the 1950s until 1973, when the US Federal Trade Commission sued twenty-six plastics manufacturers, a standards organization, and a plastics professional society for underrepresenting the flammability of cellular and foam plastics.[24] This legal and safety blow, combined with the soaring prices of the 1970s oil crisis, stymied the advancement of the highly plasticized home—save for the low-cost manufactured housing market, which is more plastic than conventional homes but less plastic than "all-plastic."

With plywood walls, fiberboard doors, laminate in-built furniture, and particle board subfloor, no housing utilizes as much polymerized wood as mobile homes. The mobile home represents both the ultimate industrialization of home construction and, through its affordability, democratization of homeownership.[25] On the higher end of the market spectrum, the Futuro epitomized the midcentury dreamworlds—of technological optimism and liberation through consumption—that brought the mobile home market from obscurity to a conspicuous figure of the rural and suburban landscape. Mobile homes are the only sustained and scaled vestige of the petrochemical fantasy of the all-plastic home. The less charismatic offspring of the Futuro continue to realize this dream in their own debased ways.

In the last quarter of the twentieth century, mobile homes settled into a social and financial position not far from where they are today: a deep double bind. The financial savings of low-cost manufactured housing, which gives those with modest incomes access to the housing market, have been offset by the social costs of being relegated to marginal land and ascribed overt and covert stigma, in addition to health costs. From the very same low-cost materials that contribute to its affordability, a pernicious cloud of formaldehyde emanates and accumulates within the mobile home. The head-spinning arithmetic of financial advantage and social and biological sacrifice is often made simple for those who can afford no other option.

Beyond Predatory Inclusion

As the largest form of unsubsidized affordable housing in the US—costing upward of fifty percent less per square foot than conventional homes—factory-built mobile homes no doubt keep roofs over the heads of tens of millions of people who might otherwise be even more housing-insecure. But the insecurities of these homes from social stigma, more costly loans with fewer protections,[26] steep devaluation, threat of mobile home park eviction,[27] disproportionate lack of water service reliability,[28] elevated mold levels, greater proximity to outdoor environmental exposures,[29] and indoor chemical exposures totalize into a daunting set of obstacles for their low-income residents. In this view, mobile homes swap the massive and singular weight of financial burden with a constellation of smaller hidden weights as residents attempt to tread water at the very least.

Our climatically destabilizing planet will only compound these problems. As mobile homes have limited walling integrity (limited insulation and poor seals), they are difficult to heat and cool, saddling residents with exorbitant energy costs. As the most energy-cost-encumbered housing type, their residents are twice as likely to bear a high energy burden as those who live in single-family detached homes.[30] Indeed, a just energy transition is farther away for mobile home residents than for any other housing type in the US, as every dollar invested in increasing the energy efficiency of a mobile home only saves three cents, a net return on investment twenty-four times lower than single-family homes.[31]

While the vast majority of manufactured home owners are lower-class white people, stigmatized as "trailer trash" due to their financial and geographic proximity to minorities, the profits that can be extracted from housing vulnerability are heightened for people of color and Indigenous people through instruments of colonial land tenure and loan risk assessment. The ways that this form of shelter can become exposure are highlighted by how retirees in the Southwest are both three times more likely than those under retirement age to live in manufactured housing and three-and-a-quarter times more likely to die from heat inside their homes than those who live in other housing types. In sprawling and sweltering Maricopa County, Arizona, twenty-eight percent of indoor heat-associated deaths occur in manufactured homes despite their only amounting to five percent of the housing stock.[32] In a destabilized climate, mobile homes are increasingly sited in the hottest census tracts and on floodplains.[33]

There is much excellent policy work happening right now to mitigate some of these risks, from regulating chattel loans and increasing eviction protections to pushing the federal Low-Income Home Energy Assistance Program to include mobile homes in their eligibility criteria. But calls to think and build beyond this form of affordable housing are seemingly nonexistent. And with increasing risks to the marginal lands that these nondense forms of housing are placed on, attempts to cultivate reconciliation with Indigenous peoples without the return of land and sovereignty indicate clear limitations to these reforms.[34]

The manifest shortcomings of European traditions of homemaking were baked into the establishment of the colonial project through the use of mobile housing for settlers, and are present today in the intimate atmospheres of some twenty-two million people who inhabit mobile homes in the United States. As the toxicity of manufactured housing is woven into their very structure (formaldehyde from hydrocarbons), their conceptual moorings (mold and energy poverty from environmentally inappropriate design), and the theft of Indigenous lands (disproportionately forcing Indigenous people into these structures), an equitable vision of affordable housing cannot stop at achieving racial parity for mobile home loans or elaborating private property protections. Land restitution and Indigenous-led architecture and planning are key avenues for "meeting lands where they are" and developing or reinvigorating place-based interventions into widespread housing insecurity that refuse to flatten human-land relations in the way that the mobile home was designed to do.[35] Massive increases in affordable multifamily housing with access to mass transportation would have crosscutting benefits, from those whose shelter is exposure to those without a home at all. Until these movements are embraced, mobile home inhabitants will remain suspended between countervailing currents of structural marginalization, toxic exposures, and the predatory benefits of low-cost shelter.

An earlier version of this essay was originally published by e-flux Architecture in 2022, and is based on "Manufacturing Home," *Journal for the Anthropology of North America* 22, no. 2 (2019): 121–124.

p222 Photo: Akasha Rabut.
p223, 224 Photos by the author.
p225 (top) Reproduced from Gilbert Herbert, "The Portable Colonial Cottage," *Journal of the Society of Architectural Historians* 31, no. 4 (December 1, 1972).
p225 (bottom) *London Illustrated News* 14 (1849): 109; reproduced from *Gazette des Beaux-Arts: Courrier européen de l'art et de la curiosité*, vol. XXXIII.
p226 Reproduced from Carl Bernhard Wadström, *An Essay on Colonization, Particularly Applied to the Western Coast of Africa ... Also Brief Descriptions of the Colonies ... in Africa, Including Those of Sierra Leona and Bulama* (London: Darton and Harvey, 1794).
p228 "Design No 21." Reproduced from D. N. Skillings and D. B. Flint, *D. N. Skillings and D. B. Flint's Illustrated Catalogue of Portable Sectional Buildings: Patented Nov. 19, 1861* (Boston: Andrew Holland, Woodcut Printer, 1862).

1. J. B. Jackson, *Landscape in Sight: Looking at America* (New Haven: Yale University Press, 2000), 222.
2. Numbers here are kept approximate to protect reseller identities from discovery by using these same public records.
3. In Texas, many of the white people I talked to used the term "Louisiana people" to mean Black people.
4. Walter Benjamin, *The Arcades Project*, trans. Howard Eiland and Kevin McLaughlin (Cambridge, MA: Belknap Press of Harvard University Press, 2002), 16.
5. Charles Peterson, "Early American Prefabrication," *Gazette des Beaux-Arts* 6, no. 36 (1948): 37–46.
6. Gilbert Herbert, *Pioneers of Prefabrication: The British Contribution in the Nineteenth Century* (Baltimore: Johns Hopkins University Press, 1978); emphasis mine.
7. Herbert, *Pioneers of Prefabrication*, 9.
8. While the US primarily fulfilled the prefab house desires with thousands of shipped houses, houses were also shipped from China (including Hong Kong), Tasmania, New Zealand, and the UK.
9. Herbert, *Pioneers of Prefabrication*, 27.
10. John Fraser Hart, Michelle J. Rhodes, and John T. Morgan, *The Unknown World of the Mobile Home* (Baltimore: Johns Hopkins University Press, 2002); Robert Kronenburg, *Houses in Motion* (London: Academy Editions, 2002), 80.
11. Kenneth J. Cooper, "As Housing Shortage Worsens, Tribes Forced to Use FEMA Trailers," *Truthout*, May 6, 2011, https://truthout.org/articles/as-housing-shortage-worsens-tribes-forced-to-use-fema-trailers/.
12. Kevin Johnson and Richard M. Todd, "The Market for Manufactured Home Loans to American Indian and Alaska Native Borrowers In Indian Country Remains Highly Concentrated," *Federal Reserve Bank of Minneapolis*, December 1, 2017, https://www.minneapolisfed.org/article/2017/the-market-for-manufactured-home-loans-to-american-indian-and-alaska-native-borrowers-in-indian-country-remains-highly-concentrated/.
13. Mike Baker and Daniel Wagner, "Minorities Exploited by Warren Buffett's Mobile-Home Empire," *Seattle Times*, December 26, 2015, https://www.seattletimes.com/seattle-news/times-watchdog/minorities-exploited-by-warren-buffetts-mobile-home-empire-clayton-homes/. The manufactured housing market experienced a securitization-driven market meltdown in the late 1990s that foreshadowed the bursting of the larger housing bubble around a decade later. The boom in risky chattel loans was made possible by large increases in the securitization of manufactured home loans—from $184 million in 1987 to $15 billion in 1999. When the national housing market bubble popped in 2007–2008, hundreds of billions of federal dollars were dedicated to rescuing mortgages from default that did not include chattel mobile home loans. Ann M. Burkhart, "Bringing Manufactured Housing into the Real Estate Finance System," *Pepperdine Law Review* 37, no. 2 (2010): 427–458.
14. Lawrence Saunders, "Roll Your Own Home," *Saturday Evening Post*, May 23, 1936.
15. Hart, Rhodes, and Morgan, *The Unknown World of the Mobile Home*, 9.
16. Janet Ore, "Mobile Home Syndrome: Engineered Woods and the Making of a New Domestic Ecology in the Post-World War II Era," *Technology and Culture* 52, no. 2 (2011): 270, 272.
17. Ore, "Mobile Home Syndrome."
18. Richard K. Green and Susan M. Wachter, "The American Mortgage in Historical and International Context," *Journal of Economic Perspectives* 19, no. 4 (2005): 96–97.
19. National Commission on Urban Problems, *Building the American City: Report of the National Commission on Urban Problems to the Congress and to the President of the United States* (Washington, DC: US Government Printing Office, 1969).
20. The ownership rate among US households rose from 43.6 percent in 1940, the last census year before World War II, to 64 percent by 1980 (Census of Population and Housing, 1940 and 1980).
21. Lawrence Mishel, Jared Bernstein, and Heather Boushey, *The State of Working America, 2002/2003* (Ithaca: Cornell University Press, 2003). Similarly, mortgage debt rose from being 15 percent of household assets in 1949 to 28 percent in 1979 and 41 percent of household assets by 2001.
22. Mortgages confer status to owners by virtue of having qualified—via credit ratings—for a mortgage/debt relationship with a bank. Constance Perin, *Everything in Its Place: Social Order and Land Use in America* (Princeton: Princeton University Press, 1977).
23. Earl W. Morris and Margaret E. Woods, *Housing Crisis and Response: The Place of Mobile Homes in American Life* (Ithaca: Department of Consumer Economics and Public Policy, New York State College of Human Ecology, 1971), 3.
24. Billie Faircloth, *Plastics Now: On Architecture's Relationship to a Continuously Emerging Material* (London: Routledge, 2015), 263.
25. Ore, "Mobile Home Syndrome," 273–277.
26. Keeanga-Yamahtta Taylor, *Race for Profit: How Banks and the Real Estate Industry Undermined Black Homeownership* (Chapel Hill: University of North Carolina Press, 2019), 35.
27. Esther Sullivan, *Manufactured Insecurity: Mobile Home Parks and Americans' Tenuous Right to Place* (Oakland: University of California Press, 2018).
28. Gregory Pierce and Silvia Jimenez, "Unreliable Water Access in US Mobile Homes: Evidence from the American Housing Survey," *Housing Policy Debate* 25, no. 4 (October 2, 2015): 739–753.
29. Esther Sullivan, Carrie Makarewicz, and Andrew Rumbach, "Affordable but Marginalized," *Journal of the American Planning Association* 88, no. 2 (August 25, 2021): 1–13.
30. Chip Berry, Carolyn Hronis, and Maggie Woodward, "Who's Energy Insecure? You Might Be Surprised," in *ACEEE Proceedings*, 2018, https://www.aceee.org/files/proceedings/2018/index.html#/paper/event-data/p393.
31. Bruce Tonn, Erin Rose, and Beth Hawkins, "Evaluation of the U.S. Department of Energy's Weatherization Assistance Program: Impact Results," *Energy Policy* 118 (July 1, 2018): 279–290. Thanks to Greg Pierce for pointing out this vital connection.
32. Mark Kear, Margaret Wilder, Patricia Solís, David Hondula, and Mark Bernstein, "Self-Isolating from COVID-19 in a Mobile Home? That Could Be Deadly in Arizona," *Arizona Republic*, May 3, 2020.
33. Dalbyul Lee and Juchul Jung, "The Growth of Low-Income Population in Floodplains: A Case Study of Austin, TX," *KSCE Journal of Civil Engineering* 18, no. 2 (March 1, 2014): 683–693.
34. Gregory Pierce, C. J. Gabbe, and Annabelle Rosser, "Households Living in Manufactured Housing Face Outsized Exposure to Heat and Wildfire Hazards: Evidence from California," *Natural Hazards Review* 23, no. 3 (August 1, 2022).
35. See Wanda Dalla Costa, "Contextualized Metrics + Narrating Binaries: Defining Place and Process in Indigenous North America," presented at the Association of Collegiate Schools of Architecture (ACSA), Santiago, 2016, https://www.academia.edu/27664592/Contextualized_Metrics_Narrating_Binaries_Defining_Place_and_Process_in_Indigenous_North_America; David S. Edmunds, Ryan Shelby, Angela James, Lenora Steele, Michelle Baker, Yael Valerie Perez, and Kim TallBear, "Tribal Housing, Codesign, and Cultural Sovereignty," *Science, Technology, and Human Values* 38, no. 6 (November 1, 2013): 801–828; Erin Marie Konsmo and Karyn Recollet, "Afterword: Meeting the Land(s) Where They Are At," in *Indigenous and Decolonizing Studies in Education: Mapping the Long View*, edited by Linda Tuhiwai Smith, Eve Tuck, and K. Wayne Yang (London: Routledge, 2019).

MAN CAVES: TOXIC MASCULINITY UNLEASHED

KARA MORGAN
PLAXA ARXA

My childhood play space was in the basement of a condominium in suburban Connecticut. The room was allowed to be messy, disorganized, and filled with loud noises. This bounded tolerance of chaos came from my mom, who as a stereotypical Virgo (perfectionist) needed to keep childish clutter out of sight. Once I outgrew Barbie and stopped leaving her dream home, car, and clothing accessories all over the floor, the basement was converted into a man cave for my mom's then-fiancé and his La-Z-Boy, tools, pint glasses, and football jerseys. Both the playroom and man cave are spaces for items associated with one's identity that don't belong in the rest of the house. Not just childhood imagination but also toxic masculinity, and its displays of aggression, competition, and leisure, must be enclosed in a space hidden from the gaze of the domestic sphere.

Over the years, I began to realize that my distaste for suburban homes was related to my identity as a white, queer, cisgender woman. Suburban and white heteronormative gender roles work together to enforce "proper" binary expression and labor tasks scripted by the patriarchal American society.[1]

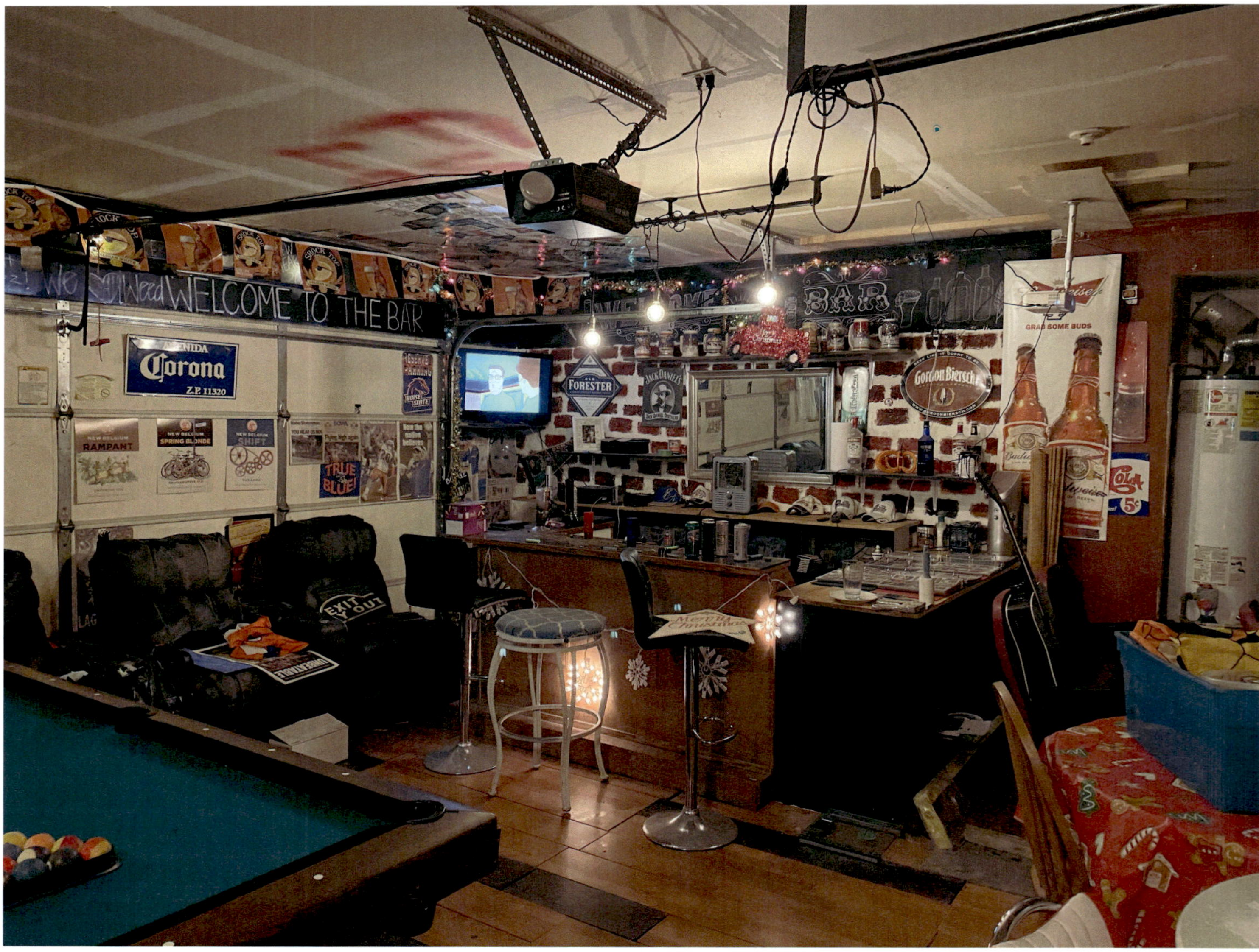

↑ Photo from the Reddit community r/Mancaves.

Heterosexual families claim the suburbs as their territory, constructing their identity within its interiors surrounded by white picket fences, decorative window shutters, and perfectly groomed gardens. As a queer bachelorette, I was eager to leave for the city in search of a lesbianic version of *Playboy*'s bachelor pad.

My flight to the city and the space carved out by my mom's then-fiancé share the same motivation: to evade the confines of the feminine. In the latter case, however, the family man seeks escape within the limits of the domestic, that traditionally feminine space, by inhabiting the forgotten, transitional, leftover spaces of a house, like the garage, basement, or attic.[2] Tied to the marriage script of the American dream, the family man instrumentalizes the suburban domestic as a form of domination even as it threatens his identity. Man caves cannot be understood outside of their relation to the totality of adjacent interior spaces devoted to the construction of femininity.[3]

From Utilitarian Space to Masculine Sanctuary

From Tim Allen's *Home Improvement* (1991–1999) and other sitcoms to DIY shows on HGTV, the portrayal of suburban white husbands and their man caves continues to spread across the televised spectrum as a model for inhabiting the suburban landscape. The presence of suburban white husbands and their man caves, exemplified in such sitcoms, has become a prevalent archetype for suburban living. These depictions showcase a recurring theme of men seeking solace and camaraderie away from traditional family structures. The evolution of suburban architecture reflects a transition from emphasizing family separation to promoting togetherness, mirroring the dynamics within these gendered domestic spaces.

Roseanne (1988–1997), for instance, portrayed a supposedly typical white working-class American family—husband and wife and three children—living in the suburbs of Illinois. The show was centered on its eponymous character, the dry-humored matriarch, and plotlines featured parenting struggles as well as family members holding down various blue-collar jobs. When arguments broke out, Dan, the husband, would withdraw to the garage. A contemporaneous sitcom, *Married ... with Children* (1987–1997), similarly depicts a suburban white middle-class family consisting of a husband, wife, and two kids living in Chicago. Most of the show's humor revolves around the husband, Al, and his bad luck, unrewarding career as a shoe salesman, and constant annoyance toward his wife, Peggy. When she discovers she is pregnant with their third child in the sixth season (1991), Al wants only to escape.[4] Trying to flee the responsibilities of a family man, he converts their garage into a second family room, complete with its own toilet, but for men only.

In the garage, both Dan and Al claim a territory segregated from the rest of the house as their retreat from family chaos. Dan's space contains his "man chair," a refrigerator stocked with beer, a dartboard, and space to work on his motorcycle. Al's space is set up more like a living room, and features wood paneling and carpet, but shares certain elements with Dan's room, including a seating area, TV, and a supply of beer. Al's language is coarser than Dan's, showing the extent that toxic masculinity can manifest inside these rooms of retreat.

> Peggy: Al, you're not really thinking about moving away from me and the baby?
>
> Al: Thinking of it? I did it! Be gone, jackals!
>
> *Al pushes the family out of the man cave and secures the door with an excessive number of locks. He is soon visited by another husband, Jefferson, who expresses his disgust toward his wife, who is also pregnant.*
>
> Jefferson: Having sex with your pregnant wife is like putting gas in the tank of a car you've already wrecked.[5]

In Akiva Schaffer's 2012 film *The Watch*, a group of neighbors form a local neighborhood watch group. The film's premise is that this fraternity of men comes together to save the world from an outer space alien takeover, but the real reason for the group's formation is that they were looking for brotherly camaraderie away from their typical nuclear family structure. In particular, Bob, played by Vince Vaughn, invites the team over to show off his man cave, which quickly becomes the main meeting place for the group and the site of shared rowdy masculine expression.

Much like communities, the home is built around various experiences where each room represents different associations to family, marriage, and domestic labor.[6] The homosocial life inside the man cave is a withdrawal from feminized domestic space. Still, it is a domestic space in its own right, where a kind of

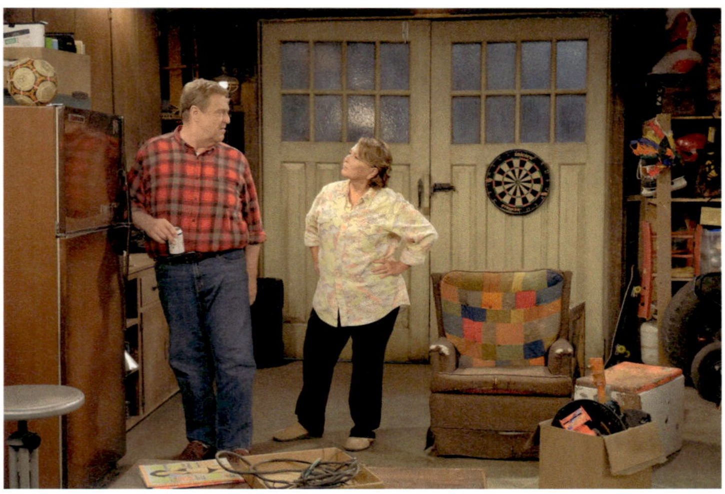

↑ Film still from the 2018 revival of *Roseanne*.

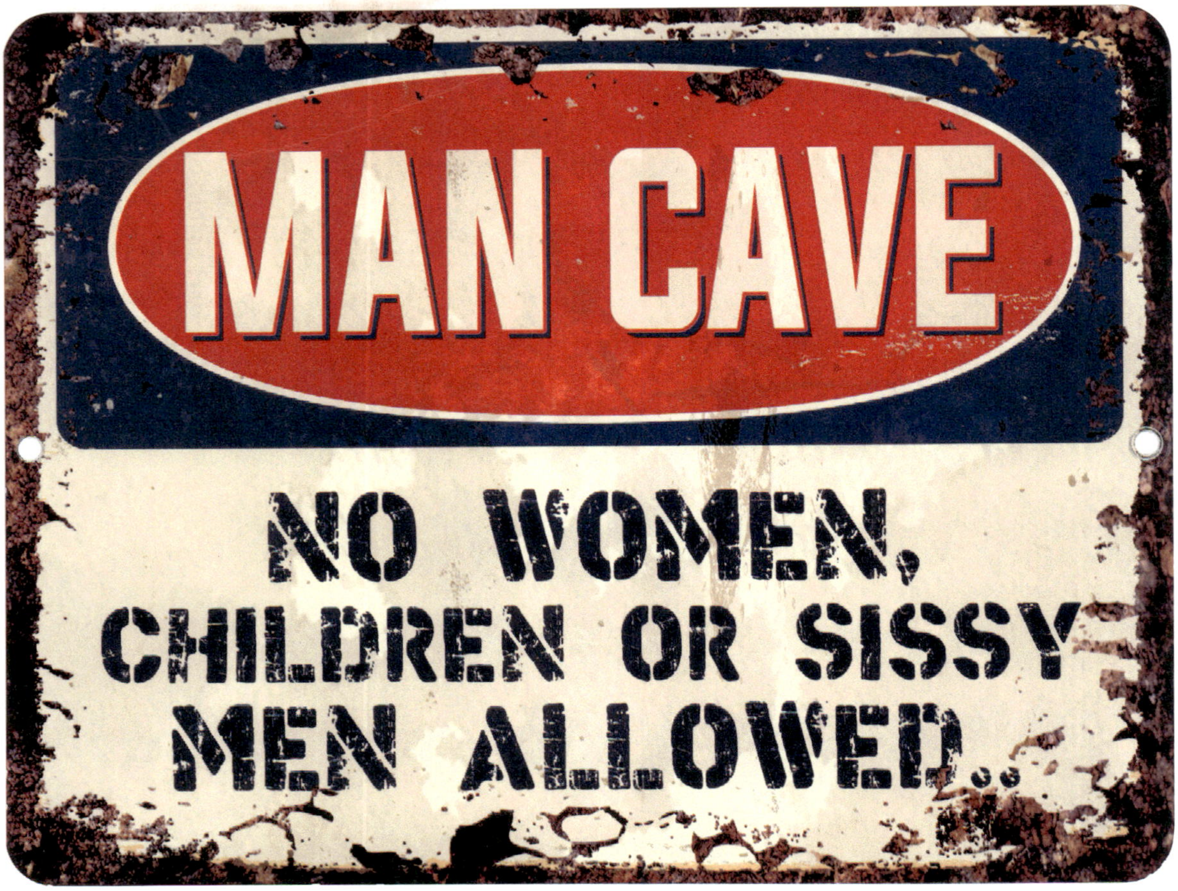

← "Man Cave" vintage-style sign.

masculine domesticity is constructed with techniques typically assigned to women within a household, including the organization, arrangement, and management of the home's interior spaces, as well as catering to aspects of nurturing, care, and homemaking. The man cave mimics a house within a house.

Though the man cave aims to be an antifeminine domestic space, the use of "feminine methods" in its creation, such as building an environment conducive to accommodating food, drinks, entertainment, sleeping areas, and even a private toilet, signifies the adoption and imitation of domestic strategies. The utilization of these methods within the man cave constructs a parallel domesticity—a sort of "counter-domesticity"—that impersonates the key elements of a home while protesting outside the typical feminine domestic sphere. This creates an alternate space that borrows from traditional womanly-associated methods to establish a distinct masculine enclave within the domestic landscape.

The push for suburban built environment moralized the family structure, and according to historian Margaret Marsh, "discourages excessive attention to one's individual wants."[7] Around the mid-1800s, middle-class domestic architecture was designed so that members of the family could be separated from each other in parlors or the idealized manly refuge, the study.[8] But starting in the early 1900s, the design of suburban houses began incorporating ideas such as "family togetherness" expressed through new concepts of space such as "living rooms" and open floor plans.[9]

Despite this openness, Elsie de Wolfe, best known as America's first interior decorator, observed in 1913 that "it is the personality of the mistress that the home expresses. Men are forever guests in our homes, no matter how much happiness they may find there."[10] And in 2016, when sociologist Tristan Bridges interviewed straight men about the meaning of their man cave in the context of their heterosexual relationship, the most common response was, "I feel like the whole house is hers. And this is a space for me."[11] Bridges followed up by asking them which spaces in the house are "hers," and in an echo of Betty Friedan's 1963 *The Feminine Mystique*, men would "list off rooms associated with domestic labor, not with leisure—the kitchen, the laundry room, the nursery, etc." The garage, the attic, or the basement are seen to not be "owned" by anyone.

The economic structure of twentieth-century America institutionalized the divide between public and private spheres by enabling a single salary to support a household, thereby privileging middle-class white families.[12] This separation also gendered the built environment, contrasting the private domestic mother against the public working father, whose remaining domestic labor functions were relegated to extradomestic spaces.[13] The man cave demarcates a domestic space within the home, yet one where labor or care-work does not take place. For men dwelling as husbands in the home—a space socially assigned to femininity—man caves work as exaggerated representations of identity. The man cave, then, is more than a retreat. It is both a canvas and symptom of toxic masculinity.

The Museum of Macho Expression

The representation of suburban husbands and their cherished man caves serves as a blueprint for navigating the suburban environment. Moreover, in today's digital age, online platforms and social media outlets further perpetuate the script of the traditional middle-class family man striving to claim territory inside the home in opposition to feminine gender or labor roles.

The magazine *Man Caves* describes its namesake spaces as inviting fantasies "all dreamed up by guys and for guys," and offers "How To" guides to personalize one's space by collecting themed elements. A specific theme—the sports bar, the pub, rock'n'roll, the tool shop, the hunting shed, etc.—is key to achieving a theatrical impression of coherence among a curated selection of more or less standard essentials: recliners, TV/entertainment systems, bar and fridge, pool table, dartboard, poker table, sports memorabilia, pin-up posters, and bar stools/extra seating.

Man caves often hint at sensations of intensity and aggression that have been excluded from the masculine/feminine gender binary framework. For example, sports memorabilia such as jerseys, autographed athletic equipment, and trophies evoke a sense of competitiveness and physical prowess. A tool shop theme reflects practical skills and a hands-on approach. Dartboards and poker tables symbolize camaraderie, competition, and strategic thinking often associated with brotherhood. And rock'n'roll is associated with rebellion and a sense of individuality. The combination of these symbols and items creates a carefully curated environment that reflects traditionally masculine interests and fosters a sense of identity and belonging within the man cave space.

Like Walter Benjamin's collector who creates a fantasy of object culture, the creator of the man cave conceives a fantasy of masculine culture.[14] The man cave can be situated in the genealogy of the "bachelor pad," a concept fashioned by *Playboy* in the 1960s to groom men into excessive consumers of goods and women by appealing to their teenage instincts.[15] According to Paul B. Preciado, "the important thing about teenagers was not his age, but his ability to consume without moral restrictions. ... The young, white heterosexual teenager was the focus of a new cultural market structured around university life, jazz and rock and roll, movies, sports, cars, and girls. ... The teenager who was not yet tied down by marriage."[16]

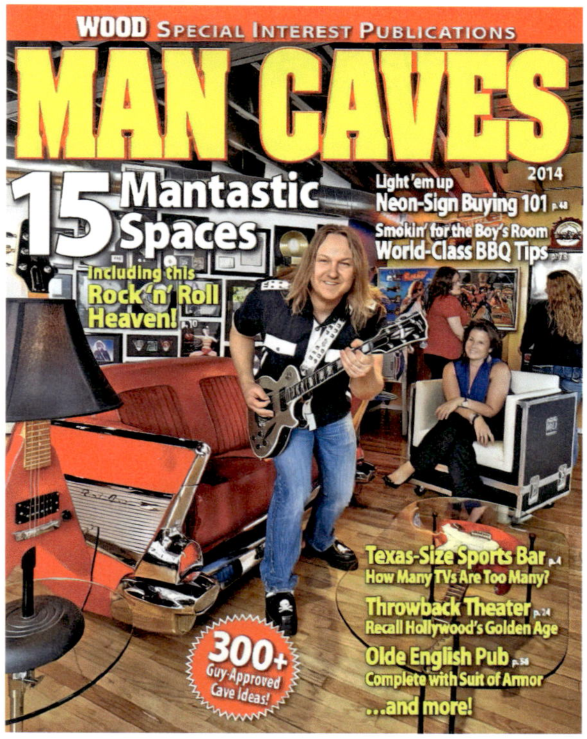

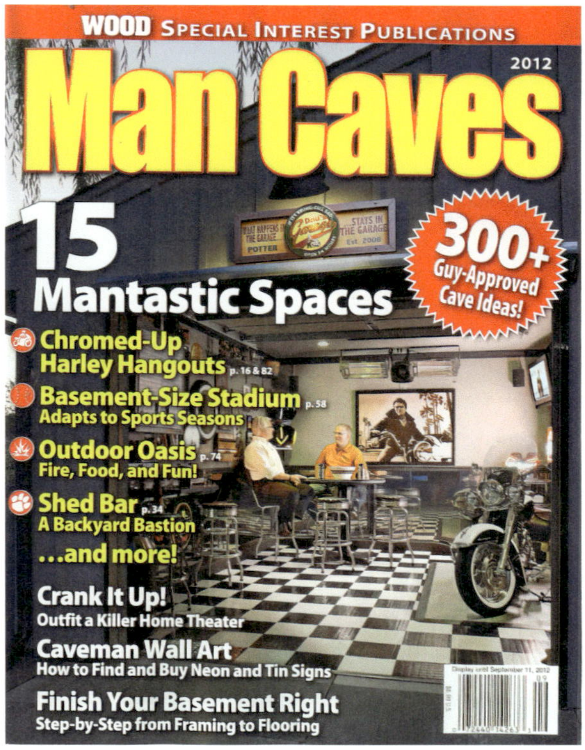

↑ *Man Caves* magazine, 2014 and 2012.

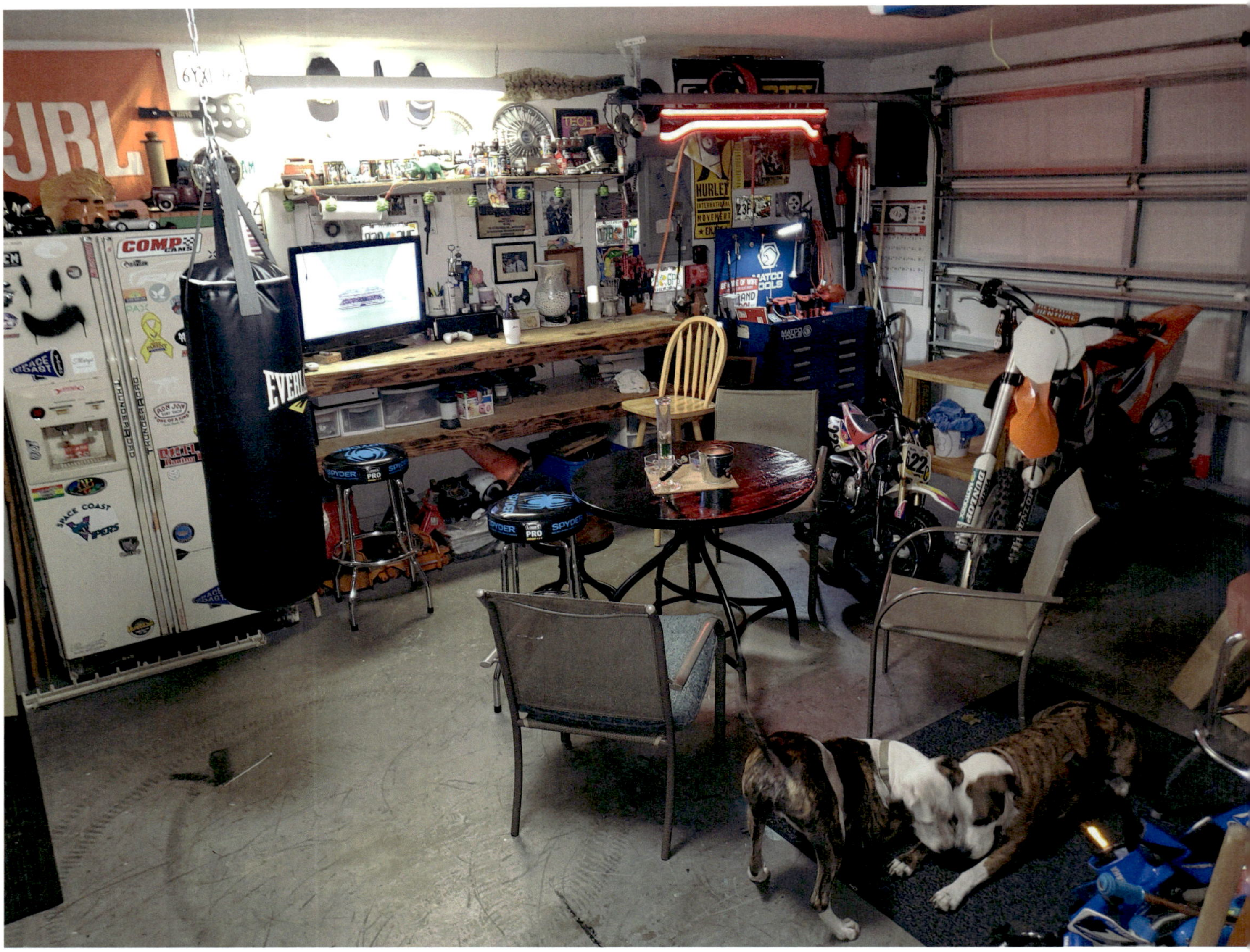

In Bridges' interviews, most men revealed that they don't actually have time for friends, and that their man caves are unfinished. When asked who they expected to use the space in the future, they did not have a clear response. In general, both the physical materiality and the social camaraderie of the man cave exist more in the realm of aspiration than in constructed reality. Jack Halberstam defines masculinity as the performative, social "connection between maleness and power."[17] With a fantasy unable to be realized, the need to express one's masculinity can spill over into the virtual spaces of forums, community boards, social media, and Zoom calls.[18]

The man cave is an archive of hypermasculine nostalgia whose existence can only be validated through the approval of other men. In 2008, retired US Army intelligence officer Mike Yost founded The Official Man Cave Site LLC, ManCaveSite.org. Man cave dreamers who pay a yearly membership fee receive a certificate and hat, access to the online forums, and exclusive discounts on other Man Cave Site LLC merchandise. Forums serve as a platform for men to show off their man caves and look for validation as others seek ideas. The exchange of ideas and comments are organized in specific discussion groups, ranging from sports and cigars to "over-the-top" sandwich recipes. The site also gives out yearly awards for the best man cave in the United States and sports the tagline, "Taking back the world, one Man Cave at a time!"

An Epidemic of Toxic Masculinity

The man cave is less an inevitable consequence of suburban gender binaries than it is the designed outcome of the repeated choice to draw on this strict binary. After all, many converted basements, attics, and garages engage nuanced gender dynamics through different spatial typologies. The built environment cultivates community moments and becomes the stage for cultural identity. But the hoarding of masculinity for social validation that takes place inside a man cave establishes a noxious codependency with the feminine domestic.

Whether the man cave is a physical or virtual expression, it stays in the gray space of fantasy between the binary of private and public realms.

↑ A photo from the Reddit community r/Mancaves.

It lives in a scapegoat utopia that allows the husband/father to ignore the work and daily responsibilities of a family. Its purgatory location—a house within a house—asserts the belief that men dilute their toxic behaviors and manly alter egos in the presence of women.

The man cave is an assertion of men's presence and dominance within the domestic space, expressing hypermasculinity through tangible possessions or territorial claims. Its defined physical environment acts as a barrier, protecting this expression of extreme masculinity from the societal pressures or expectations related to postwar family values. The man cave synthesizes an interiorized domesticity with the concept of individualized shelter to create "an almost literal attempt to control, reprivatize, render invisible, and bury not only domesticity but also women's sexuality."[19] The man cave is a place where caustic dynamics become endemic to the relationship between gender identity, material culture, and architecture. Understanding the built environment as a mechanism for gender politics reveals a contemporary social epidemic of toxic masculinity.

An earlier version of this essay was originally published by e-flux Architecture in 2020.

1. According to Dolores Hayden in *Redesigning the American Dream*, homes in American still follow the Victorian script of the home outside the city as being defined as "woman's place" while places within the city are labeled a "man's world." See Dolores Hayden, *Redesigning the American Dream: The Future of Housing, Work and Family Life* (New York: W. W. Norton, 2002).
2. Susie McKellar and Penny Sparke, eds., *Interior Design and Identity* (Manchester: Manchester University Press, 2004).
3. Abby Ferber, "Keeping Sex in Bounds: Sexuality and the (De) Construction of Race and Gender," in *Gender, Sex, and Sexuality: An Anthology*, ed. Abby Ferber, Kimberly Holcomb, and Tre Wentling (New York: Oxford University Press, 2009), 136–141.
4. The pregnancy is later revealed to be an invention from Al's nightmare (due to the real-life miscarriage of the actress). See Andreas Carl, "Some Frequently Asked Questions," *Bundyology*, May 31, 2009, http://www.bundyology.com/faq.html.
5. *Married with Children*, episode 6.0, "If Al Had a Hammer," directed by Gerry Cohen, written by Kevin Curran, aired September 22, 1991, on FOX.
6. Toon Dreessen, "How Architecture Can Bring Communities Together," *HuffPost*, May 8 2015, https://www.huffingtonpost.ca/toon-dreessen/architecture-and-community_b_7236966.html.
7. Margaret Marsh, "Suburban Men and Masculine Domesticity, 1870–1915," *American Quarterly* 40, no. 2 (1988): 165–186.
8. Gwendolyn Wright, *Building the Dream: A Social History of Housing in America* (Cambridge, MA: MIT Press, 1981), 109–111; and *Moralism and the Model Home: Domestic Architecture and Cultural Conflict in Chicago, 1873–1913* (Chicago: University of Chicago Press, 1980), 9–46.
9. Marsh, "Suburban Men and Masculine Domesticity, 1870–1915."
10. Elsie De Wolfe, *The House in Good Taste* (New York: Century, 1913).
11. C. Brian Smith, "This Guy Studies Man Caves for a Living; Here's What He's Learned," *MEL Magazine*, August 29, 2016, https://melmagazine.com/en-us/story/this-guy-studies-man-caves-for-a-living-heres-what-hes-learned-2.
12. Raia Prokhovnik, "Public and Private Citizenship: From Gender Invisibility to Feminist Inclusiveness," *Feminist Review* 60, no. 1 (September 1998): 84, 87.
13. Miliann Kang, Donovan Lessard, and Laura Heston, *Introduction to Women, Gender, Sexuality Studies* (Amherst: University of Massachusetts Amherst Libraries, 2017), http://openbooks.library.umass.edu/introwgss/.
14. The passage parallels Walter Benjamin's collector with the man cave creator—both craft fantasies around objects. It argues that interior space embodies its essence when reflecting the identity of the collector or creator. In the collector's context, the mission involves transforming objects by stripping them of their commercial value and claiming ownership. The collector can then emphasize their significance over practical utility, showcasing a pursuit of a curated, meaningful collection reflecting self-identity. Walter Benjamin, "Paris, Capital of the 19th Century," in *Walter Benjamin: Selected Writings*, vol. 3: *1935–1938*, ed. Howard Eiland and Michael W. Jennings (Cambridge, MA: Belknap Press, 2006), 39.
15. Kaitlyn Tiffany, "What Happened to the Man Cave?," *Vox*, March 4, 2019, https://www.vox.com/the-goods/2019/3/4/18246518/man-cave-boom-pre-recession-masculinity-male-friendship.
16. Paul B. Preciado, *Pornotopia: An Essay on Playboy's Architecture and Biopolitics* (New York: Zone Books, 2014), 48.
17. Jack Halberstam, *Female Masculinity* (Durham: Duke University Press, 1998).
18. See the Man Caves website, http://mancaves.com/.
19. Preciado, *Pornotopia*, 74, referencing Beatriz Colomina, *Domesticity at War* (Cambridge, MA: MIT Press, 2007).

ARCHITECTURE IN THE AGE OF STRESS

VICTORIA BUGGE ØYE

In the postwar decades a new understanding of disease was gaining ground.[1] Earlier hygiene reforms, generalized vaccination programs, and the discovery and administration of several new antibiotic treatments in the 1940s–1960s had drastically reduced the prevalence and threat of diseases such as tuberculosis, typhoid, and polio.[2] As a result, the main causes of death worldwide were no longer infectious disease but chronic illnesses such as cancer and heart disease. By the 1960s and 1970s many medical professionals (incorrectly) believed that the age of communicable diseases was largely over, and that one of the main roles of medicine would now be to treat new "lifestyle" or "affluence diseases" such as hypertension, cardiovascular issues, and stress.

The term "stress" had been coined by Canadian-Hungarian endocrinologist Hans Selye in the 1930s and entered the vernacular in 1956 with the publication of his bestselling book *The Stress of Life.*[3] According to Selye, stress was the body's response to changes or "stressors" in the environment that triggered the fight-or-flight response and required the body to readjust to remain in a state of equilibrium.[4] In and of itself, stress was a normal and necessary bodily function: Selye compared it to the immune system's response to a threat or injury by causing "inflammation or the formation of immune bodies."[5] However, if the organism did not return to its baseline condition—if it failed to adapt to its environment—the hormonal and visceral imbalance would eventually cause the body to break itself down and lead to stress-related disorders or "adaption diseases."

Selye argued that the fast pace and demands of modern society caused people to remain in a prolonged state of alertness that could eventually cause permanent physical changes. He suggested that stress was instrumental in understanding diseases such as ulcers and heart attacks, deviating from previous theories that most diseases were caused by pathogens. Discourse on stress at the time often focused on low-grade, everyday stress and its potentially detrimental effects on human health. The most dangerous stress was that which was not taken seriously, which was allowed to sit and slowly eat away at the organism. This did not necessarily require a very high level of stress, just prolonged exposure. Often the person was not even aware of their own stress. This understanding of stress, as existing in a perpetual fight-or-flight mode, was widely adopted

→ Hans Selye showing the organs of a stressed rat. Image produced for a 1955 photo story titled "Montreal Medical Scientist Explores 'Stress': Selye Gives Medicine New Direction."

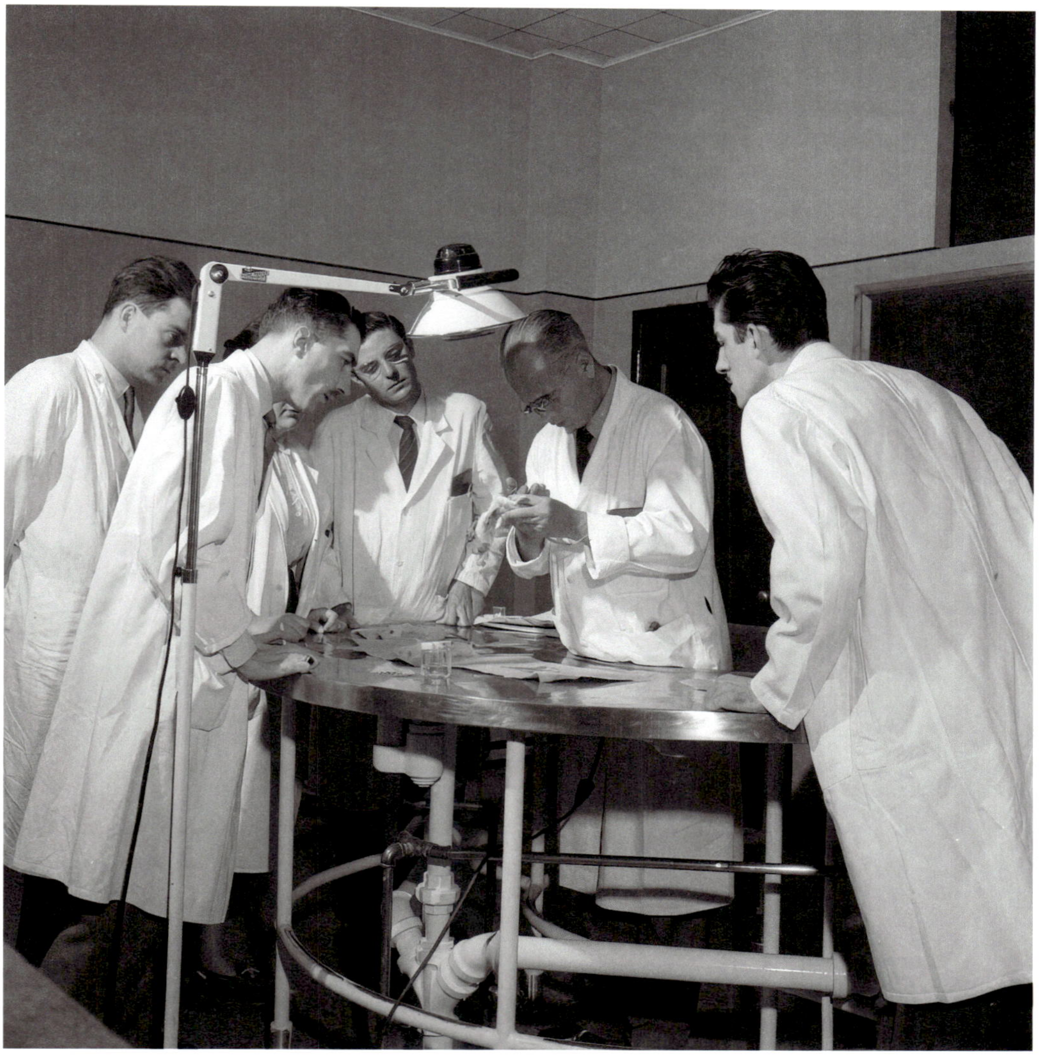

throughout the 1970s, helping to inform the health buzz and self-care cultures of that decade, the medicalization of meditation, and the revival of relaxation techniques. It also came to be seen as an idea that artists and architects could address—and even treat—through their work.

Coop Himmelblau and the Institute of Environmental Health

In the decades following the publication of Selye's book, the discourse on stress went global. At the University of Vienna, the Institute of Environmental Health was founded in 1970 specifically to assess the impact of the modern, urban environment and its stressors on human health and productivity.[6] The Institute's first study on stress and the environment was done in collaboration with the experimental architecture group Coop Himmelblau.[7] The head of the Institute, and Coop Himmelblau's main collaborator for the next seven years, was Manfred Haider, a doctor with a joint degree in medicine and psychology. Together, Haider and Coop Himmelblau worked to find ways that design could help both protect against and actively combat stress. This included the design of entire apartments, special relaxation furniture, and pop-up relaxation rooms.[8] Coop Himmelblau also designed objects that were used for experiments at the Institute.

Haider defined the new discipline of environmental health as the "correlation between environmental influences and the health and wellbeing of people." Such "environmental influences" included "the chemical as well as the physical, climatic, biological, and of course in a broader sense also the psychosocial influences."[9] Thus, if the effects of the urban environment in the early twentieth century had been understood in terms of shock and trauma—a form of sensory overload that "shocked" the senses—the urban and architectural environment was now theorized as a site that worked on the subject through a slow and often imperceptible process of deterioration, where the effects of toxins, radiation, and stress gradually accumulated, in contrast to producing an instantaneous and recognizable impact. This new sensibility marked a shift from the fast-working currents of electricity and adrenaline of the early twentieth century to the "invisible" and seeping effects of the postwar environment.

Haider's notion of environmental influences was, notably, not only a theory of *which* things influenced us in the modern environment, but *how* they influenced us. Any sensory stimulus could potentially have a greater impact when registered below the threshold of consciousness, where it could accumulate undetected. In an article on environmental health and housing, Haider writes that further research on the relationship between the environment, stress, and illness is especially warranted: "the diseases caused by stress and the living conditions associated with health problems, such as, for example, cardiovascular diseases and degenerative diseases, have not been tackled to date."[10] This link between stress and living conditions was what Haider set out to investigate in his work with Coop Himmelblau.

Airbox and Relab First meeting sometime in 1969, Coop Himmelblau and Haider united over the belief that the scientific union of architecture and medicine could potentially solve what they considered to be one of the most fundamental and pressing concerns of the day: how humans could live well in an increasingly urbanized, polluted, and stressful world. At the Institute they collaborated on several experiments. In the summer of 1972, they examined the effects of different spatial surroundings on a person's sense of relaxation. The central, driving question was how "environmental influences" could be reverse-engineered and architecture designed to relax rather than stress the

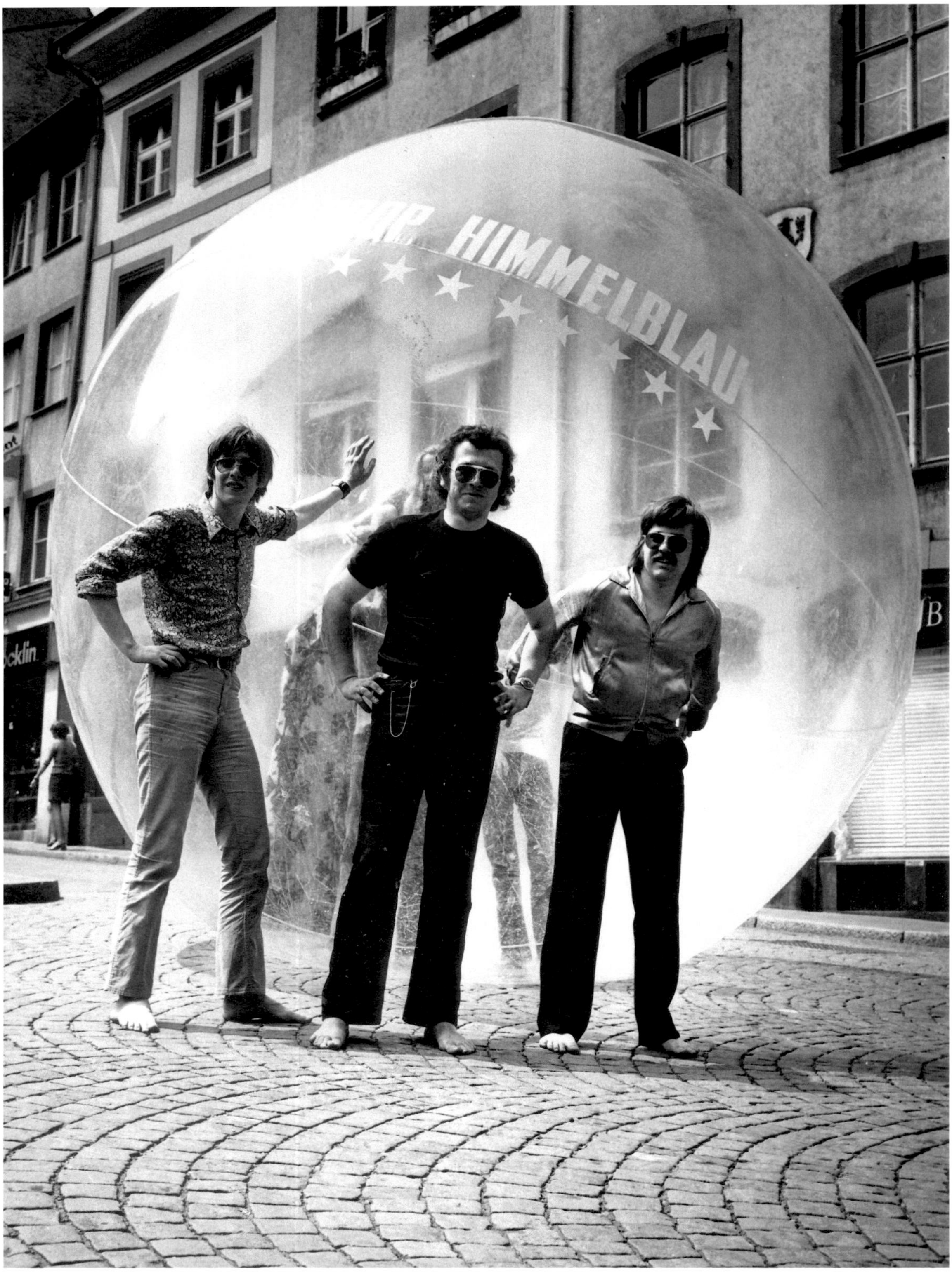

↙ The members of Coop Himmelblau posing in front of their Restless Ball in 1971. From left: Wolf Prix, Michael Holzer, and Helmut Swiczinsky.

↘ Press clipping showing the Airbox in an earlier experiment on air pollution. The original caption reads: "The pneumatic test chamber Airbox is [these days] finalized for a Viennese research institute by Austria's avant-garde architecture team Coop Himmelblau. The air tent is used for neuro- and psychophysiological experiments to investigate the effect of poisonous gases on humans."

↓ Relab shown in noninflated state in the foreground, with the Airbox in the background, 1972. Renate Wagner, who was gathering data for her PhD thesis, is seated in front of the EEG tape recorder that registered brain waves during the experiment. Standing to the right of Wagner are Helmut Höller, who helped supervise the experiments, and the Institute of Environmental Health's technician Hans Stiedl.

subject. Doctoral student Renate Wagner theorized, organized, and conducted the experiments as part of her psychology degree and recruited ten test subjects.[11] For the experiments, Wagner measured how two different inflatable environments designed by Coop Himmelblau—the spherical Relab and the cylindrical Airbox—combined with a relaxation technique developed in the United States in the 1920s called progressive relaxation, affected the test subjects.[12] These experiments sought to understand whether test subjects would be more relaxed after spending an hour inside each of the spaces. Although Wagner conducted the actual experiment,

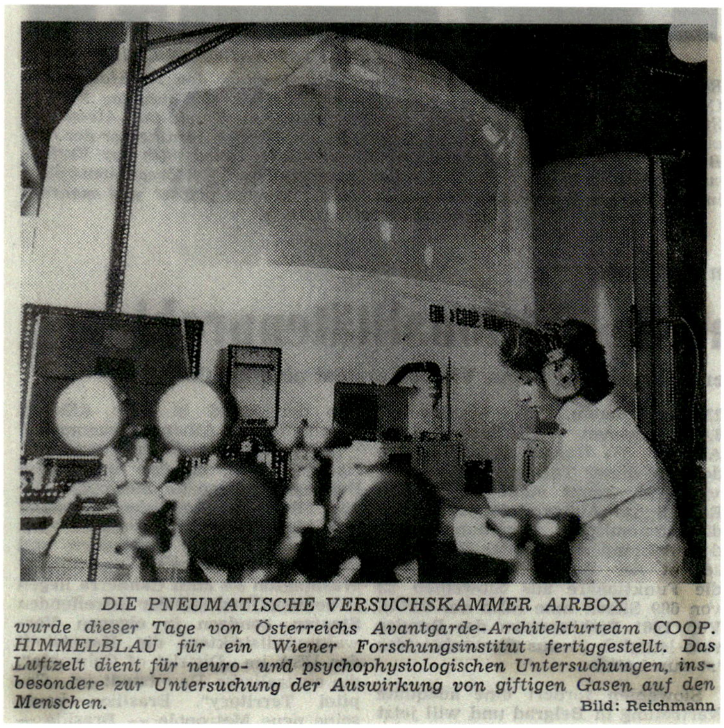

DIE PNEUMATISCHE VERSUCHSKAMMER AIRBOX wurde dieser Tage von Österreichs Avantgarde-Architekturteam COOP. HIMMELBLAU für ein Wiener Forschungsinstitut fertiggestellt. Das Luftzelt dient für neuro- und psychophysiologischen Untersuchungen, insbesondere zur Untersuchung der Auswirkung von giftigen Gasen auf den Menschen. Bild: Reichmann

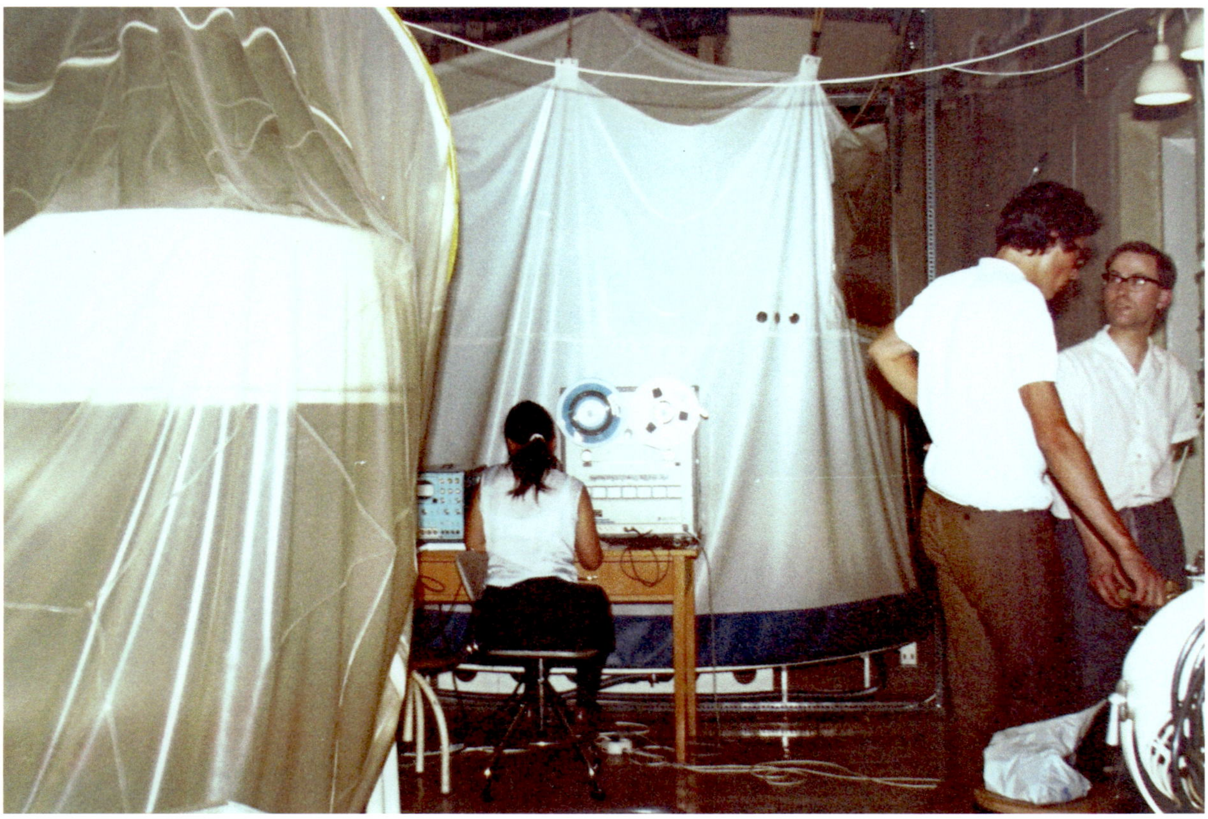

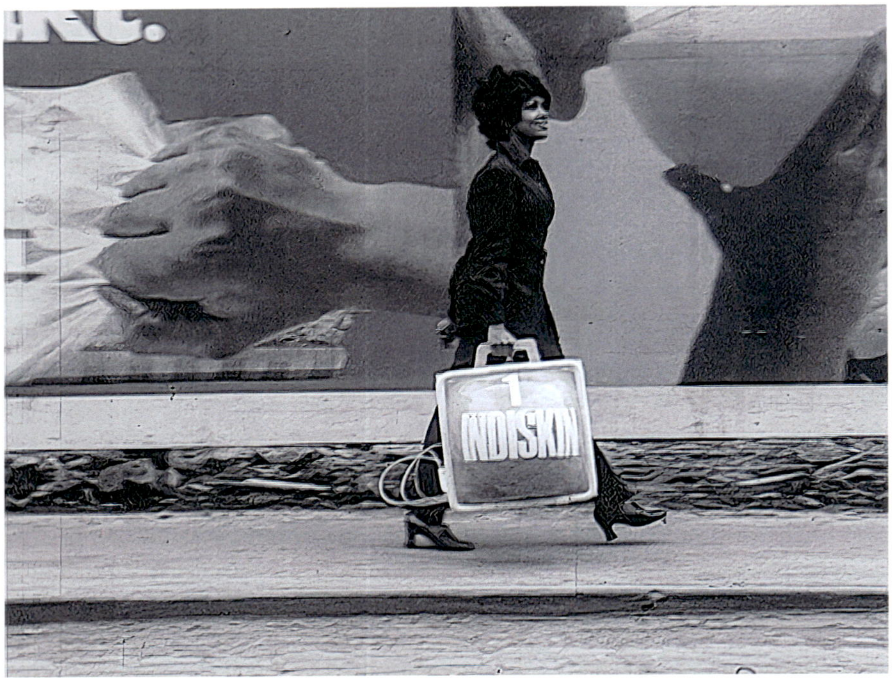

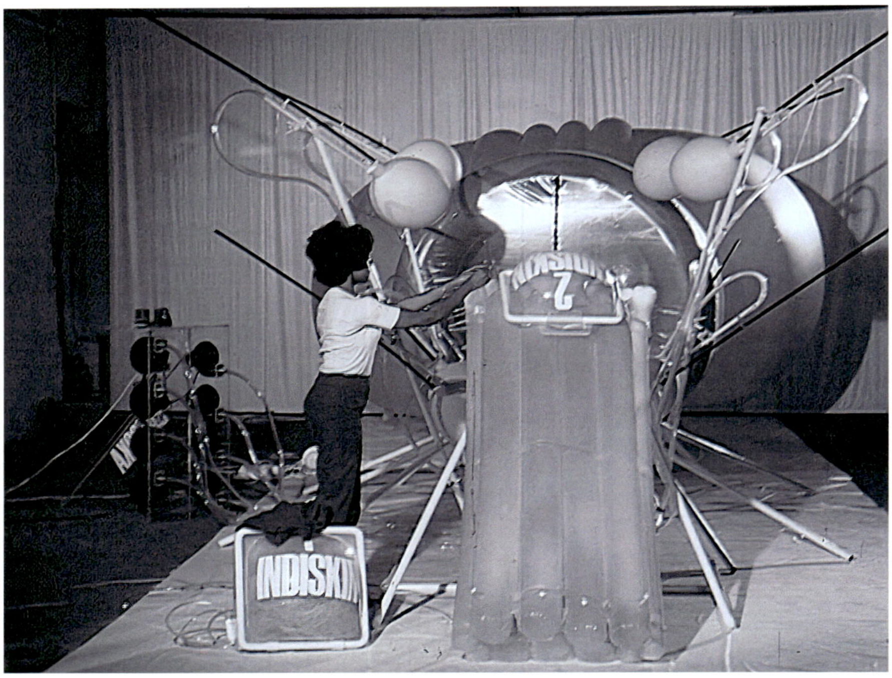

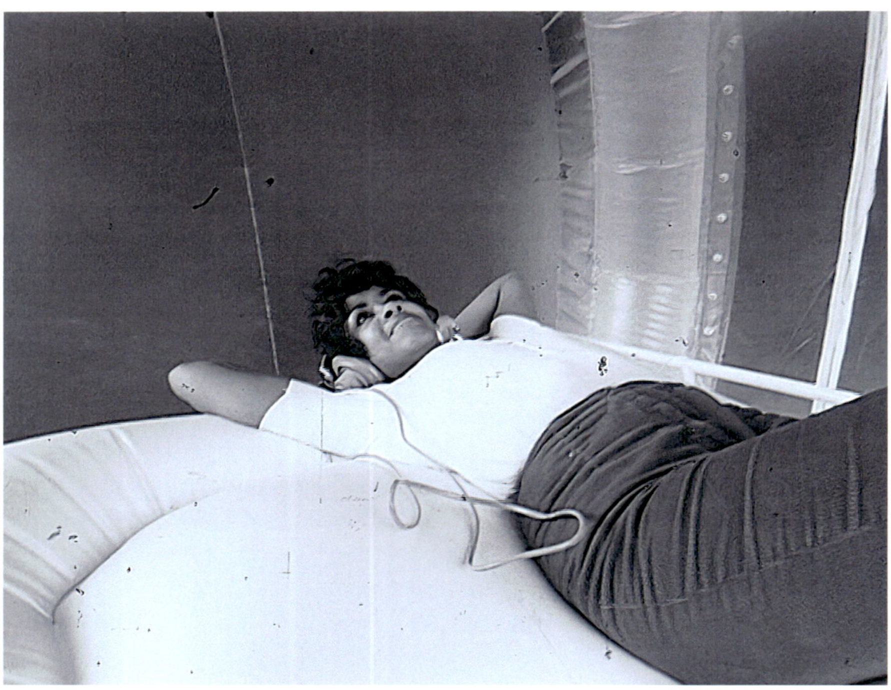

↙ Indieskin, a transportable component to be connected as part of the Insider. Stills from Michael Pilz, "Himmelblau im TV," 1970. ORF, Vienna, May 5, 1970.

the idea behind it had been a joint effort between Haider and Coop Himmelblau. For Coop Himmelblau and Haider, the existing urban environment was rarely, if ever, discussed as a neutral factor, but as a primary stressor with potentially negative effects on human life and psyche. Within this context, the notion of "relaxation" did not emerge as an independent technique, but as stress's "other"—a counterpractice to ameliorate the effects of modern, urban life.

Introducing her dissertation, Wagner immediately situated the experiments within a medicalized discourse of relaxation. She writes that "experiences from daily life, alongside the findings of clinical psychology, show how important and how difficult it is for people to achieve a relaxed state."[13] While progressive relaxation exercises played an important part in the experiment, its most distinctive aspect was arguably the two inflatables supplied by Coop Himmelblau. The inclusion of Relab and Airbox introduced an architectural and environmental factor to existing research on bodily states of relaxation and activation, a field that until this point had mostly been based on experiments performed in nondescript rooms with closed eyes. Wagner referred to the inflatables as *pneumatische Entspannungslabors*, or "pneumatic relaxation laboratories," and the name Relab was itself a conjunction of "relaxation" and "laboratory."[14] The structure consisted of a partially freestanding inflatable sphere 260 centimeters in diameter. Relab's interior steel platform connected to an exterior ladder, allowing the test subject access through a zippered entry, which was raised above ground level. Airbox was repurposed from an earlier collaborative experiment between Coop Himmelblau and the Institute on fatigue and air pollution. Airbox was cylindrical (with a height of 260 centimeters and a diameter of 300 centimeters), made from the same material as Relab and structurally supported by steel scaffolding.

In 1974, two years before Wagner completed her PhD, Haider briefly recounted the results in a short article titled "Environmental Influences in Living Spaces" in the national journal for research funded by the country's Research Association for Housing, Building, and Planning.[15] Haider referenced the work of his colleague Maximilian Piperek, a Viennese psychologist who focused on the psychological aspect of environmental health.[16] Piperek and Haider knew each other well and had even collaborated on a project in 1971 that examined the stress experienced by members of the Vienna Symphony Orchestra before and during concerts. The experiments, published in the book *Stress und Kunst*, were in part based on Haider's own research on activation and fatigue.[17] In the article that Haider was now referencing, Piperek had interviewed several people about the qualities they valued most in housing, ranging from factors such as natural light to more intangible aspects such as the feeling of safety. Piperek had subsequently categorized both physiological and psychological "needs" according to rank. The desire for some kind of shield from external stimuli had been central to the responses of several of the interviewees, and Haider understood this as a need for an "intimate zone, a concentration zone, or possibility for relaxation in the apartment."[18] For Haider, this was the kind of function that "Plastic Architecture"—as he referred to inflatables—could potentially serve, and he argued that plastics should be further investigated "from a medical and psychological point of view."[19]

The important "shielding" function of domestic architecture proposed by Piperek translated into very specific material qualities in Coop Himmelblau's design. Both inflatables had been designed with a wide enough girth to comfortably fit one person and were made from translucent plastic, which filtered light but did not allow for visual access. This translucency would provide a secluded and protective space for the test subject to relax, shielding and distancing them from the immediate environment without making them feel enclosed or claustrophobic. This was very different from the work that Coop Himmelblau presented in galleries and museums during the same period. *Astro Balloon* (1969–1972), for example, referenced and dramatized the act of self-regulation through meditation but primarily as performance art rather than therapy.[20]

Haider mused that perhaps in the near future such inflatable pop-up relaxation rooms could become an everyday feature of people's homes and apartments.[21] In a feature on Coop Himmelblau's work in the Swiss art magazine *Kunst Nachrichten*, the group also suggested that the "short-time recreational/relaxation rooms" produced for the Institute would, "after the conclusion of a series of tests," be "further developed into a use object," revealing a plan to develop "a serially produced relaxation capsule."[22] The design of this capsule would be presented in a later collaboration with the Institute, Entspannungsarchitektur 1 (Relaxation Architecture 1) in 1976, but would never go into production. Although the inflatables produced for the experiments at the Institute were relatively large (they relied on interior metal scaffolding in order to support the reclining arrangements), Coop Himmelblau had previously suggested forms of inflatables that could be more easily acquired and installed. The Insider, for example, first presented at Coop Himmelblau's solo exhibition *Count Down* at the Museum of Applied Arts in Vienna in 1969, was a personally sized inflatable that included a rotating bed, music, and light projections. Sections of the installation fit into a specially designed suitcase dispensed from a vending machine, making it a stylish accessory that

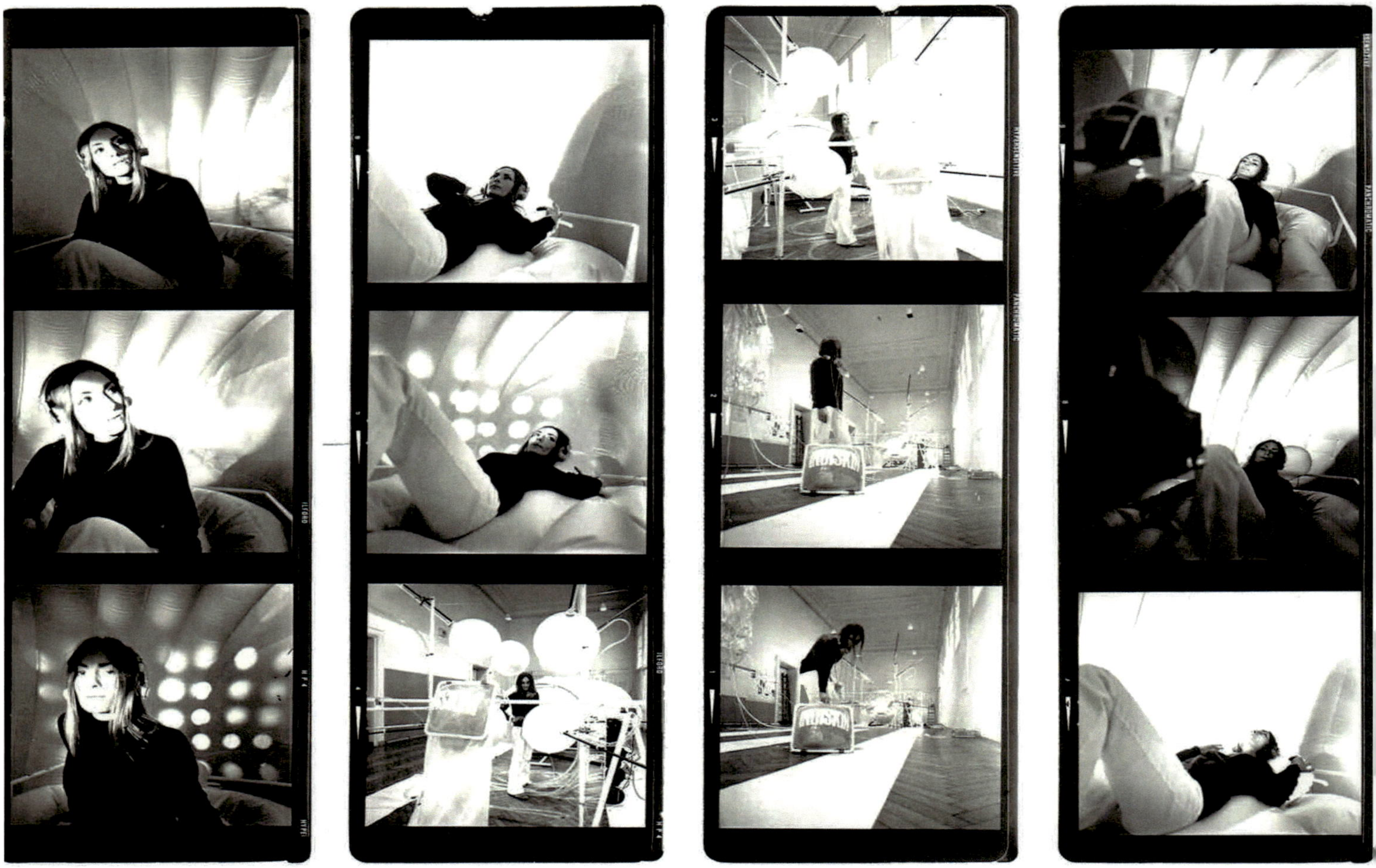

could be easily carried around and spontaneously erected if the need to relax should arise. In a recent interview, Wagner also confirmed that there were discussions about commercial production of relaxation rooms:

> [Coop Himmelblau] had designed what they called a Relab. [It was] supposedly a small environment which could potentially help people relax more than other places. I think it was even a commercial idea. Somebody said: if it comes out that it was relaxing, they could put it up in rest stations on the autobahn or wherever people need to relax for a little while before they get on with their stressful lives.[23]

Under the Influence of Environment

For her experiments, Wagner relied primarily on the activation theory of emotion, which had been introduced by American behavioral neuroscientist Donald B. Lindsley, founder of the Brain Research Institute at the University of California in Los Angeles, and Haider's mentor during a research residency there in 1962. The activation theory of emotion connected brainwave patterns with psychological states and behaviors and was used to understand the relationship between brain and performance. Specific patterns of alpha brainwaves, for example, were connected to feelings of relaxation. In the Institute's 1972 experiment, test subjects produced better alpha waves in the Relab than in the Airbox. Wagner thus concluded that its spherical form was better for relaxation.

Lindsley's research on brainwave patterns had shown that visual stimuli and focus of attention tended to block alpha waves and thus the relaxation process.[24] Wagner's experiments, which relied heavily on the scholarship of Lindsley and the connection between alpha waves and relaxation, asked the test subjects to close their eyes once inside the inflatables. Coop Himmelblau therefore encountered a dilemma when designing Relab and Airbox. They had to design structures that would, ideally, function as environmental influences without attracting any form of attentive looking from the user. With their smooth and translucent skins that blocked visual stimuli from the exterior, Relab and Airbox were designed to elicit a diffuse or peripheral mode of attention rather than a focused one. They were designed as environments that would easily recede into the background; as surroundings to literally be sensed with eyes closed, conducive to alpha waves and thus relaxation. For Airbox and Relab, becoming environmental meant retreating into the recesses of conscious attention.

This wider psychologization of the environment was due to a number of factors, including the professionalization and growth of the discipline of psychology in the decades after World War II (especially in the US, but also in Europe), the strong influence of behaviorist theories in the immediate postwar years (which stipulated the importance of environmental factors in the shaping of human behavior), and the emergence of the environment as a new field of interdisciplinary interrogation.[25] Anthropological, sociological, behavioral, and ethological research conducted in the 1950s and early 1960s all became precedents for theories of environmental perception and spatial behavior, and for the development of environmental psychology. Widely influential publications such as Edward Hall's *The Hidden Dimension* (1966) theorized that "invisible" spatial territories determined human interaction in public space and, alongside works such as Marshall McLuhan's 1967 essay "The Invisible Environment: The Future of an Erosion," suggested that the postwar environment influenced subjects through opaque and often imperceptible processes.[26]

Research on the mind, the role of attention, and the relationship between brainwave and behavioral patterns also opened up a new way of understanding channels of influence. Alpha waves required a different mode of attention that related to the surroundings in a more peripheral or environmental manner. In the world of art, the departure from object-centered aesthetics in the 1960s toward environmental and atmospheric assemblages also elicited a different mode of attention and experience. The "artwork" could remain peripheral, dispersed and out of focus, and function as ambience rather than as an object to be contemplated in and of itself. The horizontal bodily habitus in Relab and Airbox further emphasized the durational aspect of this new form of environmental influence. The slightly psychedelic experience that they were designed to produce—of melting slowly into the environment through deep relaxation—echoed other durational and performative artworks of the period, such as

← Insider presented at the Museum für Angewandte Kunst in Vienna for Coop Himmelblau's solo show *Count Down: Architekturmaschinen Testgeräte*, 1969.

↑ Image of Relab from Renate Wagner's dissertation.

↓ Coop Himmelblau, Relab (Insider 2), ca. 1972.

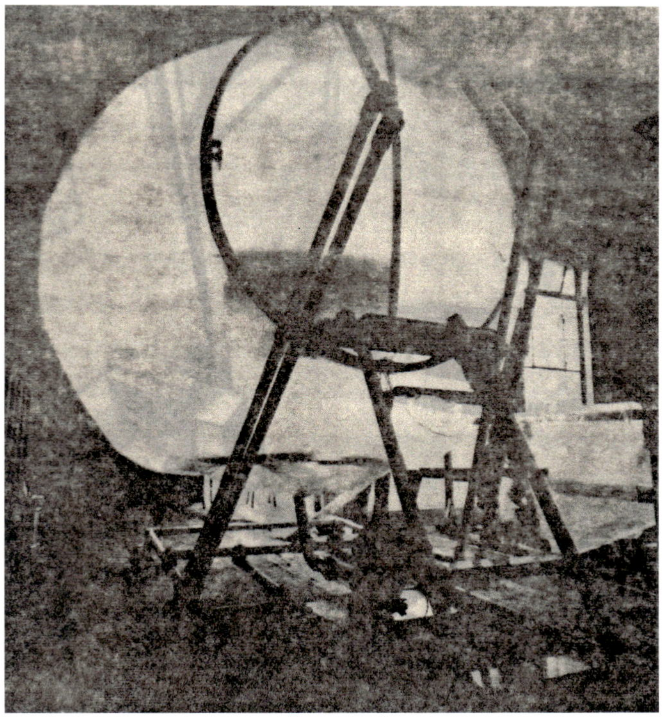

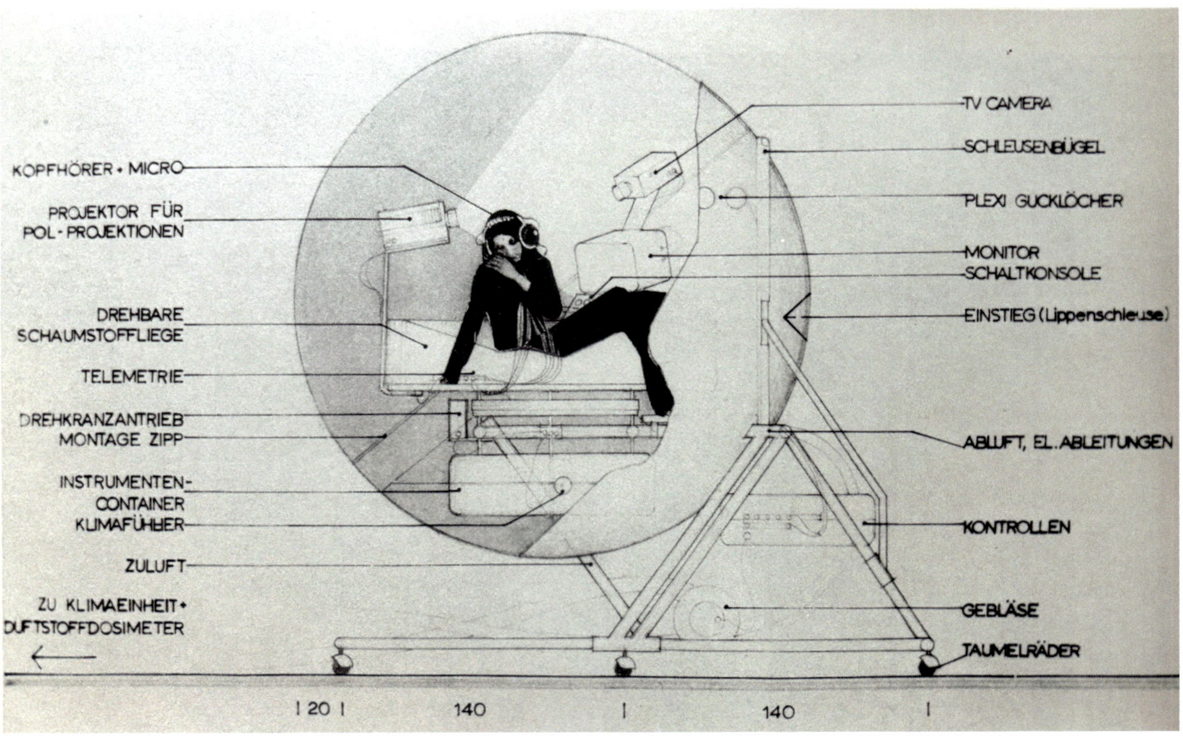

↓ Coop Himmelblau's Airbox used for experiments on air pollution. Still from "An den Boxen: Abgase und Lärm. Aktion Überleben in der verschmutzten Umwelt," screened on Austrian television. ORF, Vienna, October 5, 1970.

↘ The Airbox with Coop Himmelblau's logo is shown in the background while a collaborator, Dr. Johann Schedling, explains the experiments on air pollution. Still from "An den Boxen: Abgase und Lärm. Aktion Überleben in der verschmutzten Umwelt." ORF, Vienna, October 5, 1970.

the installations presented in the 1970 exhibition *Contemplation Environments* at the Museum of Contemporary Crafts in New York.[27] As McLuhan suggested in *Understanding Media*: "'Comfort' consists in abandoning a visual arrangement in favor of one that permits casual participation of the senses, a state that is excluded when any one sense, but especially the visual sense, is hotted up to the point of dominant command of a situation."[28]

Airbox and Relab were nested precisely in this nexus of environmental aesthetic and medical practices, peripheral and environmentalized attention, and a new ebb and flow of environmental influences. They suggest a postwar understanding of the urban environment, one that is no longer based on the late nineteenth-century idea of shock but on the slow and accumulative effects of durational exposure, and which was mirrored in the aesthetic, environmental, and medical discourses of the time. They also point toward a larger shift in ideas of aesthetic perception. The attempt to correlate spatial and neural organization effectively medicalized aesthetic experience, positing architecture as a tool against stress. At the Institute, data was gathered about environmental influences to be used as parameters for design, with the goal being to measure, quantify, predict, and script emotional and bodily responses. Foreshadowing the art world's turn to affect in the 1990s and its more recent turn to neuroscience, Coop Himmelblau's work at the Institute argued that architecture should not necessarily be evaluated by its formal or artistic merit, but rather by its ability to induce a specific psychophysiological state in the inhabitant. Or, in other words: good architecture is architecture that helps you de-stress.

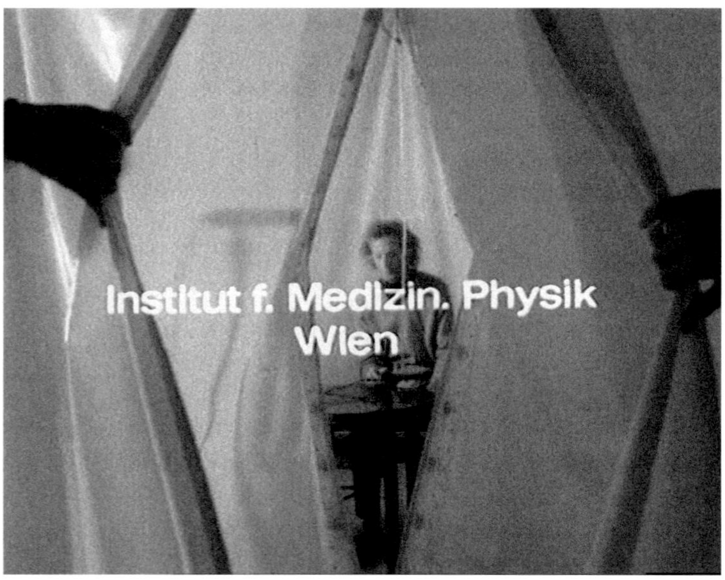

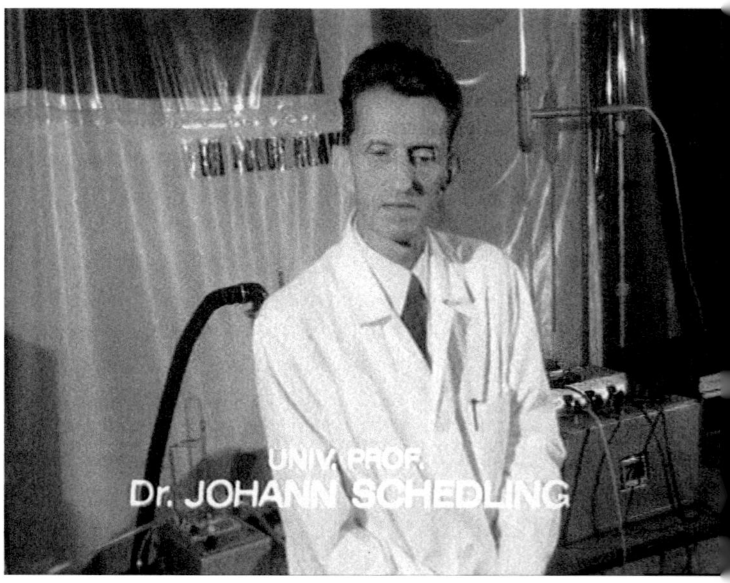

1. This essay includes sections from Victoria Bugge Øye, "'You Must Relax': Stress and Environmental Health in the Work of Coop Himmelblau, 1969–1977" (PhD diss., Princeton University School of Architecture, 2023).
2. Center for Disease Control, "Reported Incidence of Notifiable Diseases in the United States, 1960," *Morbidity and Mortality Weekly Report* 9, no. 53 (October 30, 1961): 4, https://stacks.cdc.gov/view/cdc/951; Center for Disease Control, "Reported Incidence of Notifiable Diseases in the United States, 1970," *Morbidity and Mortality Weekly Report* 19, no. 53 (August 1971): 4, https://stacks.cdc.gov/view/cdc/951.
3. See Mark Jackson, *The Age of Stress: Science and the Search for Stability* (Oxford: Oxford University Press, 2013).
4. Hans Selye, *The Stress of Life* (New York: McGraw-Hill, 1956), 95.
5. Hans Selye, "A Syndrome Produced by Diverse Nocuous Agents," *Nature*, July 4, 1936, 32.
6. For a discussion on the import of the concept of "stress" to Germany and Austria, see Patrick Kury, "Neurasthenia and Managerial Disease in Germany and America: Transnational Ties and National Characteristics in the Field of Exhaustion 1880–1960," in *Burnout, Fatigue, Exhaustion: An Interdisciplinary Perspective on a Modern Affliction*, ed. Sighard Neckel, Anna Katharina Schaffner, and Greta Wagner (Cham, Switzerland: Springer International, 2017), 51–73; Patrick Kury, *Der überforderte Mensch: Eine Wissensgeschichte vom Stress zum Burnout* (Frankfurt am Main: Campus, 2012).
7. Coop Himmelblau was founded in 1968 by Wolf Prix, Helmut Swiczinsky, and Michael Holzer. At that time, they called themselves Bau-Cooperative Himmelblau, but were also referred to in the press as Himmelblau until 1970, when they became more consistently referred to as either Coop. Himmelblau, Coop-Himmelblau, or Coop Himmelblau. Holzer left the group in 1971 and was not involved with the work at the Institute. The firm was later renamed Coop Himmelb(l)au, which is the name that the office operates under today. Since I am addressing the historical group and not the contemporary office, I use the denomination Coop Himmelblau.
8. See Victoria Bugge Øye, "The Health of Democracy: Coop Himmelblau's Entspannungsarchitektur and the Expansion of the Austrian Welfare State, 1970–77," in *Architecture and Democracy 1965–1989: Urban Renewal, Populism and the Welfare State*, ed. Dirk van den Heuvel, Sun Ah Hwang, and S. R. Monteiro de Jesus (Delft: TU Delft and Het Nieuwe Instituut, 2019), 116–124.
9. "Einwirkung aller Umwelteinflüsse und deren Wechselbeziehung mit der Gesundheit und dem Wohlbefinden den Menschen. Zu diesen Umweltfaktoren gehören sowohl die chemischen als auch die physikalischen, klimatischen, biologischen, und natürlich im weiteren Sinn auch die psychosoialen Einflüsse." Manfred Haider, "Umwelteinflüsse im Wohnbereich," *Wohnbauforschung in Österreich*, no. 1/2 (1972): 1.
10. Haider, "Umwelteinflüsse im Wohnbereich," 1.
11. Renate Wagner, "Die Wirkung von Umräumen und systematischer Entspannung auf psychologische und physiologische Indikatoren der Aktiviertheit" (PhD diss., University of Vienna, 1974), 51.
12. Edmund Jacobson, *Progressive Relaxation; A Physiological and Clinical Investigation of Muscular States and Their Significance in Psychology and Medical Practice* (Chicago: University of Chicago Press, 1929).
13. "Wie wichtig und wie schwierig die Erreichung eines entspannten Zustandes für den Menschen ist, zeigen neben den Erfahrungen aus dem täglichen Leben die Erkenntnisse der klinischen Psychologie." Wagner, "Die Wirkung," 1.
14. Wagner, "Die Wirkung," 1.
15. Haider, "Umwelteinflüsse im Wohnbereich."
16. Maximilian Piperek, "Grundaspekte einer Baupsychologie: Die psychischen Wohnbedürfnisse als Grundlage d. Bauplanung," *Schriftenreihe der Forschungsgesellschaft für Wohnen, Bauen und Planen*, no. 41 (1971).
17. Maximilian Piperek, *Stress und Kunst: Gesundheitliche, psychische, soziologische und rechtliche Belastungsfaktoren im Beruf des Musikers eines Symphonieorchesters* (Vienna: Wilhelm Braumüller Universitäts-Verlagsbuchhandlung Ges. m. b. H., 1971).
18. Haider, "Umwelteinflüsse im Wohnbereich," 6.
19. Haider, "Umwelteinflüsse im Wohnbereich," 2. The Institute of Environmental Health would later conduct research on the temporal properties of plastic as a building material. See Manfred Haider, *Der Wärmehaushalt des Menschen, verbunden mit einer Wohnumwelt aus Plastikkonstruktionen*, Schriftenreihe der Forschungsgesellschaft für Wohnen, Bauen und Planen 68 (Vienna: Forschungsgesellschaft für Wohnen, Bauen und Planen, 1976).
20. See Victoria Bugge Øye, "On Astroballoons and Personal Bubbles," *Positions*, e-flux architecture, April 17, 2018, https://www.e-flux.com/architecture/positions/194841/on-astroballoons-and-personal-bubbles/.
21. Haider, "Umwelteinflüsse im Wohnbereich," 6.
22. "Entwicklung einer serienfertigen [sic] Entspannungskapsel." Wolf Prix, Michael Holzer, and Helmut Swiczinsky, "Coop. Himmelblau zur Ausstellung in Basel, Galerie Stampa und 'Offener Saal', Kunsthalle."
23. Renate Wagner, interview with author, September 19, 2018.
24. Donald B. Lindsley, "Foci of Activity of the Alpha Rhythm in the Human Electro-Encephalogram," *Journal of Experimental Psychology* 23, no. 2 (1938): 159–171; Robert W. Lansing, Donald B. Lindsley, and Edward Schwartz, "Reaction Time and EEC Activation under Alerted and Nonalerted Conditions," *Journal of Experimental Psychology* 58, no. 1 (July 1959): 1–7.
25. See Joy Knoblauch, *Architecture of Good Behavior: Psychology and Modern Institutional Design in Postwar America* (Pittsburgh: University of Pittsburgh Press, 2020); Ellen Herman, *The Romance of American Psychology: Political Culture in the Age of Experts* (Berkeley: University of California Press, 1996); Paul Warde, Libby Robin, and Sverker Sörlin, *The Environment: A History of the Idea* (Baltimore: Johns Hopkins University Press, 2018).
26. See Larry D. Busbea, *The Responsive Environment: Design, Aesthetics, and the Human in the 1970s* (Minneapolis: University of Minnesota Press, 2020).
27. American Crafts Council, *Contemplation Environments* (New York: Museum of Contemporary Crafts, 1970).
28. Marshall McLuhan, *Understanding Media: The Extensions of Man* (New York: McGraw-Hill, 1964), 32.

CHRONIC WHITENESS

MARK WIGLEY

> Whitewash is extremely moral. Suppose there were a decree requiring all rooms in Paris to be given a coat of whitewash. I maintain that that would be a police task of real stature and a manifestation of high morality, the sign of a great people.
> —Le Corbusier, *The Decorative Art of Today*, 1925

A shocking call for compulsory whitening is made at the end of a key modernist manifesto. The pronouncement is associated with the signature whiteness of modern architecture—an aesthetic regime that was presented as a complete revolution of the built environment in the 1920s and became the unconscious default setting of everyday life. Le Corbusier didn't simply call for whitewash to be imposed by the police in the name of health. It was meant to act as a form of policing in its own right, a technology of surveillance that would put in motion an ever-expanding culture of self-policing. Whitewash exposes every dimension of life in front of it to judgment. It acts like "a court of assize in permanent session" that will "give a power of judgment to the individual," and thereby "make each one of us a prudent judge." Whiteness is both the effect and means of "cleaning" buildings, bodies, eyes, brains, and society to produce "pure," "clean," "clear," "bare," "neat," "sharp," "simple," "exact," "essential," "economical," "healthy" people, forms, and thoughts. Society, and even thinking itself, are threatened by an "epidemic" of unhealthy ornament that blurs the eye and harbors the dust and dirt that incubates disease. A "Law of Ripolin"—the brand name of the hard, impermeable,

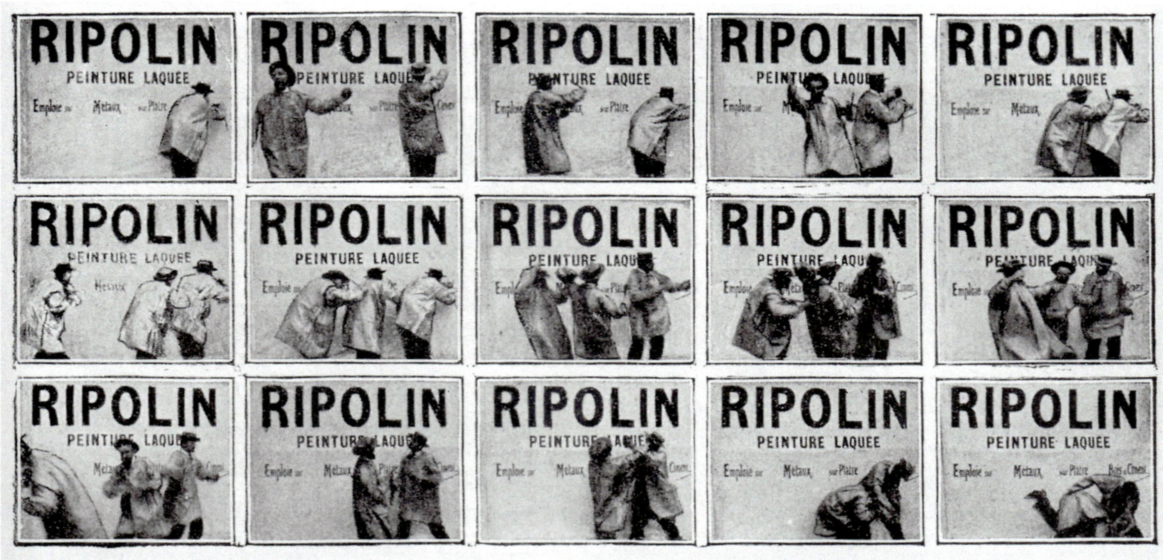

→ Stills from an advertising film for Ripolin paint made on a Paris boulevard wall by Félix Mesguich in October 1898, considered the inauguration of the advertising film genre, published in *Lectures pour tous—Revue Universelle Illustrée*, January 1900.

and washable enamel "sanitary paint" invented at the end of the nineteenth century, promoted for its antibacterial properties, and favored by hospitals—is needed to ensure that all interiors are coated in white to target any form of "dirt" or "darkness."

> Imagine the results of the Law of Ripolin. Every citizen is required to replace his hangings, his damasks, his wall-papers, his stencils, with a plain coat of white ripolin. *His home* is made clean. There are no more dirty, dark corners. *Everything is shown as it is.* Then comes *inner* cleanness, for the course adopted leads to refusal to allow anything at all which is not correct, authorized, intended, desired, thought-out: no action before thought. When you are surrounded with shadows and dark corners you are at home only as far as the hazy edges of the darkness your eyes cannot penetrate. You are not master in your own house. Once you have put ripolin on your walls you will be *master of yourself*.[1]

The white coat acts as a hinge between the visible and the invisible. Its smooth surface actively resists the unseen bacterial sources of disease.[2] It is a kind of inhospitality to disease. Yet this disinfecting medical function extends to visualizing any incomplete, imprecise, ill-considered, or overworked objects, behaviors, and even thoughts as forms of disease in their own right that need immediate cleansing treatment. Whiteness manufactures health, morality, and intelligence. A white room with a white table painted with Ripolin and topped with white porcelain is "healthy, clean, decent." The office of a modern factory that is "clear and rectilinear and painted with white ripolin" is a place of "healthy activity" and "industrious optimism." Cleaning the interior of buildings produces an "inner cleanliness" of the mind that ultimately cleanses society. Mastery of the self through the mastery of others.[3]

Le Corbusier's routinely authoritarian and often explicitly eugenic and fascist impulses, associations, and actions make him an easy target. But there are endless quieter, ultimately more controlling and insidious celebrations of whiteness in other hands. Le Corbusier is but a tip of the vast iceberg of whiteness. Indeed, what is most shocking about Le Corbusier's law, and the whole set of ideas that prop it up, is its complete lack of originality. Whitewash had been treated as a form of policing for centuries, particularly in the name of public health in the face of epidemic disease. Sick buildings, or buildings that sicken, are arguably as old as building itself. Architecture might even be the origin of human sickness and attempts to resist it, starting with whitewash. Indeed, whitewash is at the very origin of the delusion that the human is the being that can separate itself from the world.

Building Sickness

Ten thousand years ago in southwest Asia, the invention of freestanding rectilinear buildings established the Neolithic transition from small nomadic bands of hunter-gatherers foraging resources in 300–500 square kilometers to larger communities in settled agrarian villages domesticating themselves, other

↓ 10,800-year-old architecture in Kharaysin, Jordan, with newly invented right angles and polished white lime plaster floor—unpainted in the space on the right and painted with red in the adjacent space on the left.

→ Collapse of Neolithic spine initiated by tuberculosis infection, 2012.

animals, and plants in a much smaller territory. In a nonlinear process involving multiple erasures and reinventions of technologies and practices in disconnected times and places, the hunter-gathering base camp—typically consisting of semi-subterranean mud-lined oval spaces cut into a hillside with mud plaster floors and a wood and brush canopy overhead—was displaced by a new type of building constructed on top of the ground with a fully enclosed interior, internal divisions, and levels.[4] This new interior—of the building, adjacent buildings, and the surrounding domesticated environment—was a new architecture of transspecies community, a new microbial system. Pathogens thrived in this environment, and became increasingly endemic to its cultures. Infectious diseases like tuberculosis were marked for the first time as lesions on the skeletons of the inhabitants of these spaces. Human health dramatically declined. Settled humans got shorter.[5] Architecture slowly but dramatically remade the species that made it.

Yet the design of these Neolithic buildings also began to counter disease. The interior was formed by smooth white lime plaster, which disinfected while drawing all the surfaces of the newly quadrilateral system of floor, wall, and ceiling together into a continuous sealed skin.[6] Lime plaster was cutting-edge technology. Its production involved the largest single

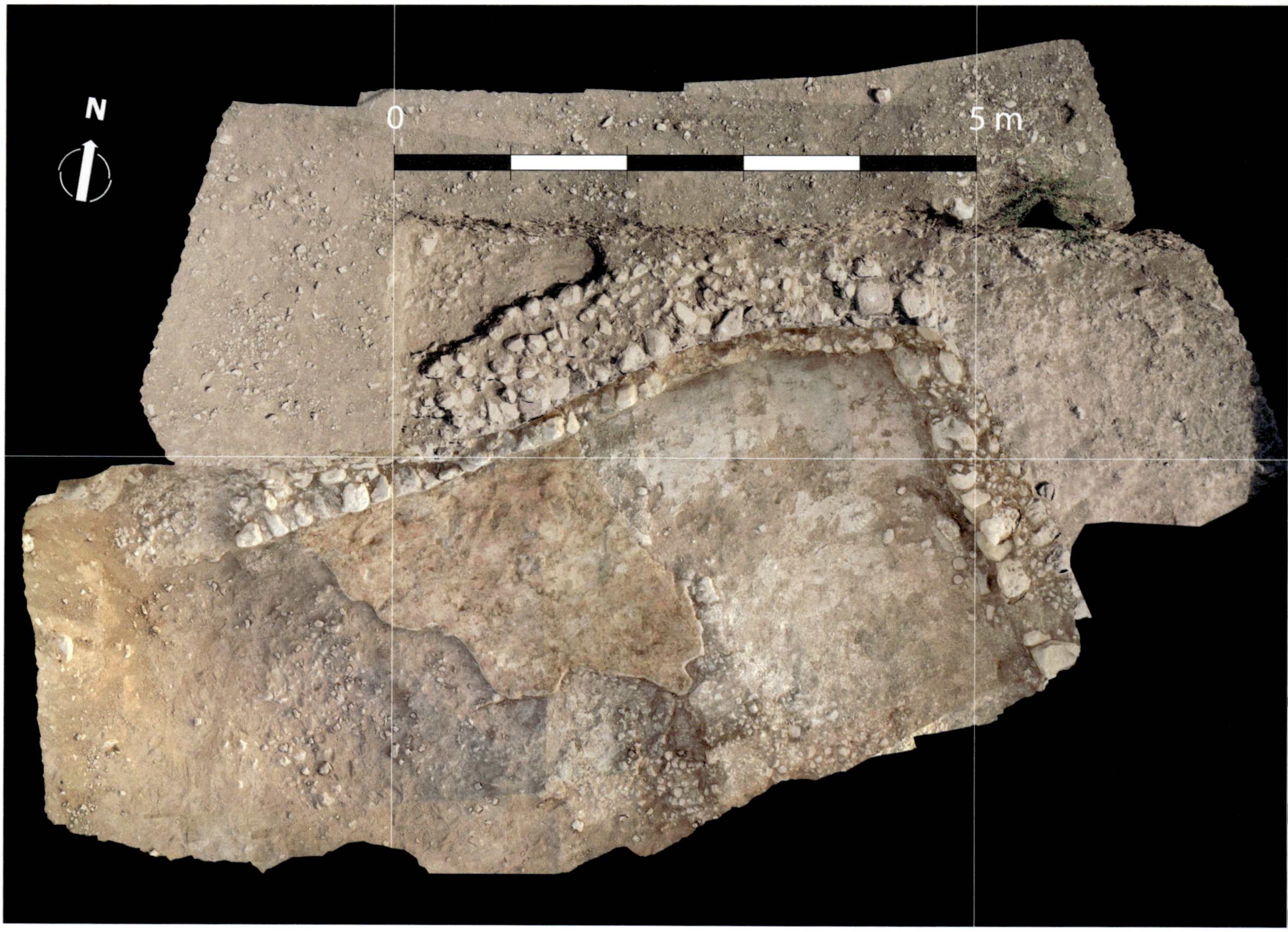

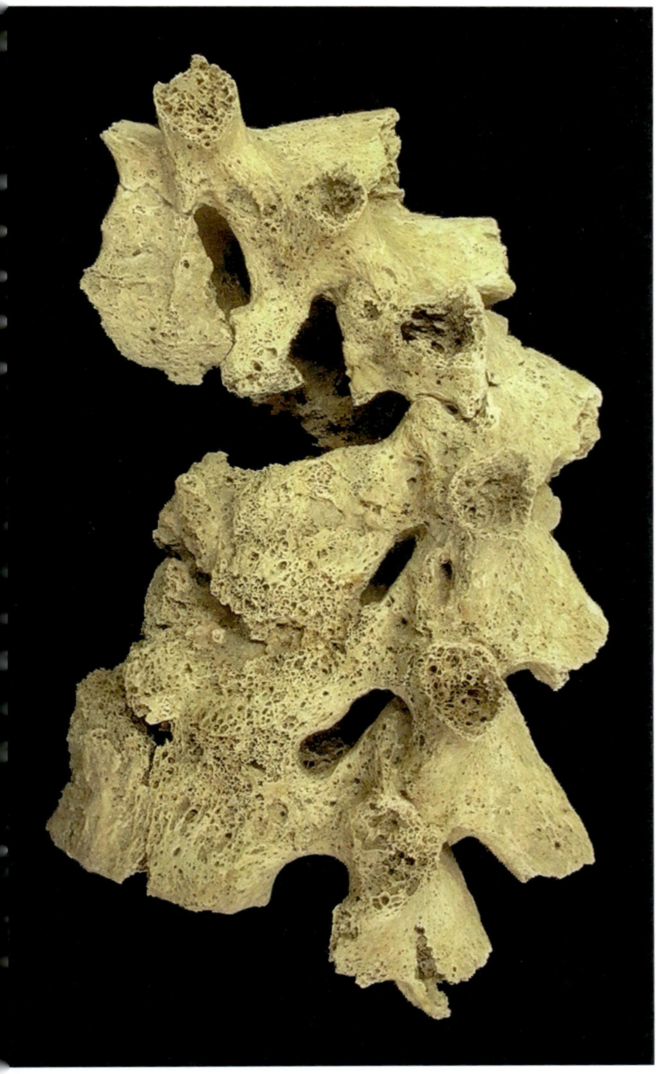

investment of collective energy in early societies. Rocks needed to be excavated, and an enormous amount of wood was needed to generate the days of extreme heat in the covered stone-lined pit that was necessary to catalyze the required chemical transformation to produce the first synthetic material. "Pure lime" manufactured a whiteness nowhere to be found in the environment. Like the newly invented right angles of buildings, it constituted a whole new environment, a visual field and way of seeing. Never simply a background, it acted as a central focus of life, crafting the daily intersection between living body and building, between life and death. Human and nonhuman bodies were buried within the white surfaces of buildings, and body parts, like skulls, were modeled in white plaster to occupy the interior as if fellow inhabitants.[7] Interiors were divided between clean and dirty zones, a distinction that whiteness made visible.[8] It is not that architecture was whitened; it was only architecture inasmuch as it was white.

Architecture has remained white ever since, shockingly white in the sense that it systematically blackens, rendering multiple forms of others visible as other, producing otherness and thereby sustaining hierarchies of exclusion and subordination. In almost all its diverse forms, times, and places, architecture represents stability, certainty, security, comfort, and order, but only through otherings, outings, and downings. The very idea of an interior is the effect of this everyday violence. Architecture is never simply complicit with authority. Authority without architecture might not even be thinkable. Yet this structural and structuring violence is rarely made visible to those it serves by so relentlessly forcing others to serve.

The whiteness of architecture pulsates. Whiteness is not a fixed thing but the idea of a fixed thing constructed by repetition. It is repeated not just through endless rewhitenings, but in the belief that each rewhitening is a whole new beginning, a return to zero. It paradoxically takes a huge labor to construct a surface that is seen to precede all making, all history even, as a nonstatement statement—the belief that whiteness is blankness (literally from the word *blanc*). To experience white as zero requires both the great effort to manufacture whiteness and a parallel labor to deny that effort. Paradoxically, then, white keeps returning as that which is supposedly already there, preceding the history it reveals.

Skin Police

The canon of so-called Western architecture is whiter than the white surfaces that punctuate the successive Egyptian, Phoenician, Hellenic, and Roman systems that fed its "foundational" texts.[9] Vitruvius's scrolls are dedicated to the question of "healthfulness" and give lengthy technical descriptions of how to make and apply lime in combination with other materials, either for structure as mortar or surfaces as calibrated layers of plaster. Architecture's whiteness, however, is not the white surfaces that accentuate any pigment or pattern added to them. The real whiteness of architecture is in its systematic exclusions and subordinations, its regimes of privilege. A white-colored architecture, therefore, does not necessarily impose whiteness, or may only do so in an uneven way. Critical discourse about whiteness risks giving the color itself the magical, universal authority being critiqued.

Leon Battista Alberti's pivotal mid-fifteenth-century treatise on architecture, *De re aedificatoria*, for example, echoes Vitruvius in starting with a long section on the question of healthy building. Vitruvius gave particular attention to the ways that design can control air, light, and water to avoid making "pestilent places" and even cure "epidemics" in otherwise "plague-ridden regions."[10] Buildings can either resist or succumb to sickness, and thereby shape the mental character and behavior of those who live there. Architecture shapes body and mind by defining the physical and visual environment. Alberti goes even further, citing the very first germ theory of contagious disease by the Roman agriculturalist Marcus Varro in 30 BCE: that plague is caused by "tiny atom-like creatures" that can float in the air and enter the

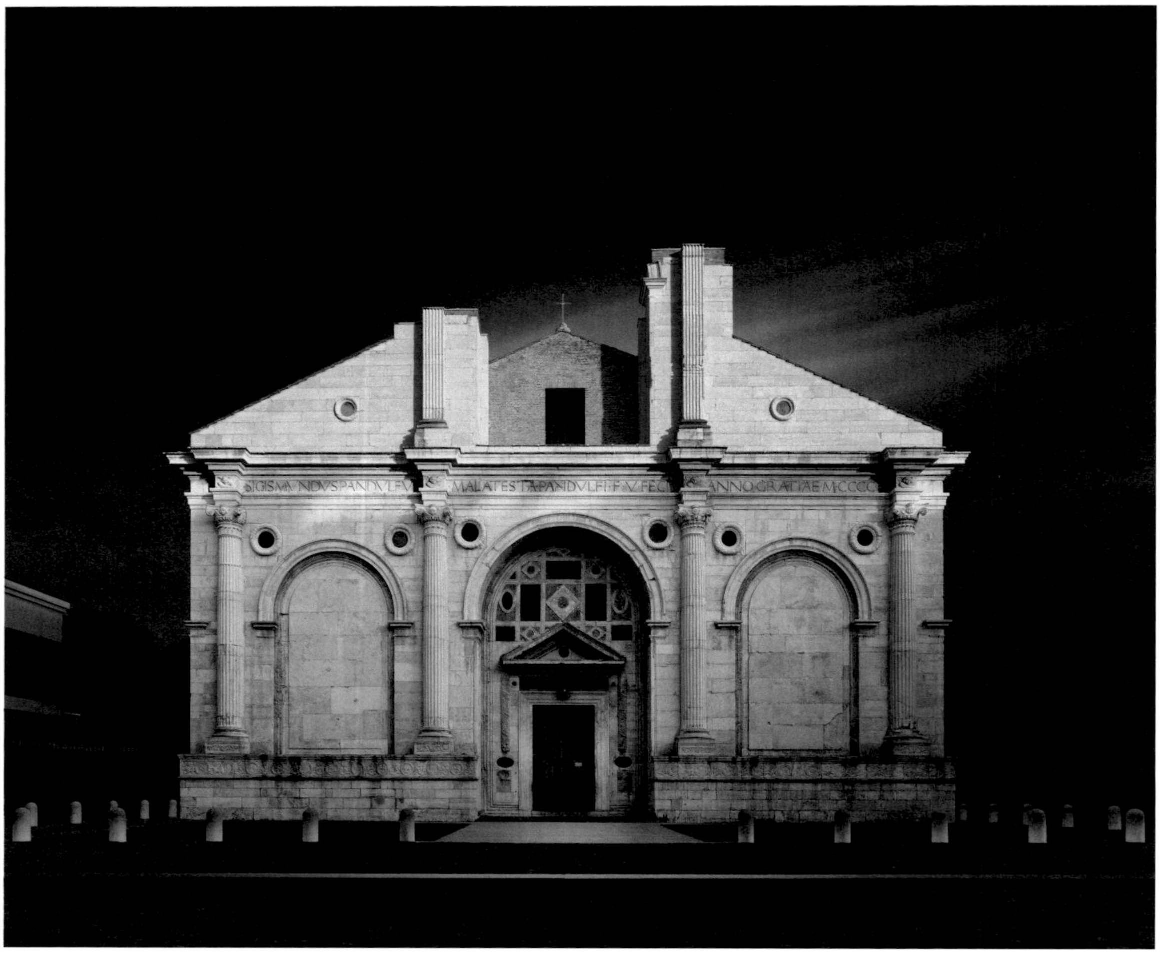

← Front facade of Malatesta Temple, 1450–1466, Rimini, designed by Leon Battista Alberti.

body through the nose or mouth. Even healthy and health-giving buildings in healthy locations can be infected by those coming from diseased places.[11] This calls for regimes of organization that extend beyond the purest air, light, and water to include a purification of contact with people.[12] These cleansing and controlling regimes are ultimately framed in terms of the idealized purity of whiteness.

Alberti's treatise gives precise instructions on how to manufacture lime plaster to produce the smoothest and whitest surface possible to "gleam with an amazing sparkle" and "achieve a sheen superior to that of marble." Purification against disease is linked with purification of the eye and mind. The last of the ten books that form Alberti's treatise invokes Cicero's argument from Plato that the distractions of ornament should be excluded from temples in favor of purity, simplicity, and the sacred color white. Not by chance was Alberti's first church building—the unfinished Malatesta Temple in Rimini, commissioned during the last years of writing the treatise—polemically white on its main facade, sides, and interior.[13] A symbol of the Renaissance, it attempted to reconstitute the classical architecture of antiquity by wrapping a new all-white skin around the outside and inside of an existing thirteenth-century Gothic church.

Alberti's writings mobilized this "renewal" of an imagined white system to explicitly misogynist ends in a discourse that unites health, cleanliness, neatness, beauty, and morality—with the control of women directly linked to the control of architectural surfaces. The body of the building, itself conceived as feminine, must be defined by what appears to be an inherent whiteness rather than an added layer. The art of layering plaster, then, is to conceal the very existence of layers so that whiteness is experienced as a given rather than a manufactured effect. Likewise, wives treated as property are prohibited from whitening their faces with chalk. The beauty of their purity has to be conveyed by their own whiteness rather than an added layer of makeup:

> You'll not poison yourself or whiten your face to make yourself seem more beautiful for me. You are white and bright enough complexioned for me as you are. Rather, like the Alberti girls, you will just wash and keep clean with water alone. My dear wife, there is no one but me for you to think of pleasing in this matter.[14]

Whiteness, understood as hygiene and control, is both what judges and what is judged. At the same time, Alberti detaches himself from his ancient Greek sources by condemning the ongoing slave trade in Florence.[15] Hierarchies of all kinds are the very ambition of his texts, and especially of architecture, but he portrays slavery as a sickness of society that extracts all it values most for itself from the enslaved.[16] A light-skinned slave would effectively be coded dark in such an extractive transformation of person to property, but the specific racializations involved in Alberti's white are not so easily recognizable by contemporary discourse based on the transatlantic slave trade from Africa that had yet to begin.[17] As a child, Alberti had been forced to leave Genoa with his father to escape the devastating plague that killed his mother. Not by chance, then, did his treatise on architecture refer to the fact that the Genoese colony of Pera (Istanbul) was always prone to the plague because the slaves brought there (mainly from the East and later from Africa) were "sick of soul and neglected of body, wasting away from idleness and filth." Yet the expansion of the Italian slave trade in the fourteenth century that increased the multiplicity of skin colors perceived as shadings relative to white within the domestic interior was precisely driven by the recent decimation of labor by the plague—as if two kinds of sickness fed on each other.[18]

What counts about whiteness is not its visibility as such but the specific concept of health, and who or what it constructs through inclusions and exclusions. There is no apolitical concept of health; no natural body or brain waiting to be cared for or abandoned by medicine and architecture that is not already an effect of those biopolitical regimes. The idea of a healthy architecture is always about the health of a small group relative to multiple others, but is routinely made in the name of all. Appeals to what would be good for the entire human species, then, are actually made as part of a project to refuse humanity to the majority. Whiteness is at the heart of this refusal. The exclusionary logic of white is that no skin is ever white enough. A white skin may make less of a mark but it still makes a mark. The skin of buildings will always be whiter than the skins of those admitted into them, let alone those who are excluded and subordinated but forced to labor on their construction and maintenance. Indeed, having a lighter skin is treated as the marker of those that most need the prosthetic defense of architecture. Whiteness is coded as a fragility requiring protection through continual acts of preemptive violence. Whiteness is not a thing but a defense and deployment of power over others.

The whiteness of architecture that is integral to the more recent four centuries of slavery, for example, is not simply in the white surfaces of buildings. Racialization participates in this longer millennial history of white, in which architecture is never simply whitened but is the very effect of whiteness.[19] Calls for racial justice are calls to undo, resist, transgress, and confuse architecture. This cannot be honored by a design community unwilling to go beyond patronizing and ultimately imprisoning forms of inclusion under the banner of diversity and ultimately demolish its own exclusionary house. Justice against the violence of whiteness is a matter of undoing the house, de-policing the borders, multiplying the possible spaces of reflection and action, and a real diversity of sustained reparations. Part of such an urgent yet sustained collective project is to confront the way the exclusionary and subordinating ideology of the white surface operates in its own absence. More precisely, it is to comprehend the lethal force of the way white flickers, as seemingly the most fragile skin assumes the force of law.

The Nonwhiteness of White

It may seem irresponsible to make such implausibly millennial, monolithic, and monocultural claims about the whiteness of architecture here, yet this is precisely how the discourse around whiteness operates and needs to be confronted. A unique kind of history and theory has to be developed to account for the extended chain of historically specific appeals to the supposedly transhistorical qualities of whiteness. The aura of the transhistorical cannot be wished away by dedicated scholarly attention to the specificities of time, place, and culture. On the contrary, specificities only expose the imagined force of the transhistorical and material effects of that imagination.

Appeals to whiteness are never singular. Each invocation of whiteness involves a repetition of repetitions of repetitions—with each pulse as it were reverberating across time and space. Whiteness in Le Corbusier's *The Decorative Art of Today*, for example, is simultaneously the most modern thing to do, the very symptom of modernity, and the most ancient of gestures. The appeal to whiteness as law is framed as an appeal to the transhistorical condition of architecture itself. As with most classical architectural treatises, every making of architecture is understood as a remaking of its origin:

> Whitewash has been associated with human habitation since the birth of mankind. Stones are burnt, crushed and thinned with water—and the walls take on the purest white, an extraordinarily beautiful white.[20]

Whitewash and humanity invent each other. Le Corbusier's argument was first published in a late 1923 issue of *L'Esprit Nouveau*, the polemical magazine that he edited with fellow "purist" painter and writer Amédée Ozenfant.[21] The text condemned the complex forms, colors, and the exoticism of contemporary decoration as intoxicating "poisons" that lack "health" or connection with a "healthy life," and prescribed the treatment of this sickness with a "purifying" trajectory toward "simplicity," a displacement of the figure of the decorator in favor of the architect. The prescription was not yet formulated as the "Law of Ripolin," but the text was immediately preceded by a celebration of stripping down multicolored interior walls to "pure ripolin" in order to think. Le Corbusier first talked about the need for a "law of whitening" (*loi du blanchiment*) in an early 1923 interview that presented it as a cleansing moral act to expunge decorative art in favor of a "purity" of body, eye, and brain:

> This is a necessity both moral and material. It is necessary to establish the law of whitening. This cleanliness makes one see the objects in their sincere truth: hence in perfect purity. Remember the term: it defines a whole discipline. It implies a certain nudity. These trifles, these small pieces of furniture, these futilities of decorative art, are intrusive and indiscreet.[22]

In the same moment Le Corbusier was making these claims, he was designing a house that was polemically white and modeled as such—the Villa Besnus in Vaucresson, made for a client who had been impressed by the all-white plaster model of the Maison Citrohan exhibited at the Salon d'automne in 1922.[23] Yet the law of white, or whiteness as law, was never about every surface being white. Already in mid-1923 when finishing the house, Le Corbusier was starting to add other colors to more celebrated projects that were originally conceived as white—the Ozenfant Atelier, Villa La Roche, and the Petit Maison for his parents on Lake Geneva.[24] These projects continued to be seen as white because of their exteriors, but were in fact "colored" on many interior surfaces. In all of Le Corbusier's polemical work with his partner Pierre Jeanneret, white was always surrounded by other colors. Indeed, Le Corbusier argued that this magnified the whiteness, radiating it outward. He repeatedly argued that a building needed other colors to be white: "To tell the truth, my house will only appear white when I have placed the driving forces of colors and values in the right places. ... The white, which makes you think clearly, is supported by the powerful tonicity of the color."[25] Paradoxically, an all-white building is unable to radiate whiteness.[26]

Furthermore, Le Corbusier's architecture was, in fact, never really white. Its surfaces were more of a cream or eggshell color.[27] While proselytizing whitewash and Ripolin, Le Corbusier was actually using neither, and instead working obsessively to find the right unpainted plaster to get a particular smooth, resilient, off-white finish.[28] Buildings don't need the whitest white or even a single white surface to be white. Just the thought that there is such a surface somewhere, acting as the background against which everything else in the world is judged, is enough. And ultimately, this surface doesn't even need to be on site somewhere; it could even be in history, revealing and judging everything that comes after it. The Law of Ripolin is only necessary as a reminder of a lost sense of whiteness.

Le Corbusier's 1925 book actually talks of "two laws": a law of whitewash and a Law of Ripolin. One is the law of vernacular architecture that all architecture has been whitewashed since the beginning of habitation—a law that doesn't have to be framed as a law since it is so habitually self-enforced. The other is the formal law requiring a modern white to reactivate the unspoken sense of the first law that has been lost. Each gets a dedicated section in the last chapter of the book, and each is represented by a photograph at the end of the argument. The first law is represented by a photograph of "Sultan Mahembe and his two sons. Three black heads against a white background, fit to govern, to dominate ... an open door through which we can see true grandeur." The second law is represented by a full-page image of the "Studio of M. Ozenfant."

The passage between these two images of white space that end and summarize the whole argument of the book is a passage from far to near, other to

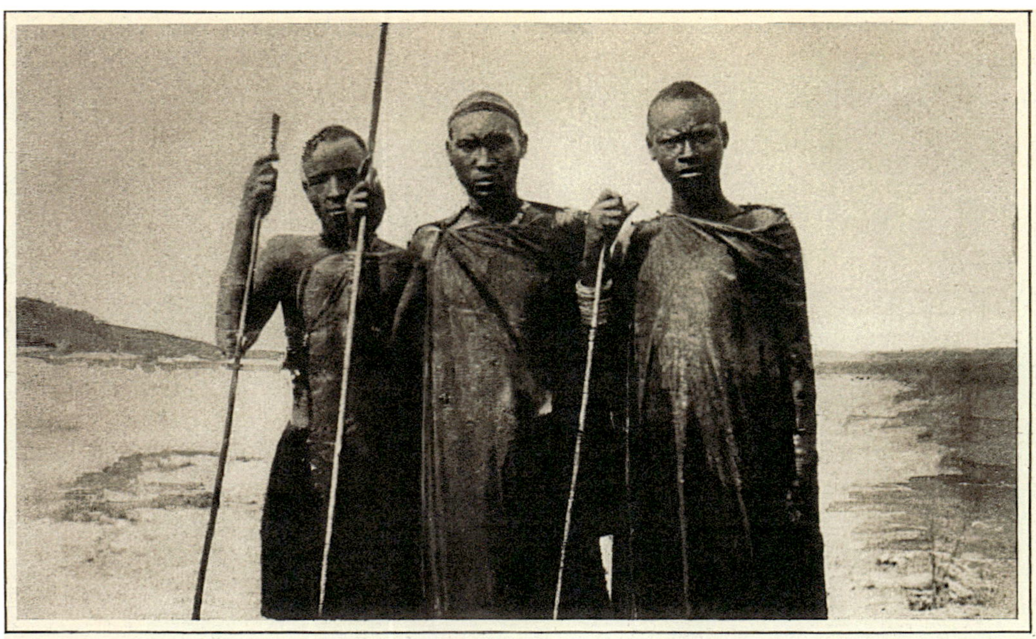

↙ Sultan Mahembe and his two sons, seen near Lake Tanganyika.

→ Le Corbusier and Pierre Jeanneret, studio for Amédée Ozenfant, 1923.

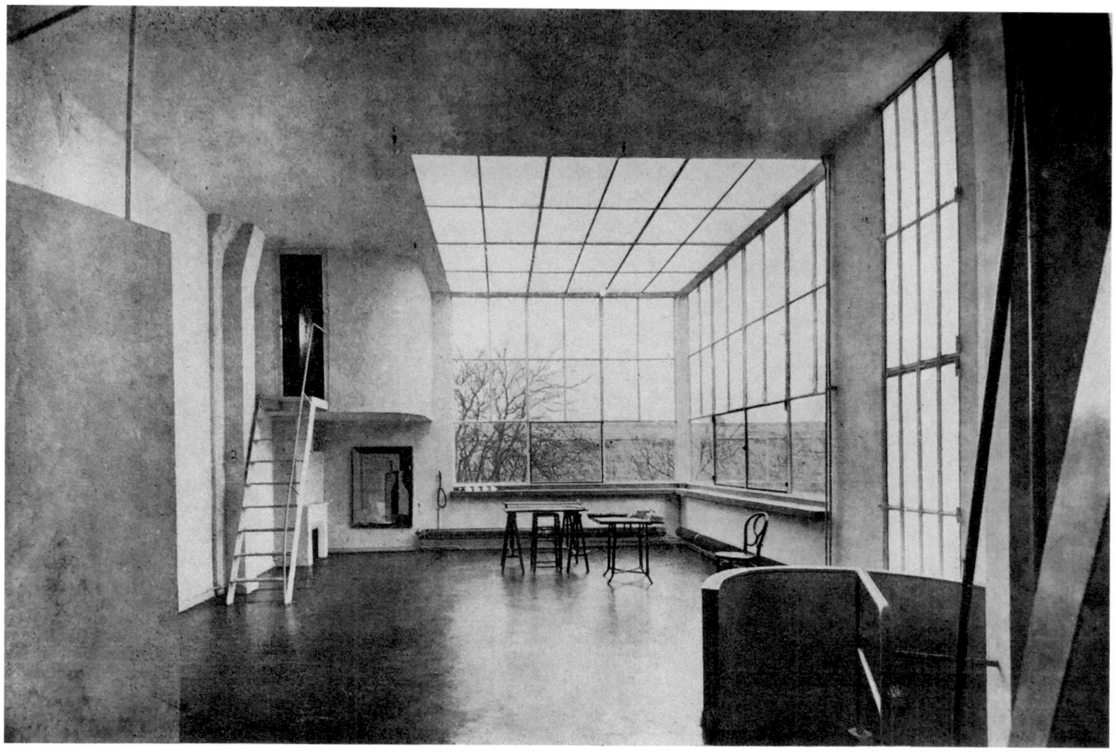

same, history to present, black to white, south to north, east to west, outside to inside, reception to production, field to laboratory. The first image appears respectful of the designated distant, external others; respectful of their status as leaders and referring to them by name. But in designating the figures as "black heads," and without feeling the need to designate Ozenfant or himself as white, or even to present Ozenfant in his habitat, Le Corbusier finally rules over the scene with a patronizing orientalist eye driven by fear of what it would mean for the figures to come inside, into the present, into the north, or even to lurk in the dark, as the dark. This act of exposure, of being exhibited against white, as if in a gallery, is already an imprisoning. The prison is invented by the photograph itself; its overexposed background renders the land, water, and sky as a seamless white space.

In the first image, the human figures are treated as an artwork on display against a "white background." In the second image, the white has become the figure. It is an image of the background becoming art, since the whiteness of the interior walls, ceiling, ladder, and fireplace seemingly fuse with the white sky seen through the windows and reflected in the floor. A white surface is suspended within white. It is as if the whiteness of the sky is becoming architecture, or rather the reverse: the slightly off-white interior is framing and producing the perceived whiteness of the sky, since skies are only rarely white. The white interior manufactures the sense of a white background—an effect that is itself framed by the nonwhite surfaces in the foreground and the floor. The darker floor that whitens the room that whitens the sky echoes the similarly darker landscape outside that marks the whiteness above it as sky. The culmination of all this is the three intersecting planes of gridded glass that produce a sense of a perfected white cubic form somehow suspended between inside and outside. Both sky and room appear relative to this idealized space. This already complex layered effect is magnified by the fact that this white-in-white or white-making-whiter space is a studio for making art, as marked by the two drawing tables bathing in the white and one of Ozenfant's purist paintings on the wall next to them.[29] It is precisely not the image of an empty space, but an image of laboring in, under, and with white. White is never a given. It is a permanent labor—an ongoing repetitive work of exclusion.

Le Corbusier had taken the matching image of Sultan Mahembe and his two sons from an article entitled "In the Heart of East Africa" published in a May 1924 issue of the Swiss weekly magazine *L'Illustré*.[30] It portrayed the region on the eastern edge of the vast Lake Tanganyika as a site of continuous violent extraction by outsiders. The title "Sultan" itself already marks the majority Muslim religion that was brought inland via the slave-trading routes linked to the sultanate established on the coast starting in the tenth century.[31] The photograph was taken by a member of a Swiss geological team that presumably had his eyes on other forms of extraction. Like Le Corbusier, the article speaks in respectful tones of the "majesty" of the local chiefs, but also shows images of tribesmen carrying the bags of the white and white-clad visitors who appear like newly arrived chiefs. The more radical implication of Le Corbusier's

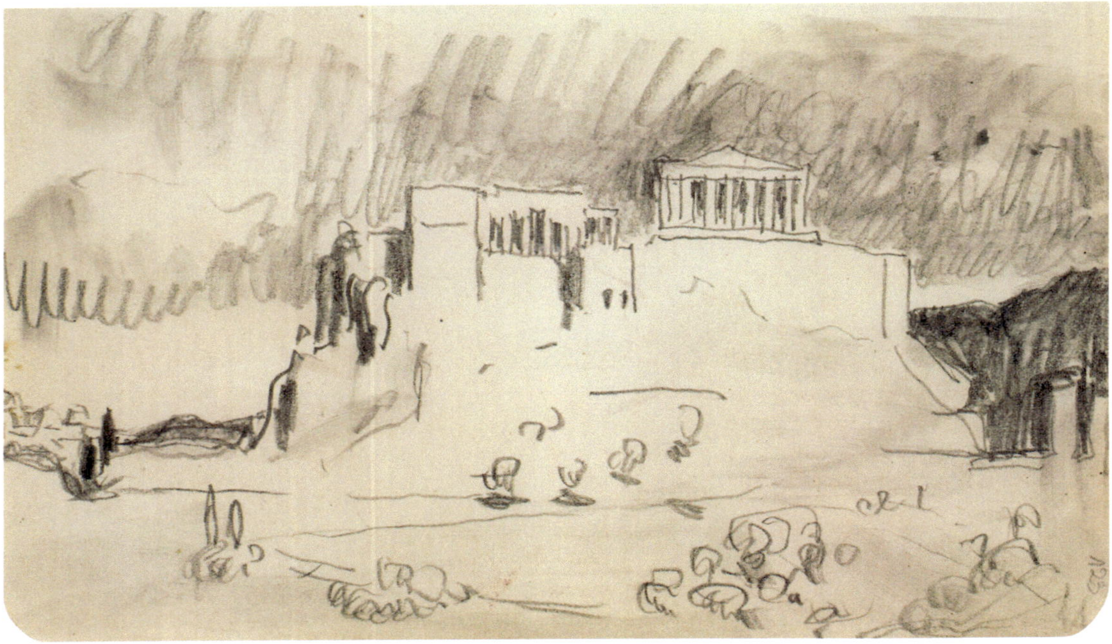

← Charles-Édouard Jeanneret, the Acropolis, Athens, September 1911.

→ Cover of *Le Petit Journal*, December 1, 1912.

use of this image and the narrative framing it is that white is a black invention that has steadily whitened its inventors or acted as a self-selecting eugenic filter. As if humans constructed the background that acts as the laboratory and engine of their own self-willed evolution by rendering them newly dark. The newly produced sense of "shades" of skin is experienced as degrees of distance from white, treated as degrees of distance from humanity and from the present.

White Fever

It was, after all, during the extended "Voyage d'Orient" of 1911 (including the Balkans and Greece, but especially Turkey) that Charles-Édouard Jeanneret, the young architect from a small mountain town in Switzerland who would a decade later rename himself "Le Corbusier," became "besotted with white" and convinced that the future of architecture was white.[32] Whiteness is discovered in the lands of the nonwhite; of those seen to be closer to deep human history and therefore to be admired and learned from. In fact, the very point of going to the East was to encounter its "great white walls" as an antidote to the self-absorbed decadence of architecture in the North.[33] The whole voyage of discovering white is dominated by the experience of its designated others. Jeanneret's travel notebooks and published narratives repeatedly offer descriptions of dirt, filth, smell, vermin, bedbugs, nausea, diarrhea, fever, delirium, disorientation, epidemic disease, and death, only to portray their erasure by the sight of "majestic," "bare," "raw," "impassive," "beautiful," "sparkling," "bright," "shining," "dazzling and astounding," "blinding," "brilliant," "great," "triumphal" white. This repeated oscillation between disease and whiteness culminates in the experience of being held for four days in a "stinking quarantine" on the island of St. George because of the cholera epidemic "sweeping all the East." After his release, Jeanneret spent two weeks in Athens daily studying and famously canonizing the Parthenon, as if the building's apparent whiteness had absorbed and perfected all the lessons of the East.

The whiteness of the Parthenon was never as simple as it appeared. The building, constructed in the fifth century BCE, was originally a fully polychromed pagan temple, which was turned into a Christian church around the fifth century CE after a devastating fire had collapsed the roof and the building was substantially reorganized. The iconoclastic use of whitewash was followed by the successive addition of painted frescos and mosaics, especially in the twelfth century. These additions were themselves whitewashed over by another iconoclastic act to turn the building into an Ottoman mosque in the mid-fifteenth century.[34] The mosque was destroyed in 1687 when a Venetian missile launched from a nearby hill detonated the massive supply of gunpowder stored inside, tearing apart the building along with hundreds of soldiers and citizens. The Venetians were unable to hold Athens because the plague arrived at the same time as they did, so the ruins of the Parthenon came to house another smaller whitewashed domed mosque that was built in the eighteenth century using many of the dispersed stones, and which was only removed once it too collapsed ten years after Greece had become independent from the Ottoman Empire in 1832. The Acropolis was a site of every form of whitewashing, and the image of its supposedly eternal abstract beauty is the precise effect of whitewashing this fact.

Even for Jeanneret, the building's white was not as transcendent as advertised. The Parthenon itself had been infected like those dying around it. Feeling ill, drinking too much resin wine in the hope

Le Petit Journal

ADMINISTRATION
61, RUE LAFAYETTE, 61
Les manuscrits ne sont pas rendus
On s'abonne sans frais
dans tous les bureaux de poste

5 CENT. SUPPLÉMENT ILLUSTRÉ 5 CENT.
23me Année — Numéro 1.150
DIMANCHE 1er DÉCEMBRE 1912

ABONNEMENTS

	SIX MOIS	UN AN
SEINE et SEINE-ET-OISE..	2 fr.	3 fr. 50
DÉPARTEMENTS..........	2 fr.	4 fr. »
ÉTRANGER	2 50	5 fr. »

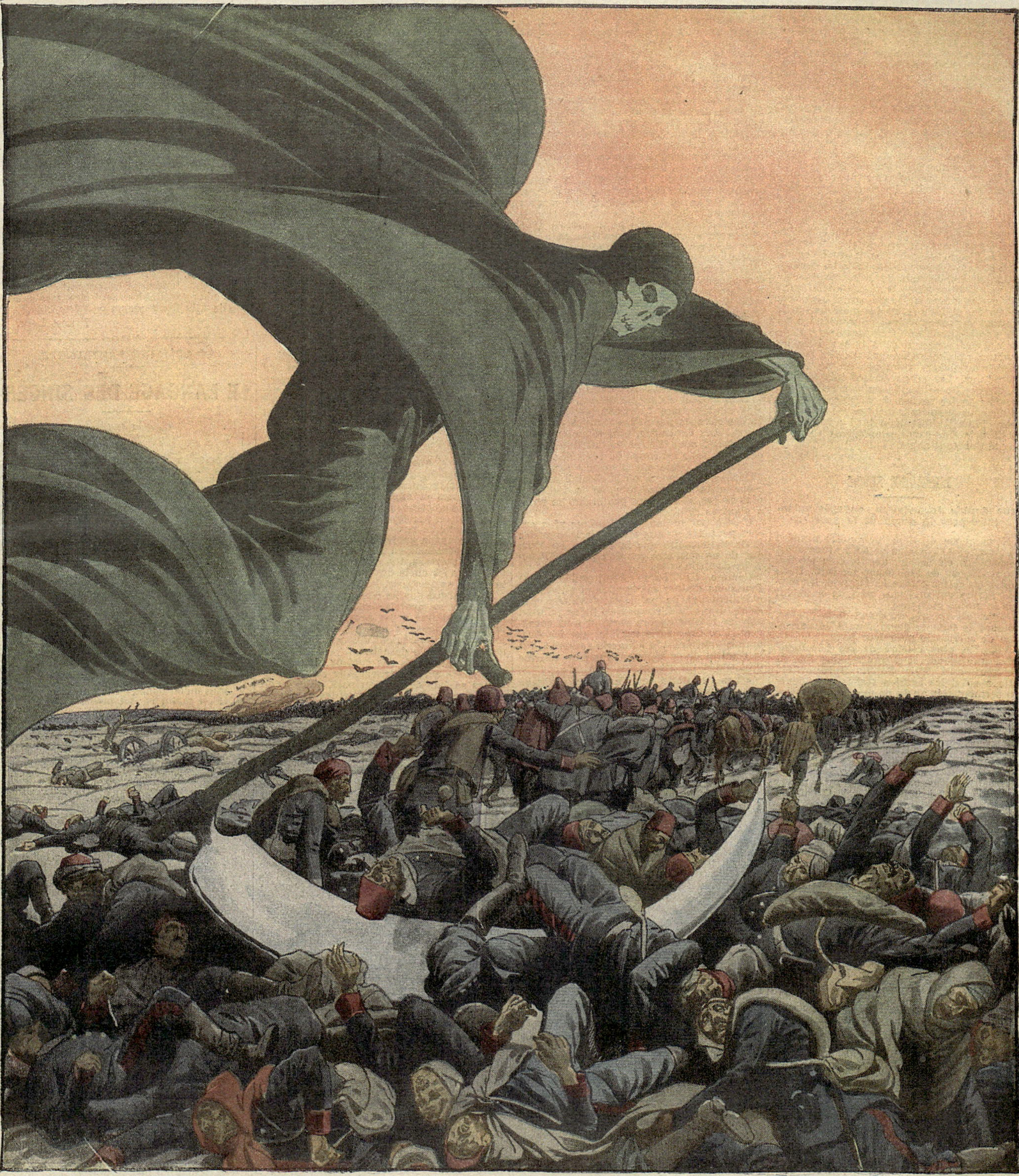

LE CHOLÉRA

of resisting cholera, and disgusted by the sight of dead bodies being transported through the streets covered in flies, Jeanneret started to see the building itself "like a corpse," with all its parts strewn across the hill. Halfway during his stay in Athens, his travel notes describe a growing aversion to visiting the building, as "every hour it grows more deadly up there."[35] Jeanneret expresses nostalgia for the more intact and mesmerizing whiteness of the great mosques and vernacular houses of Constantinople (Istanbul) that had been so inspirational during the longest stay of the voyage—and had always been imagined as the real destination of the whole trip. The combined effect of the traditional whitewashing protocols of houses and the impositions of Ottoman law on all religious spaces made whiteness an urban principle and effect defining the whole city, one that Jeanneret hoped to experience long before arriving.[36] But cholera was also raging there. The seven-week stay in Constantinople ended when he "ran off to Athens" to escape it immediately after a hundred people contracted the deadly disease on a single day. He was treated as a "young Turk" needing an onboard quarantine at the mouth of the Black Sea when leaving, but the disease seemed to be closing in on him when he finally arrived in Athens after the much longer second quarantine. Even the Parthenon had succumbed.

Jeanneret eventually acquiesced to a celebration of the building's triumphant transhistorical condition and its "monochromy!" that would be echoed countless times in his subsequent polemics and associated by readers with the supposed civilizing whiteness of the Greeks.[37] Yet this mythical base of the Western tradition and the associated cult of aesthetic and bodily purity was, for Jeanneret, a message from the East, the work of darker skins. Jeanneret explicitly rejected the "European legend" that the East is "unclean." Far from "filthy," it was "in fact, quite clean." The first symptom of cultural life and the precondition for all art is, he claimed, cleaning, and was represented by vernacular seasonal whitewashing in the East. The real disease, accordingly, is the current form of international industrial culture broadcast from Europe. The necessary purification of international design is a "recovery" of the healthy origins of architecture and culture to be found where skins are not white. Not by chance did *The Decorative Art of Today* end with a description and even a map of the tour as a "confession," citing the travel notebooks about the "deadly germ" of ornament that was even infecting the traditional whitewashed architecture of the East. It must be treated everywhere by a "cleaning out," to "return, yes, to health and thereby to beauty."

This cleansing of infection had to be applied to its very source, following the all-too-religious logic of self-purification. The East was to be treated by its own medicine. What Le Corbusier mined and extracted from those perceived as people of color is the very whiteness that marks "them" as colored in the first place, and thereby distanced from a purified modernity and a supposedly colorless superhumanity that doesn't even need to name itself white as it designs itself to rule, to be the rule. This extractive and ultimately punitive logic would become most obvious in Le Corbusier's projects in North Africa where, for example, Algerian Arabs were to be disciplined, cleansed, and subordinated by the whiteness of their own "inspiring," "so clean, so measured" vernacular architecture: "Algiers-the-white."[38] Le Corbusier's turn to white was always driven by this colonial gesture of framing, claiming, and maiming. A celebration of nonwhiteness or blackness is but the first step in a call for whiteness to overrule it.[39]

Jeanneret had explicitly disparaged the white skin of Ripolin in 1908 when writing to his first mentor, Charles L'Éplattenier soon after leaving his hometown, but emphatically embraced it when disparaging both L'Éplattenier and decorative art on his return home from the East in 1911. He then insisted that all architecture should be white, as if religiously converted by all the white houses, monasteries, and mosques he had just visited. Upon his return, he moved into the upper level of a whitewashed vernacular barn, specifying "very white walls" for the interior renovation. The 1912 house, with which the young architect bankrupted his parents, was even called the "Maison Blanche," with its cladding in hexagonal white tiles and all-white master bedroom with a blue floor for the parents opposite the all-white studio for Jeanneret himself. The house received the purifying whiteness and nudity of the East: "it was white and naked: I had traveled."[40] Yet it took another ten years for the white plaster Maison Citrohan model to fully capture the principles that would define Le Corbusier's canonical work, work that was self-consciously presented as a quasi-religious stripping away of the offensive seductions of material imagery in favor of a cleansing immateriality of white. "Let us be iconoclasts," concludes *The Decorative Art of Today*'s opening assault on the disease of decoration that "thrives and spreads as virulently as a cancer." Whitewash is at once a medical and theological-philosophical procedure—a "purification" ritual. Not simply the cleansing of diseased and disease-producing architecture, but cleansing itself, whiteness, as architecture.

Sanitary Law

Le Corbusier was in no way a pioneer of white nor claimed to be. On the contrary, the unoriginality of white was the point. The polemical arguments, models, and constructions were never the beginning of modernizing architecture but the end of a long line of white architects doing white, including, to name but a few examples, Adolf Loos, Josef Hoffmann, Joseph Maria Olbrich, Leopold Bauer, Otto Wagner, Josef Frank, Charles Rennie Mackintosh, Margaret McDonald, Charles Voysey, and Edward Godwin.[41] All had celebrated vernacular whitewash and progressively moved the sanitary smooth white surfaces of hospitals and sanatoria into all building types. Each had explicitly theorized white as such, under the inspiration of the mid-nineteenth-century sanitary reform movement led by figures like Florence Nightingale with her call for "pure, white, polished, non-absorbent cement," light, ventilation, and removal of all extraneous fittings, furniture, and ornament in hospitals and homes.

The "white" architecture of the 1920s drew on countless experiments in whitening buildings in the name of health. This included the use of Ripolin that had already become standard in clinics, hospital wards, and sanatoria rooms at the turn of the century. In 1899, for example, the Touring-Club de France, inspired by one of its 75,000 cyclist members who was a doctor, started a campaign for an easily disinfected "hygienic room" in hotels that would be Ripolin-lined with minimal furnishings and no ornament or fabrics to attract microbes.[42] Hotel rooms were treated as hotspots for contagion because travelers would inevitably pick up the feared pathogens deposited by previous unknown guests. Given the largely upper-middle-class membership of the club, this anxiety about disease was also class anxiety, a fear of the unclean other. The tourist was to be mobile yet isolated by a prophylactic whiteness that would itself travel in advance.

The Touring-Club first exhibited a prototype "white room" with toilette and bathroom spaces designed by Gustave Rives at the 1900 Exposition Universelle in Paris—strategically placed just inside the entrance of the Palais de l'hygiène and next to the display of all known pathogenic microbes in the Salon Pasteur. The design had been approved by a committee of prominent medical experts, was seen by hundreds of thousands of visitors, and was awarded the gold prize by the international jury. It reportedly looked "like a hospital room" with its complete medicinal arsenal: Ripolin paint on all surfaces; no gaps, fabrics, cornice or moldings; curved transitions between floors, walls, and ceiling; minimalist bentwood and metal furniture; and large windows. Every element was presented as a form of resistance to disease-causing microbes. The whiteness was even said to expose insects intruding into the "hygienic nest."[43] The club distributed a detailed document for hotels on how to produce a Ripolin-lined interior that reads like a manifesto for modern architecture, insisting on sunlight, air, ventilation, simplicity, and smooth washable whiteness without any gaps, protrusions, or ornament.[44] Whitewash could be used instead of the much-preferred Ripolin, they stated, but only if it was renewed each year. All surfaces had to be continually disinfected, but the whiteness would encourage cleaning, since "stains are more likely to appear." The wooden writing and dressing tables, toilet, curtains, mattress covers, and linen all had to be washable white. Even the chimneypiece had to be made of plain white marble to show all dirt and foster cleaning. The additional light that reflected off white surfaces

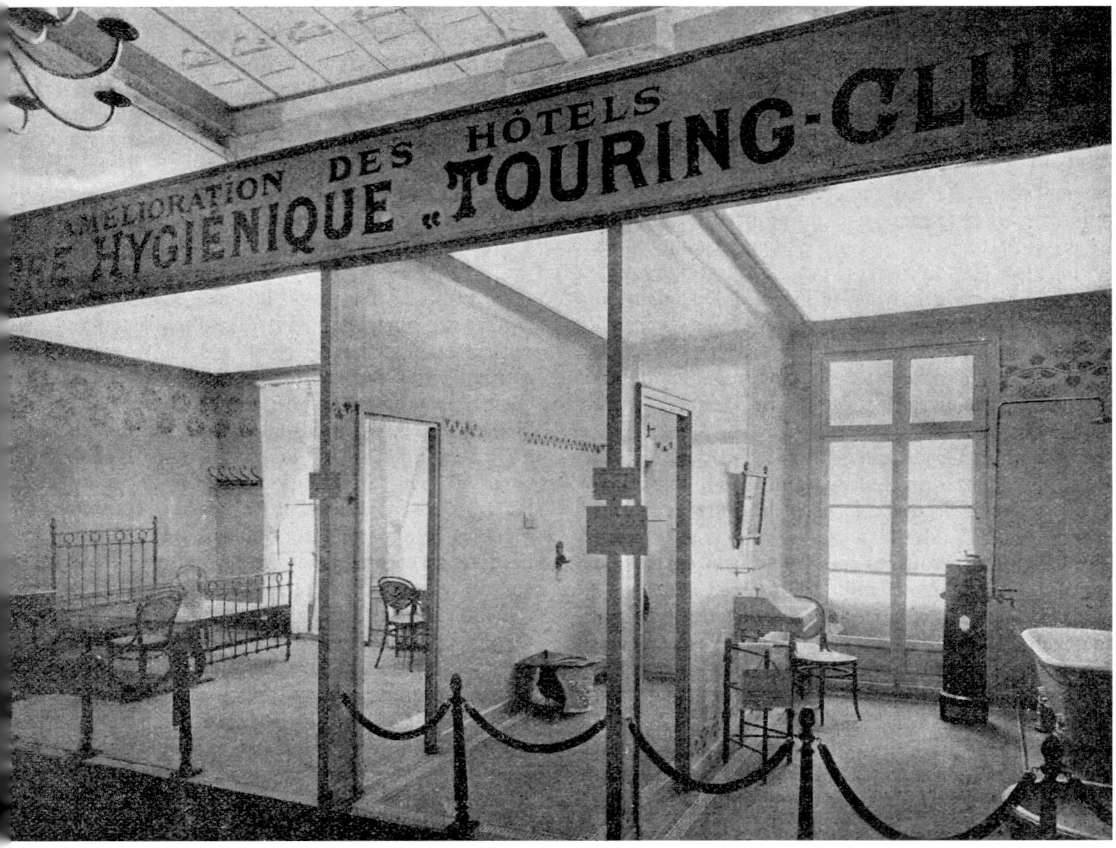

← Second model of *chambre hygiénique* designed by Gustave Rives for the Touring-Club de France, exhibited at the Exposition du Cycle et de l'Automobile in the Grand Palais, Paris, December 1902.

also supposedly contributed to mental cheerfulness, understood as a crucial part of comfort.

The Touring-Club later installed a series of such model *chambres hygiéniques* in automobile shows, congresses on tuberculosis, and international fairs. It was successful in persuading thousands of hotels to install such spaces and adopt the recommended cleaning protocols. The campaign quickly expanded to whitening all spaces in hotels. Other organizations cited the highly publicized initiative and expanded it into a call to use the same design protocols as a defense against disease-causing bacteria in waiting rooms, office buildings, barracks, trains, and department stores.[45] Newspapers, popular magazines, sport, automobile, art, and architecture magazines, international sanitary reform journals, medical journals, and books on disease control noted the "bare," "plain," "naked," hospital-like aesthetic of unornamented shiny white spaces but promptly treated it as a model for housing in general.[46] It was seen to offer a new sense of comfort by addressing the pervasive fear of contagious disease, and even a new understanding of an artistic space.[47]

Ripolin was used "everywhere," for example on the walls of the "hygienic housing" project for workers in Paris by Henri Sauvage and Charles Sarazin in 1903–1904.[48] The two architects tried to resist ending up with too much of a look of "hospitalization,"

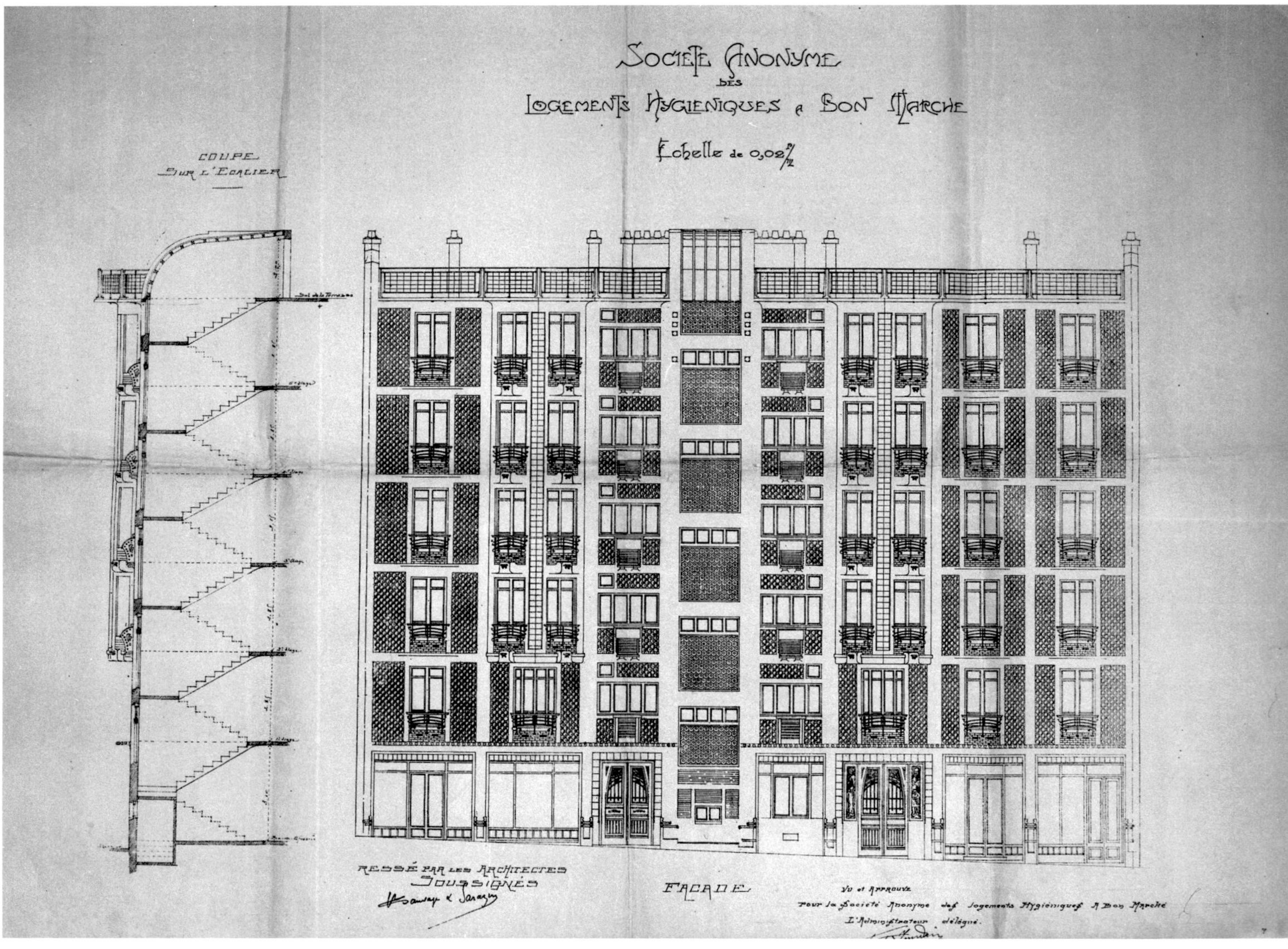

↓ Henri Sauvage and Charles Sarazin, original elevation and section of all-glass facade for "hygienic" workers' housing building, 7 rue Tretaigne, Paris, 1903.

→ Henri Sauvage and Charles Sarazin, terraced residential building clad in glazed white ceramic tiles, 26–28 rue Vavin, Paris, 1912–1913.

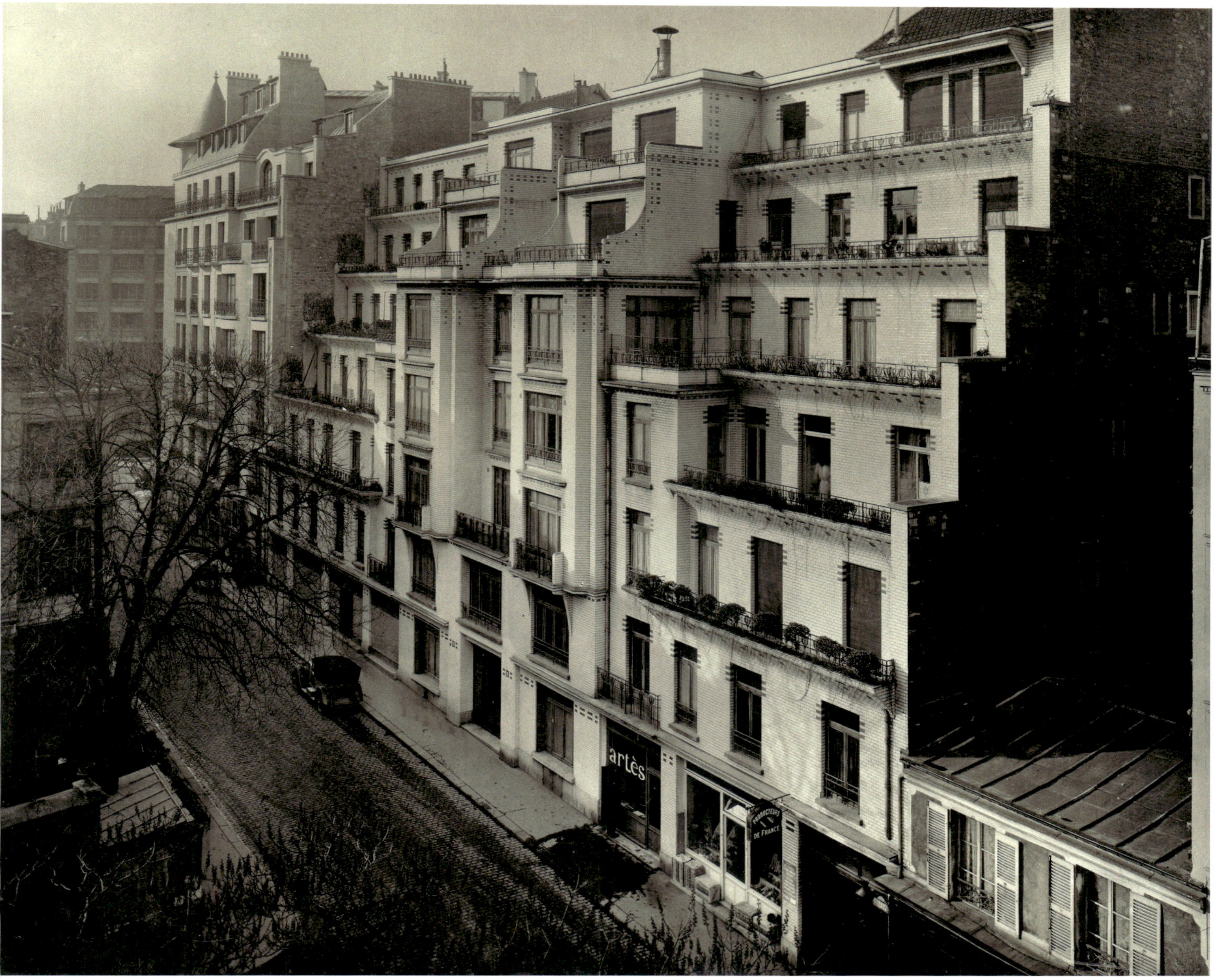

but the project absorbed the default Ripolin surfaces of hospitals and sanatoria, along with their smoothly curving intersections of floor, wall, and ceiling to facilitate cleaning, the absence of added ornament to collect dust, large operable windows for light and air, and added the innovation of a shared sun terrace on the roof. The project was originally intended to be more extreme even than any sanatorium by featuring a radical all-glass street facade with every window surrounded by webs of floor-to-ceiling hexagonal glass blocks floating in the exposed reinforced concrete structural frame to offer maximum light while maintaining privacy. The design was produced in immediate response to the new public health law of 1902 and the associated new building regulations. Architects were now encouraged to admit more sunlight and air to cleanse the housing for the poor that was itself "diseased" and acting as "nests of microbes" or even "microbe factories." The building authorities forced the replacement of the glass blocks in the apartments with bricks and the stairwell glass blocks with regular glass, but subsequent urban housing projects by Sauvage took the form of polemical all-white antimicrobial sanatoria with layers of sun terraces lined with shiny white ceramic tiles stepping back from the street.

Le Corbusier was all too familiar with these projects, and the eugenic arguments about racial purification surrounding them. Once again, the "healthy" logic of whitewash involves a revolutionary act that takes the form of a repetition. In echoing the seasonal "clean starts" of vernacular whitewashing, the intimate relation between whitewash and disease gets repeatedly forgotten and rediscovered, with convention repeatedly lost and reimposed by law. For example, in 1774, the prison reformer John Howard successfully persuaded the British government to pass a national law to scrape and whitewash all prison interiors at least once a year to counter "jail fever" (typhus). He was advised by a small network of doctors who were pioneering the contact tracing of epidemic disease like smallpox and setting up isolated whitewashed spaces for the infected in many cities, disinfecting and whitewashing patients' homes, and giving supplies of whitewash to families of the infected poor. By the end of the eighteenth century, charitable societies were inspired to go beyond the houses of the sick to focus on the "prevention of the return of the disease" by providing the labor and materials to whitewash as many houses as possible.[49] In a kind of frenzy, some crowded multiroomed poorhouses were whitewashed every six weeks and their disease-free condition was used as a model for whitewashing all workplaces and public buildings.[50] A national law of 1802 soon compelled all factory spaces to be whitewashed twice a year.

Yet the campaign to whitewash every space occupied by the poor repeatedly lapsed in the absence of disease. When Edwin Chadwick became the leader of the sanitary reform movement in the late 1830s, he argued that the emergency police actions of disinfecting and whitewashing houses during the 1817 outbreaks of typhus and the devastating cholera epidemic of 1831–1832 had to be turned into permanent law. He passed an 1838 law for enforced whitewashing in London, and then engineered the first national public health law in 1848 during yet another cholera epidemic that included continuous compulsory disinfection and whitewashing houses to "prevent or check" contagious disease. Florence Nightingale expanded the call for preventative whitewashing when taking over leadership of the movement in the middle of the nineteenth century. The call itself thus rapidly spread like a virus, first to Paris and then to urban centers across Europe and the United States, and was soon globalized through colonial networks. It was as if the networks themselves, seen as the original vectors of epidemic disease, needed to be disinfected, starting with the enforced whitewashing of ships and ports.

Every one of these repetitions of the call for a law of whitewash, like that of Le Corbusier, explicitly aims both to counter disease and to enhance the eye, clarity of thought, and morality. It is always about asserting control over the threatening other of epidemic disease as well as the laboring poor, itself coded as dark, migrant, and contagious—a disease in its own right. The interiors of houses, halfway houses, hospitals, factories, and schools were to form a kind of health net of isolated but interlinked white spaces inserted into the increasingly unhealthy industrializing city. The whiteness of these healthy and heath-giving interiors would counter, reveal, and accentuate the perceived darkness of interiors, dirt, soot, excrement, polluted water, vermin, the dirty skin of workers, poverty itself, and industrialization. Throughout this discourse of control, there is a seemingly "modern" disdain for disease-incubating ornament in favor of smooth white surfaces. As John Howard put it in 1789: "From a regard to the health of the patients, I wish to see plain white walls in hospitals, and no article of ornamental furniture introduced."[51]

The context of this comment was Howard's tour of European lazarettos for isolation from epidemic disease. After all, even the extended history of repetitions and forgettings of whitewash through the eighteenth and nineteenth centuries was itself a repetition of the protocols repeatedly established, forgotten, and reestablished in Italy between the fourteenth and seventeenth centuries in the face of devastating plagues, where a logic of separation and compulsory whitewashing was increasingly imposed by law in city-states.[52] Throughout these centuries of pulsating discourse in which architecture itself became a contagious patient that had to receive medical treatment by being rewhitened during emergency conditions, whitewash itself is symptomatically almost never discussed in the countless plague treatises and discourse of health officials that prescribe it. Whitewash is taken to be uncontroversially healthy—a cleaning, curing, preventive, and life-enhancing surface. The transhistorical resilience of whiteness paradoxically allows it to be repeatedly forgotten and revived as if it never left, as if it precedes everything and can be invoked to control anything. This is the veritable plague of architecture itself as the violent law of whiteness that lurks in the background as the all-too-guilty image of innocence. Whiteness is the real disease. Orchestrating life and death, it is the most lethal of pandemics. Chronic whiteness is organized around a millennial fantasy about the health of a certain kind of surface, one whose background is sustained by a continuous hidden labor and has to be repeatedly foregrounded, confronted, and defaced.

An earlier version of this essay was originally published by e-flux Architecture in 2020.

p250 From Juan José Ibáñez et al., "Los primeros agricultores y ganaderos. Excavaciones en el yacimiento del Neolítico Precerámico A y B de Kharaysin (Zarqa, Jordania). Campañas de 2015 y 2016," in *Informes y trabajos: Excavaciones en el exterior* (Madrid: Ministerio de Cultura y Deporte, 2019), 17.
p251 From Nicole Nicklisch et al., "Rib Lesions in Skeletons from Early Neolithic Sites in Central Germany: On the Trail of Tuberculosis at the Onset of Agriculture," *American Journal of Biological Anthropology*, October 2012.
p252 Photo Solon Malkas, 2015. © Solon Malkas.
p254 From "Au Coeur de l'Afrique orientale," *L'Illustré—Revue Hebdomadaire Suisse*, May 8, 1924.
p255 From Le Corbusier, *L'art décoratif d'aujourd'hui* (Paris: Éditions G. Grès et Cie, 1925). © Fondation Le Corbusier / ADAGP, Paris / Artists Rights Society (ARS), New York 2024.
p256 From Le Corbusier, *Voyage d'Orient: Carnets*, vol. 3, ed. Giuliano Gresleri (Milan: Electa; Paris: Fondation Le Corbusier, 1987). © Fondation Le Corbusier / ADAGP, Paris / Artists Rights Society (ARS), New York 2024.
p259 Published in *À Travers le Monde*, January 31, 1903.
p260 Fonds Sauvage. SIAF/Cité de l'architecture et du patrimoine/Archives d'architecture contemporaine.
p261 Photo Chevojon. Fonds Sauvage. SIAF/Cité de l'architecture et du patrimoine/Archives d'architecture contemporaine.

1. Le Corbusier, *L'art décoratif d'aujourd'hui* (Paris: Éditions G. Grès et Cie, 1925), trans. James Dunnet as *The Decorative Art of Today* (Cambridge, MA: MIT Press, 1987), 188.
2. Ripolin was already a default surface in clinics, hospitals, and sanatoria at the turn of the century and was explicitly understood to be inhospitable to the invisible microbial sources of disease and to paradoxically visualize that resistance with a look of hygiene. Advertisements for "Ripolin Enamel—The Most Sanitary Finish" in architectural and hospital journals in 1913, for example, cited studies on how the bacteria of cholera, diphtheria, typhus, staphylococcus, and tuberculosis do not survive as long on fifteen-month-old glossy and flat Ripolin surfaces as on other surfaces.
3. Mark Wigley, *White Walls, Designer Dresses: The Fashioning of Modern Architecture* (Cambridge, MA: MIT Press, 1995).
4. The overall transition from nomadism to a default built environment of mainly quadrilateral buildings across the whole Near East took around four thousand years through multiple parallel transitions in a polycentric mosaic of dispersed groups linked by complex networks of exchange and migration. Juan José Ibáñez, Jesus González-Urquijo, Luis César Teira-Mayolini, and Talía Lazuén, "The Emergence of the Neolithic in the Near East: A Protracted and Multi-Regional Model," *Quaternary International* 470, Part B (2018): 226–252.
5. Clark Spencer Larsen, "The Agricultural Revolution as Environmental Catastrophe: Implications for Health and Lifestyle in the Holocene," *Quaternary International* 150, no. 1 (2006): 12–20.
6. A recent excavation of Neolithic buildings from 10,800 years ago in Kharaysin, Jordan, revealed lime plaster floors made of successive layers from rough to smooth until a final layer of finer material and finished with a wash of the very finest lime plaster that is either left as unpainted white or painted on with powdered red pigment. See Juan José Ibáñez et al., "Los primeros agricultores y ganaderos. Excavaciones en el yacimiento del Neolítico Precerámico A y B de Kharaysin (Zarqa, Jordania). Campañas de 2015 y 2016," in *Informes y trabajos: Excavaciones en el exterior* (Madrid: Ministerio de Cultura y Deporte, 2019), 103–123. These buildings, lined up in rows along a terraced hillside with spaces in between them, immediately preceded the domestication of plants and animals. They are transitional in preceding the move from semi-sunken to freestanding buildings, yet are already orthogonal and internally subdivided with walls. This supports the crucial sense of quadrilateral spaces being defined by the lime plaster as distinct from a quadrilateral space that is then plastered. It took around a thousand years from the first use of lime plaster to define the interior space of buildings to it being the general practice in the whole Near East.
7. No association between domestic and family, or even household, can be assumed, nor any simple opposition between domestic and special-use buildings, everyday and ritualistic, profane and symbolic life. See Bill Finlayson et al., "Architecture, Sedentism, and Social Complexity at Pre-Pottery Neolithic A WF16, Southern Jordan," *Journal of the Council for British Research in the Levant* 47, no. 2 (2015): 8183–8188. Furthermore, no assumption can be made about how buildings were actually lived in, or not in a way that is familiar, from the archaeological remains of a building alone, but the building itself is a major part of that life rather than simply its host. Even more importantly, the first production of architecture by smooth white plaster is inseparable from building as burial. Architecture had, still has, an intimacy with death, and is even the mark and maintenance of such an intimacy that makes the very idea of daily life possible. In other words, it is never simply a host. It manufactures rather than houses. To think of architecture without thinking of the production of death is to avoid thinking about architecture.
8. The archaeologists of the earliest examples of lime-plastered interiors interpret it to mean that hygiene was an integral part of the transition from nomadism to settlement. Paleoarchaeology increasingly identifies specific parts of Neolithic buildings and then specific buildings as receiving special attention to cleaning assumed to be associated with collective rituals interlaced with burials and communal processing and storage of crops. Analysis of the floors and where they smoothly curve up into walls shows that they were regularly washed.
9. This is not to argue that whiteness is in any way inherently "Western." On the contrary, the argument here is that the way an ongoing set of cultural-intellectual-military-imperial-exclusionary traditions were forged as Western included particular appropriations of the whiteness of the ancient lime plaster architectures that can be found not only in the Near East and North Africa but also in India, China, and Central and South America. More precisely, it is about the extraction of whiteness from cultures that will be retroactively coded and subordinated by that very whiteness as Eastern and Southern.
10. Vitruvius, *Ten Books on Architecture*, trans. Ingrid D. Rowland (Cambridge: Cambridge University Press, 1999), 26.
11. So "friendship and hospitality may prove harmful." Leon Battista Alberti, *On the Art of Building in Ten Books*, trans. Joseph Rykwert, Neil Leach, and Robert Tavernor (Cambridge, MA: MIT Press, 1988), 17.
12. Alberti, referring to Plato's *Laws*, raises the possibility of organizing cities to isolate "foreigners" to avoid being "corrupted" by them and likewise to "free" gentry from "any contamination from the common people." Alberti, *On the Art of Building in Ten Books*, 192.
13. On the multiple associations of the white (new Istrian marble, repurposed spolia from numerous sites, and plaster) and the polychrome (some red and green accents) in the building, see Massimo Bulgarelli, "Bianco e colori. Sigismondo Malatesta, Alberti, e l'architettura del Tempio Malatestiano," *Opus Incertum* 2 (2016): 48–57.
14. Leon Battista Alberti, *I libri della famiglia*, trans. René Neu Watkins as *The Family in Renaissance Florence: Book Three* (Long Grove, IL: Waveland, 1994), 85. *Della famiglia* closely echoed Xenophon's ancient Greek text *Oeconomicus* in which the virtue of a woman is threatened by the "trick" of having "rubbed in white lead in order to look even whiter than she is." Xenophon, *Oeconomicus*, trans. H. G. Daykyns as *The Economist* (London: Macmillan, 1897), 244. It is not simply that a natural versus artificial whiteness marks a woman's virtue. A woman "adorned with purity" without makeup wearing a white dress is Xenophon's allegorical figure of "Virtue" in *Memorabilia*, an earlier text. On the architectural misogyny of Alberti's texts, see Mark Wigley, "Untitled: The Housing of Gender," in *Sexuality and Space*, ed. Beatriz Colomina (Princeton: Princeton Architectural Press, 1997), 327–389.
15. Alberti's articulation of the tragedy of slavery in the short story *De felicitate* (happiness) was written shortly before his *Della famiglia* on the organization of the household. On Alberti's antislavery position, see Orlando Patterson, "Freedom, Slavery, and Identity in Renaissance Florence: The Faces of Leon Battista Alberti," in *The Oxford Handbook of Freedom*, ed. David Schmidtz and Carmen E. Pavel (Oxford: Oxford University Press, 2018). *De felicitate* empathizes with the expressions of deepest pain by each of the different voices in a group of slaves, understood not as the physical violence inflicted on them but the pain of "social death" that Patterson has comprehensively traced throughout the millennial and ongoing history of slavery. Orlando Patterson, *Slavery and Social Death: A Comparative Study* (Cambridge, MA: Harvard University Press, 1982).
16. The status of women and slavery intersect in Alberti in the fact that *Della famiglia* so closely echoes Xenophon's *Oeconomicus* which explicitly linked the control of the skin with purity, health, spatial order, and a system of slavery in which the wife as property must labor but appear more

virtuous than the servants who themselves are hierarchically divided between those who are ultimately going to be freed and those who will remain enslaved. *Della famiglia* repeats the argument that the master of the household maintains control of the house (health, morality, economy) by refusing to ever appear as a slave to "his" wife. It compares the idealized household to Italy itself, noting that the authority of Italy has been undone by the "barbarian nations, distant slave people" arriving into its "very heart." Alberti even argues that Italian "virtue" played as big a role as "violence" in the previous subjugation of these "savage" others. He embraces violent authority, supported by the attempt to naturalize hierarchy, servitude, and property, while trying to reject the ultimate murderous transformation of human into nonhuman object that is the very definition of slavery.

17. A regime of subordination of perceived others was fully installed as a system of classifying shades of skin long before the "scientific" construction of race was used as the ongoing weapon of colonial domination and settler colonialism. Many of Alberti's ancient Greek sources were obsessed with the Indigenous character of Greeks, the unique status of the skins of people and objects and the need to preserve and purify it, particularly in Athens. Roman citizenship was self-consciously forged out of a diversity of geographic origins, including immigrants and freed slaves, but maintained the idea of dominance by an idealized local population embodying the character of a particular place. In the continuous paradoxical process that organizes most exclusionary systems, some designated others were successively absorbed into that population and as it were converted into agents of its mythical purity, even policing it. The Vitruvius scrolls on architecture that were reframed by Alberti's treatise include an environmental theory of geography and climate to explain the source of white skins in the north and dark skins in the south and the corresponding stereotypes of character, intelligence, health, and courage—with Rome fit to "take command" because it is neither north nor south but temperate. In fact, Vitruvius initiated the transfer of stereotypes of East versus West that were first codified in Hippocrates's late fifth-century BCE medical text "Airs, Waters and Places" into stereotypes of South versus North (Benjamin Isaac, *The Invention of Racism in Classical Antiquity* [Princeton: Princeton University Press, 2004], 84). This "proto-racism" was directly linked to the question of health since "temperate" conditions are for Vitruvius the most "healthful environment" and imply an idealized skin color intermediate between white and black. Alberti's treatise on architecture repeatedly cites Hippocrates and likewise argues that health-giving architecture provides temperate conditions.

18. After the waves of plague on the Italian peninsula starting in 1348, a 1363 decree in Florence sanctioned the importation of unlimited numbers of domestic slaves from the East to Tuscany provided that they were not Christians. The late medieval slave trade centered on the Black Sea enabled any free Christian or Muslim to legally enslave anyone who did not share the same religion. Otherness was more religious than racial, and the majority of the slaves were women. See Hannah Barker, "Egyptian and Italian Merchants in the Black Sea Slave Trade, 1260–1500" (PhD diss., Columbia University, 2014). For both Christian and Muslim, white was privileged as purity but the color-coding of slaves written into slave contracts (yellow, white, black, brown) along with ethnic coding (Tartar, Abkhazi, Circassian, Bulgarian, Russian, Turkish, Greek, Mingreli, Ethiopian) was not yet racialized in the post-transatlantic slave trade sense where the slave owner self-identifies as white and manufactures blackness as the ever-threatening and necessarily dominated other.

19. The point being sketched here is to consider the possibility that the concept and reality of "whiteness as property" exposed by the seminal essay of Cheryl Harris is not only a highly specific historical and even late phase of the maintenance of the systemic violence of slavery after its official abolition in the United States, but is also a precise, even self-conscious, echo and continuation of a millennial association of whiteness and property in which both are continuously reconfigured yet architecture is ever present as agent and effect. See Cheryl I. Harris, "Whiteness as Property," *Harvard Law Review* 106, no. 8 (June 1993): 1707–1791.

20. Le Corbusier, *The Decorative Art of Today*, 190.

21. Le Corbusier, "Salon d'automne," *L'Esprit Nouveau*, no. 19 (1923).

22. Le Corbusier, cited by Guillaume Janneau in "L'Exposition des arts techniques de 1925," *Bulletin de la vie artistique*, February 1, 1923, 64.

23. A similar white model of Villa Besnus was exhibited at the Salon d'autome in 1923. The white plaster used to make the models of the early projects was not just a medium to represent the designs in exhibitions but a primary medium in which the designing was done. See Miguel de la Cova, "Plâtre de Paris. Las maquetas de Le Corbusier y Charles Lasnon (1922–1938). Diálogos sobre la materia y la forma," *LC. Revue de recherches sur Le Corbusier* 1, no. 1 (2020): 24–37.

24. Villa Besnus may have been the only all-white building of Le Corbusier. Jan de Heer has pointed to interior sketches of the project, one dated April 1923, to raise the possibility that its interiors may have had other colors in addition to the white. Jan de Heer, *The Architectonic Colour: Polychromy in the Purist Architecture of Le Corbusier* (Rottderdam: 010 Publishers, 2009), 97. The sketches are more indicative of patterned wallpaper on one of the surfaces on the upper level than of planes of color, echoing representations of the wall coverings in earlier projects. The main studio-living level appears to be defined only by white walls and patterns in the glass panes. It is not clear how the interiors of the main spaces were finished, but it is symptomatic that Le Corbusier never published photographs of them, as if editing out interiors already regarded as insufficiently modern and only showing the all-white interiors of two levels of the stairwell to show how the exterior white continues inside, thereby preserving the polemical thought of a monochrome building entirely molded out of white.

25. Le Corbusier, "Notes à la suite," *Cahiers d'art*, no. 3 (1926): 49.

26. Le Corbusier, "A House That Is Completely White Resembles a Cream Jug," in *Almanach d'architecture moderne* (Paris: G. Crès, 1926), 146.

27. This off-whiteness of "white architecture" was a generic characteristic of canonic modern architecture. See Ivo Hammer, "White, Everything White? Josef Frank's Villa Beer (1930) in Vienna, and Its Materiality in the Context of the Discourse on 'White Cubes,'" *Built Heritage* 4, no. 2 (2020): 1–16.

28. Anna Rosellini, "La surface puriste, de 'L'Esprit Nouveau' à la villa Savoye," in *Le Corbusier: l'oeuvre* à *l'épreuve de sa restauration*, ed. Christine Mengin (Paris: Éditions de la Villette, 2017), 90–101.

29. The painting, *Still Life with Bottles*, a composition that features a similar layering centered on some white crockery, was in fact made in 1922, a year before the space.

30. "Au Coeur de l'Afrique orientale," *L'Illustré: Revue hebodomadaire suisse*, May 8, 1924, 226–227.

31. These routes were highly active in the nineteenth century up to and beyond the official prohibition of slavery in 1873. The complex histories of the region during the slave trade undo any simple oppositions between slavery and freedom, with multiple overlapping forms of servitude that continuously shift. See Philip Gooding, "Slavery, 'Respectability,' and Being 'Freeborn' on the Shores of Nineteenth-Century Lake Tanganyika," in *Slavery and Abolition* 40, no. 1 (2017).

32. "In four years, I've suffered and survived a terrible evolution. I've gobbled up an East of unity and power. ... All that bric-a-brac I treasured disgusts me now. I stumble through elementary geometry in my hunger for knowledge and eventual power. In this mad dash, red, blue, and yellow have become white. I'm besotted with white ... we would be living between huge walls as smooth as they were white. It would be so ennobling that our progress would be regular, our gestures graceful, and everything would assume color. ... No ornamentation. The whole city one color, one substance." Charles-Édouard Jeanneret, letter to William Ritter, November 1, 1911, cited in Nicholas Fox Weber, *Le Corbusier: A Life* (New York: Alfred A. Knopf, 2008), 99.

33. "This journey to the East, far from the gossamer architecture of the north, is a response to the persistent call from the sun, the wide expanses of blue seas and the great white walls of temples—Constantinople, Asia Minor, Greece, southern Italy—will be like an ideally shaped vase from which the heart's most profound feelings will flow." Charles-Édouard Jeanneret, "Quelques impressions," text dated June 6, 1911, *La Feuille d'Avis de La Chaux-de-Fonds*, July 20, 1911.

34. The whitewashing was both visual and historical in the sense that Ottoman narratives about the origin of the Parthenon recast the original building as white. In the early eighteenth century, Mahmud Efendi, a mufti of Athens, wrote a history of Athens in which Pericles, the general of the city who commissioned the Parthenon, called for an all-white building: "But we must construct an outstanding and magnificent temple, unsurpassed in quality. Its walls should be of pure white marble. The roof that will rest on the walls should be supported on beams of white marble too, and indeed so also should its ceilings and substructures be constructed of white marble." Mahmud Efendi, *Tarih-i Medinetü'l-Hukema*, cited in Elizabeth Key Fowden, "The Parthenon, Pericles and King Solomon: A Case Study of Ottoman Archeological Imagination in Greece," *Byzantine and Modern Greek Studies* 42, no. 2 (2018): 269. Efendi described the quarry from which the "pure white" marble was extracted for the building

and writes that the craftsmanship was so perfect that the building seemed to have been made of a single piece of marble, with the whiteness of the structure still evident in the richly decorated interior. He also describes Sultan Mehmet II, the conqueror of Athens, experiencing the "pure white" of the buildings on the Acropolis where he stayed. The logic, repeated by most European art historians in the early nineteenth century, is white building plus colored decoration rather than a fully colored architecture defined by its decoration.

35. Le Corbusier, *Le Voyage d'Orient* (1966), trans. Ivan Žaknić as *Journey to the East* (Cambridge, MA: MIT Press, 1987), 236.

36. Jeanneret had expected the city to have been more whitewashed because of the impressionist painting by Paul Signac he had seen in Munich and the orientalist texts that he had read before traveling, and was disappointed when he saw it for the first time: "I want Stamboul to be white, brittle like chalk, and the light falling on it to crunch as it hits it. ... Under the white light I want a white city, but punctuated by green cypress trees." Yet he increasingly celebrated the traditional whitewashing of houses and mosques, seeing it as a fading tradition and despairing that the post-Ottoman future would be without the "majestic coat" of white: "No more whitewash in Turkey for a long time to come!"

37. It is symptomatic that Jeanneret does not talk about the Parthenon's whiteness directly. He does talk about the Acropolis "becoming suddenly white" during a storm and the temple "sparkling like a diadem" against the "ink-black" mountains beyond. Some of his travel sketches captured this effect but others rendered it as a dark silhouette against a light sky. Monochrome, for Jeanneret, was precisely the capacity to absorb and radiate color. He describes the Parthenon appearing "yellow" when first seen from the boat. Closer up, the marble appears "reddish brown" by absorbing the color of the surrounding landscape, then becomes the "black pilot of marble" binding land to sky as the sun goes down. The travel notes of the preceding weeks in the Balkans, Turkey, and Mount Athos repeatedly document how white emphasizes color and color emphasizes white before finally describing and portraying colors as coming out of white itself. The day after returning to Switzerland, Jeanneret's description of future cities being all-white described how "a rainbow rises out of forms" that are "unpolluted by color" but respond to the movements of the sun. Three weeks later, he did some retrospective watercolors showing the fluted columns of the Parthenon in multicolor—as if restoring the original ancient applied polychrome of the building with a polychrome now coming from the surrounding atmosphere.

38. See Zeynep Çelik, "Le Corbusier, Orientalism, Colonialism," *Assemblage*, no. 17 (April 1992): 58–77. Le Corbusier treats the vernacular whiteness of Algiers as a lesson for all Europe but argues that Algerians have lost touch with their own invention and that the Casbah has become an overcrowded den of criminality beyond the reach of any police investigation. Architecture needs to be recleansed in a time in which vernacular culture is not maintained and "Everything withers, becomes covered with dust. White becomes gray." Le Corbusier, "Le folklore est l'expression fleurie des traditions," *Voici la France de ce mois*, no. 16 (June 1941): 27–32.

39. See Mabel Wilson, "Black Bodies/White Cities: Le Corbusier in Harlem," *ANY*, no. 16 (1996): 35–39. Le Corbusier spent his whole career obsessively describing and drawing black figures, attempting to tame "them" through confining stereotypes that undo or erase the multiplicities of blackness by "giving" singular form to it, redesigning the perceived other whose simultaneous attraction and threat is to seemingly be in touch with prehistory and the origin of design itself. Black figures are, as it were, avatars of the original designers of design, the ability to transform the material world into shelter, prosthetic extension and symbolism. Design itself has to be extracted from the other and possessed through multiple violent acts.

40. Le Corbusier, "L'Architecture et l'esprit mathématique," dated January 4, 1946, in *Les grands courants de la pensée mathématique*, ed. Francois Le Lionnais (Paris: Librairie Philosophique J. Vrin, 1948), 483.

41. This very partial list is not offered as a chain of uniquely influential individuals. On the contrary, the argument here is that the whiteness of architecture was never an individual project but a broadband networked intersection of medical, governmental, religious, architectural, and artistic discourse in which the practice of white walls was not accompanied by its theorization and could, for example, already dominate so many of the projects in an architectural publication like *Moderne Bauformen—Facaden, Interieurs, Details* in 1902 even being polemically printed whiter than the pages of the journal, without any reference being made to it. White walls multiplied unevenly. Centers of experimentation with white did visibly move, for example from England to Austria at the turn of the century, as marked by this partial set of names, without ever being, as it were, designed in the usual sense.

42. "HYGIÈNE—Tentures, rideaux, etc.," *Revue Mensuelle du Touring Club de France*, October 1899, 431.

43. "Boldly, the Touring-Club has exposed something still unheard of in France: a hotel room that looks like a hospital room. It is in the hospital that the rules of hygiene are best practiced. ... On the walls, paint, whether with whitewash or oil. And the paint clear, white, so you can easily follow the steps of a bug if by chance it sneaks into the hygienic nest where it must never penetrate." Pierre Giffard, "La Chambre blanche," *Revue Mensuelle du Touring Club de France*, September 1900, 385–387.

44. Most of the detailed formula for making a hygienic hotel room suite was immediately reprinted in popular magazines and medical journals after Gustave Rives presented the report to the Tenth International Congress on Hygiene and Demography in Paris in August 1900. Gustave Rives, "La Chambre d'hôtel au point de vue de l'hygiène," *Xe Congrès International d'Hygiène et de Démographie à Paris en 1900* (Paris: Masson, 1900), 348–360.

45. *Mémoires—Société d'agriculture, sciences, belles-lettres et arts d'Orléans* (Orleans: Georges Michau, 1901). 122–124.

46. The international jury for the Exposition Universelle already noted that the Touring-Club protocol for hygienic rooms could be "a kind of code or manual" for guiding all the inhabited spaces of houses when reprinting the protocol in full in its own report. "Chambre et cabinet de toilette hygiéniques pour les hôtels, d'après le Touring-Club," *Rapports du Jury International, Troisième Partie—Groupe XVI* (Paris: Imprimerie Nationale, 1900), 321.

47. The report on the model room in *L'Art Décoratif* made the argument (later associated with Adolf Loos and Le Corbusier) that this "healthy, fresh, and happy" ensemble composed "without artistic pretension" is paradoxically a service to art in moving beauty from complex layers of ornament toward simplicity as a new form of decoration in its own right. "Chronique," *L'Art Décoratif*, October 1900, 41.

48. "Logements hygiéniques à bon marché et maison de rapport," *L'Art Décoratif*, July-December 1904, 128–136. The building closely followed the Touring-Club protocols, even in the use of a stenciled pattern to produce, as it were, a minimal hygienic decoration to substitute for the erased cornices.

49. *The Reports of the Society for Bettering the Condition and Increasing the Comforts of the Poor*, vol. III (London: W. Bulmer, 1802), 304.

50. "Extract from an account of the expense and benefit of frequently white-washing the rooms of a poorhouse," *The Reports of the Society for Bettering the Condition and Increasing the Comforts of the Poor*, vol. I (London: W. Bulmer, 1798), 86–90.

51. John Howard, *An Account of the Principal Lazarettos in Europe: With Various Papers Relative to the Plague, Together with Further Observations on Some Foreign Prisons and Hospitals, and Additional Remarks on the Present State of Those in Great Britain and Ireland* (London: J. Johnson, C. Dilly and T. Cadell, 1791), 57.

52. In a typical plague law, houses of the sick were compulsorily emptied and whitewashed forty days later by those who had survived. Anybody allowed to enter the city had to be disinfected and their new houses whitewashed. After the epidemic, all the darkest and unventilated houses were also whitewashed. This protocol, along with quarantine at the borders, isolation of the sick, and destruction of all their furniture, clothing, and possessions, was supported by the controversial concept of contagion in which disease could be passed by touching people or objects they have touched. Buildings themselves required medical treatment. This contagion theory and the whitewashing practices associated with it were typically abandoned after each epidemic crisis passed. The protocols guiding everyday life returned to the ancient miasma theory that blamed disease on bad air alone. Yet the idea of contagion and whitewashing promptly returned with each catastrophic epidemic. The plague was only understood to have been caused by the *Yersinia pestis* bacterium carried on the fleas of rats at the end of the nineteenth century. It is now understood to have accompanied and traumatized human settlement since Neolithic times. DNA analysis links its evolution to human settlement, trade routes, and ultimately the very decline of the Neolithic. The development of interlinked megasettlements from 6,100 to 5,400 years ago that housed 10,000 to 20,000 people in dense proximity with other animals optimized the conditions for infectious disease that may have led to the collapse of those settlements. See Nicolás Rascovan et al., "Emergence and Spread of Basal Lineages of *Yersinia pestis* during the Neolithic Decline," *Cell* 176 (January 10, 2019): 295–305.

LAND
SCAP

-

ES

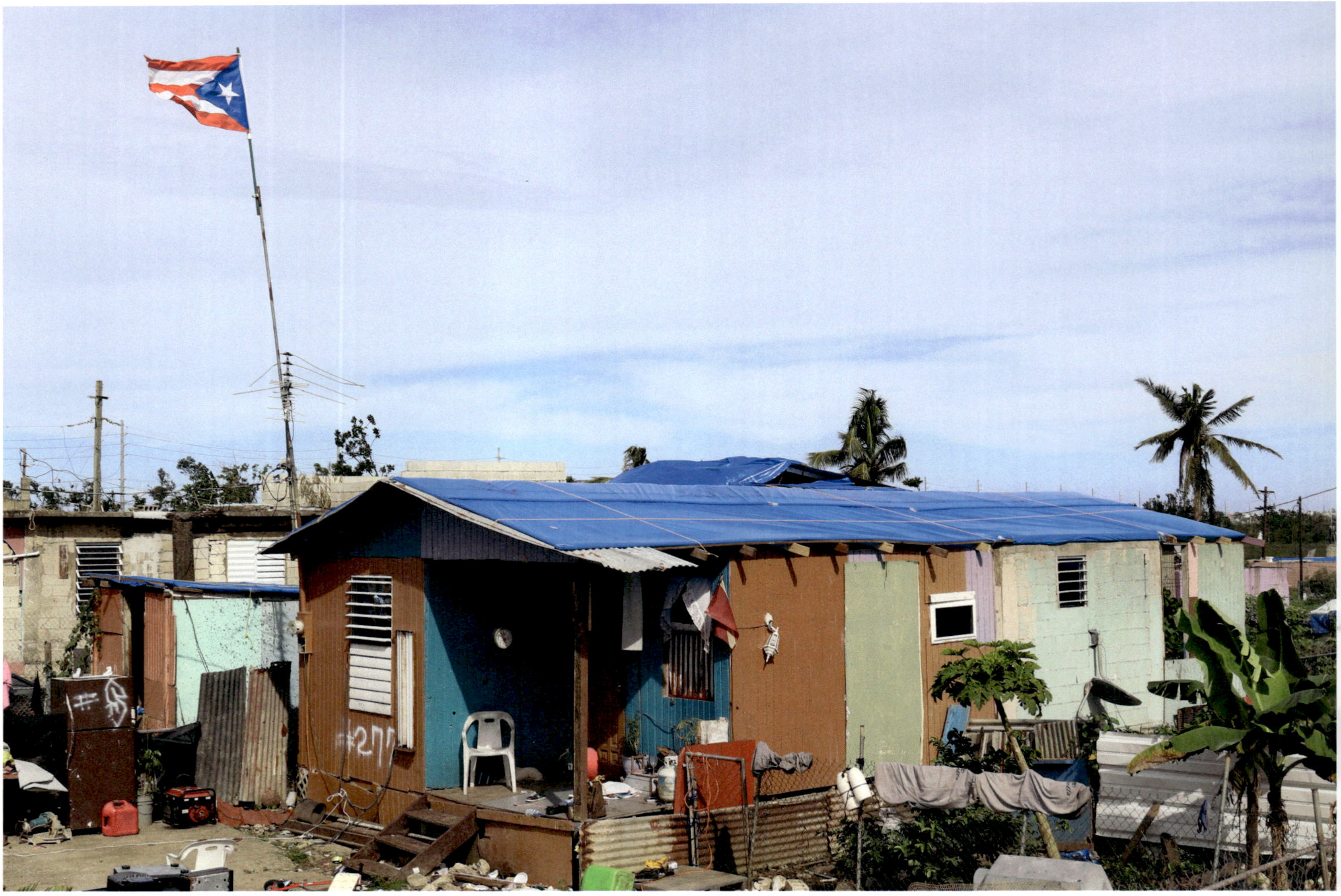

THE IMMUNO-COMPROMISED HOME

ANGELA H. BROWN

↑ House with blue tarp after Hurricane Maria, Dorado, Puerto Rico, November 29, 2017.

Le doy fuego a la Fortaleza como se supone
Y al otro día voy a la iglesia pa' que me perdonen
Mejor no quieras probar de qué estamos hechos
Aquí en El Monte heredamos el mismo pecho
Tus disculpas se ahogan con el agua de la lluvia
En las casas que todavía no tienen techo

I set La Fortaleza on fire as I should
And the next day I go to church to be forgiven
You don't want to test what we're made of
Here in El Monte we've inherited the same heart
[we are all family in Puerto Rico]
Your apologies are drowned with rainwater
In houses that still don't have a roof

—Residente, iLe, and Bad Bunny, "Afilando los Cuchillos" ("Sharpening the Knives")[1]

Houses without walls or roofs. Houses filled with plants and rainwater. Houses reduced to rubble and ash. For the Puerto Rican home, the boundary between nature and architecture is permeable and precarious. When the boundary is controlled—opening a window to let the breeze in, placing a rocking chair in a covered patio's shade—it seems as if the built and natural environments are collaborating, assisting one another. But when the balance is tipped from either side, recovery can be long and difficult.

In the last five years, the frequency and intensity of natural disasters have increased dramatically across the Puerto Rican archipelago. In 2017, Hurricanes Maria and Irma tore the roofs from homes and wreaked havoc on roads, power lines, and other essential infrastructure. Then, two years later, while Puerto Ricans were still entrenched in the process of mourning losses and rebuilding a sense of home, leaked text messages between government officials revealed gross neglect and disrespect toward women, queer people, and lives lost in the hurricane and its wake. Boricuas (Puerto Ricans) were fed up. They took to the streets, and after fifteen days of mass protests, forced the then-governor Ricky Rosselló to resign.[2] Only a few months later, a series of disastrous earthquakes caused yet more destruction on the main island's southern coast.

While forces of nature were threatening working people's houses and safety, real estate developers bought up property along the coasts and began to build luxury condos and resorts, taking advantage of low property costs and tax breaks for US citizens. Rincón, for example, a popular destination for surfing on the northwest coast of the main island, made the news in 2021 when private investors began to construct a pool on a public beach, even though a previous pool and an entire apartment complex had been destroyed by the tides of Maria.[3] Despite the known consequences of beach erosion and wildlife endangerment, the construction was approved by the government. When it came to the benefit of tourists and the moneyed elite, architectural development trumped local concerns about the natural environment, with police and security guards protecting property over people. Protestors gathered to oppose the project, and it was eventually halted.

Locals, then and now, face the double task of struggling to rebuild for themselves after nature has struck *and* resisting construction for tourists that would actively harm the environment. There are so many examples of a tipped "balance" between nature and architecture in Puerto Rico (and in the Caribbean at large) that the idea of a stable equilibrium between the two is not just naïve but delusional. Furthermore, it contributes to the doctored image of a tropical paradise that is ceaselessly fed to tourists and investors, even—or perhaps *especially*—in times of crisis. What happens if we do away with the utopian promise of a fixed equilibrium, of a controlled homeostasis? Rather than perpetuate some paradisical standard, which ignores centuries of colonial exploitation and the dependencies it has forced into place, we should consider the Puerto Rican home—from the individual house to the archipelago—to be immunocompromised.

Casa Klumb

On November 10, 2020, at around 11:15pm, a house in Río Piedras went up in flames.[4] A team of firefighters rushed to the site, but when they arrived, the majority of the house was gone. The fire had spread quickly across the already-damaged structure, leaving nothing but a charred foundation, limp sheets of corrugated aluminum, and a short flight of concrete stairs leading to a platform of smoking debris. The cause of the fire is still unknown.

The house was known as Casa Klumb, the once-residence and architectural manifesto of Henry Klumb, a German-born architect who worked with Frank Lloyd Wright in the US from 1929 to 1933 and who was invited in 1943 to serve as director of Puerto Rico's Design Committee of Public Works. Soon after moving to the island, Klumb purchased Rancho Cody, a seven-acre lot and former hacienda in Río Piedras.[5] He transformed the existing nineteenth-century building on the property into what came to be regarded as a feat of tropical modernism, and an exemplar of Klumb's approach to site-responsive architecture in Puerto Rico. Raised up from the ground, the single-story house featured an open plan with very few permanent walls and was surrounded by a lush garden that protected the interior from rain and filtered the sunlight. At the center was what Klumb called the "life core," a compact area containing the kitchen, washroom, and bathroom, from which the rest of the house unfurled, opening onto the surrounding environment.[6]

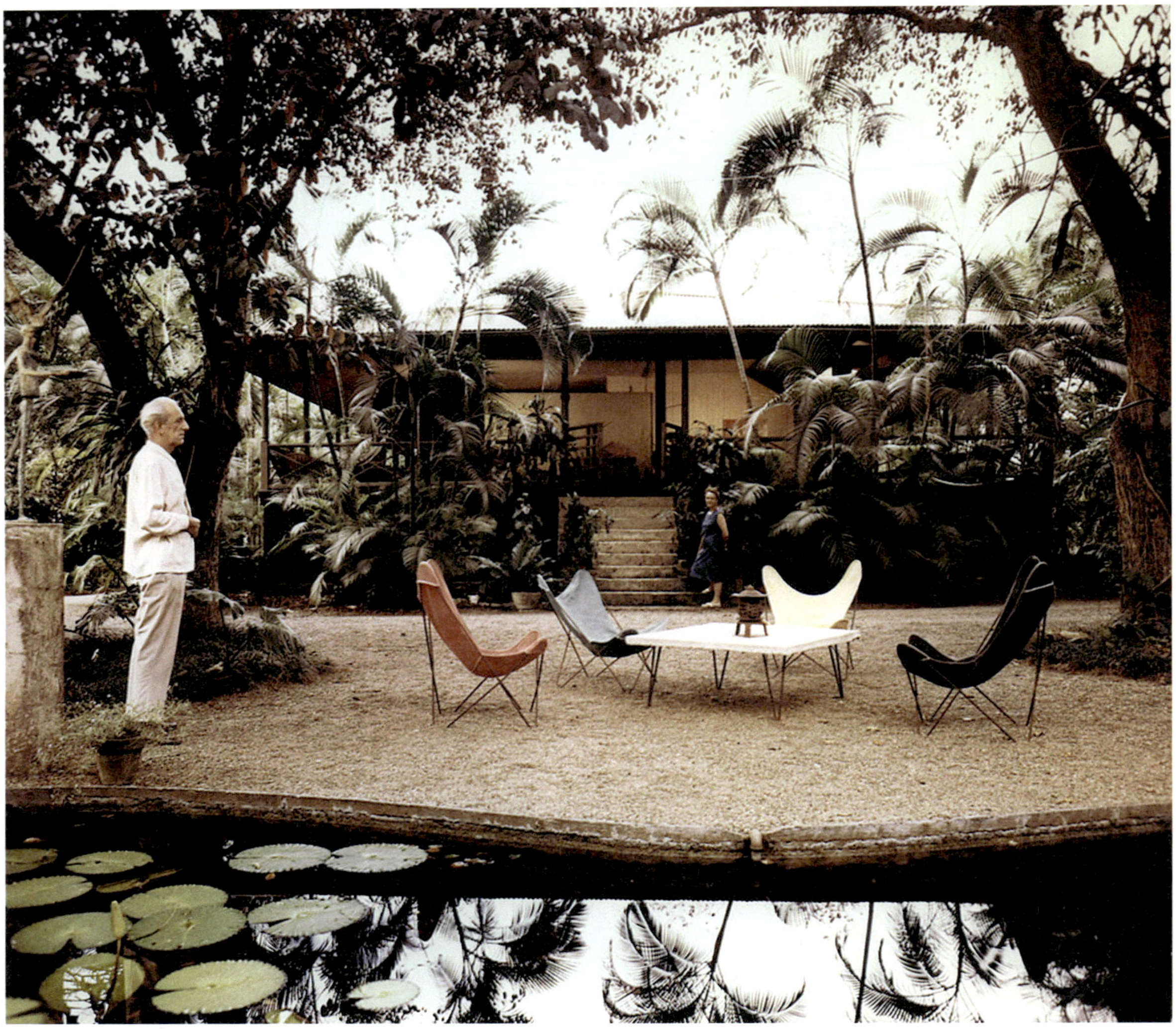

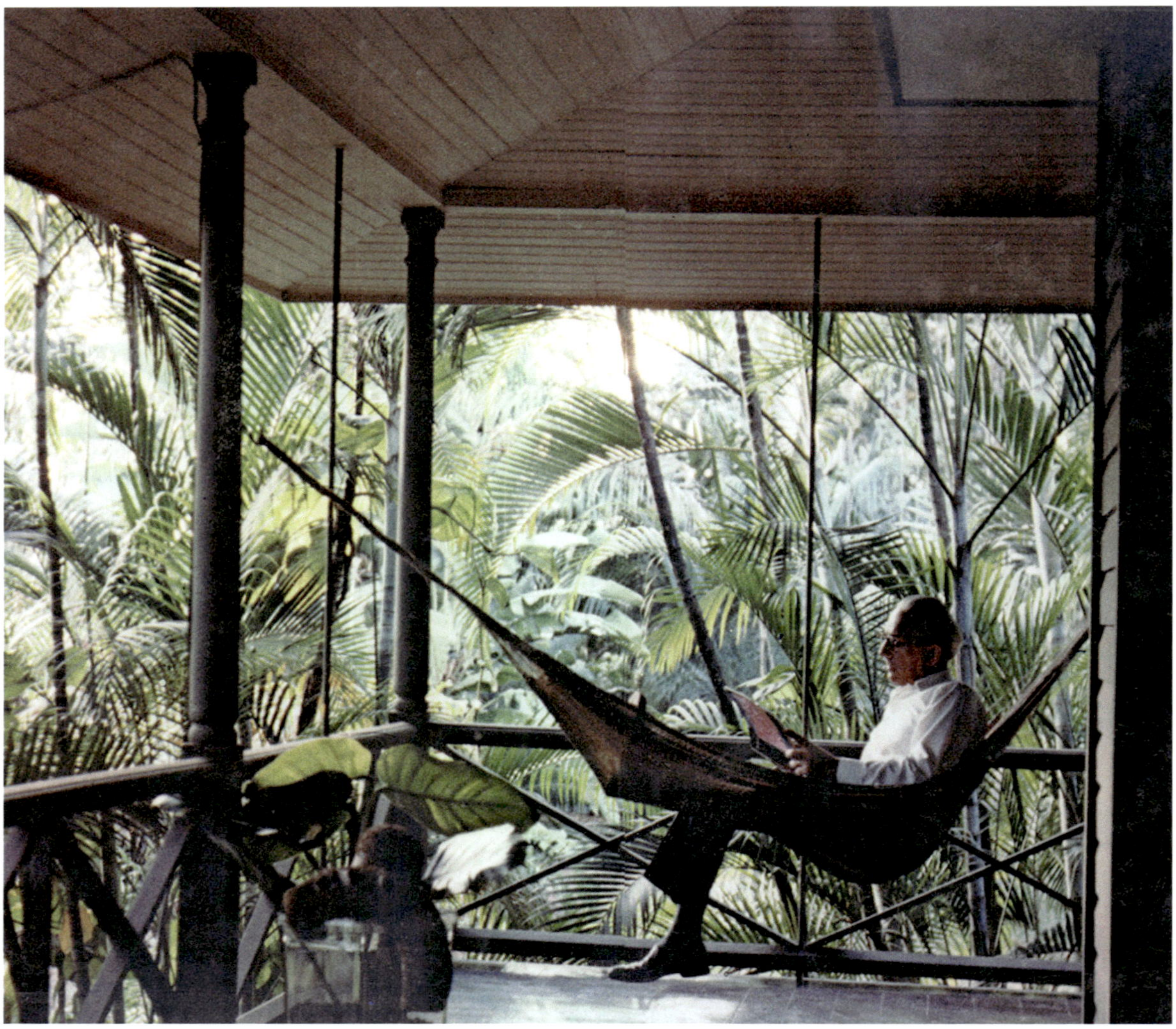

← Henry and Else Klumb in the garden of Casa Klumb.

↙ Henry Klumb on the porch of Casa Klumb.

↘ Casa Klumb, the morning after the fire. Posted on Twitter by the Colegio de Arquitectos y Arquitectos Paisajistas de Puerto Rico, November 11, 2020, 8:12am.

When Rexford Tugwell, the US-appointed governor of Puerto Rico from 1941 to 1946, invited Klumb to lead the public works committee, Klumb saw the position as an ideal way to realize his idea of architectural practice. Instead of building according to a preconceived standard, he thought architecture should be an "effort to solve problems."[7] Opposed to what he saw as the homogeneity of International Style architecture, he wanted to understand and respond to Puerto Rican values, issues, and traditions. He designed low-cost rural houses, private homes, churches, and health clinics, as well as more institutional projects such as the University of Puerto Rico campus in Río Piedras and the campuses of two major pharmaceutical companies, Eli Lilly and Parke-Davis, which were framed at the time as job-creating and economy-boosting presences on the island.[8]

Through his work in Puerto Rico, Klumb came to imagine the modern home as a space that could "[fuse] man to his environment" and "[free] his mind," allowing him to "coexist in free association with others [and] in conscious harmony with the varied moods of nature." [9] In this spirit, he conceived of the ideal Puerto Rican home as one that would keep out undesirable climatic conditions while allowing beneficial ones to enter. As a built manifesto of his philosophy, Casa Klumb functioned as a sort of epidermis, an idea that seems to have evolved out of Wright's "organic architecture."[10] The house could adapt to shifts in temperature and weather. Its built-in dining table was made of two rectangular wings that rotated freely around a post so they could be repositioned in light or shade. Horizontal glass shutters on windows tempered the sun's brightness. Chairs and a hammock on the large open porches were made of native woods and fibers and constructed in collaboration with local artisans.

Klumb and his wife Else lived in Casa Klumb from 1949 until their death in a car accident in 1984.[11] That year, the University of Puerto Rico purchased the property and hosted architecture courses and events in the space. In 1998, however, a hurricane damaged the house's kitchen and roof, which, despite Casa Klumb's inclusion on the National Register of Historical Places, were never fully repaired. In an effort to move toward a clear restoration plan, the house was added to the World Monuments Watch, and in 2014 an interdisciplinary task force, the Comité Casa Klumb, was formed. But the house's metal wiring, shutters, and roof sections were looted that same year, and more structural damage was wrought by hurricanes in 2017.[12]

Despite its articulated and controlled boundary between interior and exterior, Casa Klumb was immunocompromised from the start. The very "nature" that Klumb focused on controlling and mediating had no single identity. It was neither purely beneficial nor fully invasive. Instead, it was at once a dangerous invention, constructed and manipulated by colonial forces, as well as a site of interconnection and history, providing knowledge and healing in the hands of the local community.

Labs and Toxic Waste

The construction of nature in Puerto Rico can be traced as far back as the fifteenth century, when Spanish colonizers divided up the land in order to overwork it and the Taíno who called it home. This process picks up speed after 1952 when the archipelago (including

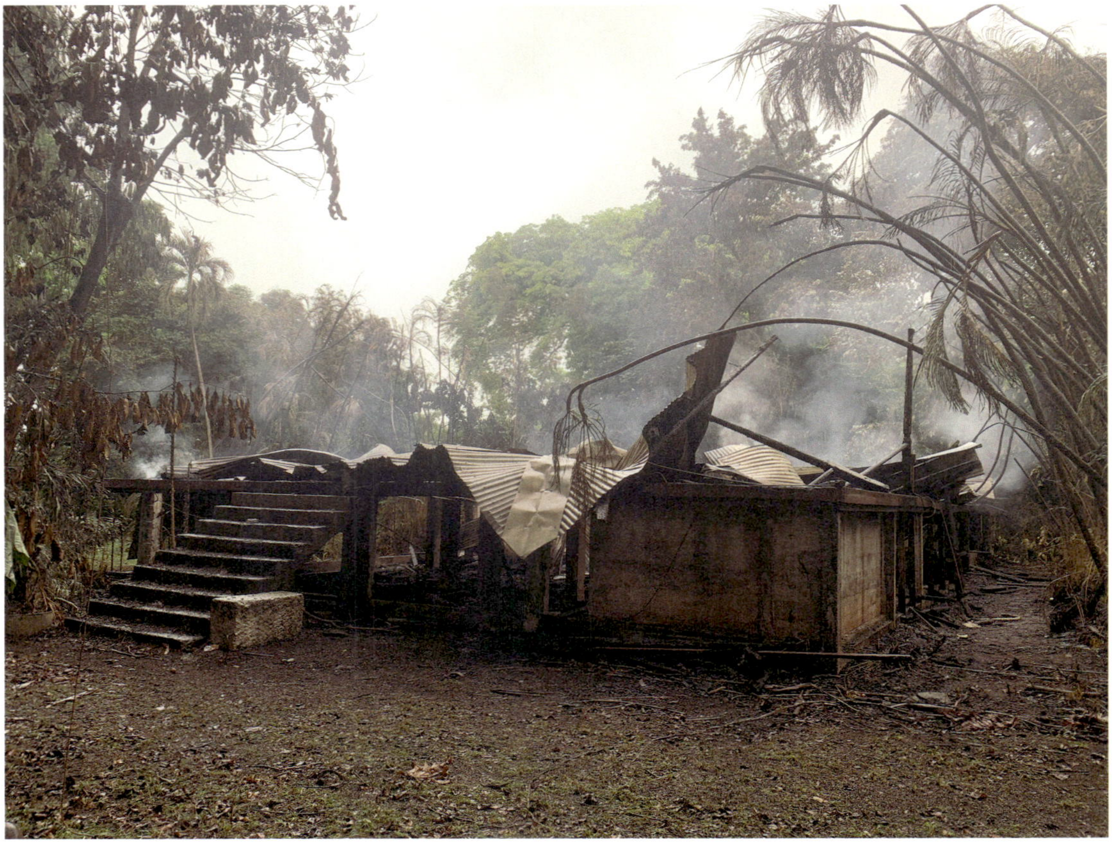

the main island plus Vieques, Culebra, Mona, Desecheo, and Caja de Muertos) was made a "commonwealth" (formally, an "Estado Libre Asociado") of the United States. With this new category in place, the US Government began to invest in a massive industrialization of both urban and rural communities, seeking to "modernize" the island's infrastructure and economy. This is the arena into which Klumb arrived. While Casa Klumb attests to the architect's interest in bridging local building traditions with modernist architectural innovations, a closer consideration of some of his institutional projects (and their wider context) reveals major contradictions lurking beneath the promises of health and modernity being made by US investors and the state more generally.

The Puerto Rican campuses of pharmaceutical companies Parke-Davis and Eli Lilly were designed by Klumb in 1960 and 1968 respectively. According to architectural historian Luz Rodríguez López, Klumb conceived of the campuses "as if they were towns," aiming to fit the buildings into a rural setting "without competing with it."[13] He reimagined the factory as an "extension of the worker's home instead of the reverse," by providing airy, open spaces with plenty of natural light.[14] This was beneficial from the perspective of pharmaceutical executives, who appreciated the fact that their campuses gave passersby "a pleasant feeling about us," and that the transparent architectural structures allowed for easy surveillance of factory workers.[15] Some of the drugs being manufactured in these factories, specifically birth control pills, were tested on Puerto Rican women in the 1950s and 1960s, often without their knowledge or consent.[16] Puerto Rican laborers were thus being encouraged to be productive in a workplace that had nonconsensually experimented with the reproductive freedom of Puerto Rican women in order to provide it as a choice to more privileged women elsewhere.

Pharmaceuticals and scientific research in Puerto Rico also had direct ecological effects. As Hilda Lloréns and Carlos G. García-Quijano have summarized, the archipelago's mid-twentieth-century modernization project—Operation Bootstrap—involved building contaminating industrial projects in "hinterland" regions away from San Juan. This has meant that many Afro-descendant communities with livelihoods based on fishing, mutual aid networks, and subsistence farming face high rates of air, water, and land pollution from oil refineries, energy plants, pharmaceutical manufacturers, and testing areas for GMO seeds and chemicals. In addition to being a tourist's idyll, "nature" in Puerto Rico is the site of extractive agriculture, slavery, and in some areas, a "waste-periphery" that gravely affects the health of people whose ancestors were forced to work the fields now being polluted.[17]

Operation Bootstrap also included experiment stations for the US Department of Agriculture and Forest Service, as well as the establishment of the Puerto Rican Nuclear Center in 1957. Consequently, El Yunque, the largest rainforest in Puerto Rico, was designated as an experimental forest rather than a nature reserve, allowing American scientists to use the biodiverse environment as a testing site, a natural laboratory.[18] One of these scientists was Howard T. Odum, who in the 1950s developed systems ecology, a study of the flow of energy and nutrients through ecosystems. In 1963, Odum was given a section of El Yunque into which he and his team used a helicopter to drop a 10,000-curie cesium gamma source (a radioactive isotope used in nuclear reactors and weapons), where it emitted radiation for over three months and destroyed foliage within a thirty-meter radius. Odum and his team then studied the forest's recovery, allowing them "to model the ecosystem's resilience under stress."[19]

To submit a body to stress, then track its ability to withstand that stress is a common tactic in imperial attempts to seize and keep power. The colonizer reports on the resilience of the colonized. One of the first iterations of this in the Caribbean was the Jeronymite Inquiry, undertaken in 1517 on the island of Ayiti (later named Hispaniola by the Spanish, and now comprising the nations of Haiti and the Dominican Republic).[20] A group of Catholic friars, charged by the Spanish Crown with administration of the island, were ordered to record the number of *caciques* (Taíno chiefs) and Indigenous peoples under their leadership who survived the devastation of European-brought diseases including typhus and smallpox. The Crown wanted to know if the Taíno could serve as an adequate labor force for the extraction of gold and, eventually, the harvesting of sugar and coffee.[21] The Taíno population declined rapidly, and in turn, the Spanish sent enslaved people from neighboring islands and the African continent, continuing to track population numbers and "resilience" to both inhumane violence and new pathogens along the way.

The historian Noble David Cook has suggested that smallpox may have been brought into Taíno homes in Hispaniola from infected Spanish clothing that was given to several Taíno interpreters to wear during a trip to Spain and back.[22] Clothing, the first layer of separation of body and environment, is one of the first historical elements of forced acculturation to European styles and norms. Seemingly banal, it nevertheless attacked both the culture and the immune systems of the Taíno. From clothing in the sixteenth century to pharmaceutical campuses and nuclear tests in the twentieth, Euro-American "gifts"—i.e., impositions of colonial ideas of health, science, and nature—weakened the Boricua home.

↓ María Teresa López (Klumb's personal secretary), Sol Aida Casanova (neighbor), and Laura Cordero Agrait (architect and former intern in the office of Henry Klumb) outside Casa Klumb, San Juan, Puerto Rico, March 19, 2014.

Gardens and Dominos

Fray Ramon Pané, a Catholic friar sent by Columbus to study Taíno culture in the early sixteenth century, noted that the Taíno called the island of Hispaniola and surrounding islands Bohío. This was a misunderstanding (the Taíno name for that island is Ayiti), but a revealing one. A *bohío* is a simple hut with dirt floors and walls and roof made of straw or palms. In the words of the Latin American Studies scholar José Juan Arrom, *bohío* is also "a synecdoche for islands that are our 'house or habitation,' our ancestral home."[23] The reverse works as well. Actions taken against the natural environment of Borikén (the Taíno name of the archipelago) are analogous with actions taken against Boricuas and their homes.

Chemical runoff and forced sterilization were certainly not Klumb's intentions. He was operating in pursuit of that healthy, ever-evasive balance between nature and architecture. His plans for low-cost schools and homes showed attunement to Puerto Rican materials, modes of construction, and community needs. But there is still much to be learned about negotiating an always-shifting boundary between nature and architecture, about living with and in contradiction.

Between 2012 and 2014, while Casa Klumb was damaged but still intact, the artist Jorge González began to think about its past and potential futures.[24] He began to work with Agustín Pérez, who had tended the gardens surrounding Casa Klumb for several decades. The gardens, designed by Klumb, were full of plants that, like the neighbors, witnessed the house in its various stages of life: from its early years as a place of gathering to its later years as an empty space, subject to nature's intrusion. Soon, González

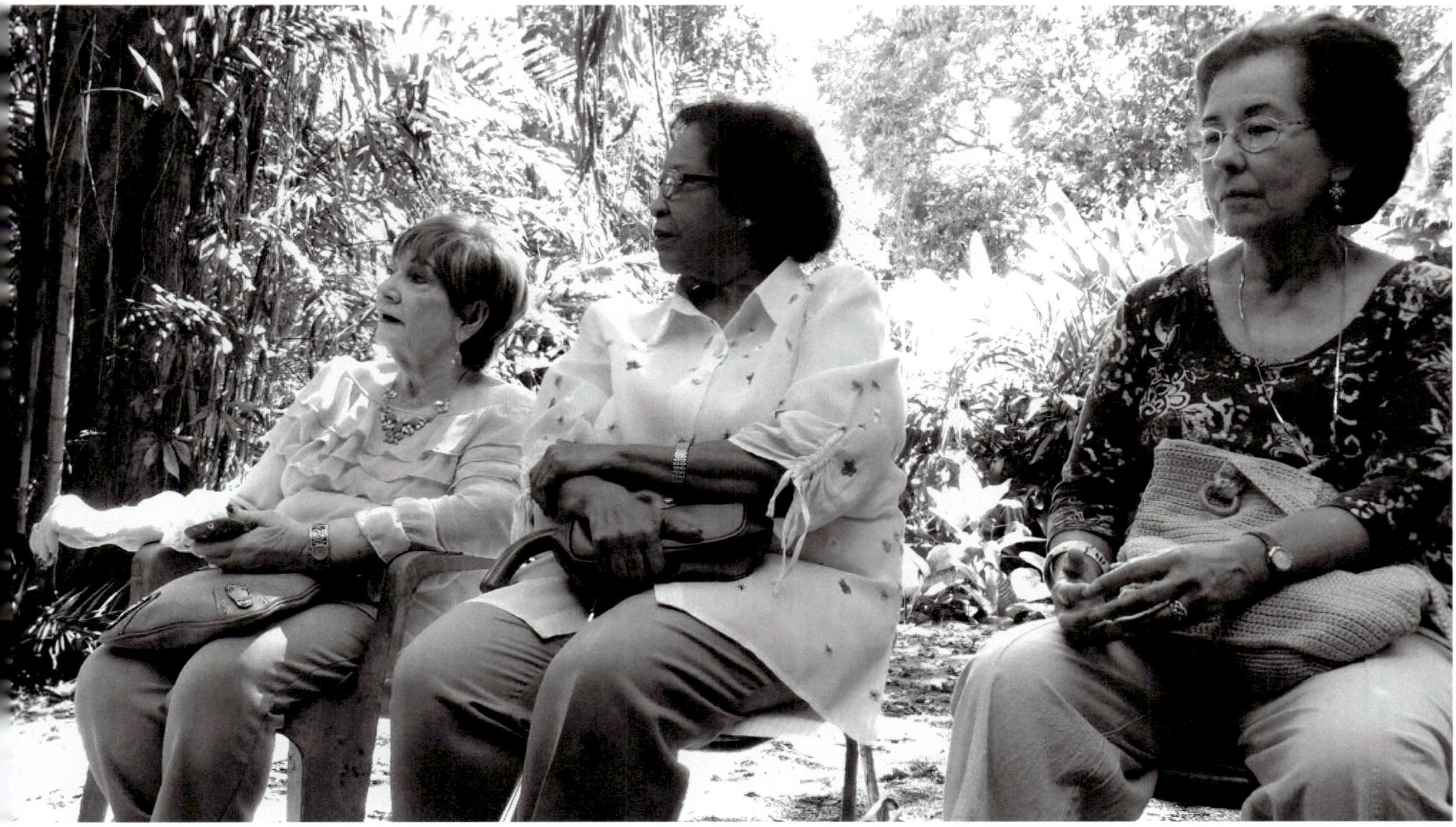

took on the role of Casa Klumb's gardener. He collected botanical specimens from the property, which were then added to the botanical archives of the University of Puerto Rico. He conducted interviews with several people in the neighborhood, whose knowledge of both flora and architecture opened alternative histories surrounding Casa Klumb. Discussing the gardens and the house with Sol Aida Casanova, who had lived in the neighborhood while the Klumbs resided there, González learned how Casa Klumb's gardens functioned as a provisional meeting place, a site for sharing knowledge about nature, and for adapting to its inevitable changes. Medicinal plants mingled with delicate orchids. As the house crumbled, the garden remained.

Considering the dynamic between her family—several members of which worked at Casa Klumb—and the Klumbs, Casanova remembered the first time Henry Klumb came to her uncle's house. He had come to play dominoes.

> The first time that Mr. Klumb went to play dominoes it was big news. Richard [his son] came all the time, but then one day my mom said "The 'old man' is coming to play dominoes at Yayo's house." The "old man" was a term of endearment for Mr. Klumb. And we said, "My God!" We didn't understand very well, because we were quite young and always playing with the idea of refusal, always saying "really?" And it was like, "Black people with these rich [white] people, the millionaires of the neighborhood?" But it was this [the idea that Mr. Klumb coming to Yayo's house would be a big deal] that I didn't understand. I am still trying to understand it. If more people understood it, we would have fewer problems in Puerto Rico.[25]

Though Yayo and other neighbors worked at Casa Klumb, helping Klumb fine-tune his vision, their contributions altered the architect's conceptions of how home and nature might be intertwined. As in dominoes, moments of equilibrium arise and provide structure. A two on one domino must be abutted by a two on another, yet its other side remains open to an alternative connection; a four waiting for a match. Experiences of class, race, and place separated the neighbors from the Klumbs, but moments arose when difference and sameness were held simultaneously at the fore, without the colonial compulsion toward a perfect resolve. Yayo pitched ideas for Casa Klumb's gardens. Else Klumb became well known in the neighborhood for her cookies. Henry and Richard came over to play dominoes.

Although the house is gone, and much of the garden's plants have dispersed from flooding, what remains of Casa Klumb is a network of Puerto Rican artists, activists, gardeners, builders, beekeepers, and botanists who have been brought together by the house and its grounds in some way. This network is highly accustomed to shifts and subversions in the fabled balance between nature and architecture. Just as the immunocompromised body must—often without institutional support—develop new means of protecting itself from pathogens and environmental triggers, the immunocompromised home is forced to transform according to potential threats and benefits. Protesters and gardeners function like antibodies and vitamins, each specializing in a particular mode of defense and sustenance. In doing so, homeostasis is pursued not as a given, universal ideal but as a term-to-be-reinvented.

González, for one, has continued to build from his experience in the Casa Klumb gardens to create the Escuela de Oficios, a platform for learning from and with Boricua artisans highly skilled in craft traditions and rural construction. As they continue to do for González, the neighbors who remember Casa Klumb have much to teach us about caring for the immunocompromised home in Puerto Rico. By playing and protesting in the unstable boundary between nature and the built environment, we might give both an anticolonial future.

An earlier version of this essay was originally published by e-flux Architecture in 2022.

1. See Felix Contreras, "A Puerto Rico Protest Song: 'Afilando los Cuchillos,'" NPR, July 28, 2019, https://www.npr.org/2019/07/28/746089844/a-puerto-rico-protest-song-afilando-los-cuchillos.
2. Simon Romero, Frances Robles, Patricia Mazzei, and Jose A. Del Real, "15 Days of Fury: How Puerto Rico's Government Collapsed," *New York Times*, July 27, 2019.
3. Tiffany Rivera, "Protests in Rincón, Puerto Rico Demand a Stop to Construction at a Beach Reserved for Endangered Turtles," *Al Día*, July 27, 2021, https://www.aldianews.com/culture/heritage-and-history/rincon-protest-erupts. See also: https://twitter.com/bgraulau/status/1418381830601035776.
4. José E. Maldonado Marrero, "The Klumb House, Historical Heritage of Puerto Rico, Destroyed by Fire," *Ey Boricua*, November 11, 2020, https://eyboricua.com/noticias/puerto-rico/destruida-por-un-incendio-la-casa-klumb-patrimonio-historico-de-puerto-rico/.
5. Heather Crichfield, Nathaniel Fúster, et al., *Klumb: An Architecture of Social Concern: Una arquitectura de impronta social* (San Juan, PR: La Editorial Universidad de Puerto Rico, 2007), 48.
6. Josean Figueroa and Edric Vivoni, *Henry Klumb: Principios para una arquitectura de integración* (Puerto Rico: Colegio de Arquitectos y Arquitectos Paisajistas de Puerto Rico, 2007), 15. Klumb's "life core" recalls what Richard Neutra called the "Block Core" facilities in his infrastructural plans for underresourced neighborhoods of wood and aluminum shacks in Puerto Rico, many of which were considered slums by the government. Richard Neutra, *Architecture of Social Concern in Regions of Mild Climate* (São Paulo, Brazil: Gerth Todtmann, 1948), 192.
7. Henry Klumb, personal papers, quoted in César A. Cruz, *Puerto Rico's Henry Klumb: A Modern Architect's Sense of Place* (New York: Routledge, 2020), 33.
8. Parke-Davis was one of the first companies to start producing contraceptive pills once the FDA had approved them. Before FDA approval, Puerto Rican women were used in clinical trials without ever knowing they were the first ones in the world to take these pills.
9. Cruz, *Puerto Rico's Henry Klumb*, 124.
10. Frank Lloyd Wright, *An Organic Architecture: The Architecture of Democracy* (London: Lund Humphries, 1939).
11. Wright, *An Organic Architecture*, 157.
12. World Monuments Fund, "Henry Klumb House," https://www.wmf.org/project/henry-klumb-house.
13. Luz Marie Rodríguez, "United States Department of the Interior, National Park Service, National Register of Historic Places Continuation Sheet, Section 8, Statement of Significance (continued), Casa Klumb, San Juan, PR," October 29, 2010, 18.
14. Rodríguez, "United States Department of the Interior."
15. Rodríguez, "United States Department of the Interior."
16. For firsthand accounts of the mass sterilization of Puerto Rican women during this period, see Ana María García's documentary *La operación* (Latin American Film Project, 1982).
17. Hilda Lloréns and Carlos G. García-Quijano, "From Extractive Agriculture to Industrial Waste Periphery: Life in a Black-Puerto Rican Ecology," *Black Perspectives*, June 22, 2020, https://www.aaihs.org/from-extractive-agriculture-to-industrial-waste-periphery-life-in-a-black-puerto-rican-ecology/.
18. Megan Raby, *American Tropics: The Caribbean Roots of Biodiversity Science* (Chapel Hill: University of North Carolina Press, 2017), 156.
19. This language has striking parallels in more recent history, as US leaders spoke often of Puerto Ricans' resilience after hurricanes Maria and Irma while failing to provide sufficient government aid. Raby, *American Tropics*, 158. Also recall Donald Trump throwing paper towels into the crowd on his belated trip to the island. David Nakamura and Ashley Parker, "'It Totally Belittled the Moment': Many Look Back in Dismay at Trump's Tossing of Paper Towels in Puerto Rico," *Washington Post*, September 13, 2018.
20. Noble David Cook, "Sickness, Starvation, and Death in Early Hispaniola," *Journal of Interdisciplinary History* 32, no. 3 (Winter 2002): 351.
21. Cook, "Sickness, Starvation, and Death in Early Hispaniola."
22. Cook, "Sickness, Starvation, and Death in Early Hispaniola," 368.
23. Fray Ramon Pané, *An Account of the Antiquities of the Indians: A New Edition*, with an Introductory Study, Notes, and Appendices by José Juan Arrom, trans. Susan C. Griswold (Durham: Duke University Press, 1999), 8.
24. Jorge González developed this project as a fellow of La Práctica, which is part of the San Juan-based artistic platform Beta-Local.
25. Sol Aida Casanova, conversation between Jorge González, María Teresa López, Laura Cordero Agrait, and Sol Aida Casanova, San Juan, Puerto Rico, March 19, 2014, unpublished transcript. Translation mine.

p268 Wikimedia Commons.
p270 © AACUPR—Archivo Arquitectura y Construcción Universidad Puerto Rico, Colección Henry Klumb.
p271 © Margarita Frontera.
p273 © Jorge González.

PLANETARY DISEQUILIB-RIUM

CLEMENS FINKELSTEIN

Arrested in motion, the personification of Earth appears precariously imbalanced. Crowned by a model of a turreted city, their muscular body twists auspiciously into the foreground. Intent on stability, their left arm forcefully presses downward, hand firmly grasping an oblong stone. The right holds out a needle-like scepter, threatening to answer any agitation in the surroundings by piercing the carnal fabric below. The overcast sky tinges the scene with a hostile atmosphere. In the background, a city emerges hewn out of the mountainous ridge to the left. On the right, naked cave dwellers depart their lithic darkness by terraforming, extracting resources. Their tool mirrors the direction of Earth's scepter as it breaks into the soil. Earth appears apathetic yet tense. The allegorical *Terra* (1587) by Jan Sadeler forcefully illustrates the foreboding entanglement of culture and nature in Western conceptions of Earth. As the mediator between natural and artificial environments, architecture crowns Earth as the synthesis of anthropic agency and emblematic caution.

Concerns of human and planetary health have always been closely entangled, growing increasingly closer at a moment when public discussions shift focus to lament the earth's transformation from a *biosphere* (a sphere of life) to a *thanatosphere*

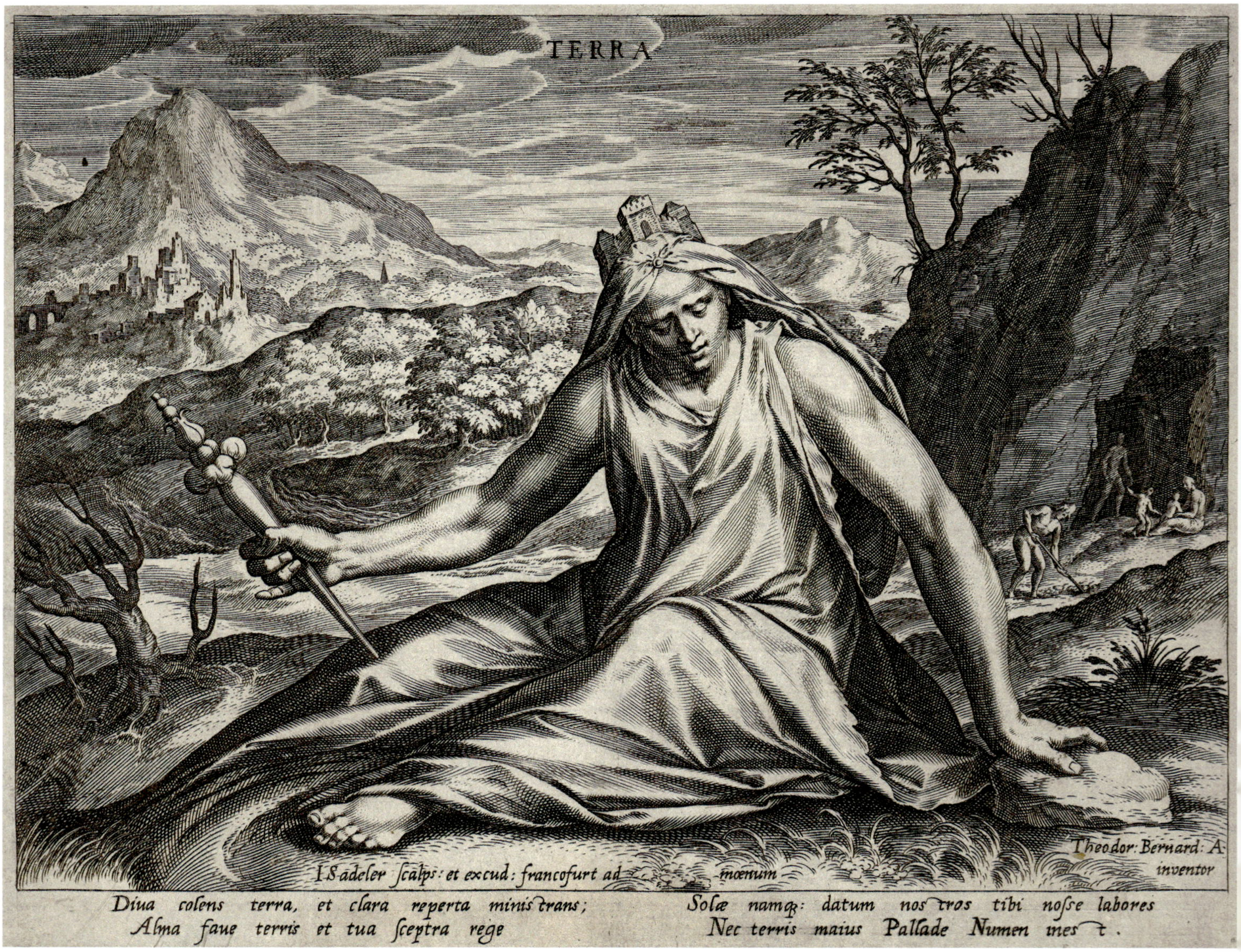
TERRA
I Sadeler scalps: et excud: francofurt ad moenum
Theodor: Bernard: A inventor
Diua colens terra, et clara reperta minis trans;
Alma faue terris et tua sceptra rege
Solæ namq: datum nostros tibi nosse labores
Nec terris maius Pallade Numen inest.

↙ Jan Sadeler (engraver), after Dirck Barendsz, *Terra (Earth)*, from the series *The Four Elements*, Frankfurt am Main, 1587.

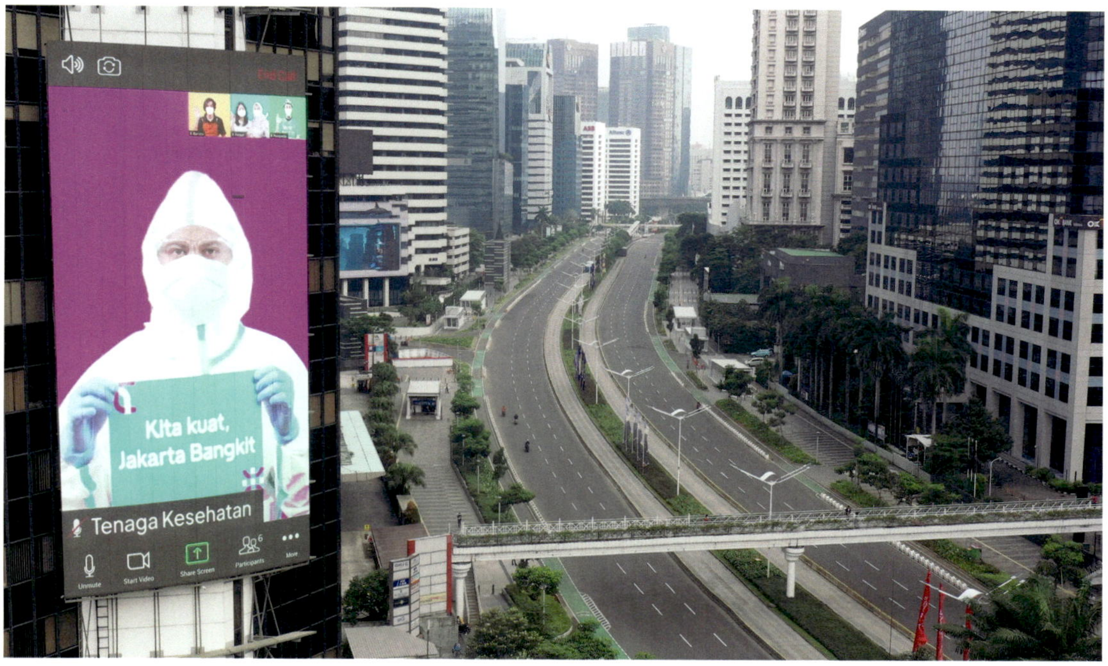

→ Empty highways amid tightening lockdown protocols to combat the novel surge in Covid-19 cases, Jakarta, Indonesia, July 2021.

(a sphere of death). Yet, instead of evolving toward equilibrium—as entangled objects do according to current physical theories of thermodynamics and quantum mechanics—their relationship has unraveled into sustained disequilibrium. Planetary infirmity is materialized through significant climatic shifts, excessive anthropogenic vibrations, the resultant corruption of its biospheric system, as well as the redistribution of its mass and axis through glacial melting.

Crucial awareness of planetary health has materialized most profoundly in periods when human agents are either temporarily removed from the intricate ecological systems they otherwise dominate or attempt to gain superior control over the planet through technoscientific innovation. Viral pathologies and their preventative measures during the height of the Covid-19 pandemic demonstrate the collective capacity of human societies to counter encroaching human sickness swiftly and effectively. Lacking adequate geopolitical protocols and actionable processes to counterbalance planetary health, however, Terra charges architecture to resume its once crowning role, balancing their heart and body.

Terra Infirma In a selfish manner befitting *Homo sapiens sapiens*, the Covid-19 pandemic bundled humanity's focus in hitherto unknown intensity on the fragile physiological envelopes that contain its beings and the organic systems that service it. Invisible viral spores transformed human bodies into supernodes of a rupturing ecology of disease, painfully dividing communities as proximity became synonymous with potential contamination. Governmental orders imposed lasting states of emergency instructing citizens to shelter in place preventatively, work from home, or quarantine those exposed. Containment measures introduced to combat the spread of the novel coronavirus emptied streets, schools, offices, and entire districts previously brimming with the bodies of human dwellers. Moderating the movement of the earth's population to mitigate the pandemic outbreak, these lockdown protocols led to an unprecedented deceleration of global transport, extraction, and construction industries. Combined, the abatement of human activity across the planetary surface slowed the vibrational agitations of the earth—its constant microseismic activity—and culminated in the greatest seismic quiet period in recorded history.

Whether extractive processes that erode the planetary crust in search of mineral resources or footsteps treading their daily paths to downtown buildings, "human activity causes vibrations that propagate into the ground as high-frequency seismic waves," explains seismologist Thomas Lecocq.[1] New subdisciplines such as urban seismology have formed to investigate the various origins of earth vibrations within cities, ranging from "footquakes," e.g., synchronous footsteps celebrating sports events or music concerts in large stadiums, to the seismic impact of architectural construction, fireworks, or subway trains.[2] In the first half of 2020, seventy-five researchers from sixty-six associated institutions globally joined Lecocq in an exhaustive analysis of the seismological effects of the Covid-19 pandemic, correlating restricted human activity measures with anthropogenic vibratory impulses—hiFSAN, or high frequency seismic ambient noise (4–14 Hz)—that constantly move the earth.[3]

Sourcing data from seismic networks located in densely populated urban areas and taking advantage of a spectrum of sensors, ranging from broadband seismometer stations to personal seismographs,

← Global temporal changes in seismic noise (daily median hiFSAN).

↓ Raspberry ShakeNet, global overview of all (online) stations, September 21, 2021.

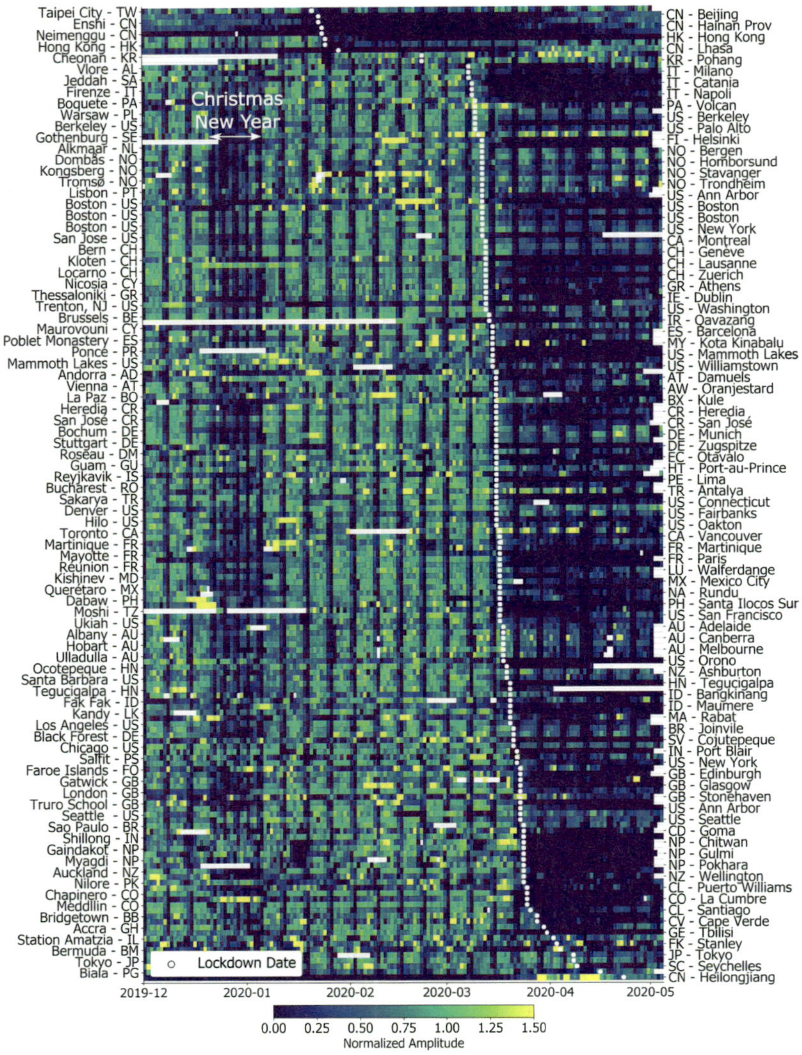

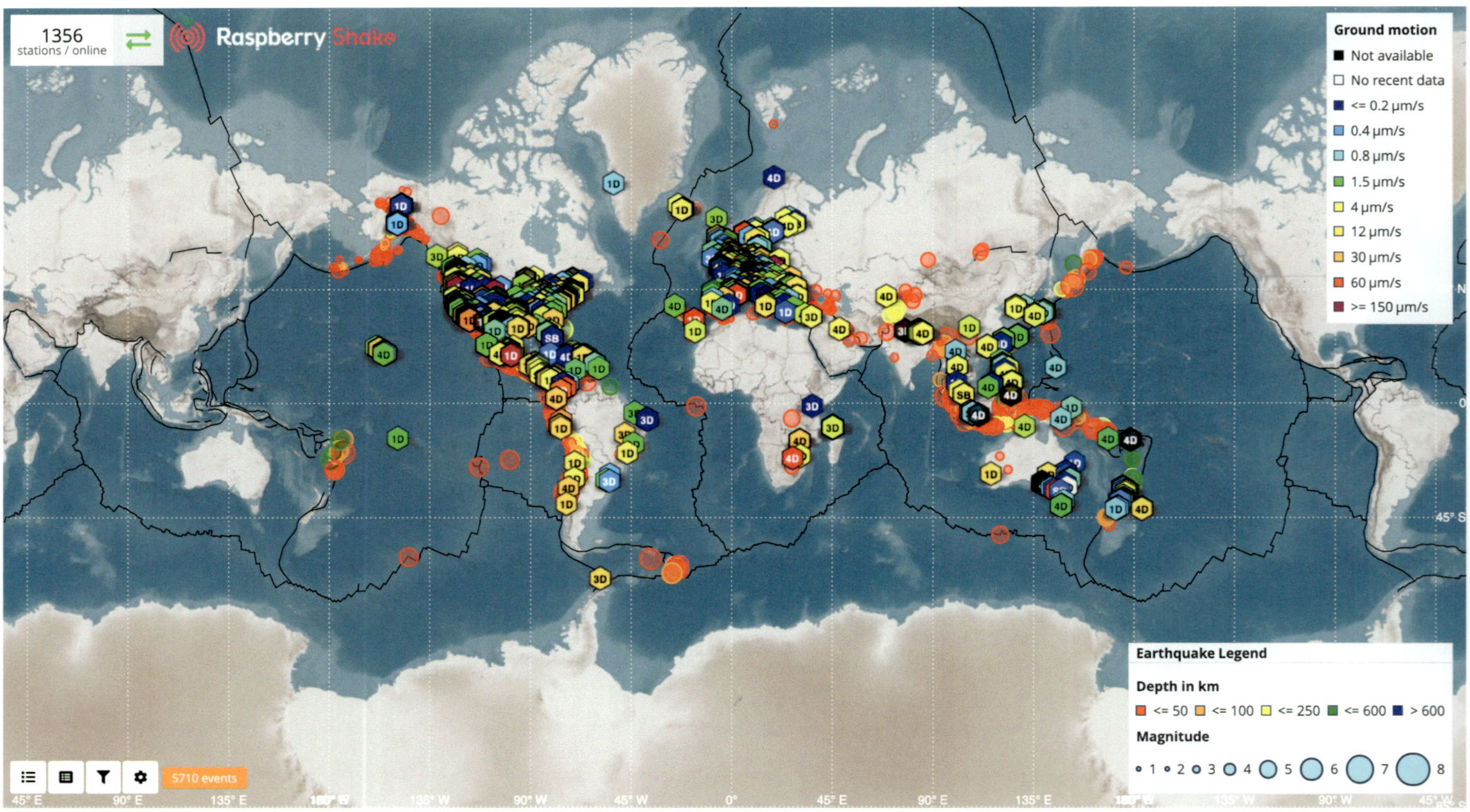

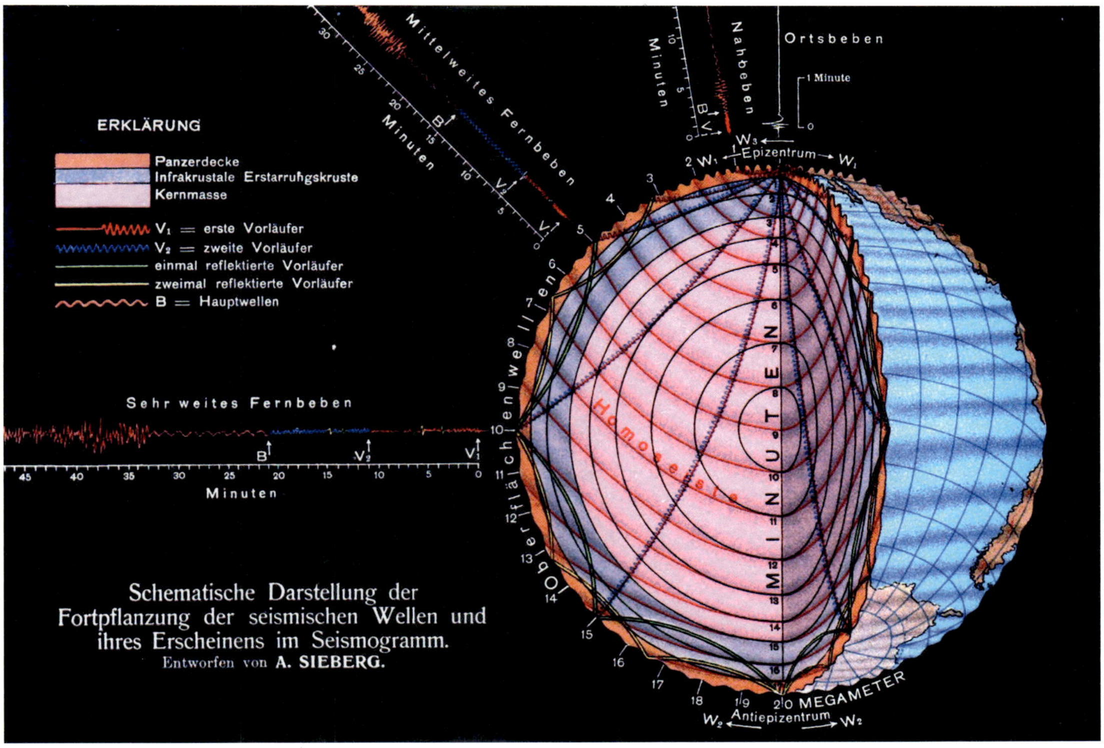

→ Schematic representation of the propagations of seismic waves and their appearance in seismograms.

they demonstrated that global metropoles such as London, Paris, Brussels, Jakarta, and Los Angeles experienced extraordinary drops, from thirty to fifty percent, in hiFSAN during periods of lockdown. The measurement of planetary ground motion and environmental infrasound activities during this "quiet period" allowed observations of microseismic events otherwise masked by the din of human enterprise and provided an unknown epistemic cache.

The liquid habitat of myriad organisms, covering seventy-one percent of the earth's surface, was similarly quieted by anti-Covid-19 protocols. Slowing commercial and touristic shipping to a significant degree led to an immediate ecological response in coastal regions all over the globe. Entire families of whales, whose echo-communicational capabilities were relieved from the deafening vibratory drone of human vessels, returned to areas they had avoided for decades. On land, various mammals, amphibians, and birds reclaimed the otherwise vibration-rich urban spaces of human dwellers that frequently displace them.[4]

Anthropogenic activity thus not only triggers defining vibratory agitations of the planetary surface; it signals planetary infirmity through resultant disruptions of the earth's biospheric systems. At the turn of the twentieth century, a distinct vibrational epistemology spurred by colonial ventures sought to unravel the interplay between human and planetary dynamics. With the aid of technologized architectural environments, scientists sought to understand the earth's geophysical intricacies and discern the reciprocal influences of planetary conditions on societal development.

Planetary Physiology: From the Heart to the Body of the Earth

On April 17, 1889, Prussian astronomer Ernst von Rebeur-Paschwitz's horizontal pendulum accidentally recorded seismic waves that originated 9,000 kilometers (5,500 miles) from the Astrophysical Observatory in Potsdam, Prussia, and forty-five minutes before his delicate device sensed them at 5:21 pm. The planetary vibrations had traveled from Japanese earthquake faults near Tokyo through the earth's crust to Potsdam at 3,060 meters per second. Their recording provided the first proof of "teleseismic" events: vibrations dissipating while deforming the planetary body that pulses, in the words of seismologist Cargill Knott, "like a beating heart."[5] As a result of this happy accident, vibrations, which were previously one of the main hindrances to precise scientific observation, became geophysics' defining epistemic tool, promising to decipher the earth's obscure interior structure. This was mirrored in architecture, with a shift in focus from insulating against exterior vibratory disturbances to isolating the "symbiotic" interior vibratory forces of the planet for study. Rebeur-Paschwitz's discovery took place in the Astrophysical Observatory designed by Paul Emanuel Spieker (built 1876–1879), which innovated the structural design of scientific observatories to provide vibration-free environments.[6] Both architects and scientists now had to distinguish between obstructive and constructive vibrations.

In the final months of his tuberculosis-ridden life, Rebeur-Paschwitz was preoccupied with "a scheme for the organized study of earthquake pulsations all over the globe."[7] Cut short in 1895 at the age of thirty-four, his vision of an international, global network of scientific observatories rehearsed well-established fantasies that sought comprehensive knowledge about the earth and its geophysical activity.[8] However, only recent technological advancements in telecommunication (e.g., electric telegraphy) and mobility (e.g., steamboats, railroads), coupled with imperial geopolitics' economic and colonial motivation, provided resources to realize this dream.

In 1898, Emil Wiechert assumed the world's first Chair of Geophysics at the Georg-August-Universität in Göttingen, Prussia. He adopted Rebeur-Paschwitz's plan and went on to establish the rural enclave as a global hub within a network of science centers that was rapidly expanding around the world, focusing on both macro- and microseismological observations.[9] Wiechert's advanced seismographs had the remarkable capability to visually amplify seismic vibrations a thousandfold, providing planetary data of unparalleled detail and consistency. Among his notable inventions was the ultrasensitive 1,000-kilogram Wiechert pendulum, which was capable of sensing vibrational agitation from halfway around the globe.

Personal infirmity drove Wiechert's interest in the vibratory frequency of the earth. His development of instruments that could "sense the deepest depths of the earth," eulogized the archaeologist Hermann Thiersch at the geophysicist's funeral in 1928, could be linked to the apparatuses that aided Wiechert's progressive hearing loss.[10] Placed on the surface of the planetary body, Wiechert's automatic seismographs were not unlike electric hearing aids or medical stethoscopes in amplifying and sensing near-imperceptible vibratory signals. Deducing knowledge about the earth's physical states, geophysicists further entangled the human and planetary body through their vibrational susceptibility.

In 1903, at the Second International Seismological Conference of the newly founded International Association of Seismology and Physics of the Earth's Interior (IASPEI) in Strasbourg, Wiechert reflected on the recent establishment of scientific outposts in the German colonies, particularly German Samoa's Geophysical "Samoa-Observatory," the empire's leading meteorological beacon in the South Pacific. Foregrounding the potential of applied geophysics, he addressed IASPEI's soaring interest in establishing a centrally coordinated and organized network of seismic sensors. Recording, measuring, and analyzing pulsating planetary vibrations would emulate what Wilhelm Röntgen had shown to be possible with the application of his X-rays: to render solid, opaque bodies transparent.[11]

"As soon as we penetrate the earth to extract the minerals necessary for our modern life," Wiechert stressed, the human enterprise may cause cataclysmic atmospheric effects that risk the health of humanity and the frequent "demise of thousands."[12] In his conference presentation, Wiechert hinged the motivation for his global scientific endeavor on the idea of *Heimatsgefühl*, a shared, common sense of *Heimat*—that German untranslatable encompassing diverse notions of home and nationality, but also original belonging. This feeling, he stressed, transcends any national, social, or racial boundaries since "just as the individual pays loving attention to the things that surround them in their daily home ... so for humanity as a whole, personal interest connects it to the special cosmic body 'Earth.'"[13] With the sober aside, "where love does not guide, material needs force attention," the geophysicist's words, however, sought to legitimize colonial expansionism with environmentalism.

After setting the capricious scene in which frail human bodies find themselves at the mercy of natural forces and planetary geophysics, Wiechert casually changed tone from magnanimous world citizen to arguing for a novel colonialism rehabilitated not by politics or economics but by science. Germany had only recently emerged as an imperial superpower and desired a greater colonial domain than allocated during and after the Berlin Conference of 1884–1885. Echoing the general German sentiment of having failed to receive sufficient "shares of the ownership on the surface of the earth," Wiechert declared in his memorandum:

> For a long, long time, we Germans sat in the cramped fatherland and viewed what was outside its borders as a strange world. That has changed today; we feel like inhabitants of the earth and send our thoughts and plans to the ships that circumnavigate the world. ... Even though we could only participate in the division of the earth among the peoples belatedly, we gained a firm foothold here and there in the distance. Our position towards the big questions of the exploration of the earth has thus become a different one. We will have to look for bases for our colonies not only politically and economically but also scientifically.[14]

Outlining Germany's pioneering role in this endeavor, Wiechert rationalized the investment of considerable assets to establish further colonial outposts based solely on their geophysical properties. Detailed observations demand at least three (as far as possible) distanced stations to determine the origin of a seismic event such as an earthquake. He thus envisioned a tripartite system of nestled stations in Africa (Togo, German Southwest Africa, and German East Africa) and the Pacific (Samoa, Kaiser-Wilhelmsland, and Qingdao).[15] These "outposts" would complement the datafication of the planet and its atmospheric systems already in progress in the "mother-stations"

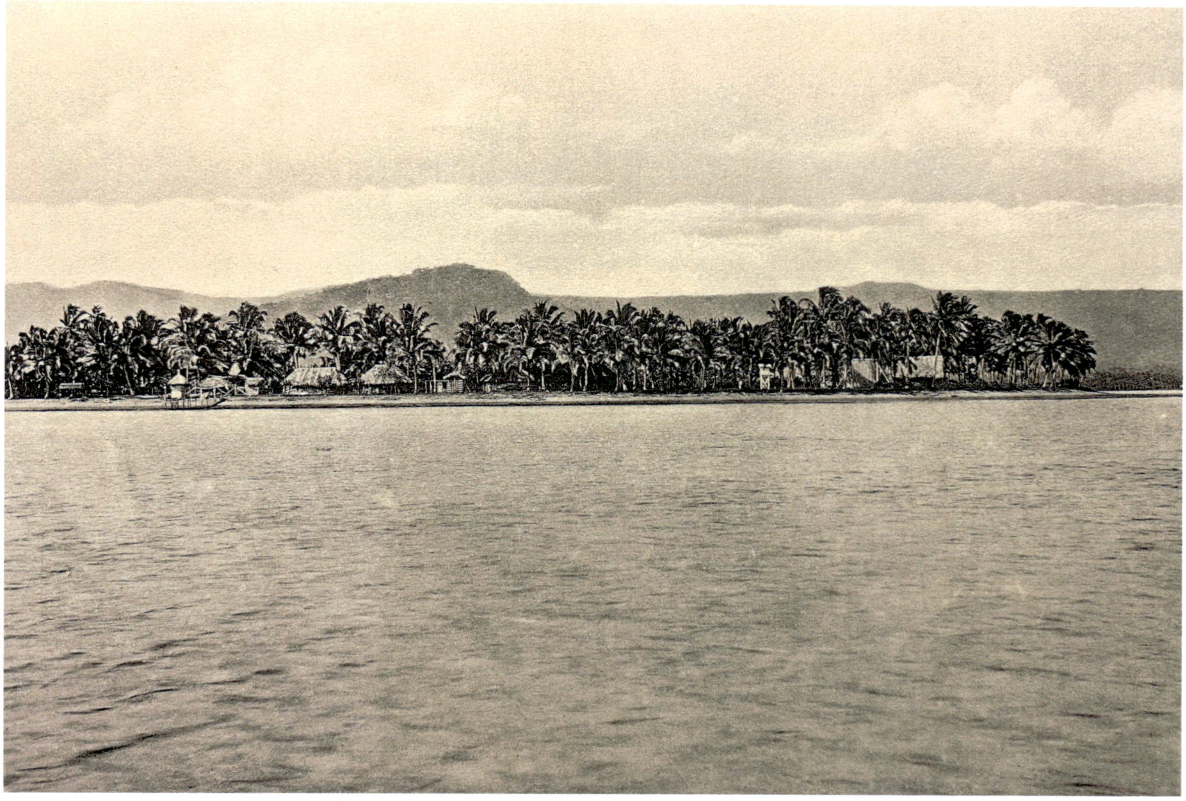

← Geophysical Samoa Observatory near Apia on Upolu, view from the lagoon (north), 1904.

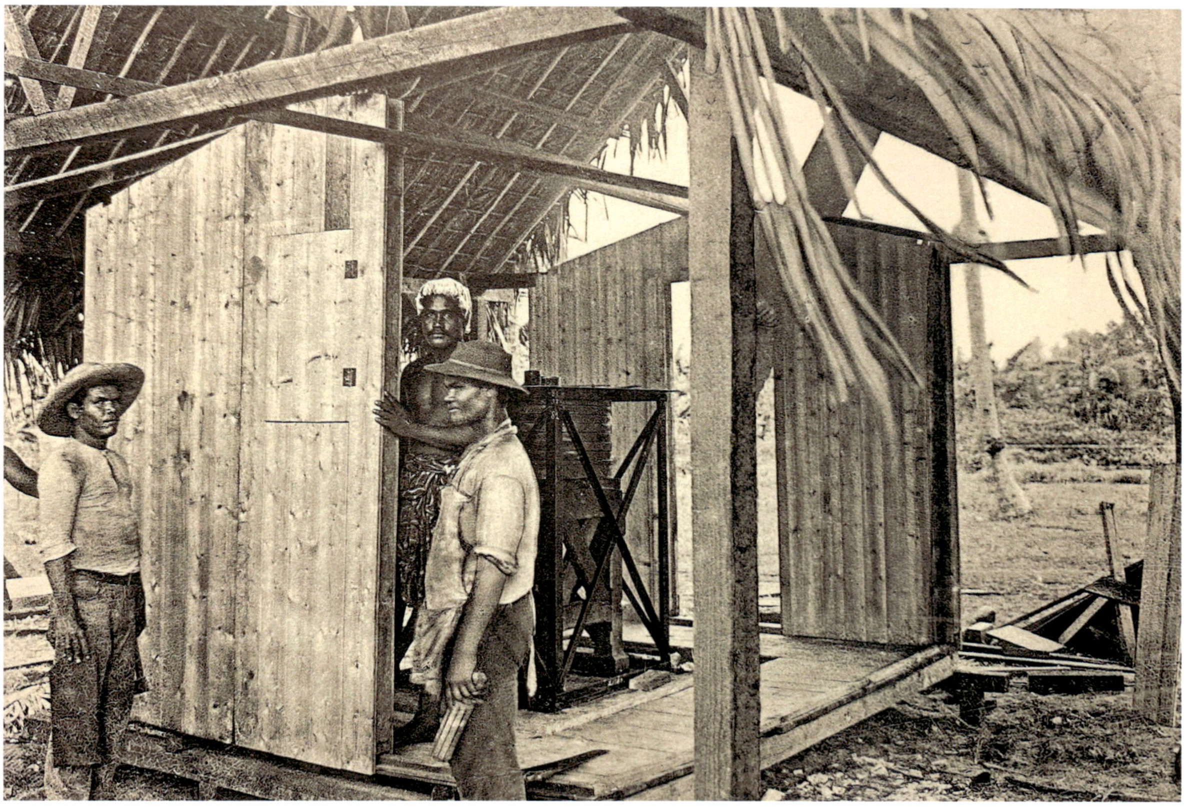

↙ Geophysical Samoa Observatory near Apia on Upolu, the seismic hut under construction by Samoan workers, encasing the seismographic unit of Wiechert's 1,000-kilogram pendulum to shelter it from atmospheric fluctuations, 1902.

of Europe, all to procure "knowledge from the deepest depths of the earth." Aided by seismic vibrations and their epistemic force, geophysics (theoretical and applied), reasoned Wiechert, would allow Germany to lay claim to the interior of the planet—which any imperial power had not yet done—and eventually provide access to its untapped well of minerals and materials through seismic prospecting. International collaboration acted as a veil for the proposed colonial catch-up and became a forceful selling point to the Imperial Government and the Royal Prussian Ministry of Education.

Confronted with various environmental zones across colonial territories, architecture was the means by which Wiechert's plans for an epistemological network could be realized. The geophysicist had previously attained considerable architectural expertise by overseeing the erection of seismological research stations such as the Earthquake Observatory in Göttingen (1902) and the designs for the prefabricated huts of the Samoa Observatory (1902–1914). The architectural units he proposed for this global network would facilitate colonial emplacement as modular system boundaries, all while isolating a regulated interior space from the uncontrollable atmospherics of the exterior.

> For each of the colonial main stations, a house is to be built, which alone contains the seismic recording devices, offering for their installation a space 2.5 meters high and at least 5 × 6 meters floor space. During the construction, care must be taken to protect the interior from rapid temperature changes and keep its walls from direct exposure to the sun and wind. It will be best to sink the house into the ground as far as the groundwater conditions and other circumstances allow. In front of the entrance, a small portal is to be installed in such a way that at least two doors must be passed through, which are never open at the same time. The doors should close adequately and be built in such a way that they provide the best possible thermal insulation. If the system of windows cannot be bypassed entirely by artificial lighting, great care must also be taken with their construction. They must have double-thick glass walls and shutters that close very well on the outside and inside. Since a person's weight affects the apparatuses already from a considerable distance, they must have very deep, free-standing pillars, or a suspended floor must be arranged for the visitors. The cost of the house is estimated at 5,000–10,000 Mark.[16]

With thirty-square-meter architectural units telegraphically connected in a planetary system of controlled environments, Wiechert's geomorphic regime ultimately aspired to cover the 510.1 trillion square meters of the earth's surface. However, the dawn of global warfare in August 1914 marked a sudden halt to the German Empire's short-lived colonial enterprise. With the progressive seizure of its territories, protectorates, and concessions, including the Samoa Observatory, Wiechert's "seismic colonialism" went unrealized. Nevertheless, its partial success during this historical period underscored the potential of vibrations to connect systemic nodes across environmental boundaries.

Endangerment Sensibilities

Over the past few years, a community of citizen scientists has emerged whose growing interest in the vibratory dynamics of the earth is motivated by linking their future health to that of the planet.[17] Affordable personal seismographs and infrasound sensors can measure and monitor planetary conditions and thus increasingly facilitate democratic empowerment and a profound communal attunement to the earth.[18] In a world grappling with climate change, biodiversity loss, and resource depletion, contemporary sensory technologies can be operationalized to build awareness of the interrelations between human, nonhuman, and inhuman entities, their intersectional environments, and the planet.[19] These sensibilities offer a means to decipher the complex interplay between human activities and planetary health.

While sensory data clouds may seek to replace Sadeler's *Terra* as a symbolic emblem of planetary infirmity in the future, nature and culture remain precariously intertwined in the twenty-first century and are still crowned by architecture as their environmental mediator. Humanity's relationship with the earth remains inherently rooted in specific geographic, cultural, and temporal contexts. While particular to these parameters, as Jennifer Gabrys has recently posited, the "planetary" knits itself together in a variegated and interrelational manner.[20] Her caution, here, serves as a critical reminder that the planetary is not an abstract, universal concept but a deeply situated and localized experience. With its disciplinary expertise in situatedness, architecture thus stands at the frontier of this planetary turn and must lead the balancing act between ailing humanity and Earth.[21]

An earlier version of this essay was originally published by e-flux Architecture in 2022.

p276 © The Trustees of the British Museum.
p277 © Shutterstock.
p278 (top) Reproduced from Thomas Lecocq, Stephen P. Hicks, Koen Van Noten, et al., "Global Quieting of High-Frequency Seismic Noise Due to COVID-19 Pandemic Lockdown Measures," *Science* 369, no. 6509 (September 11, 2020): 1338–1343. Reprinted with permission from AAAS.
p278 (bottom) Screenshot of author's account. Courtesy of Raspberry Shake.
p279 Reproduced from August Sieberg, *Der Erdball, seine Entwicklung und seine Kräfte* (Eßlingen and Munich: J. F. Schreiber, 1908), plate XXXIV.
p281 Photographer unnamed (likely Otto Tetens, the observatory's first director). Reproduced from Hermann Wagner, "Ergebnisse der Arbeiten des Samoa-Observatoriums der Königlichen Gesellschaft der Wissenschaften zu Göttingen. I. Das Samoa Observatorium," *Abhandlungen der Königlichen Gesellschaft der Wissenschaften zu Göttingen, Mathematisch-Physikalische Klasse*, vol. VII, Neue Folge, no. 1 (1908).

1. Thomas Lecocq et al., "Global Quieting of High-Frequency Seismic Noise Due to COVID-19 Pandemic Lockdown Measures," *Science* 369, no. 6509 (July 23, 2020).
2. See J. Díaz, M. Ruiz, P. S. Sánchez-Pastor, et al., "Urban Seismology: On the Origin of Earth Vibrations within a City," *Sci Rep* 7, no. 15296 (2017); Chang Che, "'Swift Quake': Taylor Swift Fans Shake Ground During Seattle Concert," *New York Times*, July 28, 2023.
3. See James N. Brune and Jack Oliver, "The Seismic Noise of the Earth's Surface," *Bulletin of the Seismological Society of America* 49, no. 4 (1959): 349–353.
4. See V. Caorsi, V. Guerra, R. Furtado, et al., "Anthropogenic Substrate-Borne Vibrations Impact Anuran Calling," *Sci Rep* 9, no. 19456 (2019).
5. Teleseismic events are earthquakes, and their vibratory effects are registered at distances more than 1,000 kilometers from their origin. Ernst von Rebeur-Paschwitz, "The Earthquake of Tokio, April 18, 1889," *Nature* 40, no. 1030 (1889): 294–295; Cargill G. Knott, "The Earthquake of Tokio, April 18, 1889," *Nature* 41, no. 1046 (1889): 32. For an elaborate account of the historical development of modern seismology as a "citizen science," see Deborah Coen, *The Earthquake Observers: Disaster Science from Lisbon to Richter* (Chicago: University of Chicago Press, 2013).
6. Paul Emanuel Spieker, "Die Bauausführungen des Königlichen astrophysikalischen Observatoriums auf dem Telegraphenberge bei Potsdam," *Zeitschrift für Bauwesen* 29, no. 1–3 (1879): 33–48; Spieker, "Die Königlichen Observatorien für Astrophysik, Meteorologie und Geodäsie auf dem Telegraphenberge bei Potsdam," *Zeitschrift für Bauwesen* 46, no. 1–3 (1894): 1–16, 203–218, 343–370.
7. Charles Davison, "Dr. E. Von Rebeur-Paschwitz," *Nature* 52, no. 1355 (1895): 600.
8. Seismology has a long tradition in Britain, where members of the Royal Society began early investigations in the 1660s. First "networks" of instruments and a seismic bulletin were established in Scotland in the early 1840s. See Roger M. W. Musson, "A History of British Seismology," *Bulletin of Earthquake Engineering* 11, no. 3 (2013): 715–861.
9. Transmitted through the planetary medium at varying intensity, macroseisms are those severe or "felt" earthquakes easily discernible by human observers. In contrast, microseisms describe the moderate or "unfelt" earth tremors whose registration depends on finely tuned scientific instruments.
10. Hermann Thiersch, "Worte des Gedächtnisses gesprochen an der Bahre Emil Wiecherts," Pers 56,3, 1, no. 16 (1928), Archives of the Academy of Sciences, Göttingen.
11. See Wilhelm Röntgen, "On a New Kind of Rays," *Nature* (January 23, 1896): 275; for transmissions of this trope in modern architecture, see Beatriz Colomina, *X-Ray Architecture* (Zurich: Lars Müller, 2019).
12. Röntgen, "On a New Kind of Rays."
13. Röntgen, "On a New Kind of Rays."
14. Röntgen, "On a New Kind of Rays."
15. Imperial German colonies around 1900: Togoland (Togo), Kamerun (Cameroon), Deutsch-Ostafrika (German East Africa, comprising present-day regions of Burundi, Rwanda, Tanzania, Mozambique), Deutsch-Südwestafrika (German Southwest Africa, part of present-day Namibia), Deutsch-Neuguinea (German New Guinea, including Kaiser-Wilhelmsland, present-day Papua New Guinea), and Deutsch-Samoa (German Samoa, present-day Samoa). Deutsch-Kiautschou (Jiaozhou Bay concession), Chefoo, and Tsingtao (Qingdao) were treaty ports, leased, as concessions, by the Qing Dynasty (all in present-day China). See Sebastian Conrad, *German Colonialism: A Short History*, trans. Sorcha O'Hagan (Cambridge: Cambridge University Press, 2012). Originally published as *Deutsche Kolonialgeschichte* (Munich: C. H. Beck, 2008).
16. Emil Wiechert, "Entwurf einer Denkschrift über seismologische Beobachtungen in den deutschen Kolonien" (1904), 316–317.
17. Madeleine Morley, "The Unheard Symphony of the Planet," *New York Times*, February 19, 2023, 15.
18. Jennifer Gabrys's Citizen Sense project (2013–) is a prime example of civic engagement and the honing of planetary sensibilities; see Jennifer Gabrys, *How to Do Things with Sensors* (Minneapolis: University of Minnesota Press, 2019).
19. Within the evolving discourse of the architectural and planetary humanities, scholars like Gabrys or Rania Ghosn and El Hadi Jazairy illuminate a profound shift in the way we perceive and interact with the earth, imploring human societies to mobilize their endangerment sensibilities and technology-aided planetary sensibilities alongside sustainable architectural making. Rania Ghosn, "World and Heritage in the Climate Crisis," in DESIGN EARTH (Rania Ghosn and El Hadi Jazairy), *Climate Inheritance* (New York: Actar Publishers, 2023), 14–16; see David Gissen, *Subnature: Architecture's Other Environments* (New York: Princeton Architectural Press, 2009).
20. Jennifer Gabrys during the opening roundtable discussion of the lecture series South Designs: Planetary Futures of the Critical Urbanisms program at the University of Basel, moderated by Kenny Cupers and Laura Nkula-Wenz (September 28, 2023).
21. This research has been supported by the Center for Digital Humanities, the Metropolis Project of the School for Engineering, and the Andlinger Center for Energy and Environment at Princeton University, the Princeton-Mellon Initiative in Architecture, Urbanism & the Humanities, the Panel on Planetary Thinking at the Justus Liebig University Giessen, and the History of Science Society.

ON THE NATURE OF PLATO'S EMBODIED CITY AND THE MAKING OF BIOPOLITICS

BROOKE HOLMES

Every city needs walls, or so Vitruvius assumes.[1] If you are going to design a city from the ground up, deciding where to locate its walls is the first order of business. These walls form, first and foremost, a military defense. But Vitruvius is also alert to the threats posed by the city's surroundings that walls cannot repel. You don't want to build on a site that is too hot or too cold, too wet or too dry. You should also avoid marshland teeming with little creatures wafting pestilence over any fortifications you build.[2] Vitruvius is drawing here on what was, by the first century BCE, a well-established tradition within medicine and natural philosophy for predicting and assessing the health of a community based on its locale. He starts, accordingly, from the assumption that the architect has to build salubrious conditions into the plan for the city if its citizens are to have a reasonable chance of flourishing.

In the *Republic*, written a few hundred years earlier than Vitruvius's *On Architecture,* Plato approaches the question of public health differently: not only from the perspective of the citizens' bodies but also, and more seriously, from the perspective of their souls. Here, perhaps for the first time in his writings, he develops a robust theory of the tripartite soul by way of his narrator Socrates. On this account, the soul is divided into the "appetitive" part, the seat of desire and appetite; the "spirited" part, which Socrates likens to a dog, vicious or loyal depending on who it obeys and how you look at it; and the part housing reason, which, Socrates argues, should rule over the appetitive and spirited parts. The psychic condition in which reason rules is what he calls "justice." Yet keeping reason on top will require, in turn, policing the affects and desires that originate in the lower parts of the soul.

To see this argument about psychic justice clearly, Socrates proposes translating it into a domain where it can be scaled up.[3] It is in this context that he introduces the city as the soul's macroscopic double. Like the soul, Socrates argues, the city has different parts: not only citizens but also, more formally, three ranked classes of citizens (the producers, the guardians, and the rulers). The city's health, too, depends on the unity of its unequal parts. But the city is not only an analogue to the soul. It is itself made up of citizens whose souls have to manage a continual influx of affects through the senses and pleasures and pains without endangering the rule of reason. Given the porosity of the embodied soul to external stimuli, the individual's psychic health is entangled with the affective life of the city. It is for this reason that Plato understands public health in terms of the shaping and regulation of both individual souls and the relations between souls.

To call the entanglement of life and politics in the *Republic* "biopolitics" registers the ambitious scope, at once vast and intimate, of Plato's "reason of the

↗ Illustration attributed to a member of the Sangallo family (Florence, ca. 1530–1545).

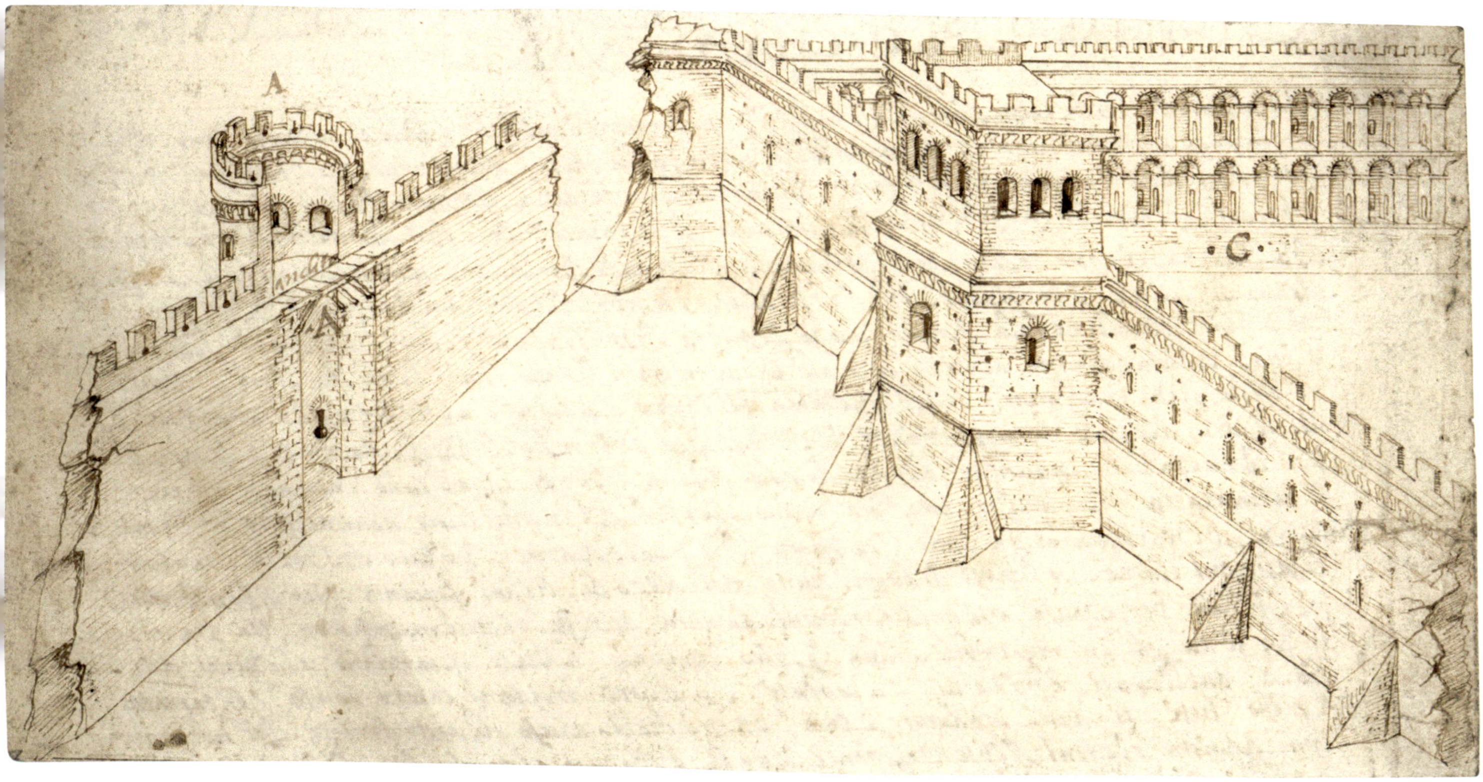

state" (as the early modern political theorist Giovanni Botero put it) in the *Republic*. At the same time, the language of biopolitics raises difficult questions about continuities and discontinuities between Greco-Roman antiquity and European modernity. The rise of biopolitics as a paradigm of analysis over the past few decades owes much to Foucault's influential definition of the modern state against premodern sovereignty in terms of the state's exercise of control over life—what Foucault called "biopower."[4] Yet the modern paradigm of biopolitics is itself shaped by the reception of the canonized texts of ancient Greek political theory, most notably Plato's *Republic* and Aristotle's *Politics*. It is therefore implicated, albeit in complicated ways, in the elaboration of a politics articulated around norms of health in fourth-century BCE Athens.[5]

One of the persistent challenges of unpacking ancient biopolitics in its relationship to modern biopolitics has been to navigate the concept of life that governs the political theory of both Plato and Aristotle.[6] Less attention has been paid to the early Greek concept of nature (*phusis*).[7] This concept was integral to the theorization of the physical body in the fifth and fourth centuries BCE.[8] In the *Republic*, Plato uses the flourishing of a body animated by a specific kind of nature as a model for both the soul and the city. The very persistence of nature as a norm in modernity makes it all too easy to naturalize nature in the ancient Greek sources rather than understand it as a historically situated, politically complex, and semantically rich concept taking form in the period when Plato is writing. By destabilizing the nature that Plato uses to stabilize the political order envisioned in the *Republic*, we are better positioned not only to interrogate its persistent legitimation of state power in modernity, but also to resist the naturalization of Greek antiquity itself as the classical origin of modern biopolitics.

Plato's understanding of nature as a norm governing human life is caught up in late fifth-century BCE debates. Above all, it is associated with the sophists, and their debates about the relationship between nature as a cause of why specific kinds of beings—human and nonhuman—behave the way they do, and the law (*nomos*) that determines what is right and just, especially in human communities.[9] In the *Republic*, as in other later dialogues, Plato primarily aims to align law and nature. In so doing, he looks to what had become the culturally dominant science (*tekhnē*) for the control of human nature in Athens by the early fourth century BCE: medicine.

Yet the nature at stake for both the medical writers and Plato exhibits something of an internal contradiction, with significant consequences for its relationship to law as well as to the techniques of control classed under the idea of *tekhnē*: namely, it is both self-legitimating and needy. On the one hand, in what will become a canonical passage from the Hippocratic text *Epidemics VI*, "untaught" nature is the model for the physician: it shows him what he ought to do in treating the patient.[10] On the other hand, the physician exists precisely because nature often fails to self-regulate. As Socrates says early in the *Republic*, it's not enough for a body to be a body: it needs the medical *tekhnē* because it is too unstable on its own.[11] The city is similarly unstable, Socrates suggests:

it must be designed, then, if it's going to be healthy; it needs constant care. Recognizing the emergent status of nature in the fourth century BCE as both the norm of health and the object of technological management holds at bay a naturalized nature—and, with it, an uninterrogated *bio-* bridging Greek origins and modern biopolitics—in our reading of Plato. In turn, we can see more closely how, in crafting human beings and a city for them to dwell in together in the *Republic*, Plato is experimenting with a concept of nature as an object of regulation by state reason while also deploying the language of nature to designate a norm that is, ostensibly, self-given and beyond contestation.

One of the ways that Plato experiments in the *Republic* with the double-sided status of nature—and, with it, ideas about health, bodies, and souls—is through the phenomenon of shared affect, or *sym*-pathy. Affects, as we have seen, are shared both between the parts of the soul *and* between the members of the city. The idea of sharing affect in both cases is premised, first, on the claim that souls and cities have different parts. If there were no difference, there would be no need to share. But difference is only one side of the coin. Parts or bodies must also hold something in common if they are going to share affects. For this reason, the fact that affects are shared can bear witness to the community that makes such sharing possible. In Book 5 of the *Republic*, Plato uses shared affect to present the unified, living body as a model for the unity of the citizen body: that is, for a "naturally" normative biopolitics. Yet this "natural" unity is heavily engineered by state reason through a far-reaching eugenics program. In other words, the (re-)production of "natural" order is seen to require the philosopher-kings acting, as Socrates says, like doctors. The need to regulate all affective exchange between the citizens to bring about psychic and civic health is especially clear in Book 10 in Socrates's critique of tragedy, in which tragedy is presented explicitly as a threat in terms of "sympathizing."

Plato's use of the verb "to sympathize" in the *Republic* is, in fact, one of the two earliest examples in Greek. The other example also comes from Plato and, more specifically, from a dialogue likely to be earlier than the *Republic*, *Charmides*. Socrates observes there that one of his interlocutors has "caught" his own aporia the way that one person yawns in response to seeing another person yawn; in other words, they "sympathize."[12] This early use of the language of sympathy to describe "contagious" yawning emphasizes the problems posed by the affective life of the ensouled body: that is, it is open to being easily influenced by the affects of others in ways that risk undermining reason's control. That Plato later uses the language of sympathy to describe the risks of tragic spectatorship suggests he understands this risk in terms of what we can call "contagious affect." Yet affects only circulate among people because they hold something in common. That what is held in common in the "sympathy" between living beings is *nature* is spelled out in the book devoted to problems "from sympathy" in the pseudo-Aristotelian *Problems*, probably written a century later than the *Republic* (where the "problems" of the title refer to phenomena that are somehow caused by nature but resist the physicists' explanations). The author of the *Problems*, who is interested in a range of problems related to "contagious affect" (such as contagious yawning as well as shared pain), glosses this nature held in common as a kind of "kinship" (*oikeiotēs*).[13] He therefore brings us back to Plato's use of shared affect to manifest the natural community of political kinship that the state eugenically engineers in Book 5 of the *Republic*.

The two sides of sympathy—as contagious affect and as a sign of natural community—reveal the unstable nature at the heart of biopolitics in the *Republic*.[14] These two different models of "shared affect" allow us to grasp the work performed in the dialogue by the ensouled physical body understood both as an internally divided object entangled in a mesh of chaotic affective relations—and thus requiring technical control—and as the paragon of complex unity. In short, sympathy presents a glimpse of how Plato imagines the body politic to be both a breeding ground for contagious affect and an organic whole. These two perspectives together disclose the natural life informing Plato's biopolitics.

The Affective Life of the City and the Soul in Plato's *Republic*

In Books 2 and 3 of the *Republic*, Socrates launches his infamous critique of the poetry that dominated education at Athens, especially Homer and Hesiod. Storytelling is the state's most powerful tool of social control in the *Republic*, capable of literally molding souls. It must therefore be used with considerable care. Socrates's attack on the poets in Book 3 targets the long-term psychic risks to the future elite of habitually molding themselves into characters rocked by disease or love. But Socrates is wary, too, of the very lability of the mimetic self, the shape-shifting character of the poet and the performer.[15]

In Book 10, Socrates turns his focus to the dangers posed to the unified soul not by acting itself but by tragic spectatorship. Socrates and his interlocutor Glaucon start off agreeing that the person whose soul is in order would never give in to excessive grief and lamentation, no matter how great the loss. But even the best of us, Socrates says, find that the rational soul relaxes its grip on the appetitive soul's desire for lamentation when we watch the sufferings of others on stage. We readily surrender ourselves to the performative grief of tragic heroes, "suffering along with the characters as we follow."[16] Socrates pathologizes this "strong pity" as the stimulation of the "appetitive" part of the soul that takes pleasure in emotion and that, prone to excess, is always at risk of overwhelming the rule of reason. Being laid open to another's suffering makes the tragic spectator more susceptible to losing control of himself in the face of his own powerful emotions (*pathē*). The exposure to the suffering of others in the theater, Socrates says, "infects" our affective life outside the theater and brings about a pathological state defined for Plato by femininity and enslavement.[17] In Book 10, then, the audience's compulsive "sympathizing" with tragic heroes is diagnosed as the problem at the root of the genre's threat to psychic unity. The affects of others on stage enter the soul or mind through the senses and compel a response. But the identification of the (once rational) spectator with the (othered) performer produced by sympathy comes at the cost of psychic disruption, thus seeding division in the city. The only option, Socrates says, is to exile tragedy.

Yet if tragedy produces a divisive sympathy, another kind of sympathy exemplifies unity for Plato. Midway through the dialogue in Book 5, Socrates is trying to wrap up his account of the ideal city and shift into a detailed description of the various pathologies to which it is eventually destined to succumb. Glaucon interrupts to point out that Socrates has failed to say anything about a critical part of any city: the family, sexual reproduction, women, and children. Glaucon's request spurs Socrates to describe another famous part of his proposal for the ideal city: first, the admission of certain women to the ranks of the guardians by way of the same educational regimen assigned to the class of boys working toward the apex of the sociopolitical hierarchy; and second, the abolition of the family, to be replaced by political kinship. The two policies go hand in hand as outcomes of Socrates's account of nature here, understood as both the nature of classes of citizens and individual natures.

Part of what is radical about this plan is that it posits that some women have the kind of nature to qualify for the guardian class. The hierarchical difference in natural capacity is thus reconfigured in terms of class rather than sex. But nature isn't sufficiently trustworthy to ensure a consistent, transgenerational reproduction of social difference. Eros is messy.[18] Sexual reproduction is messy. The city planner has to step in to stave off anarchy. Socrates, accordingly, proposes a eugenics program explicitly modeled on animal breeding.[19] This entails grouping guardian men with women of similar natures through co-ed education and coercing them to mate according to city-sponsored marriage rituals.[20] We know, too, from Socrates's account of education in Book 3 that the rulers are constantly watching the young to determine which of those assigned to the guardian class are fit to become rulers. They are also keeping an eye out for those whose births would predict a lower class but who turn out to demonstrate "natural" excellence.[21] The state thus aims to regulate sexual reproduction to stabilize a fixed social order while building in techniques of surveillance to catch out those citizens who perform contrary to what their "natural" descent would predict—and reassign them accordingly.

The aim here is the production and reproduction of the city as the citizens' only natural community. To achieve it, Socrates also has to thwart the formation of kinship within the natal family. Babies are whisked away at birth to an institutional nursery to become wards of the state, cared for under the watchful eye of the rulers. This seeks to erase the paradigmatic "natural" bond between parent and child in order to naturalize civic kinship.[22] Meanwhile, we have learned in Book 3 that everyone will be told that their memories of their childhood and education were only dreams. Experience is to be replaced with a "noble lie," that is, the myth of metals that legitimates class assignments in terms of citizens' inborn natures and casts the city as a family.[23] All citizens, according to the myth, are earthborn kin with a natural mandate to defend their motherland and love their brothers and sisters. Their souls, they are told, have been divinely fabricated out of different metals (gold, silver, bronze, or iron) that fix their position in the city's hierarchy. Like a "brave doctor," Socrates's story masks the manufacture of an unequal social order qua family with the face of nature, understood to govern both sameness and difference.[24]

Much more could be said about these proposals. Here I only want to point to the test used by Socrates in Book 5 to determine whether the technical production of kinship has succeeded in making a healthy body politic. If the eugenic technologies are successful, he says, the whole city will be united in its experience of pleasure and pain. The model of such a community is the ensouled, unified living body. For, if the finger is wounded, "the entire community stretching through the body to the soul in one system of control senses it, and this entire community suffers in pain together with the affected finger, as a whole."[25] The sharing of pain and pleasure thus bears witness to the city as a natural unity structured by hierarchy. Recall that in Book 10, pains, pleasures, and desires are dangerous because they defy reason's control. But here it is precisely because pain is unwilled that it is such a compelling sign of the unity of the citizen body, one that proves the success of *tekhnē* in stabilizing and manufacturing nature even as the "natural" living body supplies the paragon of the complex One. This sign of shared affect enables Plato to name its cause as the relationship between the parts of the whole—in this case, the relationships that make up the tissue of the city according to mythically naturalized hierarchies of power.

Unsettling the Nature of the *Republic*'s Natural Order

The city that Plato designs is decidedly not a democracy. But it is haunted by democratic politics. In Book 8, Socrates offers an anxious critique of democracy as a mess of promiscuous freedom where "those who have been bought as slaves—whether male or female—are no less free than those who bought them" and the relationship of men and women is marked by excessive equality (*isonomia*).[26] On Plato's diagnosis of democracy's ostensible pathologies, too much freedom collapses boundaries between different classes of human nature. In the *Laws*, as in the *Republic*, Plato implicates tragedy in these pathologies, offering the neologism "theatrocracy" (*theatrokratia*) as a synonym for democracy and its supposedly excessive liberties, which eventually lead to the rule of the tyrant, the embodiment of appetitive soul.[27] Whether Plato's critique of democracy is right or wrong—and whether it's a critique at all—have been much-debated questions in postwar Europe and the US. Plato's aversion to democracy was famously seen as evidence of his totalitarian inclinations by Karl Popper. The reading of Plato's *Republic* as the Ur-antidemocratic text has been elaborated more recently by, among others, Jacques Rancière, who reads the anti-Athenian perspective of the *Republic* through Socrates's investment in "natural" hierarchy. Against the Socrates of the *Republic*, Rancière theorizes democracy as the refusal of foundational order (*arkhē*) and, more specifically, the refusal of *any* order founded in the "nature" of kinship.[28]

But Plato's faith in nature, we have seen, is not so straightforward. Demetra Kasimis has argued that, by using the *Republic* to theorize the democratic ideal by way of a foil, Rancière prematurely reduces the text to its investment in "natural" hierarchy and order. She instead advocates reading the dialogue as critically "revelatory of hierarchy's various iterations, machinations, and indeterminate effects" as they operate in democracy, too.[29] By extracting democracy as an ideal thrown into relief by Plato's engineered regime of reason, Rancière, on her critique, neglects the material conditions underlying the making of democracy and the dialogue's own frame: that is, the historical Athens of the late fifth and early fourth centuries BCE on whose outskirts the *Republic* takes place, in the house of a wealthy immigrant or "metic" with no path to citizenship for himself or his children. Athens was, by this time, a birth-based democracy legitimated by the myth of autochthony.[30] Most notably, in 458 BCE, Pericles had instituted a law that required both parents to be citizens for citizenship to be granted to their children, thereby blocking interstate elite alliances. Such measures unfolded in tandem with new ideologies of race shaped by theories of the body and human nature as objects of expert medical-scientific knowledge, technical control, and care, which were all moralized by anxieties around gender, class, and sovereignty in the late fifth century.[31] According to Kasimis, Plato's myth of metals carries a subversive critique of Athens's own noble lie that its citizens were born from the earth into a natural brotherhood uniting them against noncitizens. She argues that when Plato critiques democracy, he has in mind Athenian democracy's very investment in naturalized difference qua kinship to secure political membership.[32]

In situating the dialogue as a text written in fourth-century BCE Athens, Kasimis is not registering a historicist's correction to the use of the text for the ends of political theory. Rather, she targets the "theoretical toll" exacted by the text's decontextualization and the risk of getting swept along with Plato's project of disciplining the messiness of "nature" into social stratification legitimated by nature restored as myth.[33] After all, Socrates does not hide the technological production of naturalized kinship in the dialogue itself. Nor is Athens in its practices of exclusion absent from the scene. There is a risk, too, of mistaking Plato's work of abstracting order through the manipulation of bodies and souls for a binary between nature and culture that is set in stone at the origins of Western political theory and metaphysics. Not to mark these nuances is to reinscribe the Greeks as icons of mythic origin—of philosophy, of politics, of biopolitics—and assume a classical foundation. We can instead see these texts as "nourishing food," as Andrés Henao Castro proposes to do in his recent rereading of *Antigone*, imagining Sophocles's play as the corpse of Polyneices cast to the birds who both metabolize it and scatter it to noncanonical places.[34]

We should also be careful about equating the work of demystification with the critique of naturalization, and thus, paradoxically, naturalizing a concept of nature itself. Here it is worth returning to the emergent formation of nature in the fifth and fourth centuries BCE as paradoxically both self-legitimating and needy. Plato has Socrates build an elaborate process of surveilling and correcting nature into the design of his city, thereby turning the natures of different human beings, as both individuals and as members of naturalized classes, into objects of state control. Nevertheless, he does not seem to give up on the promise that nature in the fifth century BCE offers—that is, the promise of a norm outside of convention and human institutions altogether that underwrites an account of what it means for human beings to flourish as individuals and within a political community.

Plato takes the promise of nature as a norm outside human control from contemporary medical writers and debates in fifth- and fourth-century BCE Athens that coalesced into "the inquiry into nature," as he has Socrates call it in his famous intellectual autobiography in the *Phaedo*.[35] But nature in the *Phaedo* turns out to be no ally to Plato's Socrates. For Socrates famously attacks the "physicists" for their radical materialism—their care only for bodies and mindless powers (hot, cold, wet, dry) and their failure to encode value into the nonhuman world by putting a god in charge. What Socrates wants is a cosmology that subordinates the natures of things, including human beings, to the Good as the primary cause of world order. He thus again turns to the idea of "needy" nature, that is, nature as a cause that has to be disciplined by the agents of reason.

Socrates's desire for a world ruled by the Good is addressed by Plato's cosmological epic, the *Timaeus*, probably written years after the *Republic*, although its narrative frame positions it as a kind of sequel. This time, the failures of politics practiced by embodied mortals—which eventually undo the state in the *Republic*—are subsumed into a cosmos whose own life is miraculously inviolable (the dialogue's narrator describes a cosmic animal that sustains itself in a perfect cycle of autostimulation). The account of world creation in the *Timaeus* aligns the natures of things with materialist causes that have been reassuringly subordinated to mind, reason, and divine providence. Nevertheless, nature repeatedly surfaces in the dialogue, as it does in the *Republic*, as a way of being in the world for specific kinds of things that are legitimated (or not) through being "according to nature" (*kata phusin*) or "against nature" (*para phusin*). Its force as a stable norm thus persists alongside its role as a cause requiring rational management in the *Timaeus*.

It is worth emphasizing that the normative force of nature is as much a part of the cosmological-anthropological idiom that Plato inherits as the physicists' rubric of bodies and powers. Despite Socrates's critique of the materialists for failing to think about value in the *Phaedo*, ethics was never absent from physics. When a cosmology of nature meets an account of human nature in the fifth century BCE under the pressures of an imperial, enslaving democracy's fixation on masculinized self-control as the embodiment of freedom, health and disease become *both* objects of control within a *tekhnē* of medicine *and* the ostensibly given norms that guide the physician's work. For Plato, the ethical imperative to the citizen to control the affective life of embodied soul defines the autarchy that is supposedly given to the Athenian male citizen as his birthright but in practice requires surveillance and continuous manipulation. In Book 3 of the *Republic*, Plato bears witness to the success of naturalizing medicine in this period as a regulatory (and self-regulatory) regime at Athens. Socrates frankly expresses his interest in taking over medicine's vast market in the control of human nature for philosophy's techniques of psychic care.[36] At the same time, the very proliferation of these regulatory regimes bears witness to a conceptualization of nature as animated by an elusive, nonhuman, ludic motility, or what Emanuela Bianchi has called the queer performativity of ancient *phusis*.[37]

Part of the work of situating the *Republic* for political theory and, above all, for biopolitical theory thus needs to be understanding "naturalization" itself as a polymorphous, culturally embedded, politically consequential process that persistently entangles Socrates in his efforts to imagine otherwise. We may read these entanglements as symptomatic of the limits of Plato's own grasp on human flourishing and political community, or the sophistication of Plato's use of the dialogue to read contemporary Athens critically, or theory's historical conditions. But regardless, nature cannot be taken for granted. The two sides of sympathy drive this home by helping us map the complex topology of a historically medicalized body adapted by Socrates to model the tripartite soul and then blown up to the size of a city: on the one hand, health as complex unity sustained through the regulation of affects by an immanent, dynamic, normative force of order (i.e., "nature"); on the other hand, embodiment in the physical world as a condition of precarity and porosity requiring the technical control of bodies and communities, at least until the city, like all mortal things, inevitably degenerates to the point of total collapse.[38]

The work of reading the *Republic* is imbricated in the many different histories of reading Plato, ancient and modern, that for all their differences cannot *not* mythologize him—and the Greeks more generally—as moments of origin. But what it can also do is show the seams and lay bare the decisions that go into reading Plato biopolitically, as well as the fact that decisions always get made when you craft something. That's arguably what Plato has Socrates doing in the *Republic*: showing the seams of that made object called the city. Still, this doesn't mean that Plato gives up on nature, for better or for worse, as one name of something in embodied humans that shapes their capacities to live or die, thrive or suffer. Rather, the question of imagining "natural" community is how to bridge a gap between nature as the nonhuman materiality of the self that requires discipline and care, and nature as norm that governs a usually consequential evaluation of whether a life is being lived "well" or not—and of whether a political community, or an aesthetics of collective life, or a planet, is thriving.

This question transmutes but also recurs over thousands of years across communities that have made sense of their shared world in terms of a concept of nature imbricated in Greek natural philosophy. In trying to make sense of this tenacious seriality across millennia, it is important to resist, as a model for a classicized tradition, the living being whose parts are integrated into a whole according to a master trope of health (and pathology, decline, rebirth). The risks are most obvious in the modern regimes of biopolitics that have taken a Greek origin and norm as foundational to their own claims on health and racialized practices of exclusion, expulsion, and extermination. But reifications like "the classical tradition" and "the West" also risk a less evident trust in vitalist unity. Such trust can be understood in the ways in which Plato's *Republic* has continued to condition the imagination of political community, its relationship to life, and its failures into the twentieth and twenty-first centuries. To show the seams is not simply to work through nature as something made in the fifth and fourth centuries BCE. It's to show the Greeks as made over and again, entangled in the making of the ethics and aesthetics and politics of health that still inform diagnoses of crises of public health, democratic politics, racial capitalism, and ecological collapse, neither inside nor outside biopolitics.[39]

The two sides of sympathy in the *Republic* challenge how we imagine together the difficult, provisional, and social practice of care in the face of suffering. Over the last decade, it has become easier to see how right-wing nativism in democratic politics goes hand in hand with a logic of roots. But Plato's recourse to the model of a body integrated in its parts in his work of figuring political kinship in the *Republic* also invites scrutiny of what we think is at stake when we say a community or a nation or a world is broken, divided, infected, or sick, and what we think is necessary for us to become whole or to heal.

The Socrates of the *Republic* places tragedy's contagious sympathy at the heart of his diagnosis of the ills of democratic Athens. He refers its effects to the insurgent power of what he sees as the feminized and enslaved parts within every human being, even the most rational citizen. The extant Greek tragedies are themselves caught in this cultural logic of power and abjection mapped onto gendered and raced bodies. But they are also provocative in the ways they stage the gap between suffering and the capacity to make sense of it. In that gap, characters often fail to come together. As a historical form, Attic tragedy is cultivated under conditions of hyperinvestment in law and medicine as domains for regulating collective life according to the logic of blame and cure. The plays repeatedly mark the limits of that logic. In so doing they function like aesthetic technologies for experimenting in public, by means of a highly formalized but repeatedly decentered perspectival fluidity, with the utopian possibilities, the provisionality, and the limits of the stories that people generate to sustain political life in the face of human suffering. They hold on to a space between acknowledging harm and the need for care without settling on a regime of health, disease, and cure.

The refusal in tragedy to settle on diagnoses and cures, along with the genre's rejection of the phantasy that embodied life and community can be technologically controlled, haunts the *Republic* in its quest to secure psychic and political flourishing through the regulation of state reason. Plato reads tragedy as another form of materialism, and rightly so, although his paranoid antimaterialism produces powerful distortions. But like the tragedies themselves, the *Republic* shows the seams of Socrates's creation of an aesthetics of political life. It, too, then, can help us see the seams of what we call philosophy, and art, and politics, and history, and architecture as always situated, porous, transitioning practices of collective survival that cannot and should not try to cage what they want to sustain and, in that failure, remain necessary to its persistence.[40]

An earlier version of this essay was originally published by e-flux Architecture in 2022.

1. Vitruvius, *On Architecture* 1.4.1–1.4.6, in Vitruvius, *On Architecture*, vol. I: *Books 1–5*, trans. Frank Granger (Cambridge, MA: Harvard University Press, 1931).
2. Vitruvius represents a minor tradition for explaining plague transmission (most ancient authors blamed "bad" air): see also Varro, *On Agriculture* 1.12.2–1.12.4, in Varro, *On Agriculture*, trans. W. D. Hooper and Harrison Boyd Ash (Cambridge, MA: Harvard University Press, 1934), who imagines tiny *animalia* being actually inhaled, with Vivian Nutton, "The Seeds of Disease: An Explanation of Contagion and Infection from the Greeks to the Renaissance," *Medical History* 27 (1983): 1–34, esp. 11, on Varro.
3. Plato, *Republic* 1, 368c–369a, in *Plato, Republic*, vol. 1: *Books 1–5*, ed. and trans. Christopher Emlyn-Jones and William Preddy (Cambridge, MA: Harvard University Press, 2013).
4. See esp. Michel Foucault, *The History of Sexuality*, vol. 1: *An Introduction*, trans. R. Hurley (New York: Pantheon, 1978), 135–145.
5. For the reception of ancient Greek political theory in the early modern period and in twentieth-century biopolitics, see Chiara Bottici, "Rethinking the Biopolitical Turn: From the Thanatological to the Geneapolitical Paradigm," *Graduate Faculty Philosophy Journal* 56 (2015): 175–197, 178 with nn. 17–18 on Botero. The ancient Greco-Roman dimension of modern biopolitics has been most influentially—and problematically—asserted by Giorgio Agamben, *Homo Sacer: Sovereign Power and Bare Life*, trans. Daniel Heller-Roazen (Stanford: Stanford University Press, 1998). See also Mika Ojakangas, *On the Greek Origins of Biopolitics: A Reinterpretation of the History of Biopower* (New York: Routledge, 2016). For a critique of Agamben's genealogy of life and the complicated relationship between ancient Greek *bios* and modern biopolitics, with additional bibliography, see Brooke Holmes, "Bios," *Political Concepts: A Critical Lexicon* 5 (2019), http://www.politicalconcepts.org/bios-brooke-holmes/. For a range of recent perspectives on the ancient dimension of biopolitics, see the papers in Jussi Backman and Antonio Cimino, eds., *Biopolitics and Ancient Thought* (Oxford: Oxford University Press, 2022).
6. The debate over the two primary Greek words for life, *bios* and *zōē*, has been central to critiques of Agamben's account of Aristotle's biopolitics: see esp. James Gordon Finlayson, "'Bare Life' and Politics in Agamben's Reading of Aristotle," *Review of Politics* 72, no. 1 (2010): 97–126; Holmes, "Bios"; Sara Brill, *Aristotle on the Concept of Shared Life* (Oxford: Oxford University Press, 2020), 1–34.
7. But see the important correction to Agamben's claims about Plato and "natural law" in Mika Ojakangas, "Plato and the Biopolitical Purge of the City-State," in Backman and Cimino, *Biopolitics and Ancient Thought*, 39–41.
8. For a detailed argument about how a concept of the physical body takes shape in this period, see Brooke Holmes, *The Symptom and the Subject: The Emergence of the Physical Body in Ancient Greece* (Princeton: Princeton University Press, 2010), esp. 121–191.
9. For a general overview of these debates, see now Richard Bett, "Nature and Norms," in *The Cambridge Companion to the Sophists*, ed. Joshua Billings and Christopher Moore (Cambridge: Cambridge University Press, 2023), 157–178. On the semantic zone of nature in this period, see also Gottfried Heinemann, "*Peri Phuseôs*: Physics, Physicists, and *Phusis* in Aristotle," in *Brill's Companion to the Reception of Presocratic Natural Philosophy in Later Classical Thought*, ed. Chelsea C. Harry and Justin Habash (Leiden: Brill, 2021), 13–31.
10. Hippocrates, *Epidemics* VI 5.1, in *Hippocrates, Epidemics 2, 4–7*, ed. and trans. W. D. Smith (Cambridge, MA: Harvard University Press, 1994).
11. Plato, *Republic* 1, 341e.
12. Plato, *Charmides* 169c, in *Plato, Charmides; Alcibiades I and II; Hipparchus; The Lovers; Theages; Minos; Epinomis*, trans. W. R. M. Lamb (Cambridge, MA: Harvard University Press, 1927).
13. Aristotle, *Problems* 7.7, in Aristotle, *Problems*, vol. 1: *Books 1–19*, ed. and trans. Robert Mayhew (Cambridge, MA: Harvard University Press, 2011). On the concept of kinship proposed in the text, see further Brooke Holmes, "Pain, Power, and Human Community: Empathy as a 'Physical Problem' in Pseudo-Aristotle and Beyond," in *The Body Unbound: Literary Approaches to the Classical Corpus*, ed. Katherine Lu Hsu, David Schur, and Brian P. Sowers (New York: Palgrave Macmillan, 2021), 13–56.
14. I analyze these two facets of sympathy—what I call "magnified vulnerability" and "reparative unity"—at greater length in my forthcoming book *Sympathy and the Tissue of the World: Life, Community, and Nature in the Ancient Mediterranean.*
15. Plato, *Republic* 3, 395c–395e, 396c–396e, 397a–398a. For the reading of *Republic* 10 above, see Holmes, "Pain, Power, and Human Community," 32–33.
16. Plato, *Republic* 10, 605d4, in *Plato, Republic*, vol. 2: *Books 6–10*, ed. and trans. Christopher Emlyn-Jones and William Preddy (Cambridge, MA: Harvard University Press, 2013). On the mixed pleasure and pain of watching tragedy, cf. Plato, *Philebus* 48a, in *Plato, Statesman; Philebus; Ion*, trans. Harold North Fowler and W. R. M. Lamb (Cambridge, MA: Harvard University Press, 1925).
17. On the dangers of mimesis for Plato, see *Republic* 3, 394e–396e; *Laws* 7, 814e–817a, in *Plato, Laws*, vol. 2: *Books 7–12*, trans. R. G. Bury (Cambridge, MA: Harvard University Press, 1926), with Stephen Halliwell, *The Aesthetics of Mimesis: Ancient Texts and Modern Problems* (Princeton: Princeton University Press, 2002), esp. 72–97. In the *Laws*, Plato delegates the mimesis of base characters to the enslaved or metics: citizens are not allowed to train in such forms of representation (*Laws* 7, 816e). The entanglement of mimesis and enslavement continues through the Roman period. On forced performance as a site for the exercise of domination over the enslaved in the American context, see Saidiya V. Hartman, *Scenes of Subjection: Terror, Slavery, and Self-Making in Nineteenth-Century America* (New York: Oxford University Press, 1997), esp. 17–78.
18. See esp. Plato, *Republic* 5, 458d–458e.
19. Plato, *Republic* 5, 459a–459b, 460d on infanticide.
20. Plato, *Republic* 5, 459d–460b. The men who display the best natures are rewarded with sexual access to many women in the interest of increasing their offspring (see also 468c).
21. Plato, *Republic* 3, 412e–414c.
22. See Plato, *Republic* 5, 461d–461e, on precautions against incest that reconfigure the parent-child bond.
23. Plato, *Republic* 3, 414b–415c, 416e–417a.
24. Plato, *Republic* 5, 459d reintroduces the idea of the lie as medicine used by a brave (literally: masculine) doctor.
25. Plato, *Republic* 5, 462d; cf. 464a–464b. The idea that the whole body feels the pain of the smallest part appears in a medical text from the early fourth century: [Hippocrates], *On Places in a Human Being* 1, in *Hippocrates, Places in Man; Glands; Fleshes; Prorrhetic 1–2; Physician; Use of Liquids; Ulcers; Haemorrhoids and Fistulas*, ed. and trans. Paul Potter (Cambridge, MA: Harvard University Press, 1995).
26. Plato, *Republic* 8, 562e–563b.
27. Plato, *Laws* 3, 701a. See Luce Irigaray, *Speculum of the Other Woman*, trans. G. C. Gill (Ithaca: Cornell University Press, 1985), for a classic critique of Plato's own use of scenography in the myth of the cave.
28. Jacques Rancière, *The Hatred of Democracy*, trans. Steve Corcoran (London: Verso, 2006), 40–41.
29. Demetra Kasimis, *The Perpetual Immigrant and the Limits of Athenian Democracy* (Cambridge: Cambridge University Press, 2018), 116. Kasimis is also critically engaging Arlene Saxonhouse's rich and provocative reading of Book 8, which singles out the fluidity of identity categories in democracy as the primary target of Socrates's attack: Arlene Saxonhouse, "Democracy, Equality, and *Eidē*: A Radical View from Book 8 of Plato's *Republic*," *American Political Science Review* 92, no. 2 (1998), 273–283.
30. Nicole Loraux, *The Children of Athena: Athenian Ideas about Citizenship and the Division between the Sexes*, trans. C. Levine (Princeton: Princeton University Press, 1993).
31. See esp. Susan Lape, *Race and Citizen Identity in the Classical Athenian Democracy* (Cambridge: Cambridge University Press, 2010); Holmes, *The Symptom and the Subject*, on these theories of the body and its control.
32. Kasimis, *The Perpetual Immigrant*, 95–96, 129–131.
33. Kasimis, *The Perpetual Immigrant*, 119.
34. Andrés Henao Castro, *Antigone in the Americas: Democracy, Sexuality, and Death in the Settler Colonial Present* (Albany: State University of New York Press, 2021), 17.
35. Plato, *Phaedo* 96a–99c, in *Plato, Euthyphro, Apology, Crito, Phaedo*, ed. and trans. Christopher Emlyn-Jones and William Preddy (Cambridge, MA: Harvard University Press, 2017).
36. Plato, *Republic* 3, 407a–408a.
37. Emanuela Bianchi, "Nature Trouble: Ancient *Physis* and Queer Performativity," in *Antiquities beyond Humanism*, ed. Emanuela Bianchi, Sara Brill, and Brooke Holmes (Oxford: Oxford University Press, 2019), 211–238, esp. 228–236.
38. There are also important disanalogies between soul and body that mark the limits of the health/disease model for an account of justice, virtue, and vice that I cannot discuss here. See further Sara Brill, *Plato on the Limits of Human Life* (Bloomington: Indiana University Press, 2013), esp. 111–114, on the *Republic*, and on the shifting terms of the medical analogy in Plato, Brooke Holmes, "Body, Soul and the Medical Analogy in Plato," in *When Worlds Elide: Classics, Politics, Culture*, ed. J. Peter Euben and Karen Bassi (Lanham, MD: Rowman and Littlefield, 2010), 345–385.
39. See Holmes, "Bios."
40. For superb feedback, editing, and encouragement on this essay, I am very grateful to Nick Axel, Beatriz Colomina, Demetra Kasimis, Karan Mahajan, Tony Vidler, and Mark Wigley.

p284 From "The Fortification of City Walls" (Vitruvius, *On Architecture*, Book 1, Chapter 5).

DIARY OF A DISEASE

BEATRIZ COLOMINA

→ A woman who tested positive with the coronavirus is brought to the University of Nebraska Medical Center on Friday, March 6, 2020. She was transferred from Omaha's Methodist Hospital in an isolation pod inside an ambulance.

March 20, 2020 I am in New York, "the epicenter of Covid-19," the news on TV keeps blaring, as if proud of this achievement. New York has always been excessive, so why not now? More cases, more hospitalizations, more ICU admissions, more intubations, more deaths. The news is terrifying and at the same time completely at odds with the day-to-day experience of the city, which has become so strangely quiet, so peaceful. No traffic, no construction noise, no annoying car alarms, no random screams in the middle of the night. Even the ambulances are mostly silent without cars to fight against. The birds wake us up in the morning. Who knew there were so many birds in Soho? There are not even parks around here and only a few trees. But maybe they came in as residents packed up their cars and left for their houses in the Hamptons—leaving behind a neighborhood of empty streets just like in the 1970s, when artists occupied abandoned, barely habitable lofts and there were no stores, no restaurants, and hardly anybody to be seen. These same artists, at least some of them, are still around and now much more visible with all the newcomers and tourists gone. You see them in the little Korean grocery store on the corner, with their masks on, carefully selecting their vegetables, or walking slowly with their dogs, or picking up take-out from restaurants. But it is the buildings themselves that have become the main actors again, the real occupants of the streets. The character of each one jumps out, etched in astonishing detail, constantly changing with the light. Could that beautiful abandoned New York return?

March 21, 2020 Many of our friends have left the city. They think we should leave too: "It is too dangerous to stay. Besides, they may close the city soon and you will have become involuntary prisoners."

I know. But I can't leave. I am mesmerized, glued to this place with some kind of hypnotic fascination. Andrea feels the same way. She says she is not leaving Brooklyn. We arrange to meet halfway across the bridge on a shockingly clear day. I am reminded of the blackout in New York of 2003 when she was a teenager. We were on vacation in Spain and saw it on the evening news. "Damn! We missed it," she screamed, and everyone around burst out laughing. But I knew she meant it.

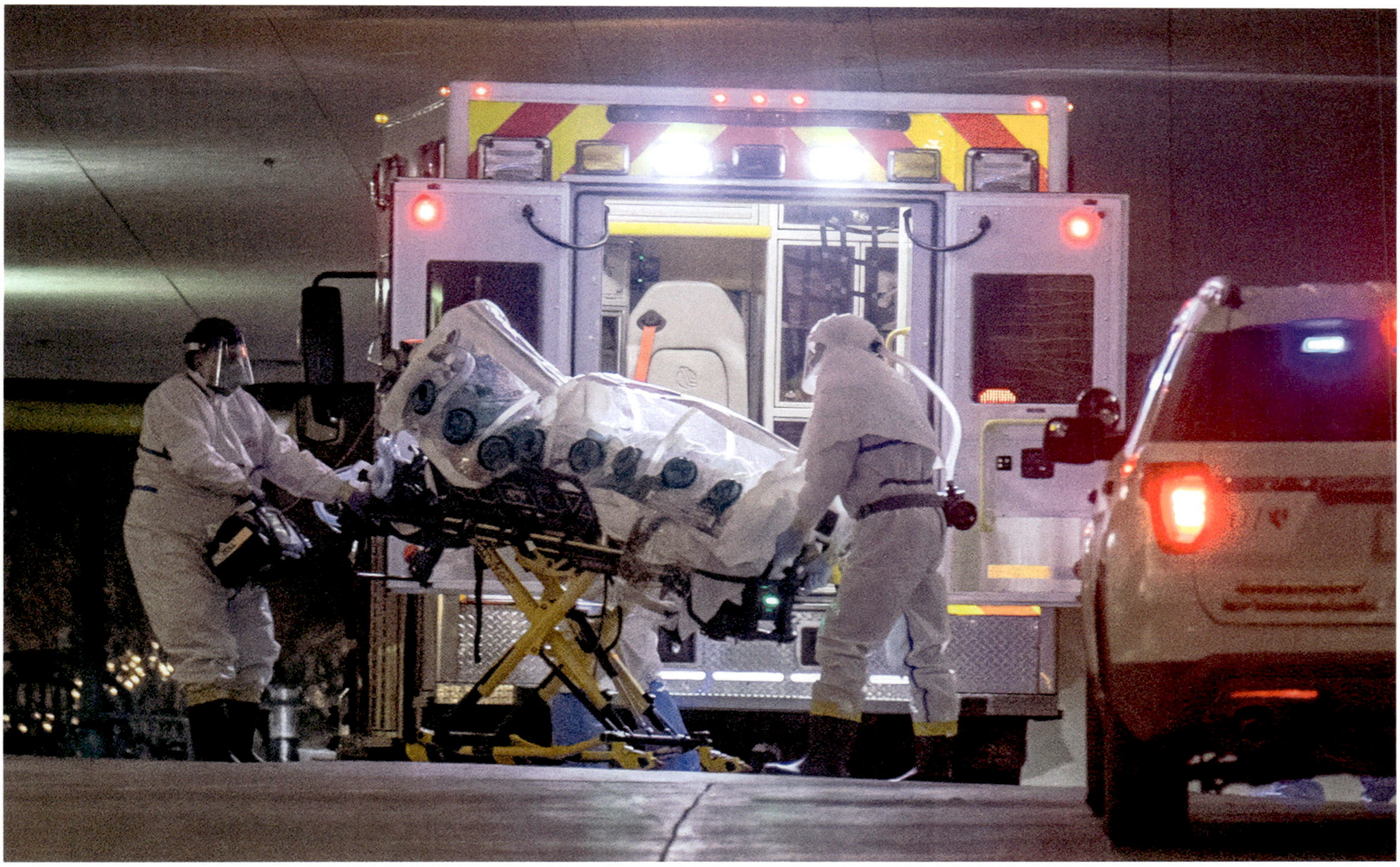

March 22, 2020 New York was still dangerous when I first arrived in 1980, but I didn't feel that way, riding the subway in the middle of the night after partying downtown. Of course, I was robbed in the streets many times, and once someone even broke into my Columbia University apartment and held me at knifepoint. But all of that felt like a tax that you now-and-then randomly paid for the enormous privilege of living in a city like this. This is also how it feels right now. It is probably more dangerous to live here than in some other places, but even with all of us isolated in our apartments, nobody can deny the immense feeling of being in this together, not isolated in some cabin in the woods—the solidarity with all those eyes you meet in the street, eyes above the masks. Everything is suddenly all about the eyes. No smiles are possible, and yet the acknowledgment you receive from passing gazes is much more profound than the nervous smiles from before, when strangers accidentally encountered your eyes in the streets or in the subway. The metropolis smile-as-mask has been replaced by surgical masks. What would Walter Benjamin say?

March 24, 2020 Being in New York right now is like being in the privileged position of a reporter on the front lines, as we were already on 9/11, when we were living only 200 meters away from ground zero and felt, heard, and smelled everything even before seeing anything. The engine of the second plane landed on the sidewalk just below our bedroom window. We saw things that never appeared on any screen. But now what is striking is what we don't see. 9/11 was a media spectacle. Covid-19 is precisely not spectacular. You don't see anything. Not even reporters, usually on the front lines of the most brutal wars and disasters, are allowed inside hospitals. There is invisible suffering everywhere. You feel it in the dense air of the streets. People are dying. But the illness, the death, is hidden. There is an architecture of this. A frightening architecture. For all the loss of barriers with contemporary media and surveillance, cameras everywhere, a huge center of our attention is completely veiled. Images of medical workers calling for equipment has become the facade of this sick architecture. They enter spaces we don't see.

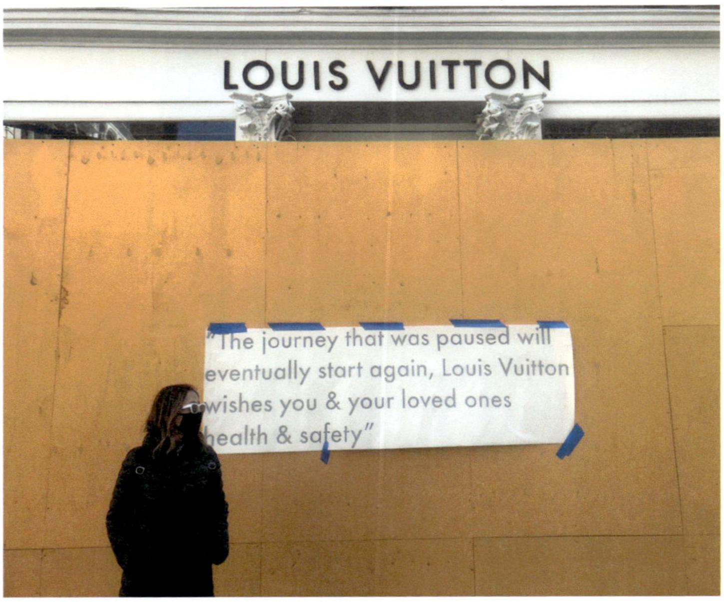
LOUIS VUITTON
"The journey that was paused will eventually start again, Louis Vuitton wishes you & your loved ones health & safety"

Beatriz Colomina in front of the boarded-up Louis Vuitton store in Soho, New York, March 29, 2020

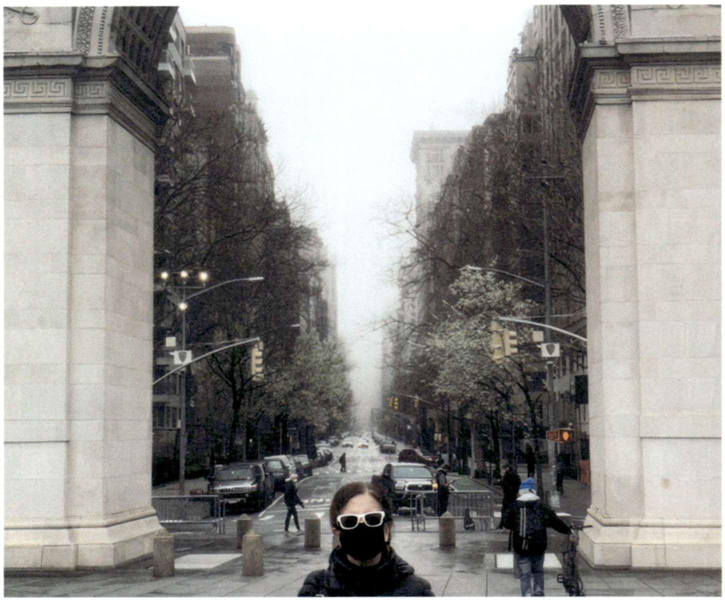

Beatriz Colomina at Washington Square Arch with an almost empty Fifth Avenue, March 29, 2020.

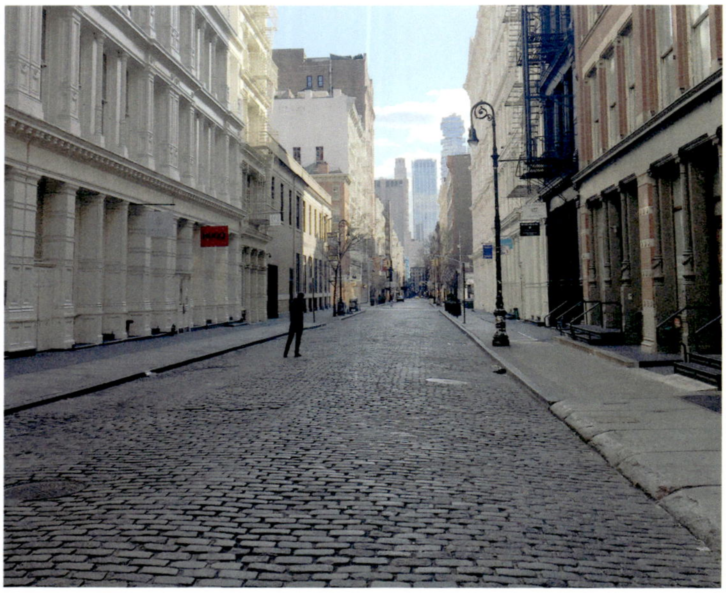

Greene Street at 4:32pm, what used to be rush hour, April 1, 2020.

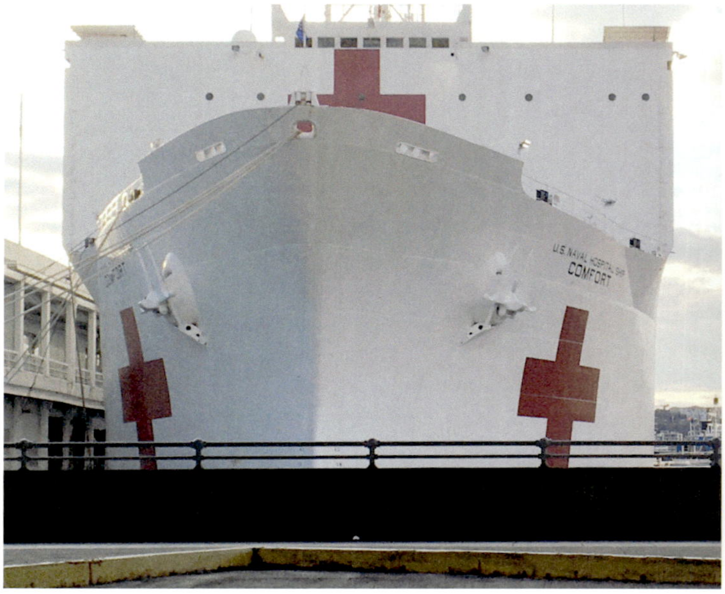

US Navy Hospital Ship Comfort, docked in Pier 90, April 1, 2020.

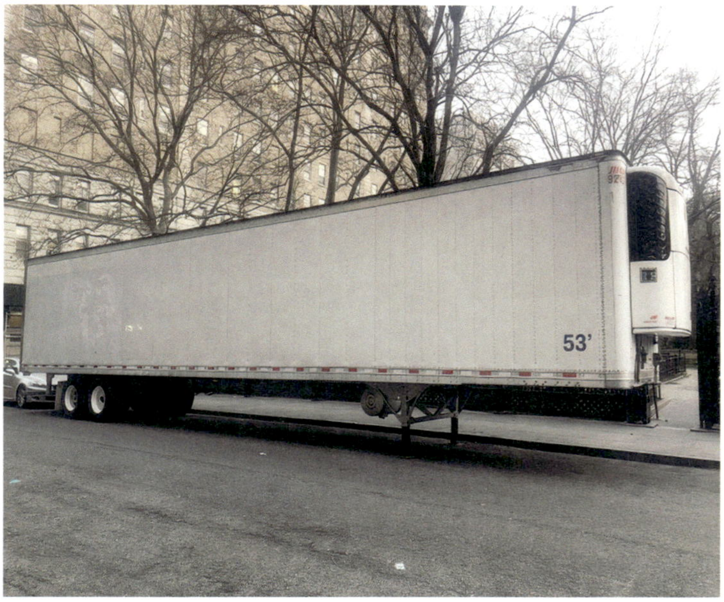

Refrigerator truck acting as morgue parked in front of hospital on First Avenue.

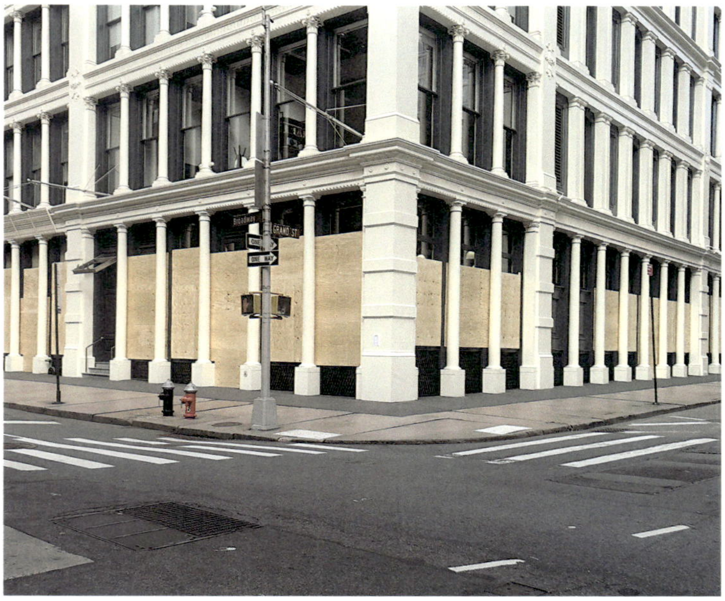

Grand Street/Broadway. Muntadas. Closed / Locked, 2020. New York.

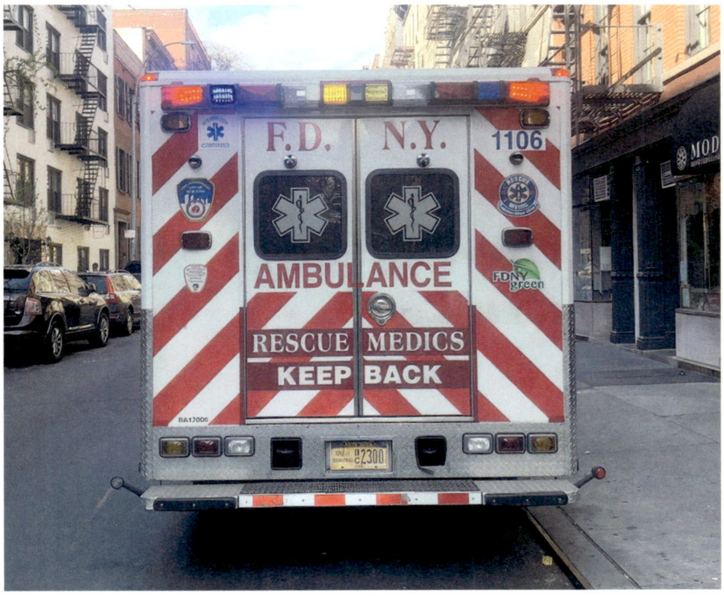

Ambulance on Thompson Street, April 12, 2020.

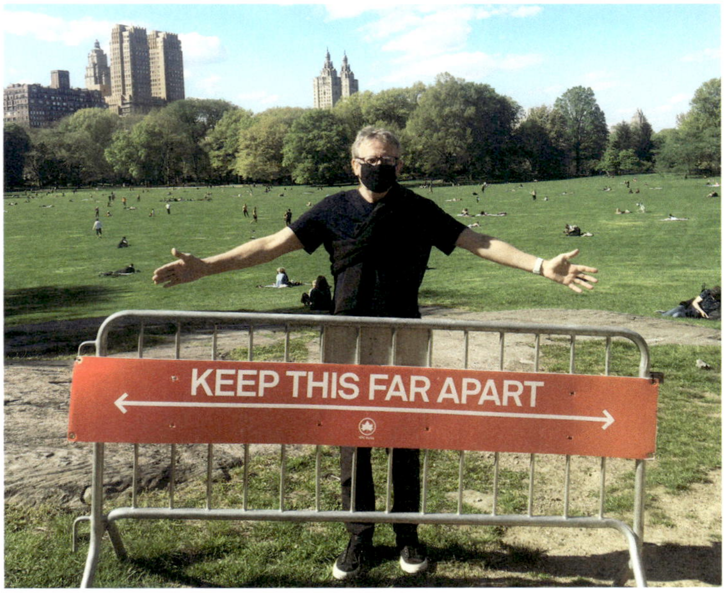

Mark Wigley in Central Park, May 7, 2020.

March 26, 2020 Michael Sorkin has died of complications from Covid-19. The whole architectural community is crying. I call a common friend and colleague. She says that today she had the first panic attack. The first? She must be expecting more. Without Michael it is harder to think.

March 27, 2020 All luxury shops around here have started to board up their windows as if a hurricane was coming. Do they know something we don't? Are they expecting civilian unrest, looting, as during the New York blackout of 1977? Or is the city just wearing a mask like the rest of us? Think of all the doors that are closed, all the blinds that are down. The city has sealed itself—everything withdrawn behind a new facade.

April 1, 2020 The *Comfort* hospital ship has arrived. Mark and I walked all the way up along the Hudson River to welcome it, but it was also very quiet, docked in Pier 90 around 49th Street, sitting behind a veil of green net in some kind of majestic silence. Nothing to see, from there down to the Javits Convention Center, which has been turned into a hospital. The Army Corps of Engineers were moving around deep in the building's vast interior like miniature figures, but still it was all very quiet. Some emergency vehicles sat idling in the streets outside, as if waiting for the unknown.

April 3, 2020 What about the regular hospitals? Could all the action be there? Today we walked for miles up First Avenue where so many hospitals are. Again, an intense sense of silence and little to see. Just some big tents that had migrated into the street to receive patients and the ominous sight of enormous refrigerated trucks parked at the curb like any other vehicle—again waiting. Not the calm eye of the storm but the calm surrounding the storm, filling the shocked city, numbing it like an anesthetic.

April 8, 2020 The veil is gradually lifting. Nurses and doctors have become reporters, broadcasting from the battlefield inside. Images are going deeper and deeper into the hospitals, to the very beds of ICU patients surrounded and invaded by beeping equipment—the only sign of breathing, of a still beating heart.

April 10, 2020 Beds, that piece of equipment usually hidden from view, are suddenly everywhere, from the front pages of newspapers to Zoom meetings. Beds are the face of this catastrophe. First it was the urgent call for more hospital beds, then beds overflowing hospitals, filling corridors and former waiting rooms. Nobody is waiting anymore. Any room of any size has become a room for beds. The whole space of the hospital has been taken over. Then beds started to make new spaces, in tents, gymnasia, parks, ships, convention centers. Haunting images of cavernous spaces with hundreds of empty beds in a grid; each with an oxygen tank and a domestic lamp—waiting beds. The questions dominating the media are always "how many beds?"; "how many are occupied?"; "how many people survived the bed?" Any bed with a ventilator has become an ICU bed, so the bed becomes the room, the architecture.

April 17, 2020 Now we are told to assume that we are all sick, to act as if we were sick, contagious, self-confined to our apartments, to our beds. The real epicenter of the pandemic is not New York but the bed.

May 1, 2020 My mother is dying in Spain. She does not have Covid. In fact, nothing is wrong with her body, except her age—ninety-seven—and with it some cognitive issues. A doctor told her a couple years ago: "You are like a vintage Mercedes car. You have your years but everything is working fine." Covid is killing her anyway. She can't go out with her friends anymore. She can't even go to church, which she never cared much about, except for the social aspect of meeting her friends, going for a walk with them afterward, for an aperitivo. "Nobody comes around here anymore," she tells me when I call. What do you mean? Cristina, one of my sisters, picked up the phone. She is there. "Yes, well, now and then one of them comes." In fact, they are always there but not all at once, trying to protect her and themselves. She does not understand what is happening and misses the human contact, the tumultuous family dinners, the kids, her friends. She has decided to let herself go.

March 28, 2020 Today we did the first Zoom cocktail party with the Spanish mafia: Juan, Blanca, Muntadas, Ivan, Andres, Mark, and me. Over gin and tonics we laughed while checking in on each other. Muntadas strikes: "I am already someone else. The only thing left of my old me is the envelope, the skin."

March 29, 2020 Since the lockdown, we have been walking the eerily empty streets for hours every day, almost in a daze, like right after 9/11, trying to understand what has happened, what is happening to this city that we love so irrationally. All love is irrational, I suppose. "The day they wounded New York," sounds in my head—the haunting lyric of Leonard Cohen's song written a few years after the Twin Towers came down. And it rang so true, as if the city was an animate being, which it is. What would he sing now?

April 4, 2020 Muntadas is in town. He wants a copy of my *X-Ray* book. We meet in the middle of an empty Greene Street with surgical gloves and masks, and like two spies we exchange publications enclosed in brown envelopes. The encounter lasts about three minutes. I see fear in his eyes. Or is it my own fear I see reflected?

April 6, 2020 I thought 9/11 was the catastrophe that would define my generation. And then along came Covid-19. In many ways 9/11 was the reverse, at least for those of us who were living in ground zero and were evacuated from our apartment, living in a hotel for what seemed like an interminable time, longing to return to our homes, to our beds. Now we are confined inside and longing to be outside, in public space.

April 12, 2020 Beds in the street, transporting the sick, have become a common and frightening sight in New York and in the media, with medical professionals completely wrapped in protective gear, like terrestrial astronauts, complete with oxygen tanks. They are like portable rooms, some encased in a plastic bubble, reminiscent of 1960s sci-fi architecture. These portable beds act as the link between the domestic bed and the hospital bed—a vast ecology of beds, then, a whole landscape.

April 15, 2020 Beds are not just in the media as the real facade of this new city; they also are media platforms, Zooming, broadcasting, FaceTiming. Bed-to-bed communication. Think of all of those connecting with friends and colleagues from bed, all the beds you see in the background of work meetings, socializing, comedy shows, at-home music concerts, etc. No bed is a secret anymore. More than anything, I keep thinking of all of those whose last contact with their loved ones is on a tablet held by a nurse.

May 18, 2020 Elena, my youngest sister, calls. She says our mother will not make it to the summer. "But have you explained to her what is happening?" I ask. "You are the doctor."

"We don't want to alarm her," she says.

I think this is worse, so I try myself, over the phone: "You know, there is a terrible virus going around, something like the 1918 flu."

"Really? Wouldn't you be exaggerating? You were always such a hypochondriac, just like your father. When are you coming?"

But I can't come. Spain has closed down completely. Yet I don't trust the airline companies that tell me nobody is flying in at all. I check online for airport activity in Valencia. An ambulance plane from Belgrade is arriving this afternoon at 7pm. That's the extent of movement in the airport today.

August 7, 2020 *Aujourd'hui maman est mort*. I am happy to be here with her. She was from a generation that was born at home, in bed, and could still die, almost a century later, at home, in her bed.

The Bed in the Age of Covid-19

More than revealing something new, pandemics expose what was already there. What Covid-19 has dramatically, even shockingly, made visible is the invisible city—not just the invisible urbanism of hypersocial microorganisms, but the invisible urbanism of inequities, hidden workers, and uneven access to care or empathy.

The new architecture of the pervasive bed is not a side effect of the pandemic but has been exposed by it. Once exposed, it might mutate again. New architectures might appear. To think about what might happen next there is an urgent need to look back and understand the intimate bonds between architecture and disease. So much of what is shocking in the current situation is what was already there but buried, overlooked, or forgotten.

Already in 2012, the *Wall Street Journal* reported that eighty percent of young professionals in New York were working from bed. The bed had already become a new kind of office. The virus has taken this to a whole new level. And is there any reason to think that we will leave the bed when all of this is over, now that we have become so much better at working in bed, teaching in bed, shopping in bed, socializing with people miles away from our beds? The bed used to be the site of intimate physical contact. Now we will only get out into the street in search of such contact.

The future city may not look so different from that of today, but all its hidden rhythms will have changed. Think of working at home, in bed even, as millions have been forced to do. What was once a fantasized future is now a reality we are unlikely, or unable, to give up. This turn indoors, which was already well underway in the last decade, is not a turn away from the city or from density. Far from an antiurban force, the virus will inspire new forms of urban density, new forms of cross-contamination. The key change will not be the shape of the city but affordable housing, education, and access to healthcare. The question will not just be the relation of the bed to work but to privacy, community, equity, mobility, race, technology, energy, labor, climate, and philosophy. The bed never simply sits in a space. It both generates space and is orchestrated by massive forces. The idea of the bed as disconnection or escape—to privacy, domesticity, rest, convalescence, and dreams—was relatively short-lived. It was always a fragile idea, riddled with contradictions. And now it is gone.

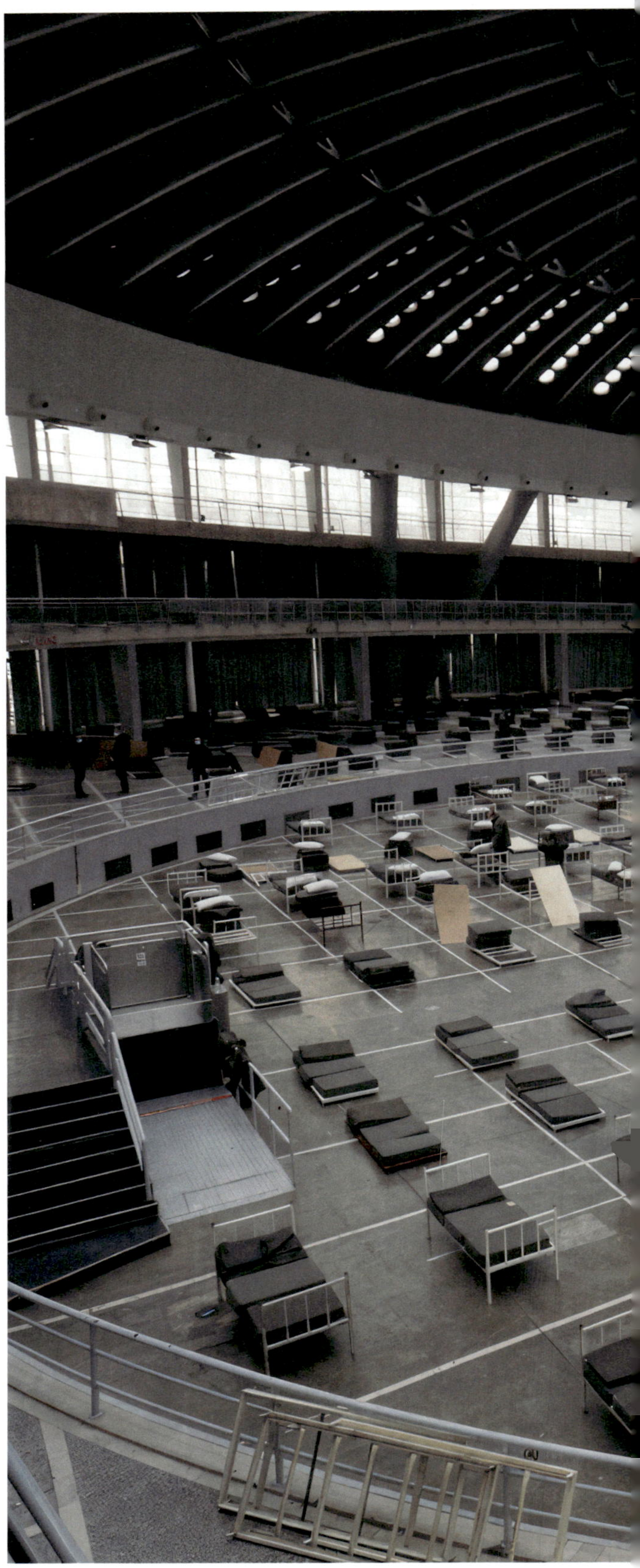

↗ Serbian soldiers set up beds for treatment of possible Covid-19-infected patients inside of the Belgrade Fair, Serbia, March 24, 2020.

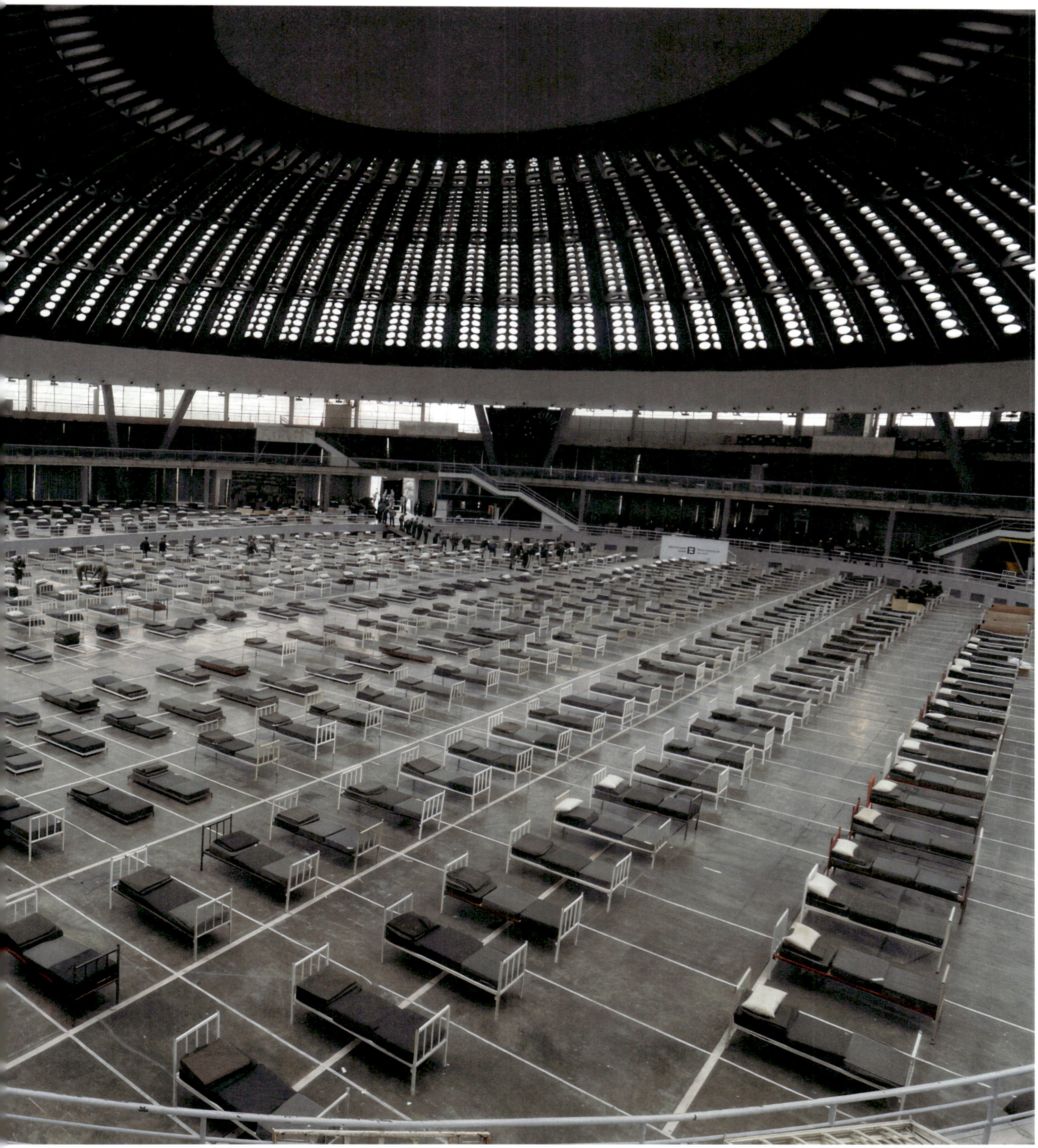

An earlier version of this essay was originally published by e-flux Architecture in 2020.

p293 Chris Machian/*Omaha World-Herald* via AP.
p294 (top left, top right), 295 (top left, bottom left) Photo: Mark Wigley
p294 (bottom left, bottom right), 295 (bottom right) Photo: Beatriz Colomina
p295 (top right) © ARXIU/AM. Muntadas Archive Association.
p298–299 Photo: AP Photo/ Darko Vojinovic.

LANDS OF CONTAGION

IVÁN LÓPEZ MUNUERA

Sylvia Rivera's Home On the bleak spring morning of April 6, 1996, the TV station WPQG interviewed Sylvia Rivera at her home in New York. The camera focused on her rescued plants, her plush toy bear, her salvaged furniture, her little altars with photographs of her chosen family, and her outfits hanging in the improvised walls of her shack—a fragile structure made with broken doors, some plastic, and cardboard. Rivera's home was in Lower Manhattan at Pier 45, which faced the Hudson River on one side and the wrecked West Side Highway on the other, at the very end of Christopher Street. After a brief period away from Manhattan, Sylvia came back to the piers in 1992, when the body of her friend, the African American sex worker and activist Marsha P. Johnson, was found floating in the Hudson on July 6.[1] It was where Rivera labored for decades as a sex worker, lived, and socialized with other members of the LGBTQIA+ community (mostly racialized, gender-nonconforming people like herself), and the "homeless" population that actually found a "home" on that piece of land.[2]

Rivera was a Puerto Rican trans activist who changed LGBTQIA+ history through her involvement in the Stonewall riots and her fight for the rights of

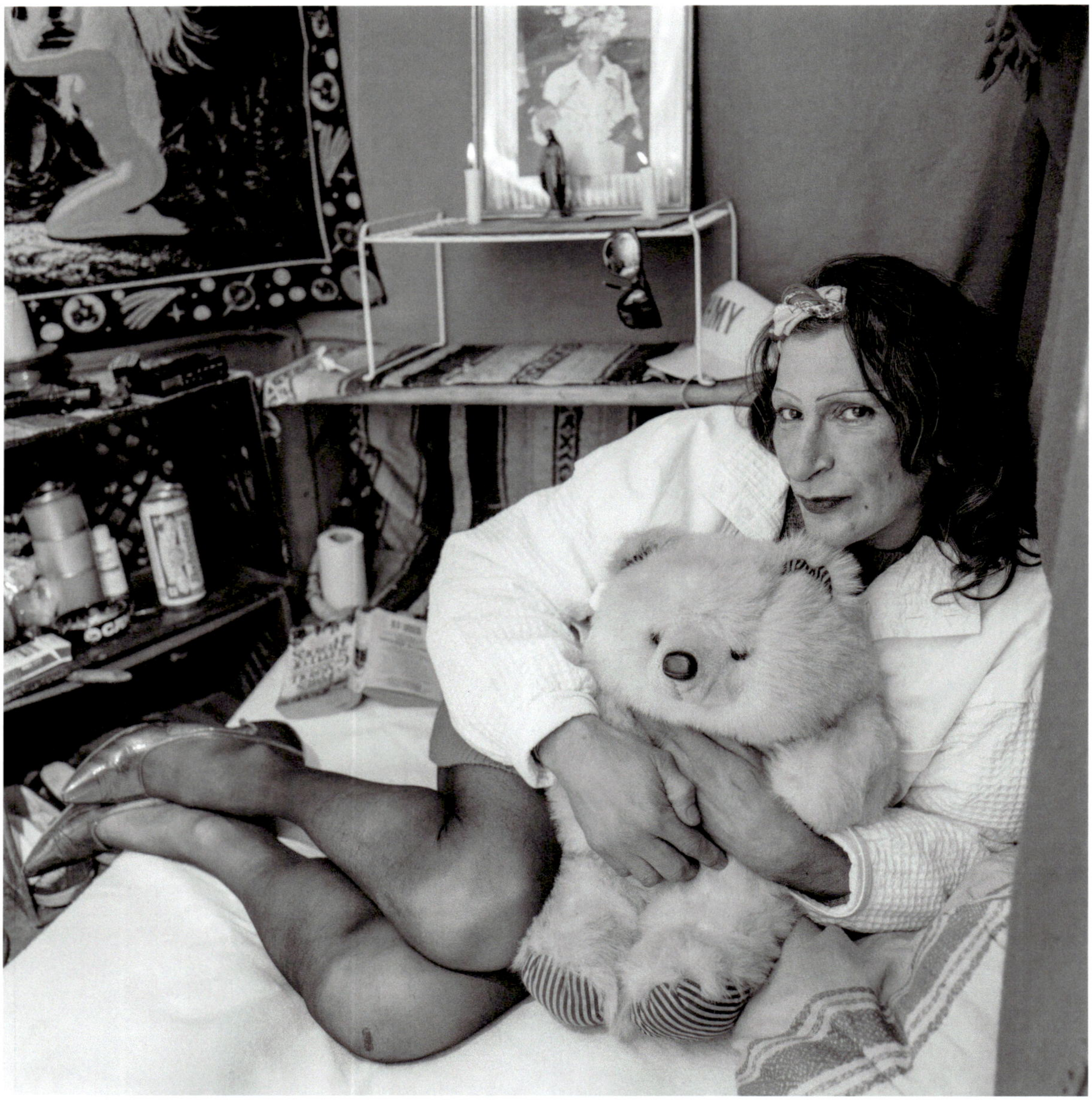

← → Sylvia Rivera at home, 1996

sex workers, incarcerated people, and the homeless. Her house, along with a dozen other dwellings where more than thirty people lived, was destroyed that morning in 1996 by the Hudson River Park Conservancy, a subsidiary of the New York State Urban Development Corporation, as part of the clearance operation to build the Hudson River waterfront (from Battery Park City to 59th Street). The Hudson River waterfront project, designed by Signe Nielsen from Mathews Nielsen Landscape Architects and Quennell Rothschild Associates, included a boulevard, trees, a seven-lane highway, and paths for bikers, joggers, and skaters. Conceived as a continuous extension of greenery, the park buffered the presence of the highway, which was intended to complete the large-scale plan of facilitating the daily commute of white-collar workers to and from the suburbs and their predominantly single-family detached dwellings. The New York State Urban Development Corporation saw in the piers a sacrificial milieu of impurity and devaluation. Rivera described the event as follows: "It's called a sweep. Not even a fucking eviction. A sweep, like we're trash."[3]

The clearance operation of the piers took place under the New York Slum Clearance Commission and the law's utopian verbiage of "sanitizing" an environment that was referred to as dangerous, unhealthy, insalubrious, and unsuitable for human life. "For more than a year," one report from the Commission wrote, "people who live in apartments near the homeless colony have complained of rotting trash, stray cats, and bonfires smoldering in the night."[4] But for Rivera that was just an excuse, epitomized by a Thanksgiving dinner they organized years before that was shut down by the New York Police Department (NYPD), when neighbors complained they were cooking a turkey and pumpkin pie in an oven made from a file drawer and a fire. The neighbors were disgusted, but for Rivera, "these guys, they might just look like dirty homeless people to you, but to me, they were my family."[5]

The demolition of the piers showed the violent clash of two contrasting forms of urbanism, differentiated by the way they shaped collective contagiousness. For Rivera and her community, the piers were a place where bodies and a riverfront architecture turned permeable by the accumulative effect of decay, wall-cutting, makeshift additions, and material abandonees were entangled as interconnected components of a single medium constituted

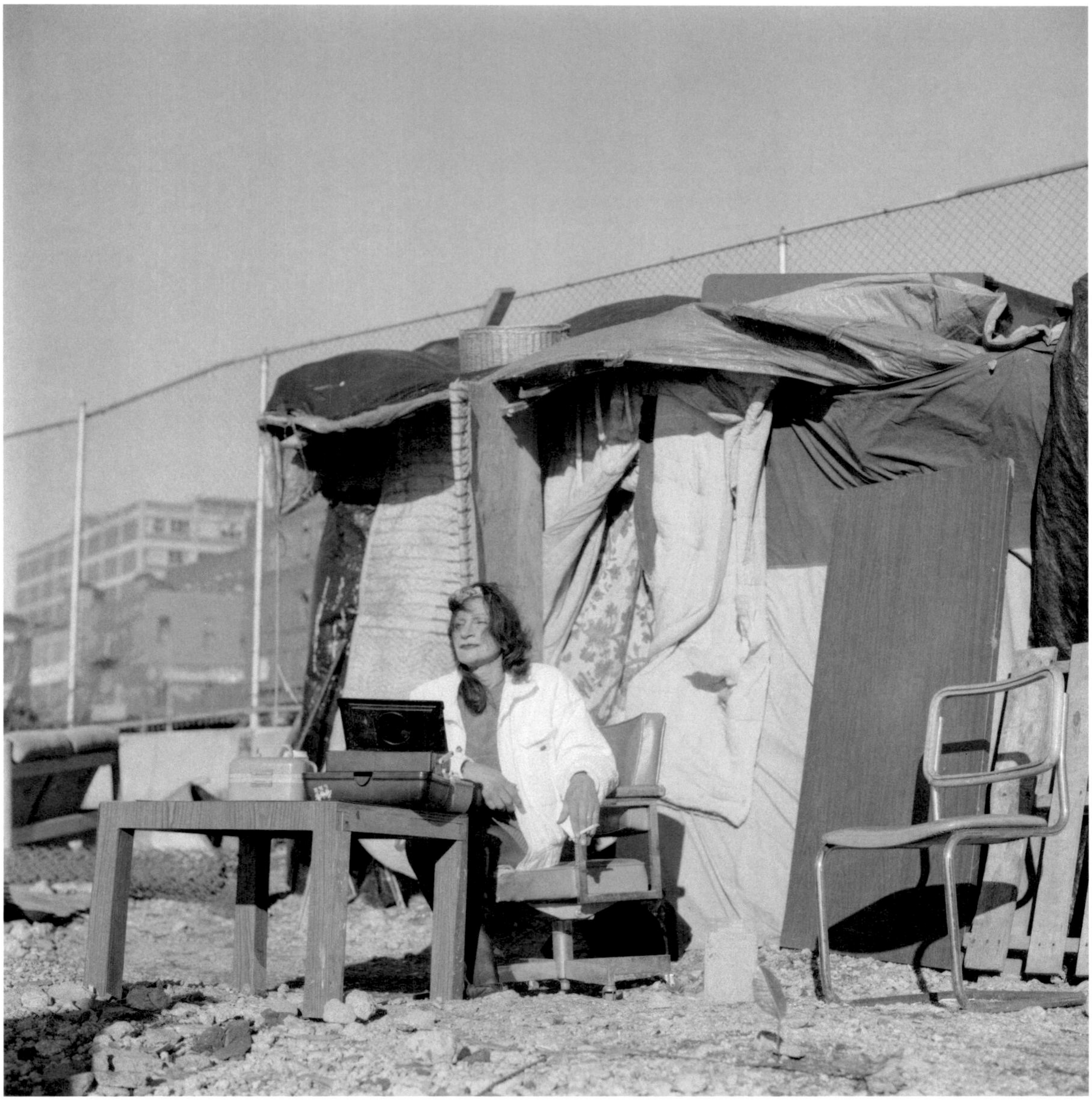

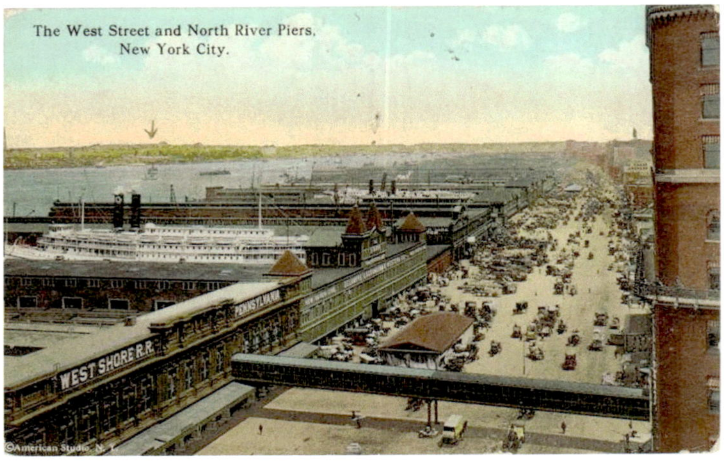
The West Street and North River Piers.
New York City.
WEST SHORE R.R.

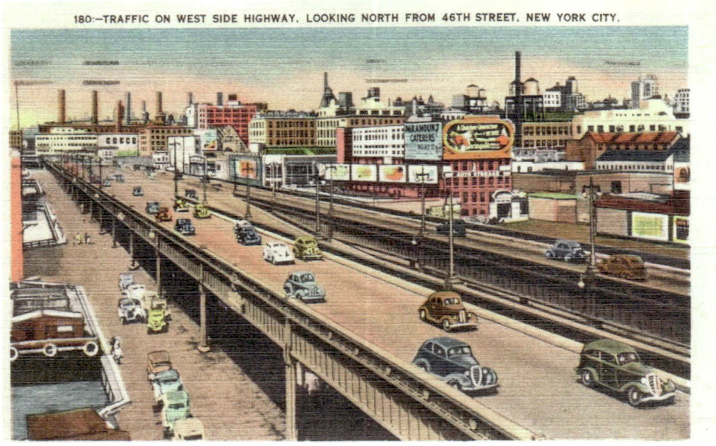
180:—TRAFFIC ON WEST SIDE HIGHWAY. LOOKING NORTH FROM 46TH STREET, NEW YORK CITY.

↑ Postcard of the Hudson River Piers, 1916.

↓ Postcard of the West Side Highway, ca. 1930.

by porousness. The other form of urbanism, promoted by the Hudson River Park Conservancy, was exemplary of the growth of the petrochemical industry that since the 1940s had established an oil-based territoriality: encapsulated humans in distant and segregated suburban, car-dependent, and family-block-based milieus. The former came from the understanding of the piers as a relational system based on nonbinary transness and mutual dependency,[6] while the latter was based on a prophylactic view that considered the piers as a promiscuous, disease-driven space that had to be erased. Before their redevelopment, the piers were "dirty" because they were porous, contagious, permeable to otherness: to the otherness of other human bodies; to the otherness of an environment and its decaying architecture; to the otherness of saliva, blood, and semen.

Blight City Since the 1910s, the Christopher Street piers were synonymous with queer cruising. The multiple buildings of the shipping companies located in the area, with their dark, hidden spots populated at night by men who had sex with men, were the perfect place for sexual encounters otherwise prosecuted under the sodomy laws of New York State. With the forfeit of the piers by the army and ocean liners after 1945, the progressively derelict infrastructures intensified their life as a complex ecosystem for alternative ways of living that included multiple bars in the adjacent West Village, from the Stonewall Inn and Julius's to the leather-friendly Ramrod and Keller; community spaces like the Women's Liberation Center and The Center; bookstores like Labyris; and queer associations like the Mattachine Society.

The piers were not alone in the creation of an ecosystem that allowed alternative ways of living to flourish, nor in their description as an unsanitary and boorish environment. Downtown Manhattan at large was known during the 1960s as "the Wastelands of New York," an epithet that came from the immense body of manufacturing buildings that were eventually abandoned during the city's deindustrialization in the 1970s and 1980s.[7] This was accompanied by a recession that hit the city especially hard in the late 1960s, when its working-class industrial base was transformed into a corporate and service-based economy and New York State Governor Nelson A. Rockefeller, together with city planners, implemented policies to frame Manhattan as a place for work, but not living. As former director of Creole Petroleum, proposals spurred through Rockefeller's mandate (1959–1973) took the private car as the center of urban development. The car allowed encapsulated human bodies to arrive into the city from the suburbs and park in a garage beneath their offices (like SOM's Lever House or Mies van der Rohe's Seagram Building) without ever having to walk in the streets.[8]

The rhetoric used by public and private officials to get rid of the piers was suffused with medical metaphors, particularly in their use of discourse around "blight" to secure political and judicial approval. As Wendell Pritchett explains, blight "was a disease that threatened to turn healthy areas into slums. A vague, amorphous term, blight was a rhetorical device that enabled advocates to reorganize property ownership by declaring certain real estate dangerous to the future of the city."[9] Lewis Mumford even referred to blight as a "cancer" that should be removed.[10] At the same time, these discussions were imbricated with racial depictions and xenophobic targets. Indeed, most of the constructions beleaguered by this operation were inhabited or used by Black people, Latin Americans, migrants, and displaced communities.

Way before the Hudson River waterfront project tore down Rivera's home, numerous plans were afloat to "cleanse" this part of the city. Already in 1941, Robert Moses proposed the infamous Lower Manhattan Express Highway (LOMEX), which would have connected New Jersey to Brooklyn and demolished large parts of SoHo, the piers, the West Village, and the Lower East Side. The project, which involved architects and urbanists like Shadrach Woods and Paul Rudolph and was based on studies commissioned by the Ford Foundation, was only canceled in 1985 after decades of demonstrations led by Shirley Hayes, Jane Jacobs, and the Committee to Save the West Village, among others. But from the early 1940s to the mid-1980s, the destiny of all that was in the way of LOMEX almost seemed inevitable: "Civic organizations, advocacy groups, and political actors, including Robert Moses, New York University (NYU), the City Club of New York, and the United Hatters, Cap and Millinery Worker's Union, argued that these buildings were, at best, obsolete for modern industry and, at worst, dangerous to their inhabitants and neighbors."[11] When a section of the West Side Highway collapsed in 1973, the enterprise to get rid of the piers at the end of the West Village intensified. Videos like Gordon Matta-Clark's *Day's End* (1975) reinforced the idea that this part of the city was "empty," just a relic from a glorious industrial past.[12]

The piers, however, thrived with life. As Grace Dunham pointed out, they were "a place where gay men, trans people, and sex workers all gathered to participate in social, sexual, and political life.

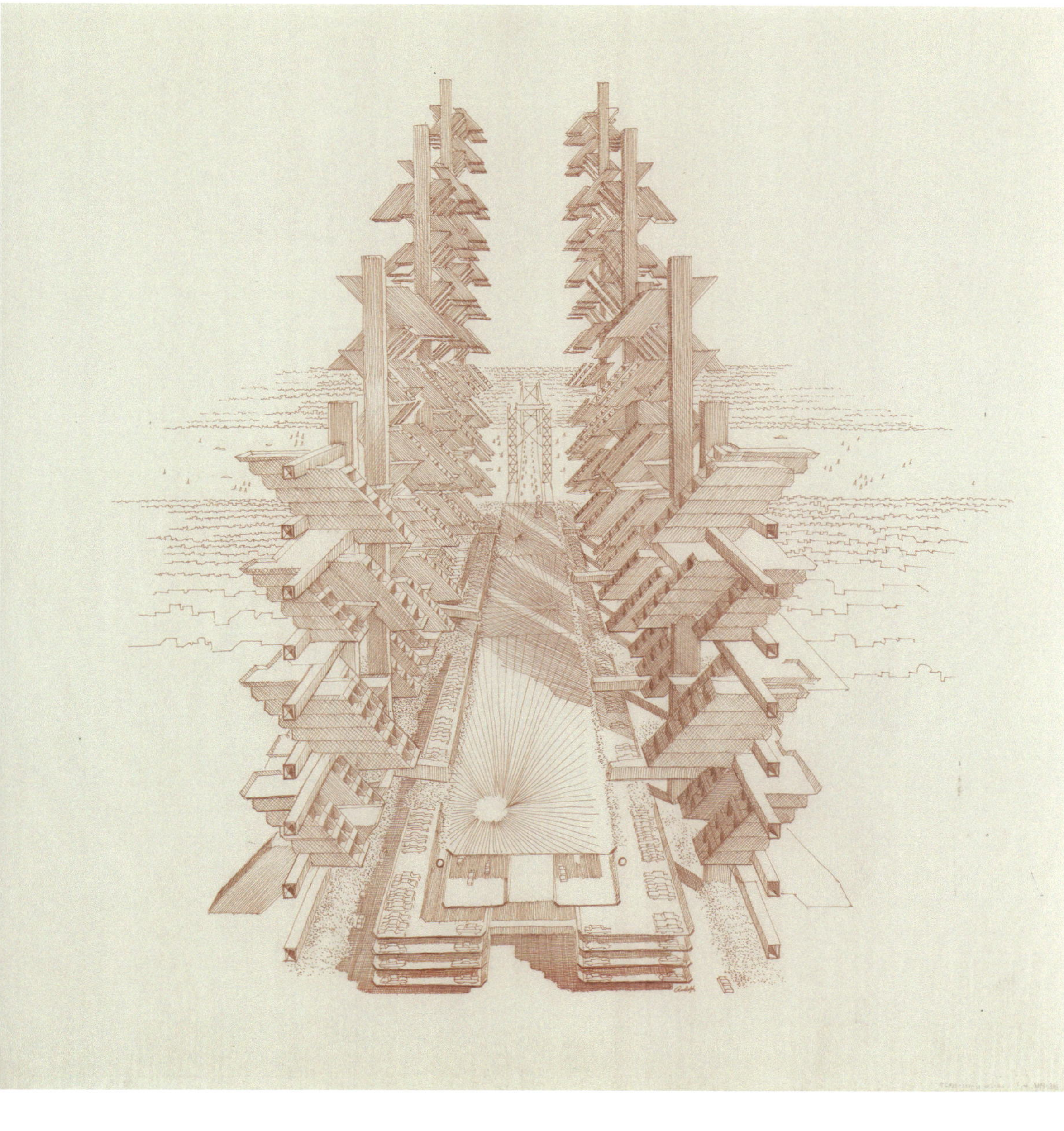

← Paul Rudolph, Lower Manhattan Expressway, New York City. View to Williamsburg Bridge. Rendering, ca. 1970.

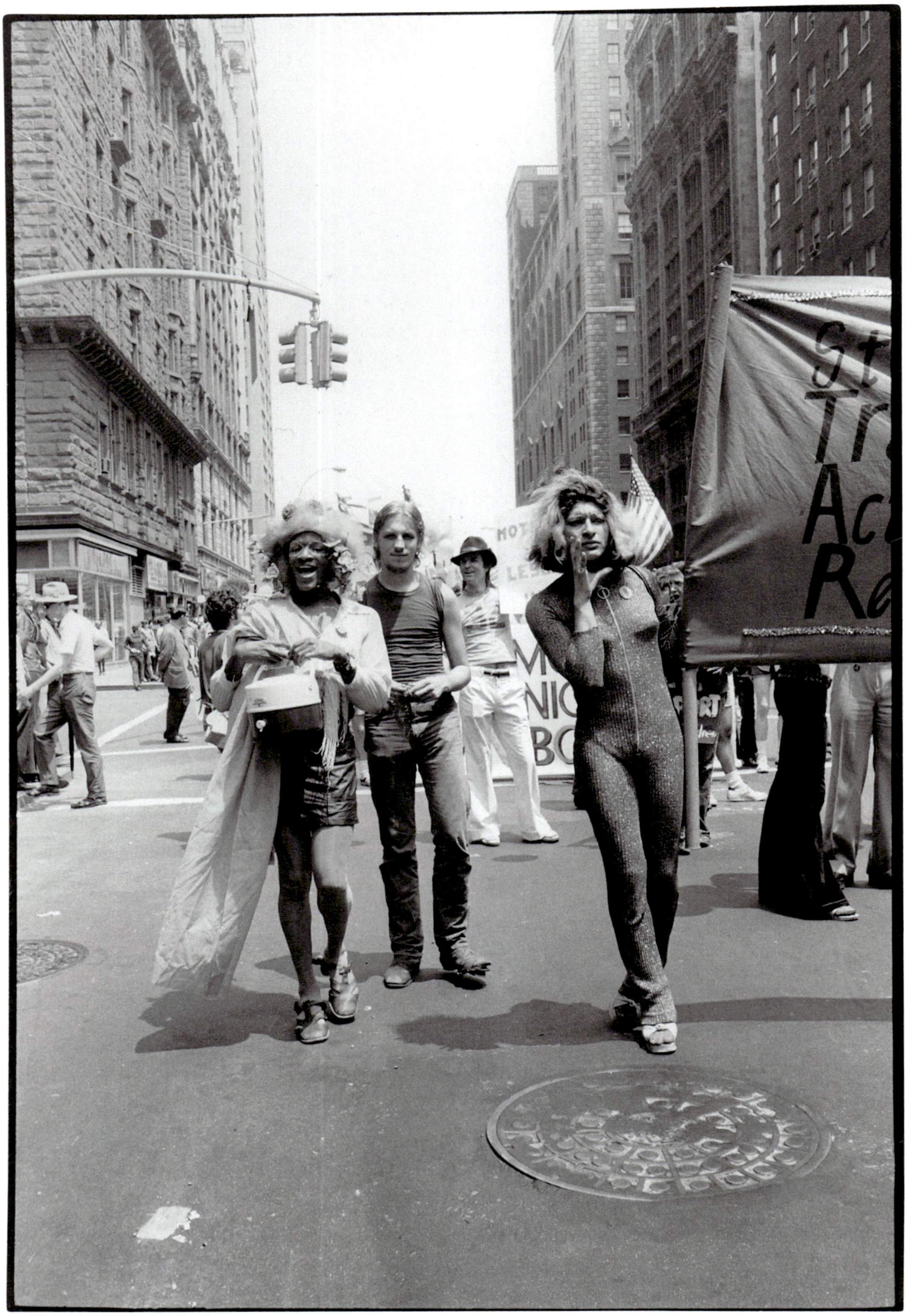

← Leonard Fink, *Street Transvestites Action Revolutionaries at the Christopher Street Liberation Day March* (Marsha P. Johnson and Sylvia Rivera pictured), 1973. The LGBT Community Center National History Archive.

→ Leonard Fink, *Onlookers Walk Beneath the Pier*, 1981.

↘ Leonard Fink, *Leonard Fink Explores the Pier*, 1979.

They provided a refuge away from NYPD surveillance, which specifically targeted low-income queer and trans people and trans people of color."[13] Here this community engaged in sexual activity, sunbathed at the docks, and cared for and educated each other. They also embarked on cultural projects inspired by their environment, as is clear in the art of Alvin Baltrop, Shelley Seccombe, Rudy Grillo, David Wojnarowicz, and Leonard Fink.

The notion of the piers as insalubrious areas that needed to be wiped out gained traction in the 1980s during the peak of the HIV/AIDS crisis, when different spaces frequented by the LGBTQIA+ community in New York (cruising areas, saunas, bathhouses, bars, nightclubs) were targeted as "public health" menaces. This categorization of "unhealthy" environments revived pervasive narratives from the nineteenth-century hygienist movement that

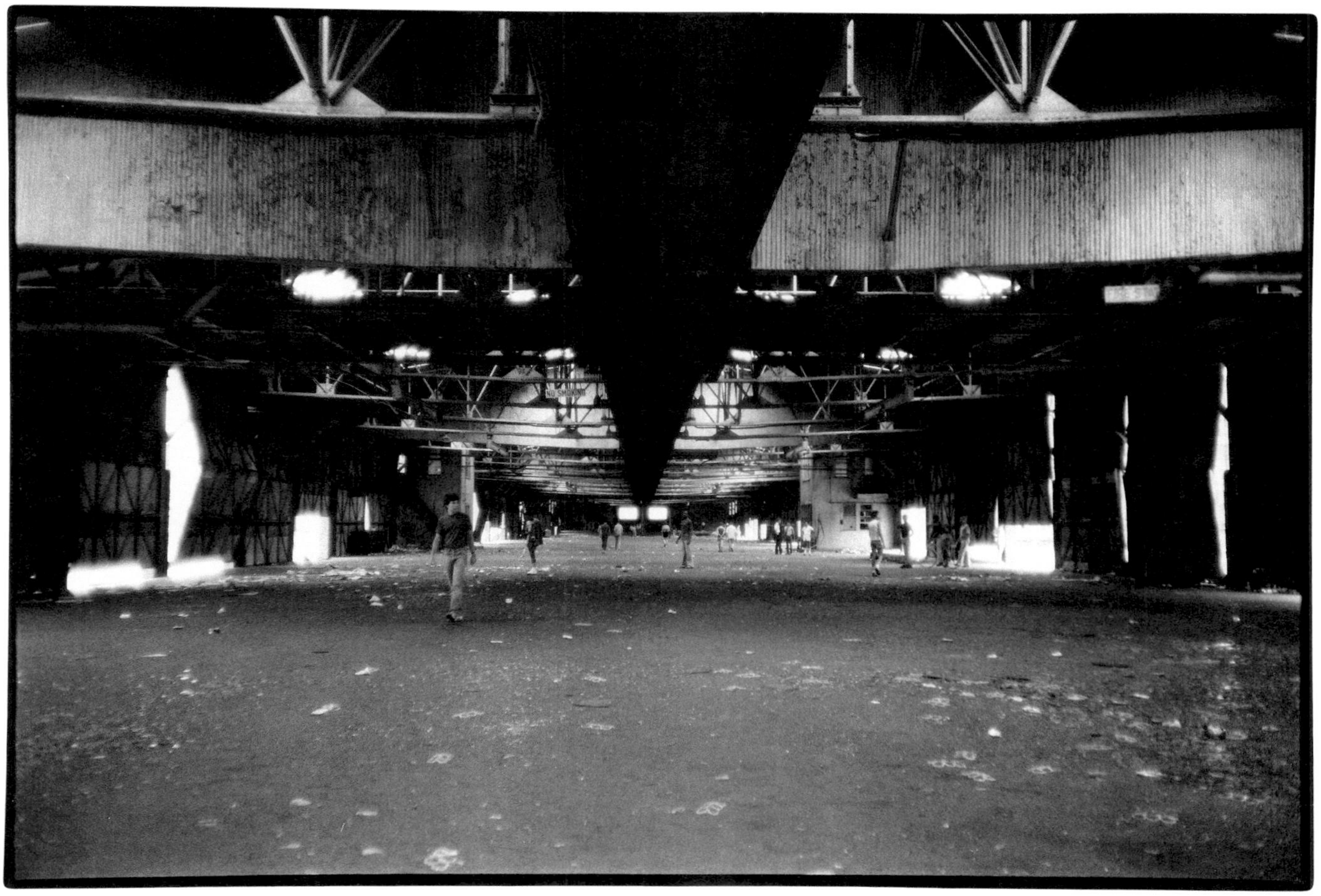

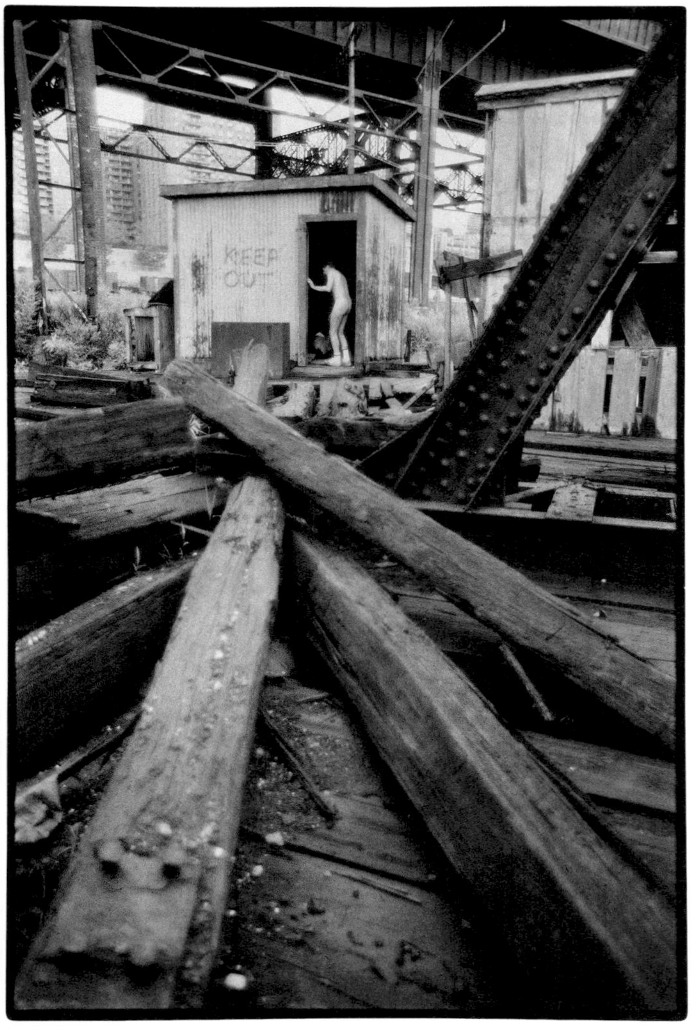

traced a false connection between disease and the appearance of the urban environment. This narrative concerning the piers was active in New York City until the early 2000s, when Mayor Michael Bloomberg and Governor George Pataki opened the Greenwich Village segment of Hudson River Park on May 30, 2003. The highway was finally demolished, the waterfront was built, and a series of gates were erected to keep Pier 45 closed after 1am to avoid concentrations of the people who had made the piers a blooming environment years before. The previous residents of these spaces were just routine casualties.

This new proposal for the Hudson River Park opted for a unitary, straightforward, and apparently open but constantly surveilled set of facilities, where constant circulation (by car, skate, bike, foot) is central and frames the conception of the piers as a passing point. This contrasts the labyrinthic and fragmented former setting, with multitudes of hidden spaces that provided a sense of privacy and safety for the persecuted queer community. It substituted a technosocial assemblage based on contagiousness—where human bodies were part of an extensive environment, shaping it and being shaped in return—for a technocratic solution—where the previous inhabitants were obliterated and erased through an urban operation that conceived them and their built environment as unhealthy and useless.

STAR

The history of the piers runs parallel to the history of the LGBTQIA+ movement in New York. The piers were where Sylvia Rivera and Marsha P. Johnson decided to locate the first installment of Street Transvestites Action Revolutionaries (STAR) in 1970 to fight for trans sex workers' rights. This was a year after the Stonewall riots, which both Rivera and Johnson took an active part in, though their participation was not immediately recognized.[14] Segments of associations like the Gay Liberation Front and the Gay Activist Alliance that were coordinating actions to fight homophobia in New York excluded them for being trans and "parodying" womanhood. This exclusion was galvanized during the 1973 Gay Pride Rally in New York, where Rivera tried to speak to the audience congregated in Washington Square. At the beginning, none of the organizers allowed her to do so. When she finally was able to, pushing her way to the microphone, she said: "I have been beaten. I have had my nose broken. I have been thrown in jail. I have lost my job. I have lost my apartment for gay liberation. And you all treat me this way? What the fuck's wrong with you all?" She asked the movement to support racialized trans sex workers and incarcerated people instead of just focusing on cis "men and women that belong to a white middle-class club." As she was booed by the demonstrators and forcefully removed from the stage, she shouted "Revolution now! Gay power!"[15]

This episode highlights the tensions between what was happening in the built environment of New York's wastelands and the LGBTQIA+ movement at large. Rivera and the pier community were pushing for a space of mutual dependency, a radical queer ecology that confronted the structural exclusion of people like them (gender-nonconforming, racialized, sex worker, homeless). Meanwhile, the audience that congregated at Washington Square proposed what Lisa Duggan calls the new homonormativity: an ideology based on the negation of alternative forms of living and the acceptance of a heteronormative framework for the LGBTQIA+ community based on a white domestic privacy and the freedom to consume.[16]

Feeling left behind by the movement, Johnson and Rivera founded STAR to provide a roof and social support for underage and homeless LGBTQIA+ sex workers in New York. They first conceived of STAR as an itinerant institution inside a trailer parked at the piers. STAR's van was the opposite of NYC officials' conception of the automobile. It was not about detaching their users from their surroundings, but connecting them, to act as a medium of contagiousness that could shape a form of kin. Teenage sex workers slept inside while Johnson and Rivera worked at night, bringing back breakfast in the morning. But one day, when Johnson and Rivera approached STAR with groceries, they saw the trailer moving. Apparently, somebody reclaimed it and drove off with all of their belongings, as well as "one stoned queen" sleeping inside, who woke up several days later in California.[17] They then moved STAR to an abandoned building at 213 East Second Street for a small amount of rent paid to the mob figure Michael Umbers. They renovated the building and threw parties to fundraise. But the owners of the building acted in malfeasance. After the renovations—once it was habitable—they were evicted.

A New Kin

Rivera continued her fight over the years. This struggle only intensified during the HIV/AIDS crisis of the 1980s, when she advocated for the rights of sex workers, the incarcerated, and trans and homeless people, who were all hit especially hard by the epidemic. At the time, the United States government, along with the mainstream media and several health agencies such as the Centers for Disease Control and Prevention (CDC), sought to identify and confine potential risk groups, who came to be known as the 4H's: homosexuals, heroin addicts, hemophiliacs, and Haitians.[18] Members of these groups were ostracized and deprived of typical considerations during the outbreak such as protocols of announcement, transparency in information, research, and measure-taking. Meanwhile, the communities that congregated around the piers, and the piers themselves, helped spread information about AIDS, made transparent the available data, and offered care among affected communities. Groups and associations like STAR, ACT-UP, Gay Men's Health Crisis, and Gran Fury were essential in this effort. A form of kinship was created that was not based on traditional understanding of lineage (consanguinity, phylogenetic relationships, traditional family structures), but on the way they engaged with a virus (HIV) and a disease (AIDS) through activism.[19]

HIV acted as both kin and the apparatus by which kinship among its carriers was created. Furthermore, not all of the people involved carried the virus or shared the same positive status, and even if they did, there were multiple thresholds in the viral load: undetectables, HIV-positive with no AIDS, false positives, etc. Thus, the bonding between community members was more than biological. What they shared was a chosen kinship: an understanding of their relationship with HIV and AIDS different from the one embraced by medical authorities, media, and government officials.[20] This environmental activism, where kin was formed through the relationship between humans, nonhumans, and their ecosystems, happened in places like the piers.[21]

The piers were not unique in the way they were depicted as a menace for collective health. At a time when "men only" spaces for dancing were still illegal, and New York legislation required clubs to have at least one woman for every three men, bathhouses created an escape from the constant scrutiny of authorities and from homophobic attacks on gay men who were caught having sex in public or private spaces. Bathhouses were found throughout the city, from Everard's at West 28th Street and St. Mark's in the East Village to Mount Morris in Harlem. HIV/AIDS was shaped in the dispute between two urban forms of contagiousness: one that would render the pandemic into both a medium and kinship, where the spread of the virus among humans would be coupled with the relational artifacts prevention and care depended on; and another that repressed the visibility and circulation of the virus as a medium and would develop efforts to isolate it in socially stagnated, segregated capsules of marginalization.

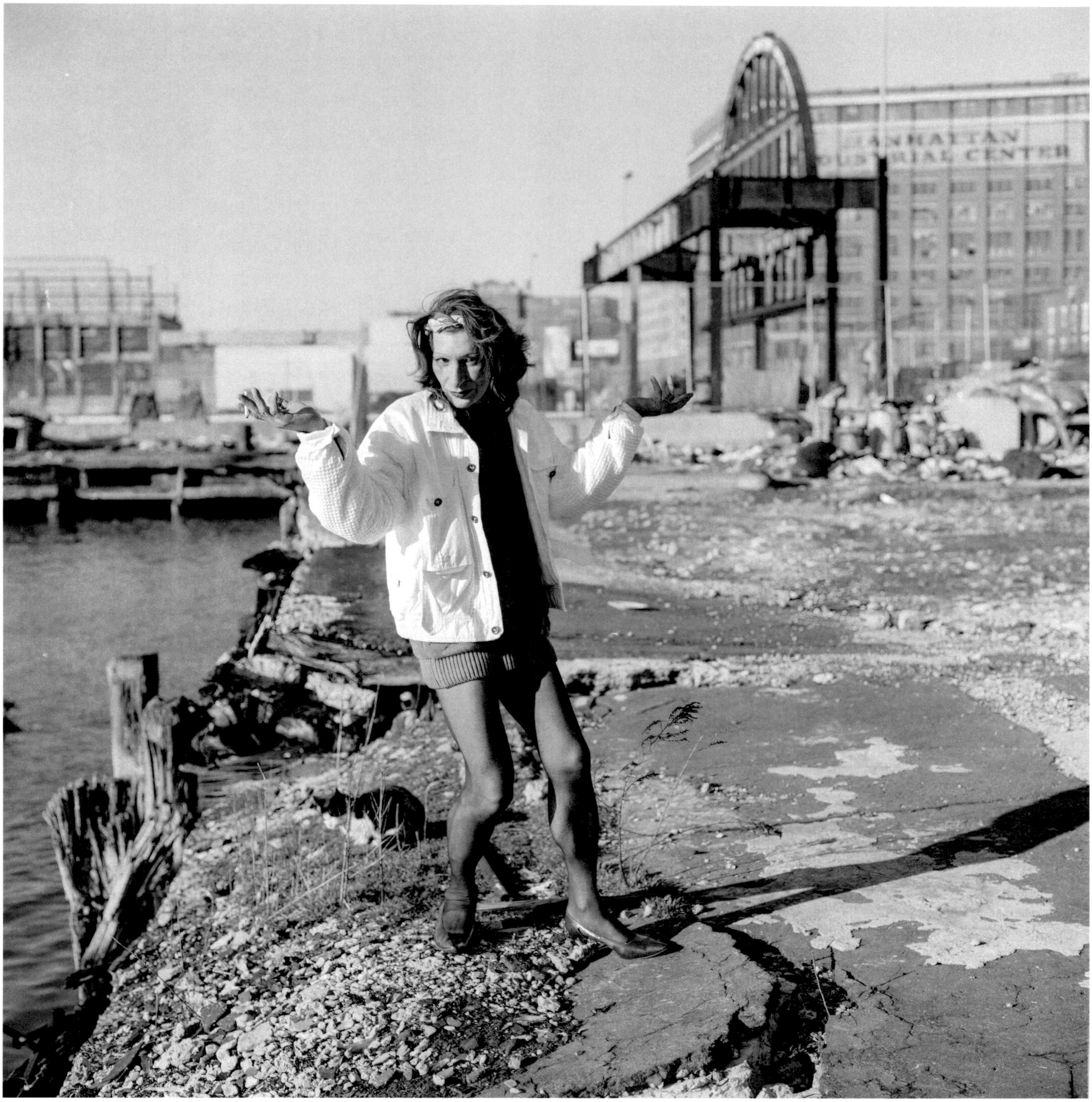

↓ Sylvia Rivera at the piers in 1996.

A Certain Environment-Specific Villain

The political importance of the piers, along with nightclubs, bathhouses, and saunas, and the contagious activism the racialized trans and queer communities sustained there, were tested during the early years of the epidemic.[22] As sociologist Steven Epstein pointed out, "AIDS became a 'gay disease' primarily because clinicians, epidemiologists, and reporters perceived it through that filter, but secondarily because gay communities were obliged to make it their own" with their responses and organized groups.[23] AIDS's first name, GRID (Gay Related Immune Deficiency), as well as the common "gay plague" and "gay cancer" epithets, strengthened the idea of a specifically gay disease related to a certain environment-specific villain.[24] Journalists, following the views of public health authorities, blamed the epidemic on gay promiscuity and the places gay people frequented.[25]

This theory was adopted by doctors like Yehudi M. Felman of New York City's Bureau of Venereal Disease Control, who declared that the disease's cause "could be the bugs out of the pipes in the bathhouses" or poppers (amyl nitrite), a recreational inhalant popular among members of the queer community.[26] This claim had terrible consequences for the activist spaces and urban fabrics that confronted the epidemic. During the decade to come, most of the saunas and bathhouses that operated in New York were forcibly closed after local health officials tagged them as places of "high-risk sexual activities."[27] The remnants of Pier 45 were demolished. The activist history of these places was "cleared."[28]

There's So Many Fucking Buildings in This Fucking Manhattan

Studies of epidemics tend to focus on the metaphor of the healthy body as being attacked by an external agent. But the interconnection of bodies, other bodies, viruses, bacteria, microbes, architectures, technologies, and environments is intrinsically founded in their contagiousness. Ultimately, heterogenous corporality composes a type of urban form, one that exceeds its understanding as the unfolding of infrastructures, land uses, and buildings. Instead, it becomes a mode of collective embodiment that challenges the exceptionality of the human flesh as much as its individuality, understanding it as both infiltrating and being infiltrated by viruses, buildings, technologies, regulations, and policies.

When Sylvia Rivera shouted to the authorities "stay away from my house!" while being evicted in 1996, "house" not only referred to the physical construction of her home. She was confronting teleological progress with the project of a technosocial assemblage based on contagiousness and mutual caring that could push for a queer ecology and defy normative narratives of race, sex, gender, and nature.[29] The territorialization of epidemics, identities, and citizenship not only shapes the built environment, but the built environment shapes them in return. Architecture thereby assumed the form of an expanded spatial practice that involves a set of material, bodily, economic, social, cultural, and ecological questions. When Rivera was trying to save her home from demolition, she exclaimed, "there's so many fucking buildings in this fucking Manhattan."[30] What New York City was losing with the demolition of Pier 45 was not just a series of dwellings. It was losing a complex ecosystem of coexistence within a specific environment of mutual dependency that recognized its contagious nature.

1. Johnson's death was ruled an accident/suicide. But Marsha's friends and trans activists, especially Victoria Cruz (from the New York City Anti-Violence Project), fought this version through the years and through an increasing amount of evidence, saying she never wanted to die, and that the previous night witnesses saw her in a state of distress because she was being harassed by men—something common among New York sex workers, especially those like Johnson, an African American gender dissident. Maybe she was murdered or perhaps she accidentally fell into the freezing waters of the Hudson. Sylvia, who was not living in New York at that time, came back to Manhattan to honor Johnson's death, maintain her memory, and fight to reopen the case along with others until the authorities agreed to change the cause of death to "undetermined causes."

2. Part of the information about Sylvia Rivera's life in the piers comes from a recorded interview with Randy Wicker in 1992.

3. WPQG News, New York, April 6, 1996.

4. David Stout, "Eviction Day along the Curb of a Dead Road," *New York Times*, April 3, 1996.

5. Stout, "Eviction Day."

6. Here transness is, as Jack Halberstam points out, the understanding of the body as fragmentary and internally contradictory, remapping gender and its relations to race, place, class, and sexuality. Jack Halberstam, *Wild Things: The Disorder of Desire* (Durham: Duke University Press, 2020). Also C. Riley Snorton, *Black on Both Sides: A Racial History of Trans Identity* (Minneapolis: University of Minnesota Press, 2017); and Andrés Jaque, *Superpowers of Scale* (New York: Columbia University Press, 2020).

7. City Club of New York, *The Wastelands of New York City: A Preliminary Inquiry into the Nature of Commercial Slum Areas, Their Potential for Housing and Business Redevelopment* (New York City: City Club of New York, 1962).

8. Proposals like Fuller and Shoji Sadao's Manhattan Dome (1964) went even further, cutting Lower Manhattan off from the rest of the island, encapsulating the rest of it under a dome; or the encapsulation of an autonomous atmosphere in the Ford Foundation building (Kevin Roche, 1967).

9. Wendell E. Pritchett, "The 'Public Menace' of Blight: Urban Renewal and the Private Uses of Eminent Domain," *All Faculty Scholarship* [Penn Carey Law] (2003): 1199.

10. This was the term that Lewis Mumford used in an article published in 1962. Lewis Mumford, "The Skyline: Mother Jacobs' Home-Remedies," *New Yorker,* December 1, 1962.

11. Aaron Shkuda, *The Lofts of SoHo: Gentrification, Art, and Industry in New York, 1950–1980* (Chicago: University of Chicago Press, 2016), 15.

12. Lola Hinojosa, "Gordon Matta-Clark's *Day's End* (1975)," description for MNCARS website.

13. Grace Dunham, "Out of Obscurity: Trans Resistance 1969–2016," in *Trap Door: Trans Cultural Production and the Politics of Visibility* (Cambridge, MA: MIT Press, 2017), 91.

14. Popular narratives said that Johnson was the one who ignited the riots by throwing a brick at the police. As a reminder, Marsha carried a cardboard brick at every gay pride.

15. This moment put together the "enunciated" and the "enunciation," as Walter Mignolo would say, opening the possibility of decolonizing the LGBTQIA+ movement.

16. Lisa Duggan, "The New Homonormativity: The Sexual Politics of Neo-Liberalism," in *Materializing Democracy* (Durham: Duke University Press, 2002). Also Martin F. Manalansan IV, "Race, Violence, and Neoliberal Spatial Politics in the Global City," *Social Text* 23, no. 3–4 (Fall Winter 2005): 84–85; and the crip-queer alliances explored in Ignacio G. Galán, "Disabled Domesticities and the Politics of Bathrooms: Architectural Enactments of Interdependence," in *Architectures of Care: From the Intimate to the Common*, ed. Brittany Utting (London: Routledge, 2023).

17. Martin Duberman, *Stonewall: The Definitive Story of the LGBTQ Rights Uprising that Changed America* (New York: Penguin Random House, 2019), 309–310.

18. "Current Trends Prevention of Acquired Immune Deficiency Syndrome (AIDS): Report of Inter-Agency Recommendations," *Morbidity and Mortality Weekly Report* 32, no. 9 (March 4, 1983): 101–103.

19. The idea of a chosen kin is based in part on Donna Haraway's notion of "staying with the trouble" of living with and in relation to nonhuman others (in this case, HIV and AIDS), which are kin in the sense of "something other, and more than entities tied by ancestry or genealogy." See Donna J. Haraway, *Staying with the Trouble: Making Kin in the Chthulucene* (Durham: Duke University Press, 2016).

20. For more on HIV/AIDS kin and its architecture: Ivan L. Munuera, "HIV and AIDS Kin: The Discotecture of the Paradise Garage," *Thresholds* 48 (Spring 2020): 133–147.

21. This can be seen in scenes from *Paris Is Burning*, directed by Jennie Livingston (1990; Academy Entertainment and Off White Productions), partly recorded at Pier 45.

22. On May 31, 1987, President Reagan finally declared AIDS a public health emergency, giving his first major address on the disease. It was at an outdoor speech in Washington organized by amfAR, the American Foundation for AIDS Research.

23. Steven Epstein, *Impure Science: AIDS, Activism, and the Politics of Knowledge* (Berkeley: University of California Press, 1996), 55.

24. This idea continued even into the late 1990s with authors like Gabriel Rotello, who blamed urban, gay, sexual culture for causing AIDS and the continued spread of HIV infection. Gabriel Rotello, *Sexual Ecology: AIDS and the Destiny of Gay Men* (New York: Dutton, 1997).

25. Of course, the "gay" community encompassed a diverse segment of the population as it has already been shown (trans, queer, gender-nonconforming, etc.), but at that time, the media, medical community, and official institutions flattened that diversity into one single group: gay people. See Michael Bronski, "AIDing Our Guilt and Fear," *Gay Community News*, October 9, 1982, 8.

26. David France, *How to Survive a Plague: The Story of How Activists and Scientists Tamed AIDS* (New York: Alfred A. Knopf, 2016), 37.

27. Maurice Carroll, "State Permits Closing of Bathhouses to Cut AIDS," *New York Times,* October 26, 1985.

28. In order to recover this and other histories, it is essential to highlight the work of the NYC LGBT Historic Sites Project, active since 2015, and the efforts of its founders and directors, Andrew Dolkart, Ken Lustbader, and Jay Shockley.

29. Andil Gosine, "Non-White Reproduction and Same Sex Eroticism: Queer Acts against Nature," in *Queer Ecologies: Sex, Nature, Politics, Desire* (Bloomington: Indiana University Press, 2010), 149–150.

30. WPQG News, New York, April 6, 1996.

An earlier version of this essay was originally published by e-flux Architecture in 2020.

p300, 301, 307 Photo: Valerie Shaff.
p303 Library of the Congress.
p304, 305 The LGBT Community Center National History Archive.

THE VIRUS: FIGURE AND INFRASTRUCTURE

ELIZABETH A. POVINELLI

I Not what is critique. Not what is a concept or a book. But perhaps, why this critique, this concept, this book? Why *Geontologies* (2016) and its obsessions with Life and Nonlife, with its figures of geontopower hovering in the space between Gaia and ground, after *Economies of Abandonment* (2011), *The Empire of Love* (2006), and *The Cunning of Recognition* (2002)? Every one of my books emerges from a limit condition in the previous one, as this limit condition encounters new discursive material currents and arrangements of the present. In this present, a world engulfed by a virus violently severed from its customary relation with the nonhuman world and, as it seeks new settings, killing and maiming those who already bear the embodied imprint of racist and colonial histories, what is the afterlife, the limit of the concept of geontopower and one of its figures, the Virus?

Concepts and their figures are born genealogically, of unexpected alignments of entangled regions of interests. Geontology was first introduced as a concept in 2012 at the Australian National University as part of the Annual Meeting of the Consortium of Humanities Centers and Institutes' "Anthropocene Humanities" symposium. The invitation to participate was my initiation into the concept of the Anthropocene. My previous book, *Economies of Abandonment*, had dived deep into the critical literature on biopower—Arendt and her Greeks, Foucault and his figures, Agamben and his two modes of potentiality, Mbembe and his spectacles of postcolonial necropower, Esposito and his positive and negative biopolitics—in order to focus on a certain moment, or condition, in the life of alternative social projects; those moments, or those conditions in which a social project is neither something nor nothing, but rather a violent oscillation in the torrents of late liberal power. When I was invited to present a talk at the symposium, I was struggling, in the wake of *Economies of Abandonment,* to articulate a space of governance that didn't preclude, even as it subsumed, biopolitics. How could one celebrate an otherwise that is located within landscapes where the "wavering of death" defines a space that does not wonder about the practices of endurance within it, let alone the dynamics therein by which such otherwise might thicken to a something, find itself as such, and then deepen and extend before the weight of late liberal governance discovers and crushes it?

This critical focus on what felt at the time to be a callous celebration of pure potential within zones that shutter rapidly and violently, or ever so slowly, between life and death, prompted me to reflect on my early work, on what started all these books, namely, a request by the Indigenous women I first met at Belyuen, Northern Territory, in 1984, for whom I credentialized myself as an anthropologist so that we could jointly analyze a *berragut* (white settler) mode of governance. This mode of what I would come to call late settler liberalism went by the name of "Aboriginal self-determination." The senior woman from Belyuen that I was working with primarily encountered this mode of governance via the 1976 Northern Territory Land Rights Act. This Act claimed to recognize and embrace Indigenous difference but in practice demanded that Indigenous people shape themselves into form conducive to settler colonialism—to be different enough that settler colonialism could tell itself that it was recognizing difference, but not so different as to threaten the communicative or moral reason of the settler state. In *The Cunning of Recognition*, I argued that the statement that animated state-sanctioned Aboriginal self-determination has "become a form of difference for us that makes no difference to us." The form of difference settler colonialism enjoys most is stories that Indigenous people are forced to tell about their relationships with not only the more-than-human animal world, but more compellingly, their mineral and meteorological existence.[1] The reason that settler law and publics could enjoy this difference was because Indigenous analytics of the deep interdependencies and formations of existence did not seem to touch the epistemologies and ontologies governing settler reason. Settled reason was safely entombed in its schizoid divisions of Life and Nonlife, while providing them *entrée* into *jouissance*—the experience of transgressing their own geontological limit without threatening the benefits of geontopower. By *Economies of Abandonment*, I was more interested in how an otherwise endured these conditions, suggesting two strategies that had a companion relation to late liberal recognition—espionage and camouflage—that I now see as the mode of the figure of the Virus.

It was out of these diverse conditions that *Geontologies* attempted, on the one hand, to assault a critical blindness within the scholarship on biopower, namely geontopower, and on the other, to find a critical language to account for the moment in which a form of power long operating in the open in late settler liberalism was now becoming visible globally under the name of the "Anthropocene" and "climate change." The book's intention was not to found a new ontology of objects, nor to establish a new metaphysics of power, nor to adjudicate the possibility or impossibility of the human ability to know the truth of the world of things. Nor was geontopower offered as a new formation of power replacing biopolitics. Instead, it sought, in the spirit of Mbembe's approach to necropolitics, to demonstrate how geontopower has long been foundational to critical thought, the governance of difference, and the extractive machinery of capitalism and its markets. The attribution of the inability for various colonized people to differentiate the kinds of things that have the sort of agency, subjectivity, and intentionality that emerges with life has been the grounds for casting them into a premodern mentality and a postrecognition difference. In short, *Geontologies* meant to provide a fuller account of the shape of a set of critical discourses and figural images coming into view as the presuppositional nature of geontopower cracked.

With these intentions in mind, *Geontologies* introduced a set of figures that I claimed had always accompanied but now were assuming a greater discursive space from the four figures of biopower. The four figures of sexuality emerged, as Foucault noted, from "four great strategic unities which, beginning in the eighteenth century, formed specific mechanisms of knowledge and power centering on sex."[2] These strategic unities (a hysterization of women's bodies; a pedagogization of children's sex; a socialization of procreative behavior; and a psychiatrization of perverse pleasure) were the effects of a host of other permutations of power as Christiandom refigured the Greek uses of pleasure and a new science of life refigured confessionary sexuality. The "myriad of clashing forces" in successive forms of government from the Middle Ages to the eighteenth century refigured previous "great forms of power" that had "functioned as a principle of right that transcended all the heterogeneous claims."[3] The clash of forces, then, was not the clash of armies but currents that crossed mobile relations of power, operating among and slipping between the equilibriums and disequilibriums of any arrangement. This is what gave rise to new forms and arrangements that were only necessary retrospectively—the hysterical woman, the masturbating child, the Malthusian couple, and the perverse adult. These are the figures biopower diagrammed and made available for liberal concern. But lurking among them were other arrangements, forms, and figures; ghostly specters liberalism glimpsed at the corner of its eyes, appearing as feverous symptoms of some aspect of themselves they could not put their fingers on. Although *Geontologies* named three figures that geontopower makes us speak of, manage, fear, assault, and embrace—namely, the Desert, the Animist, and the Virus—the diverse terrains of late settler liberalism are populated by hosts of other actual and immanent others.

Rather than exits from geontopower, the Desert, the Animist, and the Virus were meant to be diagnostic and symptomatic of the ways in which those who have benefited from geontopower respond to its potential incapacitation. They weren't meant to refer to deserts, animists, or viruses in themselves, as forms of existence subject to geontopower, but rather as the reassertion of geontopower's governance over existence. It is because of this that I chose the figure of the Virus rather than the Terrorist, even as the Terrorist lies within the broad imaginary of the Virus. When thinking of the Virus as a figure of geontopower's loss of self-evident legitimacy, I tried to forestall the celebration of it as a radical exit from geontopower. As I noted, "to be the Virus is to be subject to intense abjection and attacks, and to live in the vicinity of the Virus is to dwell in an existential crisis." I also noted that capitalism is the epitome of the Virus, as well as the major producer of it.

II Covid-19 has made these cautions terrifyingly clear. The rhetorics of war, the replacement of discourses on citizenship with those of civilians, the reemergence of a militant white supremacy in the US and Europe, and the hardening of nationalisms that have attempted to block those demonstrating how colonizing capitalism *is* the Virus, have all facilitated the virus's spread and account for its differential impact on Indigenous, Black, and Brown people. The actual virus, then, has become a figure of geontology's failure to govern in such a way that the values of capital extraction flow primarily to the white North, while the toxicities produced along the way remain within the primarily Brown and Black global South. In other words, the relays between the figure of the Virus and the actual Covid-19 virus have become increasingly rapid and ever more important to disentangle.

Rhetoric and practices of war have accumulated around Covid-19. In New York, Governor Andrew Cuomo strained to come up with new metaphors of war, battle, and combat. "This is a war. We have to treat it as a war." Cuomo was hardly alone in his imaginary stance against Covid-19. Costanza Musu provided an overview of the international rhetorics of war that enveloped national responses to the circulation of the virus, from Queen Elizabeth II's evocation of the Second World War ("we will meet again") to UN Secretary-General António Guterres's claim that "This war needs a war-time plan to fight it."[4] Strongmen from Victor Orbán in Hungary and Rodrigo Duterte in the Philippines to Xi Jiping in China mobilized internal campaigns of political oppression under the guise of fighting the heroic battle against Covid. These rhetorics of war are also a feature of the figure of the Virus. In *Geontologies*, I noted that the central imaginary of the Desert was the *carbon imaginary* (the scarred homology between biological concepts such as metabolism and its key events of birth, growth-reproduction, and death, and philosophical concepts such as event, *conatus/ affectus*, and finitude), the central imaginary of the Animist is the *indigenous society* (in perfect balance with Nature), the central imaginary of the Virus is the *terrorist*. The *terrorist*, like the *carbon imaginary* and the *indigenous society*, is a spectral projection of geontopower. They are disavowals of their internal relationship to geontopower and abjections onto those who have suffered from it. The terrorist is a projection onto anticolonial and anticapitalist movements and a disavowal of the terror of the history of colonial capitalism present in the global form of late settler liberalism. In this discourse of disavowal, the Virus-as-terrorist lurks among us, unseen, camouflaged, taking advantage of the freedoms afforded by late liberal capitalism. Its viciousness is in equal proportions to its invisibility. It is the inverse of everything late liberal capitalism stands for.

Covid-19 is neither a friend nor enemy of late liberal capitalism or those who seek to live its refusal. It neither seeks to kill nor extend its dominion. Instead, radically agnostic to its form, Covid-19 is the result of capitalism's continuing colonization of the entirety of existence and extends throughout the infrastructures of late liberal markets and their defenses. We know this. We also know that Covid is only "a virus," the Covid-19 virus, in an abstract sense; that is, the geneticists' sense that there are Covid and variants of Covid, rather than a community of viruses who do not view each other as members of the same family. Should we conceptualize the virus that lived as an internal node of an entanglement of bats and their environs, Covid-19 is the residual of capital's colonization of that arrangement.[5] We cannot know what its future form in whatever new entanglement it expresses itself will be. What we do know is that its present operation—its new form of dwelling—is diagnosing the structures and contours of power of the ancestral presence of geontopower.

To see how the actual virus is diagnostic and symptomatic of geontopower, we need to understand how the figure of the Virus-as-Terrorist blocks this analytic. This is, after all, what the figures of biopolitics and geontopower do. They huddle just inside the door between the given arrangement of geontological governance and its otherwises, trying to block entrances and exits to anyone and anything that attempts to reshape its interiors and exteriors. Figures may be symptomatic of the crumbling of geontopower, but they are still diagrams of it. Instead of approaching the current pandemic within this geontological imaginary, we need to see it as yet another form of toxicity that colonialism has seeded.

Toxicity technically refers to those substances that are biologically noxious or poisonous—those things that have the capacity to disrupt biological function. But the relationship between toxic and nontoxic things is not a line so much as a degree. All substances have within them the capacity to become toxic; all substances can move from medicine to poison, hero to scapegoat.[6] Even the purest of waters can be toxic to humans if taken in sufficiently large doses. Thus, medical discussions of toxicity typically emphasize the means by which toxins enter the body and the amount a body can process safely before becoming overwhelmed. Climatic overheating, while technically external to the body, can disrupt internal biological functions as profoundly as any toxin. High temperatures don't literally boil the blood, but they put cardiac functions under serious stress even in the healthiest individual. They raise the level of ozone and other pollutants (such as pollen and other aeroallergens) which can dramatically affect pre-existing cardiovascular and respiratory diseases. In this way, the heat index of rising temperatures and humidity is part of a more general expansion of uninhabitable zones. What surprise, then, that the advice of certain policy experts for mitigating the effects of climate change sounds eerily like older advice for interacting with chemical toxins, not to mention Covid-19: don't let them in (seal yourself off with air-conditioning and air purifiers) or remove yourself from contaminated areas (join the great climate migration).[7]

We might also see viruses and their differential effects as traces of capitalism's extractive exhaustion of any form of existence it encounters. In this sense, toxicity refers not merely to the overwhelming and exhausting of the body's immune system—which can cause more damage than the virus itself—but the exhaustion of the human and more-than-human world. An exhaustion of the violent extraction of labor as a life force from enslaved men and women in the Caribbean that powered the emergence of liberal capitalism, as well as the extraction of minerals from soils, which the anticolonial writer and activist Amílcar Cabral understood as a fundamental aspect of Portuguese colonial enrichment.[8] Toxicity as a form of extractive exhaustion is a material sedimentation. Covid-19's devastation of poor, Indigenous, Black, and Brown communities is a horrifying analytic of this historical toxic sedimentation.

Certainly, Covid-19 is not our friend. But it is not our enemy either. Covid-19 is a manifestation of the ancestral catastrophes of colonialism and slavery. It is a manifestation of the continual destruction and dispossession of existence by the massive extraction and recombination machine of late liberal capitalism. In other words, structural racism and colonialism and their devastating effects on the health of Black and Indigenous bodies and their environments existed long before Covid-19. The catastrophe of climate collapse, toxic exposure, and viral pandemics are not *à venir*. These are the ancestral catastrophes that began with the brutal dispossession of human and more-than-human worlds and a vicious extraction of human and more-than-human labor. These dispossessions and extractions birthed liberalism and capitalism, and alongside them, a massive machinery that disavowed their structural violence. The rhetorics of war and the figure of the Virus-as-Terrorist directs attention away from late liberal capitalism as the quintessential Virus, the quintessential Terrorist, the source of this horror we are experiencing. We are told, instead, to view the virus within the framework of what I called in *Empire of Love* "ghoul health," namely, the global organization of the biomedical establishment and its imaginary around the idea of the big scary bug, the new plague. Ghoul health is, in other words, the prefigure of the concept of the Virus. It is the bad faith of geontopower in which the real threat is not the virus but the contemporary global division, distribution, and circulation of health. It is the bad faith that we are living unevenly.

1. Elizabeth A. Povinelli, "Do Rocks Listen? The Cultural Politics of Apprehending Australian Aboriginal Labor," *American Anthropologist* 97, no. 3 (September 1995): 505–518.
2. Michel Foucault, *The History of Sexuality*, vol. 1, trans. R. Hurley (New York: Pantheon, 1978), 103.
3. Foucault, *The History of Sexuality*, 87.
4. Constanza Musu, "War Metaphors Used for COVID-19 Are Compelling but Also Dangerous," *The Conversation*, April 8, 2020, https://theconversation.com/war-metaphors-used-for-covid-19-are-compelling-but-also-dangerous-135406.
5. Maciej F. Boni, Philippe Lemey, Xiaowei Jiang, et al., "Evolutionary Origins of the SARS-CoV-2 Sarbecovirus Lineage Responsible for the COVID-19 Pandemic," *Nature Microbiology* 5 (2020): 1408–1417.
6. Jacques Derrida, "Plato's Pharmacy," in *Dissemination*, trans. Barbara Johnson (Chicago: University of Chicago Press, 1981), 63–171.
7. As Andrea Bagnato notes, with "the establishment of new networks of free circulation" and "permanent urban spaces" also came "unwelcome matter like viruses and bacteria," revealing "the misguided nature of Western aspirations to bring order and civilization to the rest of the world." Bagnato, "Microscopic Colonialism," e-Flux Architecture, December 2017, https://www.e-flux.com/architecture/positions/153900/microscopic-colonialism/.
8. Filipa César, "Meteorisations: Reading Amílcar Cabral's Agronomy of Liberation," *Third Text* 32 (2018): 254–272.

An earlier version of this essay was originally published by e-flux Architecture in 2020.

NUCLEAR HOMES AND IRRADIATED LANDSCAPES

MAXWELL SMITH-HOLMES

On October 1, 1998, subcontractors with the US Department of Energy set up a "situation room" in downtown Richland, Washington, to monitor a mysterious breach at the Hanford Nuclear Reserve.[1] The incident began when health monitors recorded a bizarre spattering of the radioactive isotope strontium-90 in a mobile office trailer. Geiger counts shot up near a light switch, a piece of silverware, and a cutting board. Further investigation turned up "specks" of radiation darting through the air. Then, contamination seeped beyond the trailer: first in spat-out chewing tobacco, then on a worker's dirty laundry, and eventually inside homes and garbage bins up to eighty miles from the nuclear facility. Three weeks later, officials determined that toxic material had spread after fruit flies laid eggs in concrete vats of nuclear waste. When the eggs hatched, swarms of irradiated flies found their way into the food and clothing of plant personnel, who then carried traces of radiation back home.[2]

Radioactive isotopes leaked out of the plutonium plant's policed borders and segregated waste management systems through the bodies of entomological hosts that flew over fences, burrowed in garbage, and nested in human homes. The public-private cleanup effort that followed the incident deployed insecticide "spot treatments" at contaminated sites throughout the region, installed a tent-like physical barrier around waste pits where flies might have laid their eggs, and enclosed the nuclear complex within a "2.5 hectare (6.2-acre) radiological buffer area (RBA)."[3] The contamination was considered neutralized only after 106 workers' urine and feces tested negative for bioaccumulated radiation and 210 tons of garbage were moved from the municipal dump to "low-level burial grounds" at the nuclear compound.[4]

The official response to the spread of radioisotopes throughout the Columbia River Basin emphasized the breakdown of a supposedly healthy distribution of chemicals across a regional topography of militarized borders. Substances containing unstable nuclei became toxic only once they leached into adjacent spaces and spilled over thresholds.[5] In internal communications between management and workers at the nuclear facility, toxic exposure was cast as a product of the nuclear facility's physical borders rather than a threat to human or ecological health. In an October 12 memo titled "CONTAMINATION SPREAD QUESTIONS AND ANSWERS," management attempted to allay workers' concerns by explaining that "contamination outside of a control zone is of concern because it isn't supposed to happen ... any contamination outside of controlled radiation areas is unacceptable."[6] Workers were advised that direct contact with strontium-90 at levels present in the fruit flies amounts to the same level of radiation as a dental X-ray. To stay safe, one

→ Robert Del Tredici, *Madonna of the Glove Box*, 1993.

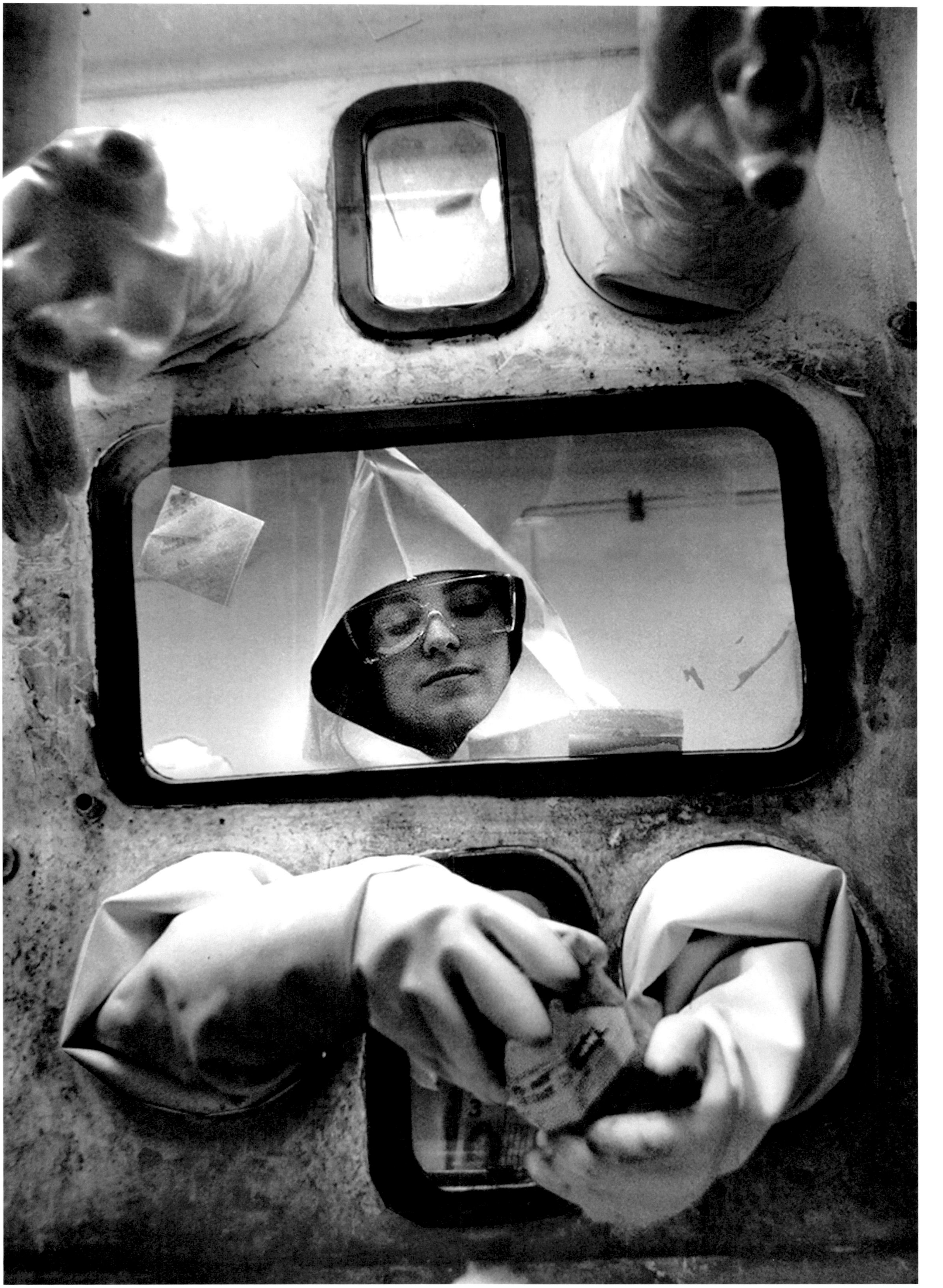

only needed to "carry their food in closed containers," and "not leave fruit, cookies, or other unwrapped food out in bowls or on tables."[7]

The toxic artifacts left behind by the twentieth-century nuclear industry exhibit a grim epistemological and spatial indeterminacy that static architectural forms simply cannot contain.[8] For government contractors, the flies themselves were less alarming than the way they breached the border between contaminated and uncontaminated zones. The lasting impacts of nuclear production highlight how toxicity has selectively concentrated injury on vulnerable landscapes and their inhabitants. Some of the most infamous episodes of toxic architecture occurred at the "Nuclear Reservations" established by the Manhattan Engineering District (MED), commonly known as the Manhattan Project, the top-secret World War II program to rapidly develop an atomic bomb for the United States. At these sites, architecture became imbricated with toxic containment through four distinct scales: the factory, the town, the home, and finally, the human body.

Occupation In 1942, General Leslie R. Groves was put in charge of building out the Manhattan Project after having successfully managed the design and construction of the Pentagon building.[9] Groves's highest concern was "security," by which he meant rigorously controlling knowledge about the bomb-making program. In a particularly illuminating instance, Groves rejected his predecessor's name for the MED, the "Department of Substitute Metals," because he worried it stood out among the US Army Corps of Engineers' (USACE) various departments and "would arouse the curiosity of all who heard it." Instead, Groves opted for the misleading geographic designation, "Manhattan Engineering District," which sounded just like any other of the Corps's engineering districts.[10] Even before the government recognized that toxicity might ooze past the militarized borders of the Manhattan Engineering District, Groves instituted discursive formations that sought to contain nuclear chemicals, controlling information rather than contaminated matter.

At the center of these efforts were the three "nuclear reservations" established within the United States for manufacturing atomic bombs, including the two ultimately dropped on Hiroshima and Nagasaki: Los Alamos, New Mexico; Oak Ridge, Tennessee; and Hanford, Washington. In constructing these reservations, wartime secrecy dictated that the USACE evict existing residents and build new cities for MED employees. The Hanford site is currently the most contaminated place in the United States, "laced with more than 450 billion gallons of liquid nuclear waste." According to the geographer Shannon Cram, "Under the direction of the US Department of Energy (DOE), Hanford is currently engaged in the largest and most expensive environmental remediation project in human history."[11]

Hanford, which began operating in the autumn of 1944, was chosen as a plutonium production facility because Army Corps generals and DuPont de Nemours & Company, the private firm contracted to operate the plant, viewed the area as a preexisting "waste land" with access to abundant hydroelectric power. Contrary to one general's contention that Hanford was "an area with almost no people, very

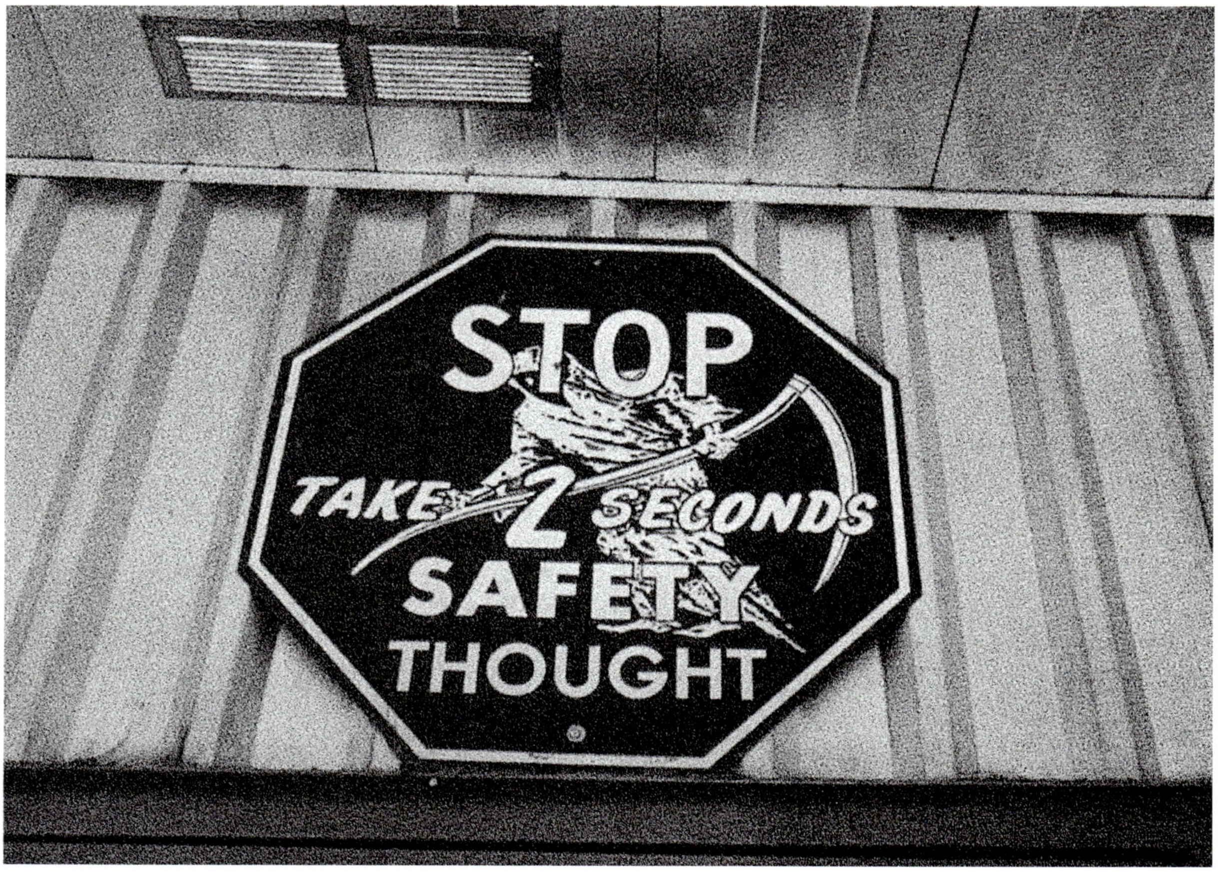

↙ Robert Del Tredici, *Safety sign at the Hanford Nuclear Reservation*, 1993.

→ Johnny Buck (left) and Frank Matthias (right) in Priest Valley, 1943.

↘ Hanford Map, 1943.

↓ Map of the US showing key Manhattan Project sites.

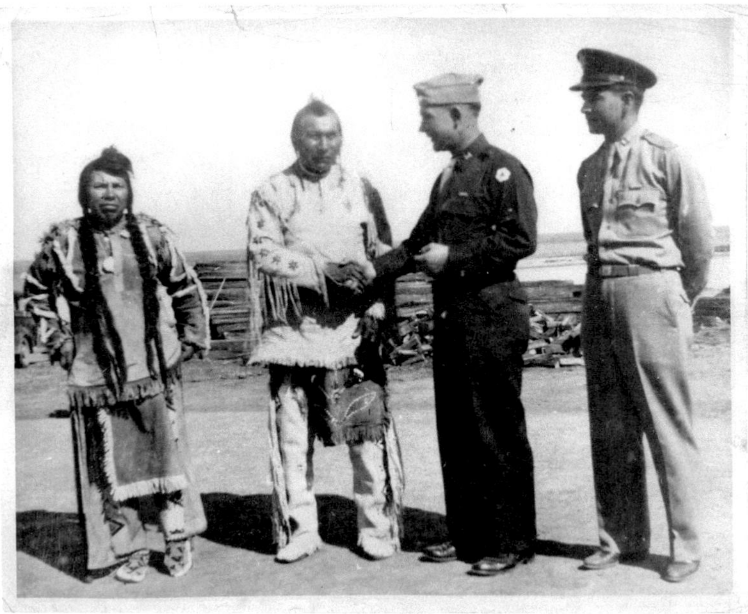

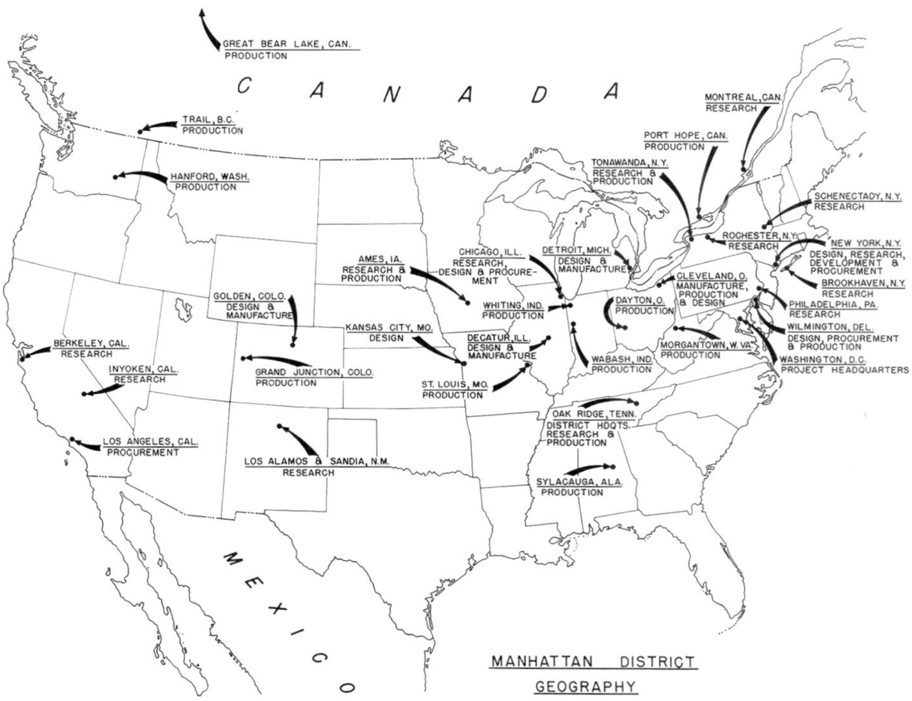

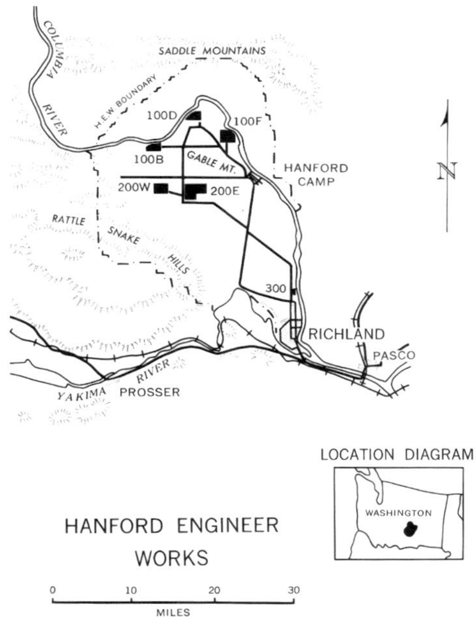

undeveloped," the Indigenous Yakama, Nez Perce, Umatilla, and Wanapum communities lived or frequently traveled within the 586 square miles of the site.[12] And in 1903, in order to provide irrigation to an influx of settler farmers in the Columbia Basin, the Hanford Power and Irrigation Company established and operated a town later advertised as a curative landscape for individuals suffering from poor health.[13]

A photograph from 1944 shows the Wanapum leader Johnny Buck shaking hands with Frank Matthias, the Army Corps general who oversaw the day-to-day construction of the Hanford site. Their comportments point toward the exclusionary logics of military-industrial containment cutting across the landscape just beyond the photograph's frame. On the left, Buck and his associate stare straight at the camera wearing traditional clothing, while on the right, Matthias and his lieutenant stand in profile, in crisp army uniforms. The photograph was taken to commemorate the general's supposed generosity in allowing the Wanapum to continue fishing in the Columbia River after the area had been fenced off from the public to promote secrecy. The glares of the Wanapum men suggest that the Army Corp's presence at Hanford was far from consensual. After the bomb fell on Nagasaki in 1945, the government revoked the Wanapam's right to fish in the Columbia, statedly for reasons of national security.[14]

Factory Groves wanted to replicate the Pentagon's fortress-like layout at Hanford. The Pentagon *parti* involved a disorienting facade to obscure the building's internal organization, which itself comprised a repeating series of enclosures laid out like a bullseye. At Hanford, the nuclear reservation was similarly designed, with the most secretive plutonium production installations located in the center of a 200-square-mile cordoned-off "sanctum" known as the "100 Area." Beyond this guarded core, the reservation included a 700-square-mile zone containing slightly less sensitive production installations, the "200 Area" and "300 Area." Ten miles from these plutonium factories were accommodations for workers and their families as well as a new shopping district. The distribution of different types of workplaces and homes at great distances from one another was integral to an ultimately failed attempt to ensure that, in Groves's words, "accidents in any one area should not affect the operation of the remaining units."[15]

The original USACE plan called for three river-cooled nuclear reactors in the 100 Area, a pair of chemical separation plants in the 200 Area, and a fuel fabrication facility in the 300 Area. The production line started at the southeast corner of the central manufacturing sector in the 300 Area, where uranium mined from the Shinkolobwe Mine in Belgian Congo was processed into fuel rods.[16] These rods were then transported to the 100 Area, where engineers used nuclear reactors to induce fission, transforming uranium rods into plutonium slugs. After cooling in a pool that drained toxified runoff into the Columbia River, the plutonium slugs were brought to the 200 Area, where the material was concentrated and eventually shipped to Los Alamos, New Mexico, for assembly.[17]

Maintaining a tight grip on the flow of information went together with increasing efficiency on the production line. When entry-level technical employees started at Hanford, they were informed of their tasks but not told why or how their work meshed with other production processes. Details about associated health risks were also omitted. Workers were required to keep their jobs secret from one another, sharing only the minimum information required to maintain productivity quotas. And wherever feasible, physical enclosures separated workers by task, compartmentalizing the distinct functions of the assembly line.[18]

Within each subfacility and across the entire campus, architecture coincided with a gradient of risk that exposed women and less educated workers to higher levels of radiation. DuPont initially refused to hire female plant operators because of concerns about the effects of radiation on childbearing, tacitly acknowledging the plant's dangers.[19] Labor shortages in 1944, however, led DuPont to begin hiring women to work in the 300 Area producing uranium slugs, where they were advised not to wear protective gloves so as not to hinder fast hand movement. Former 300 Area workers commonly suffer illnesses related to uranium exposure including cancer, heart disease, and numerous mysterious undiagnosable ailments.[20]

Town Between 1943 and 1945, Hanford required between 94,000 and 132,000 construction workers, many more than the local population was able to supply.[21] Masses of itinerant workers were recruited from around the country and housed in Camp Hanford, a temporary settlement limited to unmarried men located six miles from the construction site at a railroad junction in a preexisting settlement of 125 people.[22] To maintain secrecy, the camp was subdivided into gated zones, with workers only permitted access to their assigned section.[23] The camp's spatial division was complemented by its internal security force, which regularly interviewed inhabitants to screen for communist sympathies or potential espionage.[24] Only in 1944, and under pressure from the Fair Employment Practices Commission, did DuPont begin hiring Black construction workers, who were housed inside a separate fenced division that contained smaller barracks and fewer amenities than white workers' residential districts.[25]

Camp Hanford was a hotbed for depression, alcoholism, and violence. The settlement quickly became a toxic workplace, not only in the sense of occupational health hazards, but also by eroding the everyday well-being of its employees.[26] Meanwhile, DuPont sought an entirely different situation in its design for a town, Richland Village, which was to house mostly permanent technicians and their families.[27] DuPont was familiar with operating company towns, and its executives viewed the Hanford contract as an opportunity to build a model settlement that would promote the company's conservative ideology.[28] To design the town, military generals and DuPont executives selected the lowest-bidding local architect, G. Albin Pehrson, whose proposal synthesized the military's spartan vision with DuPont's middle-class tastes. Design proceeded rapidly, and by the spring of 1945, the Manhattan Project had rebuilt the "little rural hamlet of Richland" into a "bustling industrial community."[29]

Pehrson researched the area to determine its necessary facilities, devising precise figures for the appropriate number of hair salons, funeral parlors, restaurants, hardware stores, and other suburban necessities. In his writings, Pehrson accommodated the military mission to his own democratic ideals:

> High morale cannot be achieved by crowding skilled and veteran workers into inadequate dwellings. Neither can it be predicated upon salary, position or caste distinction. No village

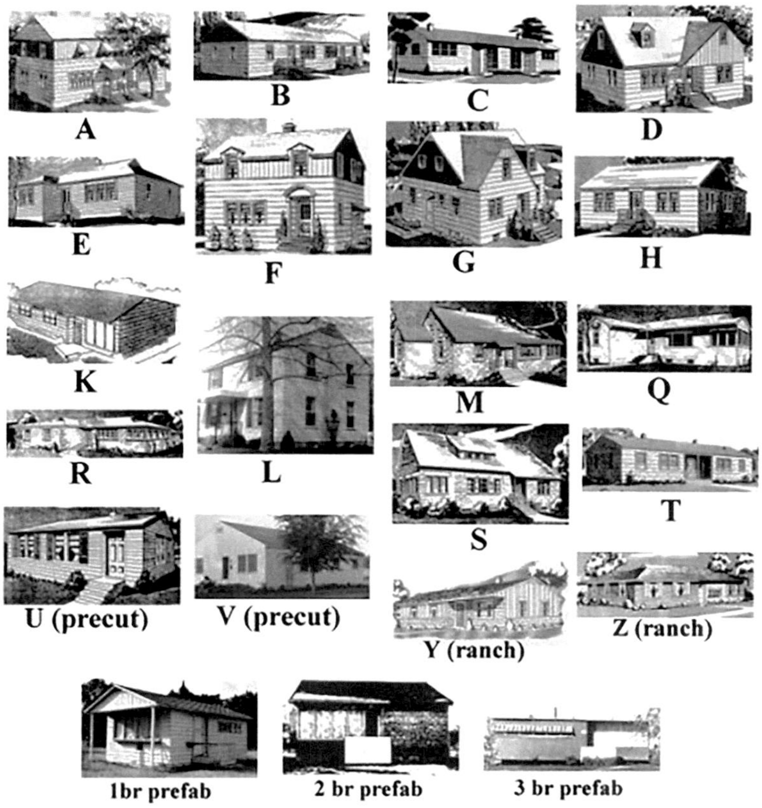

← G. Albin Pehrson, Alphabet Houses, 1943.

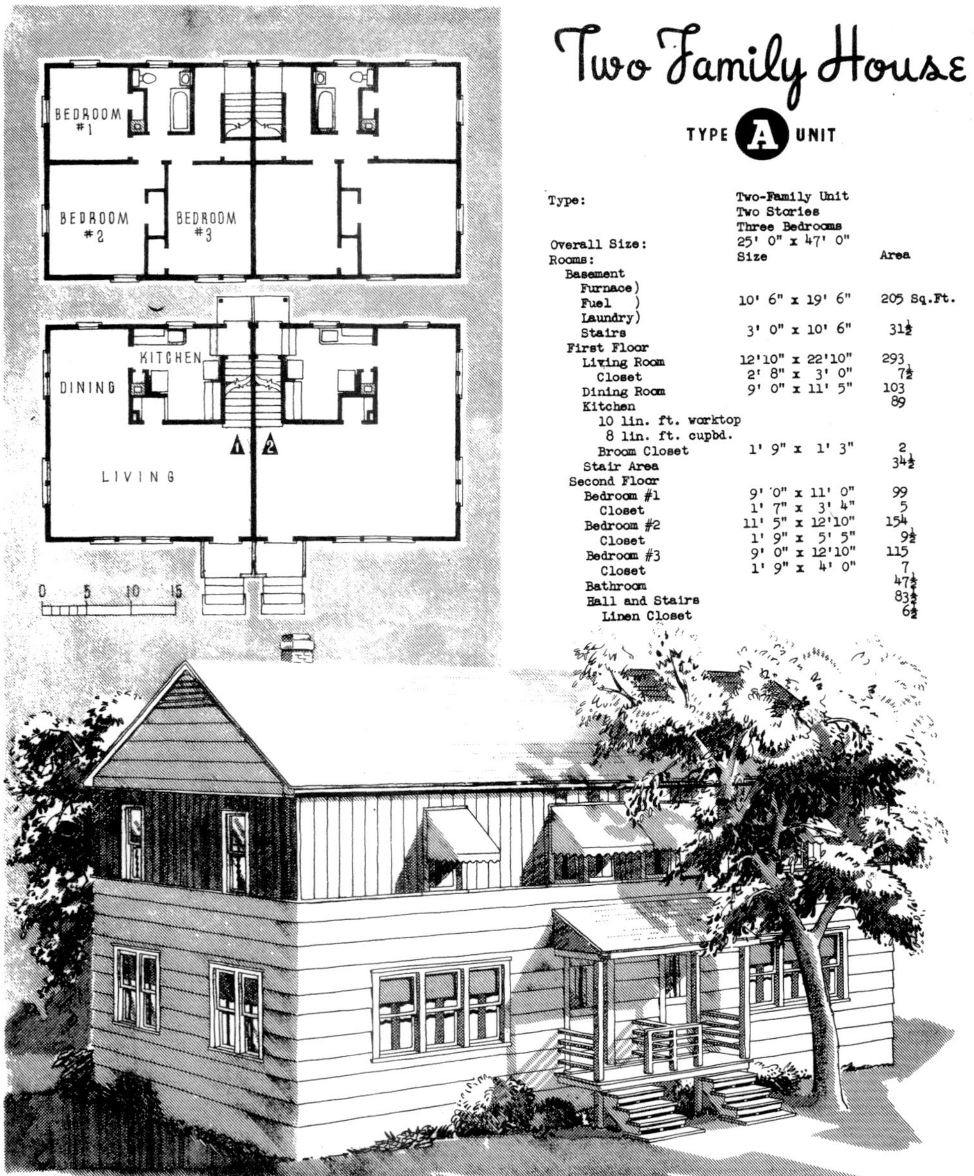

Two Family House

TYPE A UNIT

Type:	Two-Family Unit Two Stories Three Bedrooms	
Overall Size:	25' 0" x 47' 0"	
Rooms:	Size	Area
Basement		
Furnace) Fuel) Laundry)	10' 6" x 19' 6"	205 Sq.Ft.
Stairs	3' 0" x 10' 6"	31½
First Floor		
Living Room	12'10" x 22'10"	293
Closet	2' 8" x 3' 0"	7½
Dining Room	9' 0" x 11' 5"	103
Kitchen		89
10 lin. ft. worktop		
8 lin. ft. cupbd.		
Broom Closet	1' 9" x 1' 3"	2
Stair Area		34½
Second Floor		
Bedroom #1	9' 0" x 11' 0"	99
Closet	1' 7" x 3' 4"	5
Bedroom #2	11' 5" x 12'10"	154
Closet	1' 9" x 5' 5"	9½
Bedroom #3	9' 0" x 12'10"	115
Closet	1' 9" x 4' 0"	7
Bathroom		47½
Hall and Stairs		83½
Linen Closet		6½

↓ G. GAlbin Pehrson, Type A Unit, 1943.

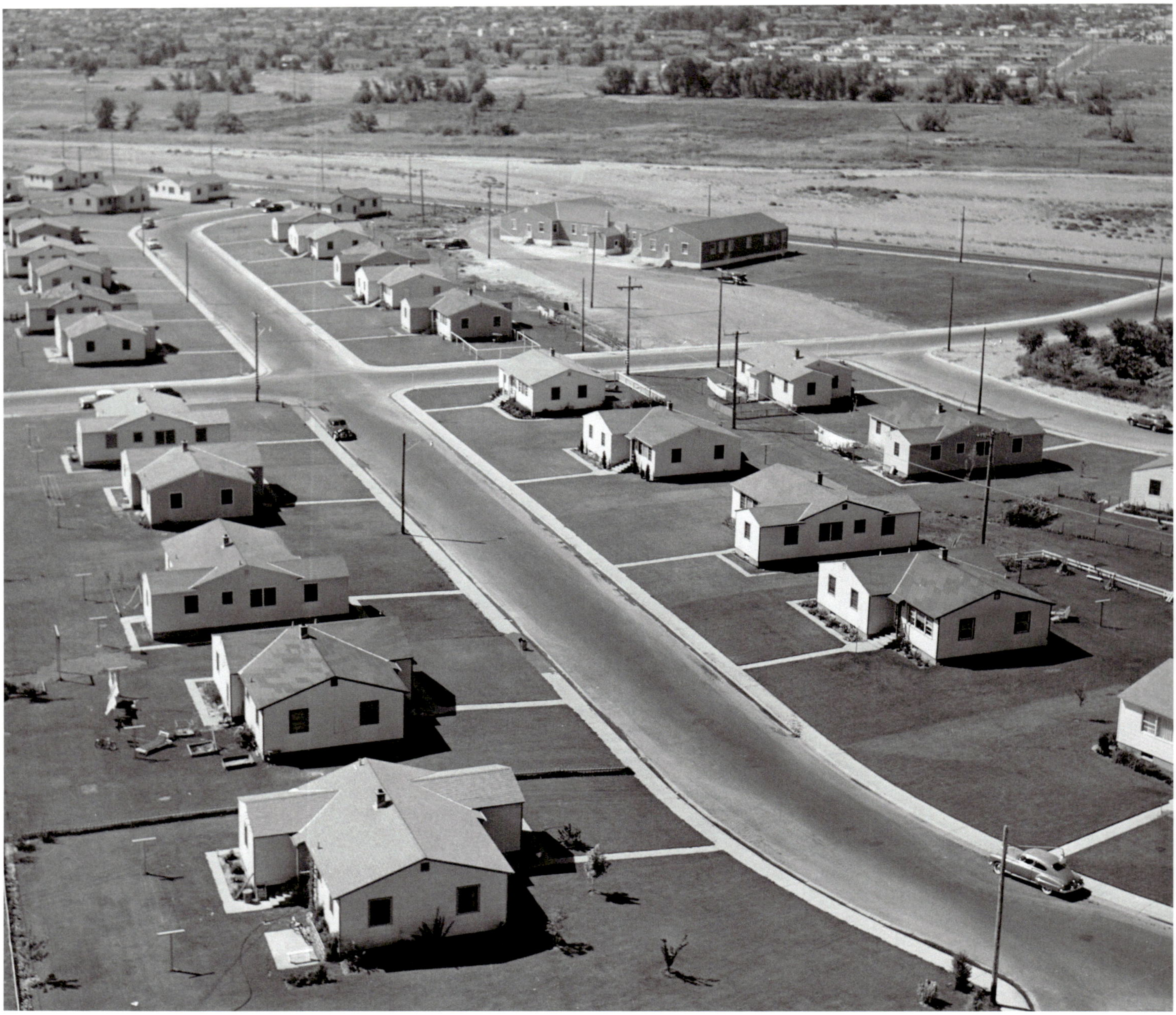

can eliminate such distinctions entirely, for it is the American tradition to aspire ... and where [the top] men locate will undoubtedly be considered favorable territory; but in so far as the planners could arrange these matters, all types of houses [were] scattered throughout the project.[30]

Pehrson designed homes for the highest-ranking officials along bluffs overlooking the winding Columbia River while smaller, less materially and functionally intricate homes for lower-ranked workers were arranged throughout tidy neighborhoods. The village's downtown was designed as a shopping loop intersected by streets that led to housing clusters. Pehrson's plan included bus routes to transport residents between the village, the downtown, and Hanford's workplaces.[31]

House The housing stock comprised a limited series of types that all mediated wartime austerity with suburban comfort. The most elaborate homes, reserved for top brass military families or DuPont managers, were styled after familiar forms of American domestic architecture. The small two-bedroom B duplex resembled a ranch house, and the D unit was modeled on a Cape Cod.[32] Less distinct homes such as A, H, and L might be seen as permutations on the same rectangular plan. The array of letter home plans aligned with Pehrson's philosophy that architecture should reflect class distinctions as an incentive for social mobility.

In Richland Village, the commodiousness of dwellings corresponded with families' performance of the virtues of hard work, citizenship, and family. Yet, in terms of day-to-day life for the inhabitants, military-industrial efficiency ended up impinging on domestic comfort. Limited housing types allowed the military to rapidly deploy domestic space and facilitate the wartime bomb effort, but such economy resulted in visual monotony, poor material specifications, and unreliable shelter from the elements. Officially, Richland Village's homes and other installations were never intended as permanent constructions. Many of the structures were prefabricated units trucked into place. However, DuPont's executives always intended to keep Hanford running after the war.[33] This veil of impermanence allowed DuPont and the US Government flexibility as the risks of environmental contamination slowly came into public view.

Human In 1942, the MED incorporated a new Medical Section led by a doctor from the Eastman company in Rochester who understood industrial medicine as a tool for improving bottom lines. Reporting to military generals, the Medical Section helped mitigate security leaks and negative press coverage by monitoring the health of workers and their communities, as well as the quality of the environment around MED facilities.[34] It made good on both the military's need for secrecy and DuPont's drive for efficiency by narrowly defining illness by its most severe and immediately onset cases. This "medico-legal" criteria for workplace injury failed to account for the slow violence of toxic waste, let alone the durational buildup of radioactive isotopes inside human bodies that manifest random, unpredictable symptoms.[35] By only acknowledging the very worst and imminently diagnosable cases of radiation poisoning, the Medical Section effectively transposed the plutonium plant's walls of secrecy onto the body.

Beginning in 1944, workers at Hanford were required to wear employee identification badges that doubled as personal radiation dosimeters. Each badge displayed an employee's photograph, their security credentials, and payroll number on a printed card above a ten-layer-thick stack of radiation-sensitive film, all encased in a clip-on plastic box. Once a week, the badges' film sheets were submitted to the Medical Section and "developed" to measure workers' individual levels of exposure against a rubric of permissible risk.[36]

Just as architectural modernism looked to an ideal human figure for a system of social organization, the nuclear age sought its own universal human as a model for life on a toxic planet.[37] Once nuclear physicists turned their attention from making an atomic bomb to addressing the lasting impacts of its production and detonation, new models of the human body were created as baselines for a range of policies intended to regulate the effects of long-term radiation exposure. In 1949, the International Commission on Radiation Protection developed the "Reference Man" based on statistical anatomy that

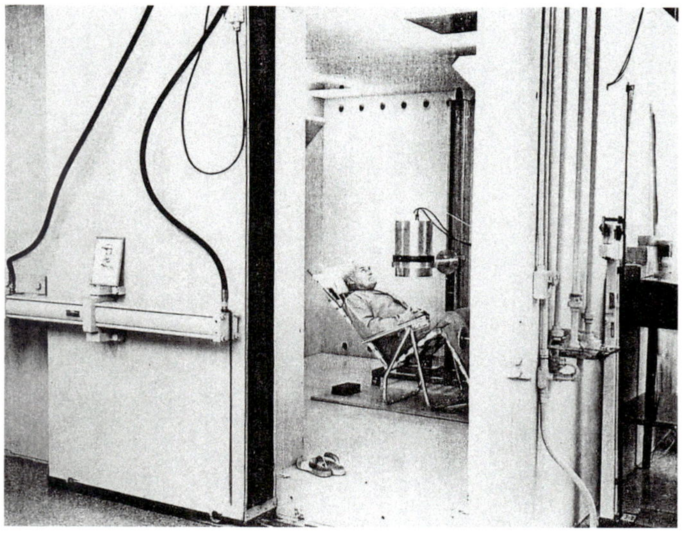

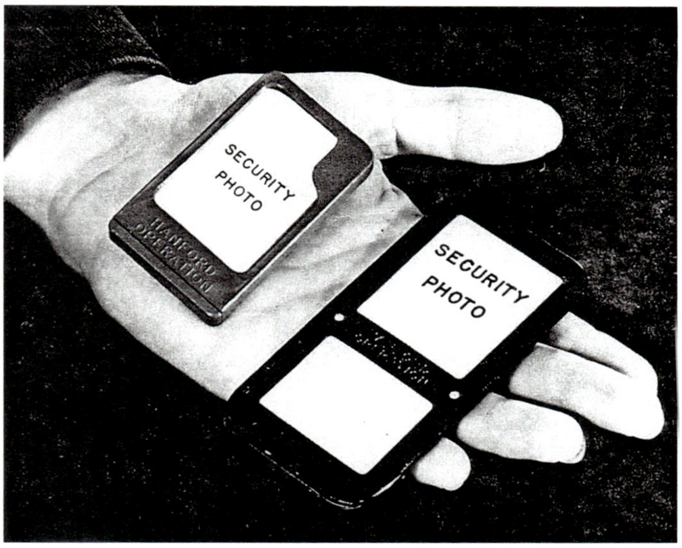

↑ Body dosimeter used at Hanford.

↓ Two models of the radio-sensitive Hanford security badge and a diagram of their assembly.

← Richland Village Alphabet Houses. On this street, M, Q, and R type houses, two, three, or four-bedroom houses with full basements and oil heat.

← Food pathways for intake of radionuclides.

↙ The "adult male" phantom and "representation of a human torso used to model radiation doses."

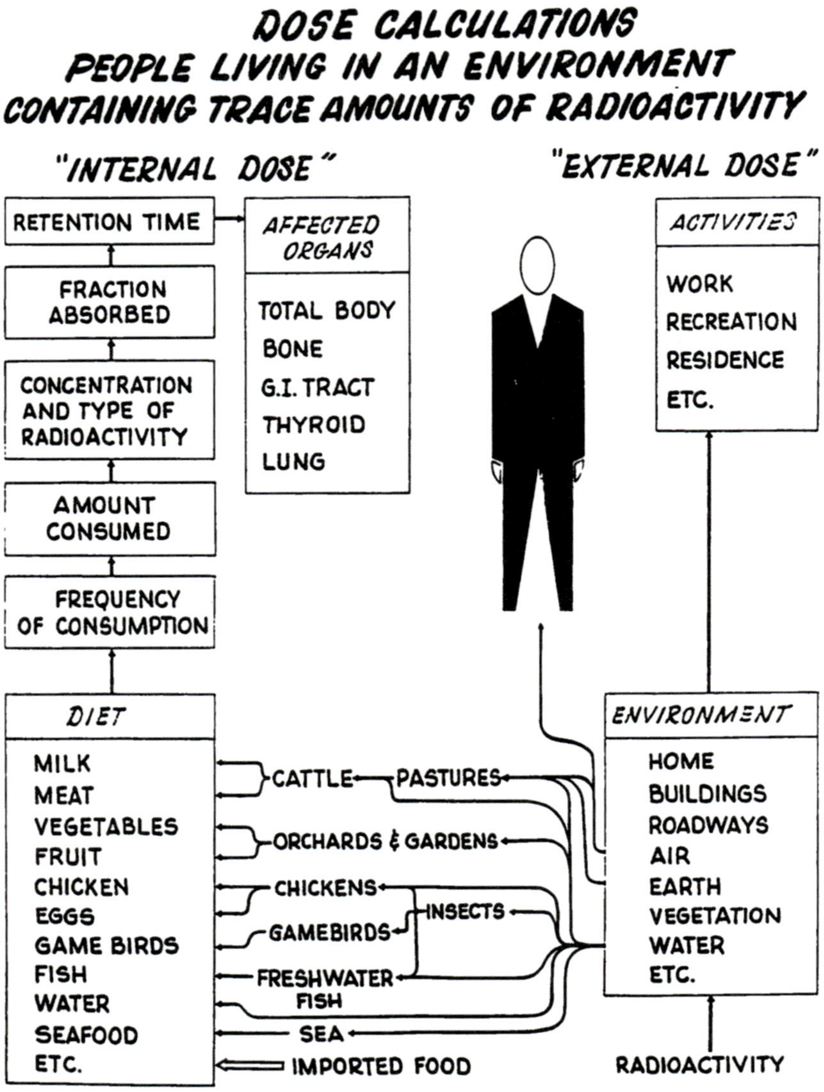

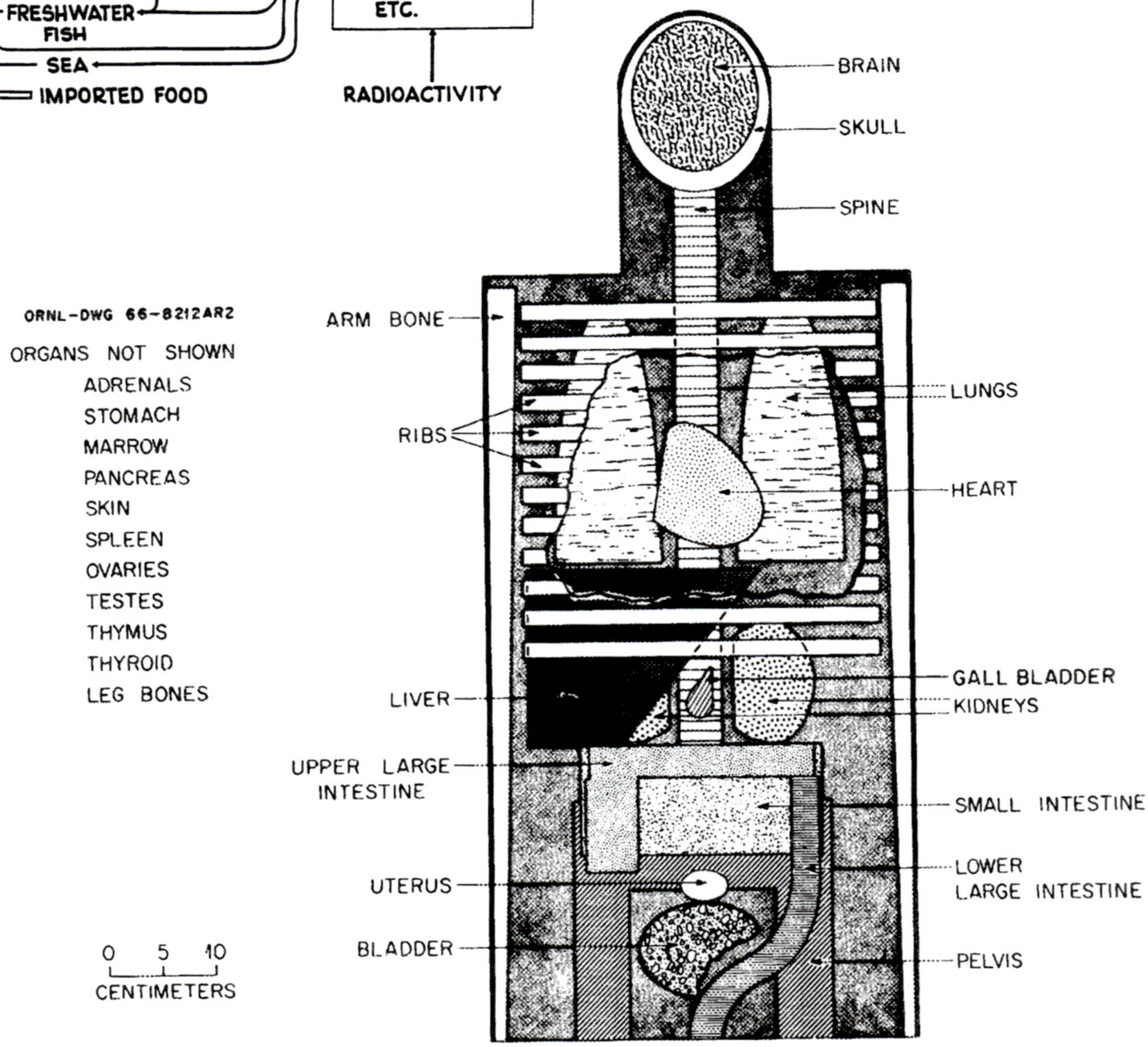

accounted for the kinds and quantities of food people eat, their bodily excretions, how they exercise, and the volume of air they breathe, among other biological factors.[38]

Reference Man's narrow model of humanness rehearses the separation of Indigenous communities from their ancestral land initially enacted by the Hanford nuclear reservation, and the Yakama Nation, Nez Perce Tribe, and the Confederated Tribes of Umatilla Indian Reservation (CTUIR) have rejected their assimilation into these statistical frameworks. In 2008, the CTUIR's Department of Science and Engineering proposed an alternative set of physiological benchmarks informed by the tribes' lived experiences. In response, the US Department of Energy and EPA claimed that legislating Hanford's remediation based on Native American bodies and cultures would be biologically "impossible."[39]

Exposure

Hanford's various techniques to mediate contamination broke down in early December 1949 when the Air Force and Hanford health physicists purposefully released one ton of radioactive "green fuel" into the skies above the surrounding Columbia Basin. The operation was designed to test a new type of nuclear surveillance by measuring concentrations of fission products in the atmosphere. Without warning, communities up to 200 miles away were exposed to radioactive iodine-131.[40] Toxic particulates ended up in the air, waterways, and soil, and in the tissue of plants and animals, where it eventually bioaccumulated, ricocheting through ecosystems. Concentrations of radioactive iodine-131 have been known to cause virulent thyroid cancer, one of the illnesses most prevalent near Hanford today.[41] Because of the extreme timeframe required for radionuclides to decay into less harmful substances, the toxic effects of the green fuel experiment will be felt for millennia.

The "green fuel" incident exemplifies how, after the war, the threats confronting Hanford shifted from an enemy combatant to an irradiated environment. In this way, the Manhattan Project's techniques of spatial control were reinvented as stopgap measures against the more abstract dangers of poisonous ground, water, and food.[42] As if following Vitruvius's suggestion to dissect the livers of animals living around potential building sites to check for any threats to biological life lurking in nonhuman nature, government health technicians regularly shot coyotes, "highly territorial creatures," and examined their thyroids as a rough measure of the concentrations of radioisotopes coursing through the region's ecosystems.[43]

Remediation

Remediation is a mode of containment that casts landscape as both cure and disease. It presumes a landscape that is too polluted and dangerous for human habitation, but that can be cured—through more wilderness, more vegetation, more ecological activity. In 2000, President Bill Clinton created the Hanford Reach Monument as a national wildlife refuge, legally barring humans from ever again inhabiting the site. Paradoxically, this also means that a higher level of contamination is allowed there because it excludes human life.[44]

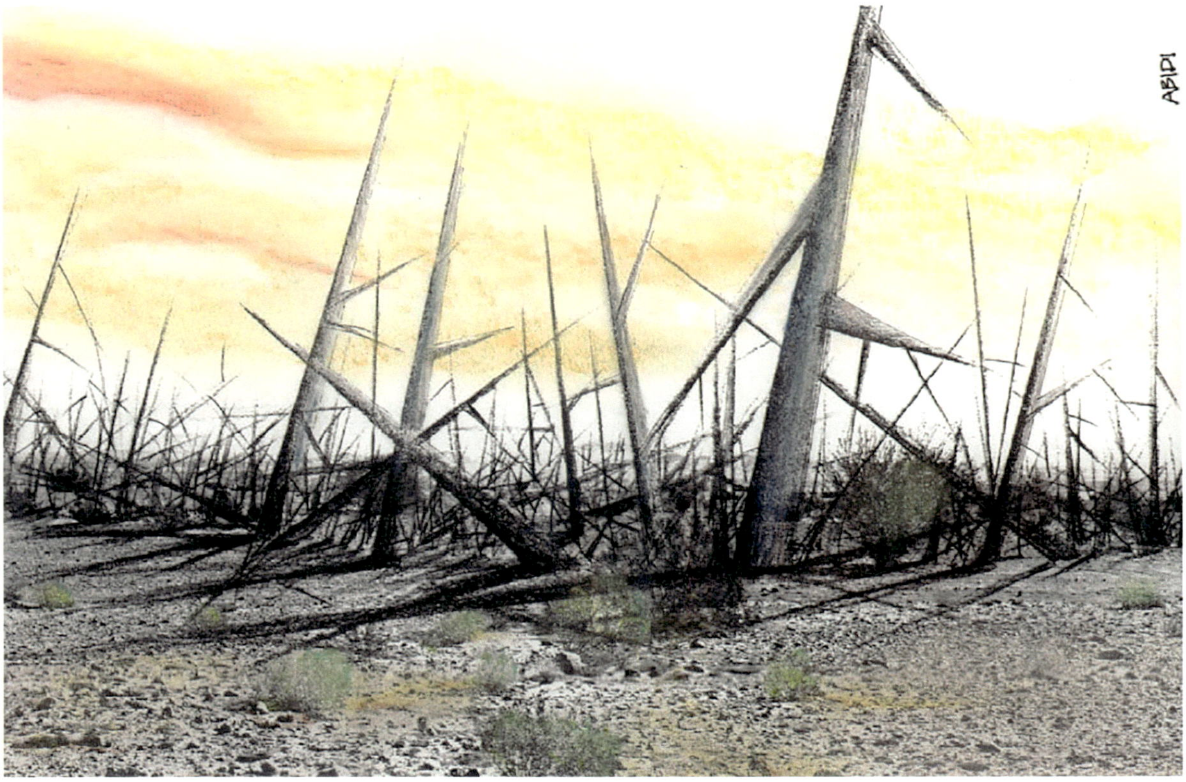

↑ Michael Brill and Safdar Abidi, *Landscape of Thorns*, 1992.

Hanford has been depopulated through its designation as a wildlife refuge, but its remediation must continue for a timeframe outlasting any reliable predictions of the future. Thus, environmental remediation at Hanford not only involves concrete-lined "burial sites" and the use of plants to leach radionuclides out of the ground, but also a variety of techniques for projecting the ethos of toxic containment into an inconceivably vast temporal horizon. Hanford's remediation bends space and time to entwine the radioactive past, the ecological present, and an unwieldy multimillennial future.[45]

Beginning in the 1980s, the US Government has conducted research in the field of nuclear semiotics to develop means of warning future humans about the dangers of toxic environments. Because future societies may have lost touch with language and history, these warning markers attempt to communicate prelinguistically to an imagined humanoid species with only elemental cognitive capacities. For example, a proposal by architects Safdar Abidi and Michael Brill cited within a US Department of Energy report for a field of spikes atop buried nuclear waste is premised on the idea that such a disturbing landscape would forebode danger to any sentient creature. Another proposal for a system of nuclear semiotics published by the Sandia National Laboratory in 1996 illustrates multiple permutations on the spike field, including a version in which spikes mark each of the world's radioactive burial sites by puncturing through a giant map of the earth.[46]

A 1984 report on a future warning system for the Hanford site imagines a perimeter of obelisks indicating the locations of buried waste and the hazards of eating vegetation growing on site. In the sequence of inscriptions, radiation trefoils resemble apples plucked from the Garden of Eden. By the final panel, one of three human figures has collapsed while two remain standing, indicating a probability (rather than guarantee) of serious injury.

At Hanford, spatial and discursive techniques of toxic containment interweave multiple scales and histories of twentieth-century nuclear production. By cleaving injurious matter from healthy bodies, nuclear and postnuclear forms of risk mitigation distribute the normative limits of the human subject in relation to a toxic planet. Operating at the scale of the landscape, the town, the workplace, the home, and the body itself, toxic containment has unequally shaped the conditions of life based on entrenched colonialist stratifications. At Hanford, landscape and architecture are both cure and symptom; they are the sources of ecological and human fragility as well as the promise of a new life on a toxic planet.

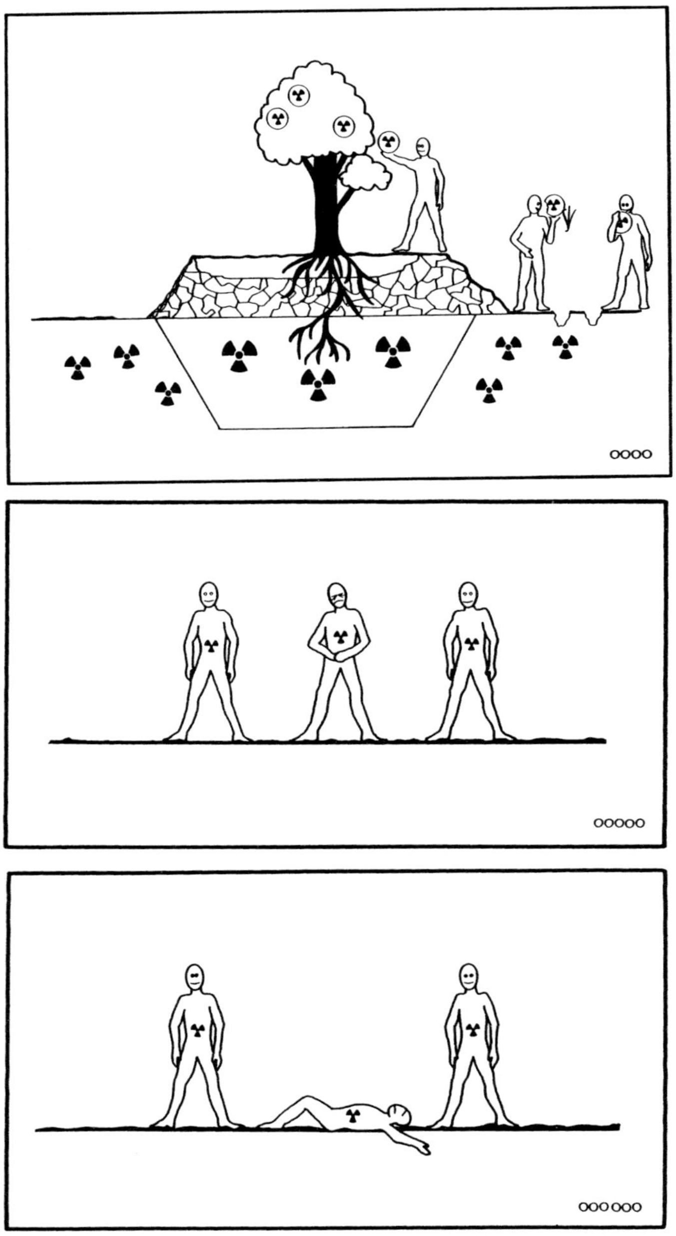

↑ Fourth, fifth, and sixth panel inscriptions on proposed buried waste surface markers.

An earlier version of this essay was originally published by e-flux Architecture in 2022.

1. D. J. Connell, "Fall 1998 200 East Area Biological Vector Contamination Report," Fluor Daniel Hanford, Inc., Richland, WA, March 17, 1999, F-5, https://doi.org/10.2172/781591.
2. This incident is documented in detail in "Fall 1998 200 East Area Biological Vector Contamination Report." My analysis of these events is informed by Shannon Cram's "Wild and Scenic Wasteland: Conservation Politics in the Nuclear Wilderness," *Environmental Humanities* 7, no. 1 (2015): 99–101. A suite of essays by Cram on Hanford have been instrumental to my thinking about Hanford, including, "Becoming Jane: The Making and Unmaking of Hanford's Nuclear Body," *Environment and Planning D: Society and Space* 33, no. 5 (October 1, 2015): 796–812. Cram's research on Hanford has more recently been published as *Unmaking the Bomb: Environmental Cleanup and the Politics of Impossibility* (Oakland: University of California Press, 2023).
3. Connell, "Fall 1998 200 East Area Biological Vector Contamination Report," 5–8, 1–6.
4. Cram, "Wild and Scenic Wasteland," 99–100. These details are documented in Connell, "Fall 1998 200 East Area Biological Vector Contamination Report," A-1, xiv. These details are also included in Cram, "Wild and Scenic Wasteland," 99–100.
5. To borrow a phrase from Mary Douglas, they become "matter out of place." Mary Douglas, *Purity and Danger: An Analysis of Concepts of Pollution and Taboo* (London: Routledge & K. Paul, 1980), 36.
6. Connell, "Fall 1998 200 East Area Biological Vector Contamination Report," F-20.
7. Connell, "Fall 1998 200 East Area Biological Vector Contamination Report," F-7.
8. This way of thinking about nuclear toxicity is influenced by Soraya Boudia et al., "Residues: Rethinking Chemical Environments," *Engaging Science, Technology, and Society* 4 (June 28, 2018): 165–178, https://doi.org/10.17351/ests2018.245; Angela N. H. Creager, *Life Atomic: A History of Radioisotopes in Science and Medicine* (Chicago: University of Chicago Press, 2013); Meredith TenHoor, "Toxic Geographies," ed. Caroline Acheatel et al., *Perspecta*, no. 53 (2020): 218–233; Gabrielle Hecht, *Being Nuclear : Africans and the Global Uranium Trade* (Cambridge, MA: MIT Press, 2014); Lawrence Buell, "Toxic Discourse," *Critical Inquiry* 24, no. 3 (1998): 639–665. Another prominent example of scholarship on the meaning of toxicity, from within the discipline of architectural history, can be found in the Aggregate Architectural History Collaborative's project on, "Toxics," *The Aggregate Website* 8 (December 2020), http://we-aggregate.org/piece/toxics.
9. Peter B. Hales, *Atomic Spaces: Living on the Manhattan Project* (Urbana: University of Illinois Press, 1997), 3.
10. Hales, *Atomic Spaces*, 35. Hales's quotation of Groves can be found in Jesse A. Remington and Lenore Fine, eds., *The Corps of Engineers: Construction in the United States* (Washington, DC: US Government Printing Office, 2003), 659.
11. Cram, "Wild and Scenic Wasteland," 90.
12. Hales, *Atomic Spaces*, 23; Cram, "Becoming Jane," 803; see also Kate Brown, *Plutopia: Nuclear Families, Atomic Cities, and the Great Soviet and American Plutonium Disasters* (Oxford: Oxford University Press, 2013), 32–36.
13. Hales, *Atomic Spaces*, 19.
14. Brown, *Plutopia*, 36.
15. Hales, *Atomic Spaces*, 45; quote from Groves on same page.
16. Gabrielle Hecht provides an illuminating account of the global uranium trade that relied on African mines for the raw materials of nuclear industry. African nations are mostly denied both the geopolitical exceptionalism of nuclearity as well as the international legal frameworks for redressing nuclear injury. According to Hecht, Shinkolobwe Mine remains unremediated and a source of "radiation-induced" disease. See *Being Nuclear*, 193, 336. The Shinkolobwe Mine has recently received attention in mass media as a significant site in the aftermath of the Manhattan Project; see Frank Swain, "The Forgotten Mine That Built the Atomic Bomb," British Broadcasting Corporation, August 3, 2020, https://www.bbc.com/future/article/20200803-the-forgotten-mine-that-built-the-atomic-bomb.
17. "Projects & Facilities—Hanford Site," accessed November 22, 2021, https://www.hanford.gov/page.cfm/ProjectsFacilities.
18. See Brown, *Plutopia*, 47.
19. However, such reservations were animated more by ideology than a genuine concern for women's health. Brown, *Plutopia*, 46.
20. See Brown, *Plutopia*, 47–48.
21. Brown, *Plutopia*, 342, n2.
22. Vincent C. Jones, *Manhattan: The Army and the Atomic Bomb* (Washington, DC: Center of Military History, United States Army, 1985), 451.
23. Hales, *Atomic Spaces*, 102–103.
24. Brown, *Plutopia*, 22.
25. Brown, *Plutopia*, 27.
26. As scholar Kate Brown has argued, systematic racial segregation was implemented in the site by USACE generals who believed that limiting the rights of Black employees was necessary to ensure the morale of the white workforce. Brown, *Plutopia*, 24, 27. For more on the relationship between toxicity and workplace reform in the nineteenth century, see Buell, "Toxic Discourse," 651.
27. The ideal residents of Richland Village, as the community would be named, were white, middle-class, college-educated, childrearing families. See Hales, *Atomic Spaces*, 96.
28. DuPont opposed government planning, social welfare spending, and, generally, most New Deal programs. Additionally, the company's executives believed that suburbia was good for business by incentivizing middle-class consumerism. Ironically, DuPont's profits largely depended on government largesse through military contracts like the one for Hanford. Brown, *Plutopia*, 38–40.
29. Jones, *Manhattan: The Army and the Atomic Bomb*, 457, quote on 459-460.
30. G. Albin Pehrson, "Report on the Hanford Engineer Works Village," November 1943, 42; quoted in Hales, *Atomic Spaces*, 96.
31. Hales, *Atomic Spaces*, 97–100.
32. My reading of Pehrson's plans is informed by Hales's description in *Atomic Spaces*, 97.
33. Brown, *Plutopia*, 40.
34. Hales, *Atomic Spaces*, 278.
35. Hales, 273, 284; Rob Nixon, *Slow Violence and the Environmentalism of the Poor* (Cambridge, MA: Harvard University Press, 2011), 10.
36. On toxicity's relationship to numerical standards, scientific instrumentation, and bodily politics, see Mel Y. Chen, *Animacies: Biopolitics, Racial Mattering, and Queer Affect* (Durham: Duke University Press, 2012), 191.
37. Fabiola López-Durán, *Eugenics in the Garden: Transatlantic Architecture and the Crafting of Modernity* (Austin: University of Texas Press, 2018), 188.
38. Cram, "Becoming Jane," 800. Reference Man is an example of the mathematical "phantoms" used by physicians and radiobiologists to analyze the risks of radiation or other hazards to human bodies. "Physical phantoms are made of solid materials which are radiologically equivalent to human tissues." George Xu, "An Exponential Growth of Computational Phantom Research in Radiation Protection, Imaging, and Radiotherapy: A Review of the Fifty-Year History," *Physics in Medicine and Biology* 59, no. 18 (September 21, 2014): 3.
39. Cram, "Becoming Jane," 806.
40. Brown, *Plutopia*, 169.
41. Brown, *Plutopia*, 57, 69.
42. In *Unmaking the Bomb*, 15, Shannon Cram elucidates the transference of wartime containment strategies to the contemporary remediation effort underway at Hanford in much greater depth than is possible in this brief essay.
43. Hales, *Atomic Spaces*, 149; Vitruvius, *The Ten Books on Architecture*, trans. M. H. Morgan (Cambridge, MA: Harvard University Press, 1926), 20.
44. Cram, "Wild and Scenic Wasteland," 90.
45. Hanford's remediation implies a warping of space and time in the same way that Peter Galison describes another large-scale remediation effort aimed at the toxic byproducts of the Manhattan Project's atomic production processes at the Waste Isolation Pilot Plant in Carlsbad, New Mexico. Peter Galison, "Foreword: What Are Technical Lands?," in *Technical Lands: A Critical Primer*, ed. Jeffrey S. Nesbit and Charles Waldheim (Berlin: Jovis, 2022), 18–27.
46. For a thorough study of US post-nuclear markers, see Julia Bryan-Wilson, "Building a Marker of Nuclear Warning," in *Monuments and Memory, Made and Unmade*, ed. Robert S. Nelson and Margaret Olin (Chicago: University of Chicago Press, 2003), 183–204.

p315, 316 Robert Del Tredici / The Atomic Photographers' Guild.
p317 (top) Click Reilander Collection, Yakima Valley Libraries' Northwest Reading Room, Yakima, Washington.
p317 (right) Hanford Engineer Works/United States Department of Energy.
p317 (left) National Archives and Records Administration.
p319, 320 Hanford History Project, Washington State University, Tri-Cities.
p321, 322 (top) Reproduced from R. H. Wilson, *Historical Review of Personnel Dosimetry Development and Its Use in Radiation Protection Programs at Hanford: 1944 to the 1980s* (Richland: Pacific Northwest Laboratory, February 1987).
p322 (bottom) Reproduced from M. Cristy and K. F. Eckerman, *Specific Absorbed Fractions of Energy at Various Ages from Internal Photon Sources* (Oak Ridge: Oak Ridge National Laboratory, 1987).
p323 Kathleen M. Trauth, et al., *Expert Judgement on Markers to Deter Inadvertent Human Intrusion into the Waste Isolation Pilot Plant* (Albuquerque: US Department of Energy, 1993).
p324 Reproduced from *Message Development for Surface Markers at the Hanford Radwaste Disposal Sites* (Washington DC: US Department of Energy, 1984).

RADIOACTIVITY IN THE SAHARA

SAMIA HENNI

Colonialism contaminates and kills human and nonhuman lives. This was the case with the French nuclear weapons program in the colonized Algerian Sahara. Detonated between February 1960 (approximately five years after the outbreak of the Algerian Revolution and four years after the beginning of the exploitation of Algerian oil) and February 1966 (approximately four years after Algeria gained its independence from France), France's atomic bombs spread radioactive fallout and caused irrevocable contamination across Algeria, Central and West Africa, and the Mediterranean (including southern Europe).[1] The French colonial regime stated that it exploded four atmospheric nuclear bombs and thirteen underground atomic bombs in the Algerian Sahara, and experimented with other nuclear technologies and weapons in its atmosphere. The archives of these events are classified and closed to the public.[2]

The four atmospheric bombs were named Gerboise bleue, blanche, rouge, and verte (Blue, White, Red, and Green Jerboas) after a small jumping desert rodent and were detonated in Reggane (also written Reggan), in the Tanezrouft plain of the Algerian Sahara, approximately 1,150 kilometers south of Algiers, between February 1960 and April 1961. For their part, the underground bombs were named after gemstones: Agathe (Agate), Béryl (Beryl), Émeraude (Emerald), Améthyste (Amethyst), Rubis (Ruby), Opale (Opal), Topaze (Topaz), Turquoise, Saphir (Sapphire), Jade, Corindon (Corundum), Tourmaline, and Grenat (Garnet), and were detonated at In Ekker (also spelt In Ecker or In Eker), on the Hoggar mountain of Taourirt Tan Afella in the Algerian Sahara, approximately 600 kilometers southeast of Reggane, between November 1961 and February 1966.[3]

These atomic detonations were conducted despite the approval of Algeria's referendum on self-determination by seventy-five percent of voters on

↘ Centre saharien d'expérimentations militaires (CSEM, or Saharan Center for Military Experiments) in Reggane, built for the atmospheric nuclear bombs detonated between 1960 and 1961. Photographs by Jean-Michel Pinaut, date unknown.

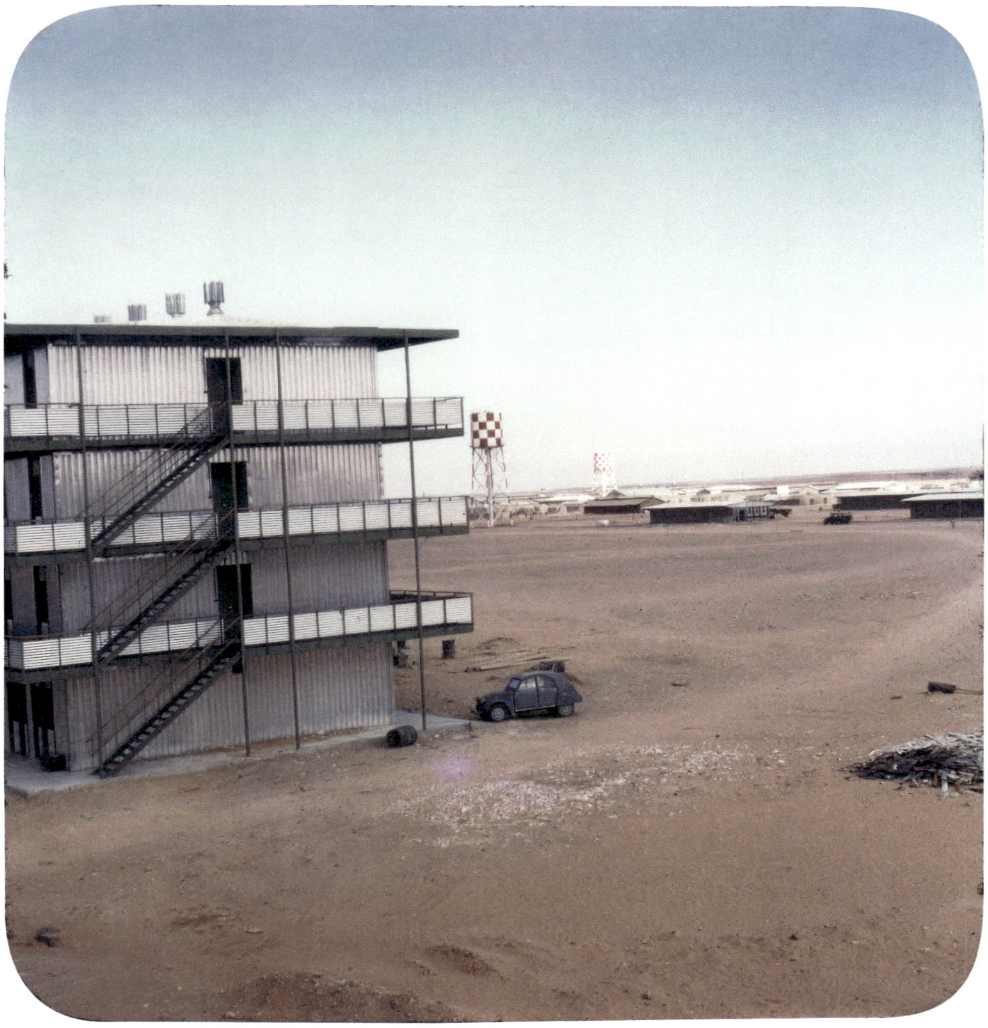

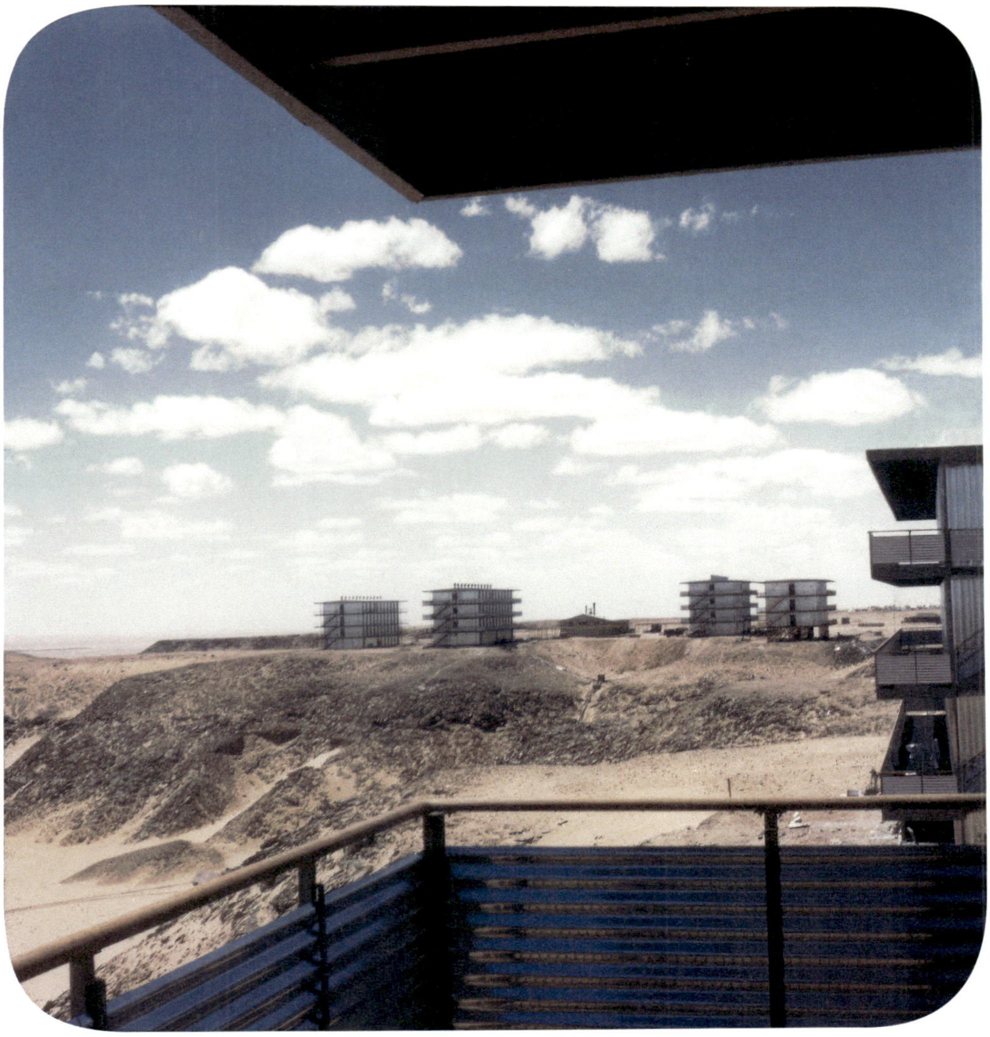

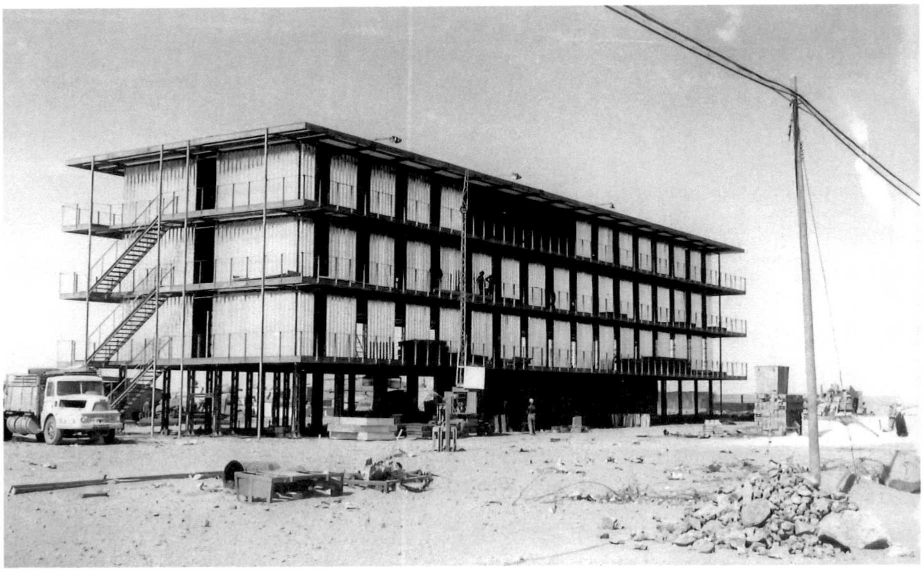

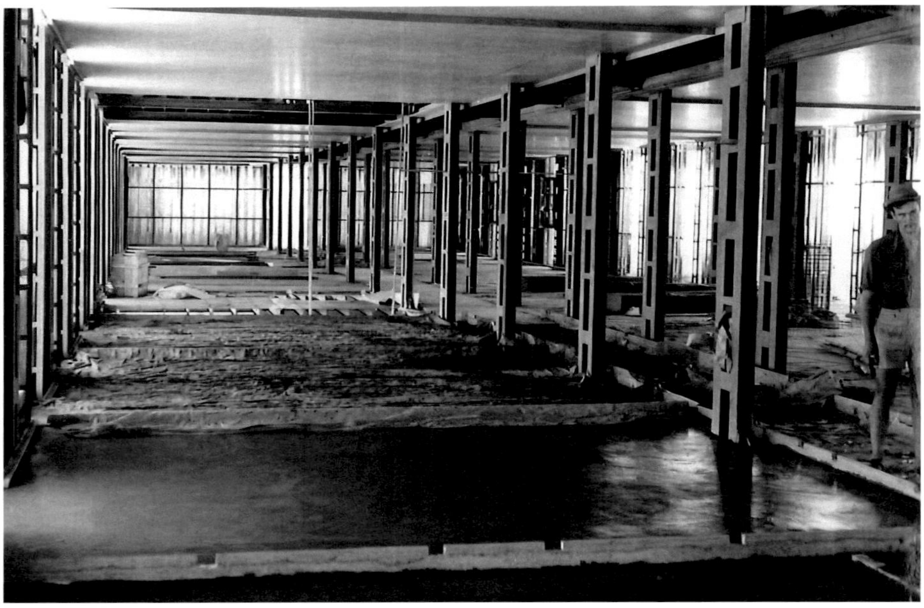

↙ ↘ The construction of the Centre saharien d'expérimentations militaires in Reggane. Photographs by an unknown author (French veteran), donated by M. A. and M. G, 1959–1960.

January 8, 1961, and the ensuing independence from France in March 1962 after 132 years of French colonial rule. Signed between the Provisional Government of the Algerian Republic and the French Fifth Republic, and presided over by General Charles de Gaulle in Évian-les-Bains, on March 18, 1962, the peace treaty—known as the Evian Accords—formalized the independent status of Algeria and institutionalized the "cooperation" between the two countries.[4] The Evian Accords allowed the French army to continue using its nuclear sites in the Sahara after Algeria's independence for a period of five years.

To carry out its secret nuclear weapons program in the Algerian Sahara, the French colonial regime built two military bases: the Centre saharien d'expérimentations militaires (CSEM, or Saharan Center for Military Experiments) in Reggane, and the Centre d'expérimentations militaires des oasis (CEMO, or Oasis Military Testing Center) in In Ekker. An estimated twenty thousand people (civilian and military) worked or served in the Saharan nuclear bases between 1960 and 1966.[5] It is unclear whether the Saharan people who worked on the construction of CSEM, CEMO, or the firing tunnels are included in this estimation. However, the French colonial regime estimated that a sedentary population of forty thousand lived in the area where the atmospheric bombs were detonated, mainly in the oases and the Touat valley north of Reggane. In this estimate, there is no mention of the nomadic and seminomadic populations of the Algerian and other parts of the Sahara.[6] The construction of CSEM and CEMO and France's nuclear weapons program had devastating effects on the construction workers, as well as on the Saharan people, who continue to live on their land and suffer contamination by radioactive matter.

Building for Atmospheric Nuclear Bombs

Together with the support of various civil and military services, CSEM was a French joint organization that prepared and executed nuclear bombs tests in Reggane. It reported to the French Ministry of the Armed Forces (General Staff of the Armies, Technical Office) through the General Joint Commander of Special Weapons. CSEM was designed to host around ten thousand civil and military personnel expected to work on the detonation and measurements of atmospheric nuclear bombs. The site comprised four functional areas: Reggane-ville (Reggane Town); Reggane Plateau, the living base or residential compound comprised of underground laboratories and ateliers; Hamoudia, a forward operating base; and the Zone des points zéro (Ground Zero Zone), where the bombs were to be detonated.[7]

By the spring of 1960, most of the construction work planned for CSEM had been completed, amounting to 82,000 square meters of buildings, 7,000 square meters of underground works, 100 kilometers of roads, 1,200 cubic meters of water per day, three power plants and 4,400 kilovolts of power, more than 200 kilometers of underground cables and pipes, and 7,000 cubic meters of reinforced concrete in the Ground Zero Zone.[8] Reggane Plateau was located about twelve kilometers east of Reggane Town, and the Ground Zero Zone was situated approximately fifteen kilometers south of Hamoudia and fifty kilometers southwest of Reggane.[9] All areas were connected by paved roads.

Located near the existing town and oasis of Reggane, Reggane Town consisted of three existing settlements: the Bordj Estienne, which served as the living quarters for the CSEM commanding colonel, General Staff officers, and visiting officers and engineers;[10] the Senegalese Bordj, which housed the military engineers and their large fleet of cars; and the Bordj of Saharan Affairs, which housed the region's civil administration services and gendarmerie.[11]

The offices of the CSEM colonel and his officers were situated in newly constructed Reggane Plateau. The base was strategically built on a rocky plateau bordered by a twenty-meter-high cliff, facing and elevated above the vast flat area that extends toward Hamoudia and the Ground Zero Zone. Designed to accommodate approximately ten thousand people, Reggane Plateau housed the program's troops, airfield, laboratories, workshops, and equipment depots, as well as its technical premises, a hospital, and an aerodrome with a runway of 2,400 meters. The residential and administrative buildings were located to the west of the plateau and arranged parallel to the north-south axis of a large (150-by-100-meter) *place d'armes*, around which lay a swimming pool, foyer, and cinema. To the south, there were sports facilities

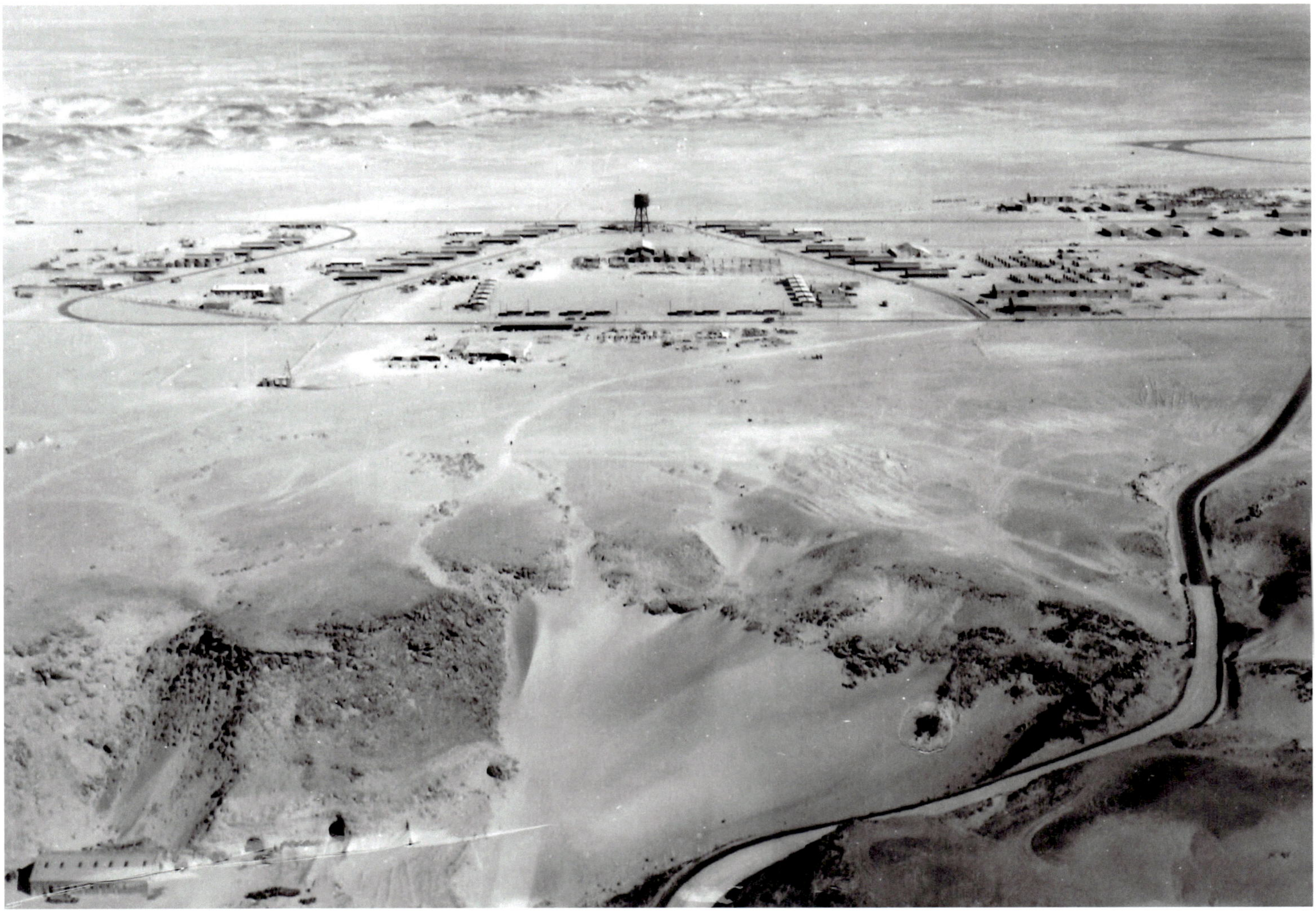

(e.g., football pitches, basketball courts, tennis courts, etc.).[12]

On February 16, 2010, a classified report titled "Volume 1: The Genesis of the Organization and Experiments in the Sahara (CSEM and CEMO)" was leaked, partially published, and commented on in the French daily newspaper *Le Parisien*:

> Reggane's construction site allows the Special Engineering Works Department to develop and test two construction processes adapted to the country's climate. The so-called "Saharan" single-floor pavilions and the prefabricated three-floor metal buildings. These two types of construction, which in fact derive from the same principle, namely the use of cavity walls with air circulation, have from the outset been studied according to their air conditioning.[13]

It was also believed that the three-story metal buildings offered better natural ventilation of the rooms and protected the occupants of the upper floors from the sand and dust that is almost constantly carried into the Saharan region by wind. Furthermore, this spatial arrangement was expected to increase the density of the buildings, decrease the effect of heat reflection from the ground, and reduce the cost of roads and air conditioning systems.[14] There are no available accounts that confirm or deny this argument. However, it is difficult to imagine that a metallic structure is well adapted to high summer temperatures that reach 50°C during the daytime.

Building for Underground Nuclear Bombs

Before and throughout the detonations of France's first atmospheric atomic bombs in Reggane, three other countries—the Soviet Union, Great Britain, and the United States—began negotiating the ban of atmospheric nuclear weapon tests. The resulting Treaty Banning Nuclear Weapon Tests in the Atmosphere, in Outer Space and Under Water was signed in August 1963 by those nations (not by France) and prohibited all atomic detonations except for those conducted underground. French colonial and military authorities had first begun searching for a mountainous site in 1958 to develop a nuclear weapons testing program below ground. This was further motivated by negotiations for Algeria's independence and numerous protests against nuclear weapons in independent African countries and elsewhere.[15]

Under the French Minister of the Armed Forces, the Commission provisoire de recherche de sites souterrains pour expérimentations nucléaires (Temporary Commission for the Search for Underground Sites for Nuclear Experimentations) was established in September 1958, enabling French scientists and officers to examine and analyze various sites in mainland France and elsewhere as possible sites for underground nuclear testing. Areas included the Crête de Pranetz, the Tête de Cluasis, and the Martin Alp in the Briançonnais region; the Grand Groyer, the Crête de la Boulière, and the Cime de Pal in the Alpes de Provence region; and Corsica.[16]

Although the geological characteristics of some sites were suitable, none were selected. Instead, the Temporary Commission designated the Hoggar mountains, in the Algerian Sahara, as its new nuclear weapons testing site. Bruno Barrillot, the cofounder of the Observatoire des armements—a French independent nonprofit center for expertise and documentation founded in 1984 in Lyon—argued that "the choice of this site, where there were areas of pasture, was made in the 'colonial' tradition, that is to say, without asking the opinion of the local populations."[17] Within the granite massif of Taourirt Tan Afella, near In Ekker, the Temporary Commission excavated tunnels and detonated thirteen underground nuclear bombs from 1961 to 1966.

To host the civil and military employees responsible for the preparation and detonation of these bombs, French colonial authorities decided to build another military base, the Centre d'expérimentations militaires des oasis (CEMO, or Oasis Military Testing Center), in July 1960. CEMO comprised a living base called Camp Saint-Laurent in northern In Amguel, near Oued Takormiasse; an airbase located fifteen kilometers north of In Amguel; a forward operating base in In Ekker; and a residential camp at the foot of the eastern flank of the Taourirt Tan Afella mountain called OASIS I, approximately thirty-five kilometers from Camp Saint-Laurent.

OASIS I was designed to house the mineworkers and the personnel of the Direction des applications militaires (Directorate for Military Applications). It was, however, too close to ground zero of the underground blasts, some of which were uncontained. OASIS I was contaminated by the bomb codenamed Béryl, detonated on May 1, 1962.[18] As a result, a second residential camp, OASIS II, was built. The forward operating base was located between Camp Saint-Laurent and OASIS I on an existing French military base known as Bordj In-Eker, which was extended and transformed.[19]

Covering 170,570 hectares, CEMO housed approximately 2,000 employees, including 90 officers, 300 noncommissioned officers, and 750 civil servants, engineers, technical staff, and miners. The construction of OASIS I started in September 1960 and ended in February 1961. The renovation and extension of Bordj In-Eker began in July 1960 and continued through different phases, even after Algerian independence in July 1962. The construction of the living base began in October 1960 and was completed a year later, in October 1961. OASIS II was built during the first quarter of 1963.

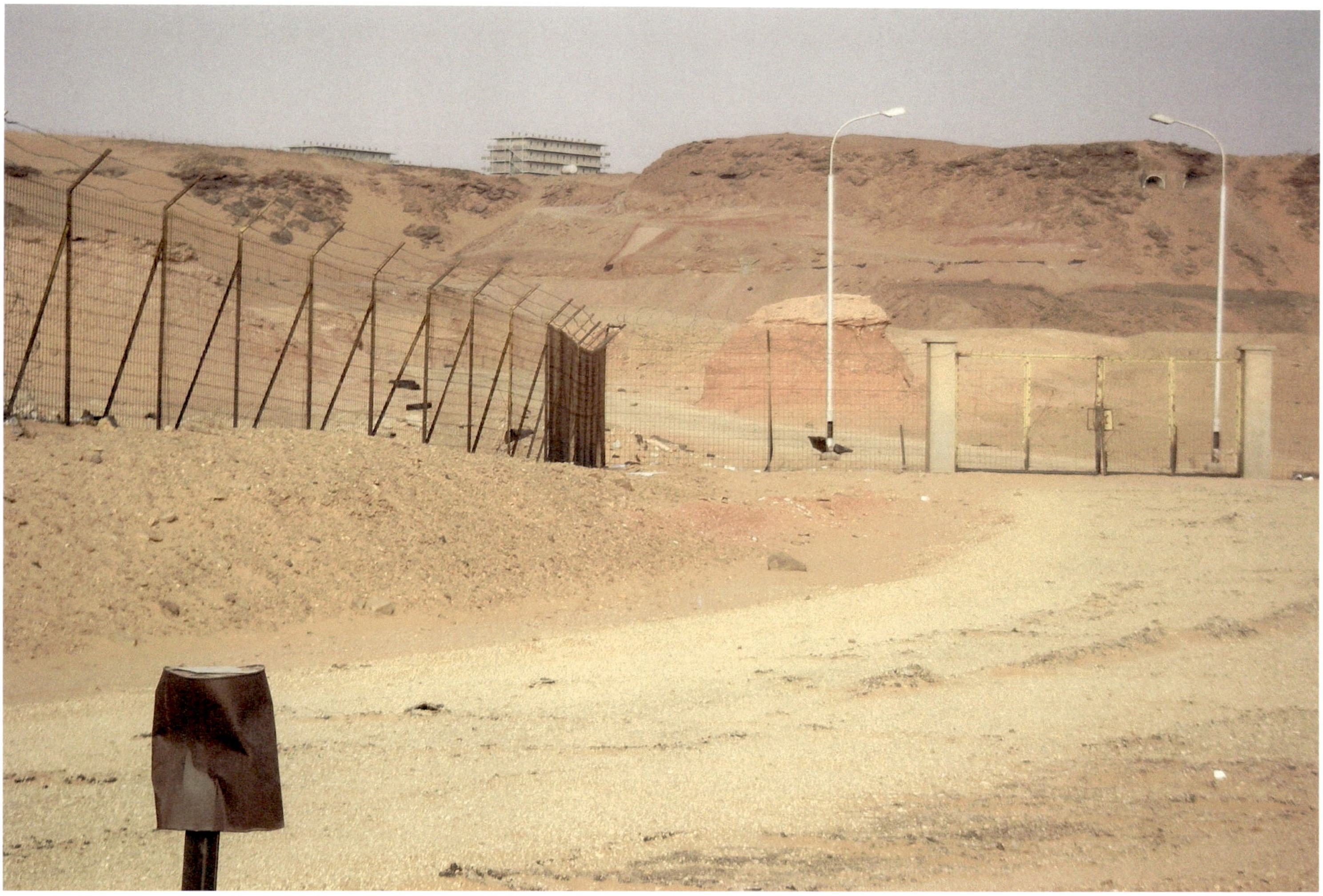

↑ Photographs by Bruno Barrillot, cofounder of the Observatoire des armements, taken during a visit to France's nuclear sites in Reggane and In Ekker in the Algerian Sahara with the filmmaker Larbi Benchiha and his team in November 2007.

Hiring and Labeling Saharan Workers

The workforce responsible for constructing the buildings and infrastructure of France's first atmospheric nuclear detonations in the Sahara included Algerian populations. According to Charles Ailleret, leader of the Commandement interarmées des armes spéciales (Special Weapons Joint Command), the entity responsible for the realization of the built environments for the bombs, "one cannot speak of the construction works carried out on the base and the firing field without mentioning a category of labor, which was both a very effective means of the construction of the installations and an essential element of the legends of the operations."[20] This category was named the Population Laborieuse du Bas-Touat (PLBT, or Working Population of Southern Tuat).[21]

The exact numbers of these workers are unknown. Referring to their assigned appellation and the financial aspects of the labor force, Ailleret stipulated that "the considerable accounts that the employment of thousands of workers justified were henceforth drawn up using the PLBT, a term which meant indigenous Saharan hired by the Center."[22] These thousands of workers were indispensable to the realization of France's secret construction works in the Sahara.

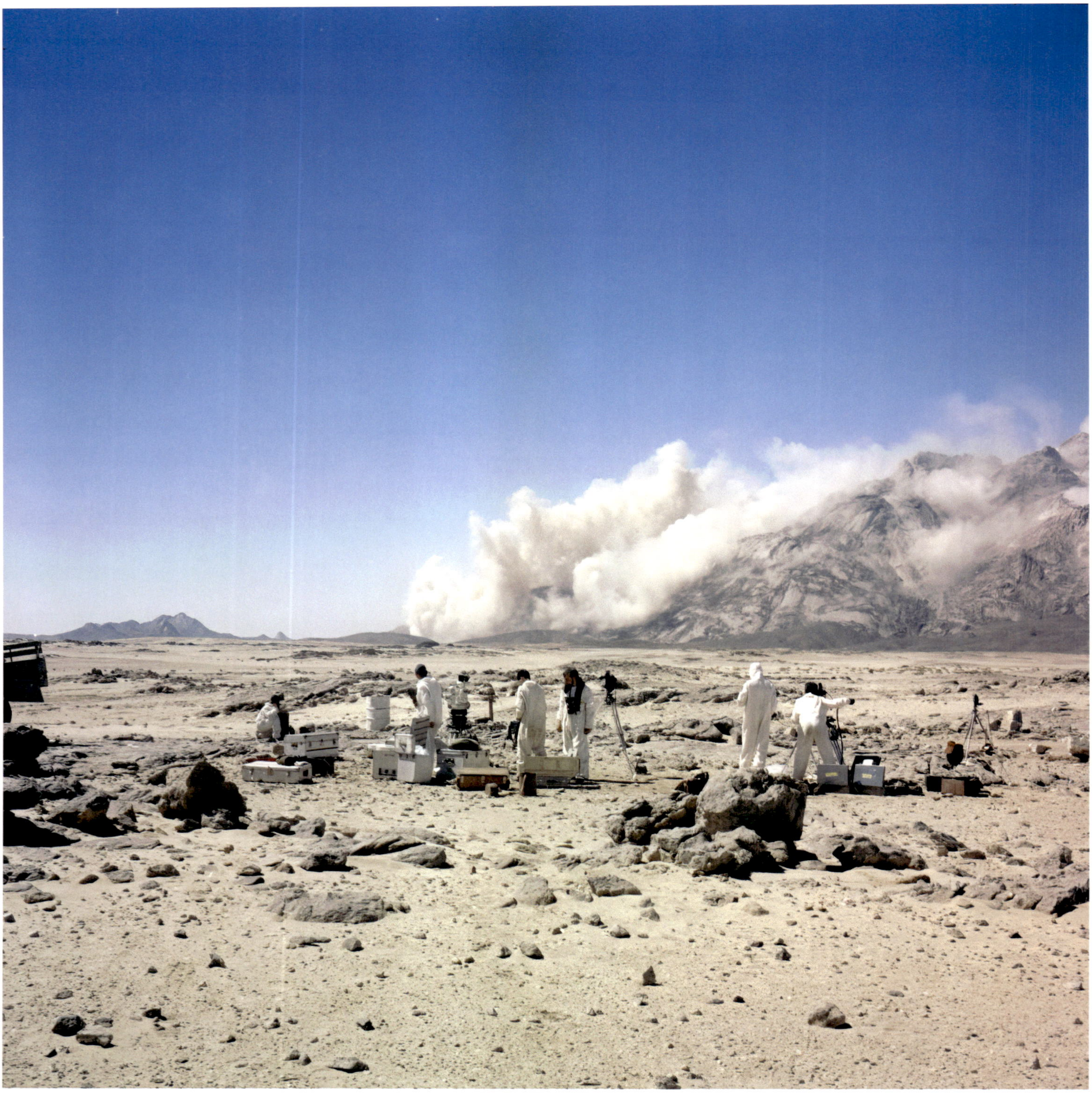

↑ Radioactive cloud resulting from an uncontained atomic underground bomb in the Taourirt Tan Afella mountain, In Ekker, 1963. According to the original caption, the bomb might have been either Émeraude (Emerald) of March 18, 1963, or Améthyste (Amethyst) of March 30, 1963.

Ailleret stated that when French officers requested an additional labor force to execute the works, they demanded more PLBT, adding that, toward the end, no one knew what this abbreviation stood for.[23]

The Algerian workers from the Tuat region were employed for various kinds of construction work, especially where the construction machines brought to the Sahara by French engineers could not be used due to their inadaptability to the soil of the Sahara. A French officer who led construction work on a building site said that Tuat workers "were employed for handling the construction sites and as far as I was concerned, they loaded and unloaded the trucks with the construction materials."[24] Another French officer claimed that they were contracted to build the main paved road between Reggane Plateau and Hamoudia, reporting that "the construction works were conducted by night for approximately one month with the participation of a hundred PLBTs."[25]

With the expansion of building sites and the increasing number of construction activities, the so-called PLBT workers were insufficient and additional personnel were necessary, prompting French colonial administrators to look to other regions of the Sahara in Algeria and elsewhere. The appellations for these newly hired Saharan workers changed, reflecting, as with the Tuat region, the area from which the workers came, including the Population Laborieuse du Tchad (PLT, or Working Population of Chad), Population Laborieuse du Djebel (PLD, or the Working Population of Djebel), and Population Laborieuse des Oasis (PLO, or Working Population from the Oases). The workers lived in self-built shelters near the construction sites. Like French personnel working in CSEM and CEMO, they were exposed to radiation. None of the Saharan workers received any medical follow-up after their participation in the construction jobs.[26]

Contaminating and Killing Lives

In June 1992, thirty-two years after the detonation of France's first atmospheric nuclear bomb in the Sahara, the French environmental activist and member of European Parliament representing the French Green Party, Solange Fernex (1934–2006), interviewed various Saharan workers who had been employed in Reggane and In Ekker, as well as Algerian nuclear survivors. The interviews were conducted to raise awareness of the ongoing consequences of French nuclear weapons in the Sahara. The testimonies covered various topics, including the working conditions, contract terms, lack of protection during and after the detonation of the nuclear bombs, lack of information about the impact of atomic weapons, diseases and symptoms they suffer from, memories of the explosions, dangers they faced after the explosions, the invisibility of radioactivity, lack of trust in the French and Algerian authorities,

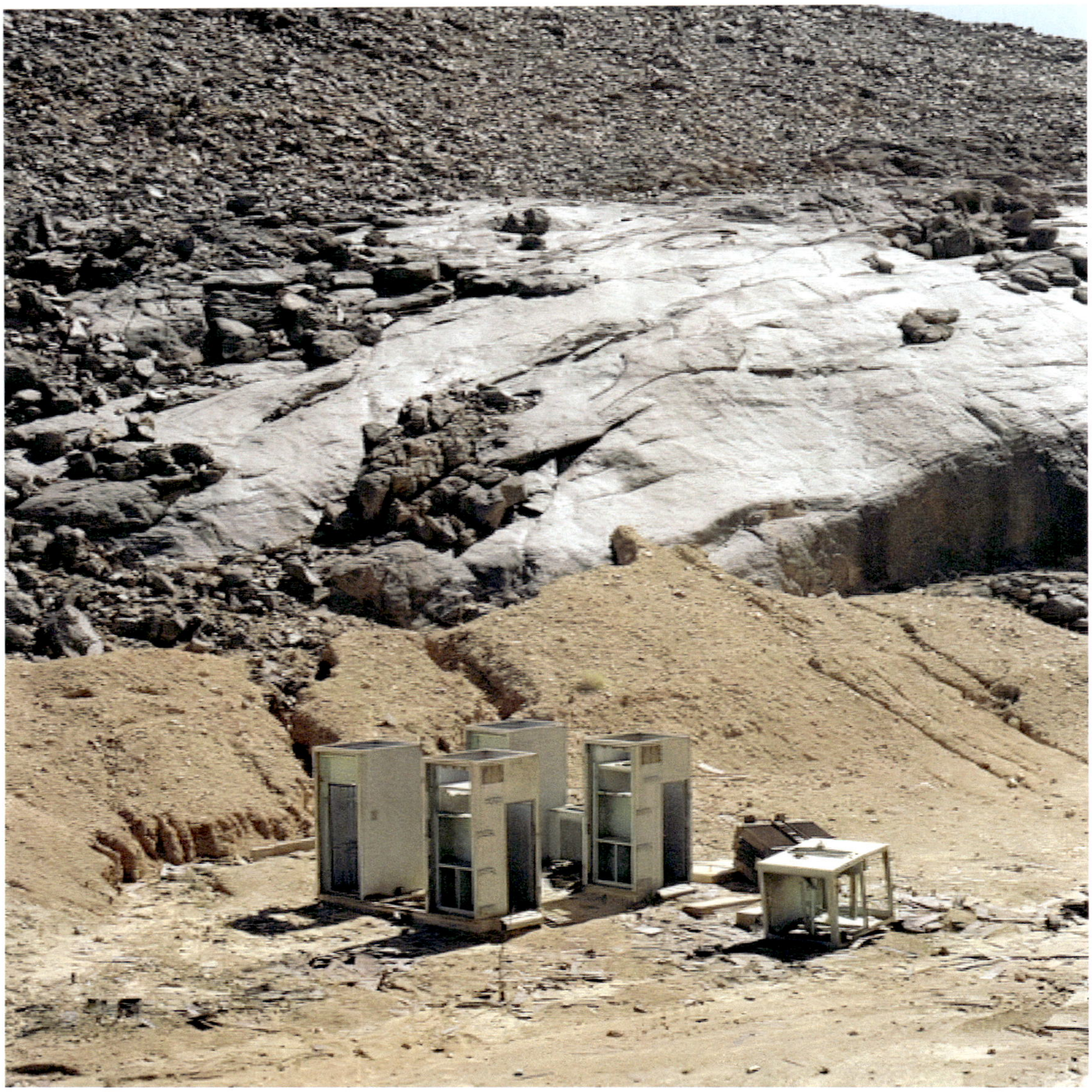

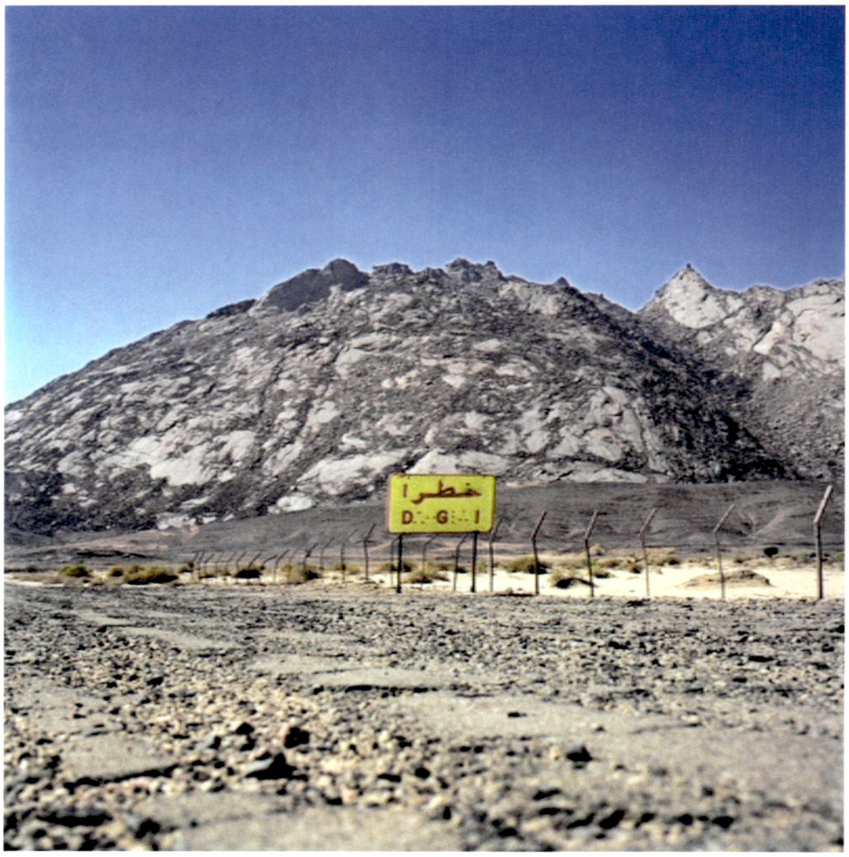

↗ Stills from *AT(h)OME*, directed by Élisabeth Leuvrey, 2013, based on the photographic work and investigation of Bruno Hadjih, and produced by Les Écrans du Large.

→ Centre d'expérimentations militaires des oasis (CEMO, or Oases Military Testing Center) in In Ekker, 1963.

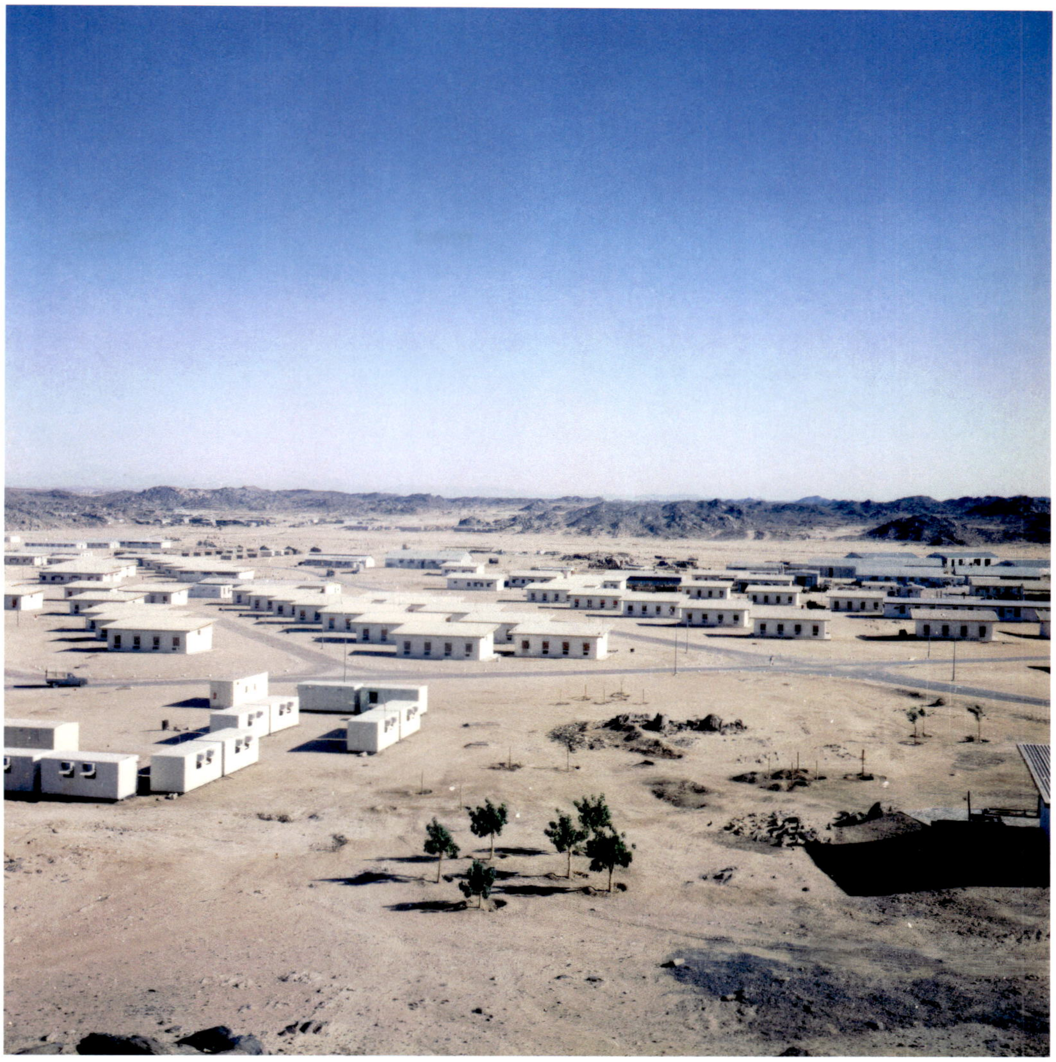

arable lands that had become unproductive, widespread infertility in the region, lack of medical follow-up, living with fear, and death.[27]

One of the interviewees asserted that "in the base, the French and the Algerians were segregated. They each had their accommodation, food, etc."[28] Another nuclear victim, who worked as a team leader between 1961 and 1966, said: "we dug tunnels into the mountain, then we built the road (tar). Each team was composed of thirty people. There were a lot of bases. ... The only days on which we did not work were Sundays. Only men lived there. ... I know several people who worked with us who are sick."[29] This man also told of his own health condition and those of his spouses and brother. He was born around 1940, married twelve times, and had eight children. However, after 1967, none of his spouses were able to get pregnant; he was unable to have children after he worked on the installations of the atomic bombs. Furthermore, he suffered from eye and stomach diseases. His brother, who had also worked on the installations, was sick as well. The brother first developed lung disease, then his blood was contaminated. When the interview was conducted in 1992, he had no hope left.[30]

In recalling the explosion of one of the atmospheric nuclear bombs, another former worker explained: "I was in Gao, in Mali, and we heard the explosion. In fact, we felt the earth tremble and we heard like a dull noise. The noise was heard as far as Tessalit"—roughly 770 kilometers south of Reggane.[31] At the time, he was told that caravans were crossing the desert while the bomb was detonated and perished, but he could not provide any details. He was also aware of the nuclear site or the ground zero in Reggane, especially the existence of underground laboratories. He claimed that "it was the French army who dug them. The people of Reggane performed the heavy work." The interviewee, referred to as Moustapha, commented on the conditions of the Reggane bases after the explosions and the departure of the French civil and military authorities:

> after the explosion, they [the French] enclosed the site with barbed wire and left it like that. But most of the barbed wire was pulled out by the copper traffickers who came from the region of Béchar and sold it in Morocco. They took the electrical installations to recover the copper.[32]

This contaminated metal was sold not only in Morocco but also in Algeria and other parts of the Sahara. Moustapha contended that Algerian copper traders filled petrol tanks with large cables twenty centimeters in diameter used by the French, which they transported on trucks and sold in Adrar and Béchar. He also mentioned the health conditions of the traffickers and their inability to have children.[33]

Another interviewee detailed the conditions in which copper cables were retrieved from the installations after 1967 when the French army left the site. He also described common symptoms of people who had been in direct contact with these contaminated cables, including infertility, headaches, stomachaches, hair loss, muscle stiffness, fatigue, and premature aging. Many people he knew who trafficked copper died at an early age. He noted: "O, dead at the age of thirty-two; P, dead at age thirty-eight; Q, deceased aged forty-five years; R, deceased at the age of fifty years; S, dead at the age of thirty-one." Other men became seriously ill: "there's an old man in the hospital here and who is still sick. I also know T, around fifty, who is still sick. Ahmed himself is still ill, his brother is still sick too." The interviewee, referred to as Interview no. 3, alleged that "the doctors here do nothing and say nothing. They just take the strain and that's all." He described in detail the miscarriages that the spouses of some of these men had suffered, as well as the short lives of the babies who were born and died, stating that "the first spouse had a child who lived six months. The second had a child who lived a year and died."[34]

Building for France's nuclear weapons program in the Sahara was deadly. The resulting architecture that is still occupying Sahara landscapes continues to contaminate, if not kill, human and nonhuman lives. The thousands of Saharan people who built the facilities that produced the irreversible contamination of their own land without their knowledge and consent continue to suffer from the humanitarian and environmental disasters of radioactivity. In 1966, France moved its nuclear weapons testing program from Algeria to another territory under French rule: the Mururoa and Fangataufa atolls in colonized Tahiti Nui (French Polynesia), in the southern Pacific Ocean.[35] Despite objections and protests, the French colonial authorities detonated nearly 200 atmospheric and underground nuclear bombs there between 1966 and 1996, further toxifying colonized and noncolonized environments. This occurred despite the 1963 Treaty Banning Nuclear Weapon Tests in the Atmosphere and the 1968 Treaty on the Non-Proliferation of Nuclear Weapons, neither of which France is a signatory to. In spite of the undeniable effects of nuclear weapons, France refused to sign or ratify the 2017 Treaty on the Prohibition of Nuclear Weapons.[36] Beyond the Sahara, both radioactive architecture and matter continue to contaminate and slowly exterminate the lives and territories of people in Moruroa and Fangataufa atolls.

p327 © Jean-Michel Pinaut/ Service cinématographique des armés (SCA) / Établissement de communication et de production audiovisuelle de la Défense (ECPAD)/ Défense. p328, 329, 331 Courtesy of the Observatoire des armements (www.obsarm.org). p332, 335 Photographer unknown. Collection Fonds général 1914–1991/F 63-115 © Service cinématographique des armés (SCA) / Établissement de communication et de production audiovisuelle de la Défense (ECPAD)/ Défense. p334 (top) Courtesy of Élisabeth Leuvrey.

1. On France's nuclear history, see, for example, Gabrielle Hecht, *The Radiance of France: Nuclear Power and National Identity after World War II* (Cambridge, MA: MIT Press, 2009). On Algeria oil's history, see, for example, Roger Faligot, Jean Guisnel, and Rémi Kauffer, *Histoire politique des services secrets français de la Seconde Guerre mondiale à nos jours* (Paris: la Découverte, 2012).
2. A repository of private and public archives is available in Samia Henni, *Colonial Toxicity: Rehearsing French Radioactive Architecture and Landscape in the Sahara* (Amsterdam: If I Can't Dance and Framer Framed; Zurich: edition finkm, 2024).
3. On the atmospheric and underground bombs please see, for example, Samia Henni, "Jerboasite: Naming French Radioactive Matter in the Sahara," e-flux Architecture: Half-Life, December 2022, https://www.e-flux.com/architecture/half-life/508392/jerboasite-naming-french-radioactive-matter-in-the-sahara/.
4. On the Evian Accords, see, for example, Benyoucef Ben Khedda, *Les accords d'Evian* (Paris: Publisud-Opu, 1986); Olivier Long, *Le dossier secret des Accords d'Evian: une mission suisse pour la paix en Algérie* (Lausanne: éditions 24 heures, 1988).
5. Corinne Bouchoux and Jean-Claude Lenoir, "Rapport d'information fait au nom de la commission sénatoriale pour le contrôle de l'application des lois (1) sur la mise en oeuvre de la loi n° 2010-2 du 5 janvier 2010 relative à la reconnaissance et l'indemnisation des victimes des essais nucléaires français," Extraordinary Meeting of 2012–2013, Senate, September 18, 2013, 61, https://www.senat.fr/rap/r12-856/r12-856.html.
6. Bouchoux and Lenoir, "Rapport," 11.
7. Bruno Barrillot, *Les irradiés de la république: Les victimes des essais nucléaires français prennent la parole* (Brussels: Éditions GRIP, 2003), 19–20; General Michel Boileau, "Rapport [confidentiel défense] sur les essais nucléaires français (1960–1996). Tome 1: La genèse de l'organisation et les expérimentations au Sahara (C.S.E.M et C.E.M.O)," French Ministry of Defense, Paris, 1996, 58–68.
8. Boileau, "Rapport sur les essais nucléaires français," 46–47.
9. Barrillot, *Les irradiés de la république*, 19–20; Boileau, "Rapport sur les essais nucléaires français," 57–71.
10. The French army used the term *bordj* to refer to a military citadel. The *bordj* is the word for Ottoman military citadels during the regency of Algiers, Tunis, and Tripoli.
11. Boileau, "Rapport sur les essais nucléaires français," 58–59.
12. Boileau, "Rapport sur les essais nucléaires français," 60–62.
13. Boileau, "Rapport sur les essais nucléaires français," 61. "Le chantier de Reggane permet à la Direction des Travaux Spéciaux du Génie de mettre au point et d'expérimenter deux procédés de construction, adaptés au climat du pays. Les pavillons dits 'sahariens' à simple Rez-de-chaussée et les immeubles métalliques préfabriqués à trois étages. Ces deux types de construction qui dérivent en fait du même principe, à savoir l'utilisation de murs creux à circulation d'air ont dès l'origine été étudié en fonction de leur climatisation."
14. Boileau, "Rapport sur les essais nucléaires français," 62.
15. On diplomatic tensions and African protests, see, for example, Roxanne Panchasi, "'No Hiroshima in Africa': The Algerian War and the Question of French Nuclear Tests in the Sahara," *Journal History of the Present* 9, no. 1 (2019): 84–112.
16. Boileau, "Rapport sur les essais nucléaires français," 120–121.
17. Bruno Barrillot, *Essais nucléaires français: L'héritage empoisonné*, 4th ed. (Lyon: Observatoire des armements/ CDRPC, 2012), 69.
18. Barrillot, *Essais nucléaires français*, 69.
19. Barrillot, *Essais nucléaires français*, 69.
20. Charles Ailleret, *L'aventure atomique française* (Paris: B. Grasset, 1968), 325. "On ne saurait pas parler des travaux effectués sur la base et le champ de tir sans mentionner une catégorie de main-d'œuvre qui fut à la fois un moyen très efficace de la construction des installations et un élément essentiel du folklore des opérations."
21. The Tuat region borders Reggane. It contains a series of oases, which extends over 160 kilometers, from the district of Bouda in the north to Reggane in the south.
22. Ailleret, *L'aventure atomique française*, 326. "[C]omme les comptabilités considérables que justifiait l'emploi de milliers de travailleurs furent désormais rédigées en utilisant comme unité le P.L.B.T., terme qui voulait dire indigène saharien embauché par le Centre."
23. On how the French named the colonized Algerian population, see, for example, Samia Henni, "From 'Indigenous' to 'Muslim:' On the French Colonial Assimilationist Doctrine," e-flux Architecture, Positions, 2017, https://www.e-flux.com/architecture/positions/160964/from-indigenous-to-muslim/.
24. Christine Chanton, *Les vétérans des essais nucléaires français au Sahara, 1960–1966* (Paris: Harmattan, 2006), 65.
25. Chanton, *Les vétérans des essais nucléaires français au Sahara*.
26. Chanton, *Les vétérans des essais nucléaires français au Sahara*.
27. Chanton, *Les vétérans des essais nucléaires français au Sahara*, 1–9.
28. Solange Fernex, "Essais nucléaires en Algérie. Interviews de juin 1992" (Paris: ECODIF, 1995), 4.
29. Fernex, "Essais nucléaires en Algérie," 5.
30. Fernex, "Essais nucléaires en Algérie," 5.
31. Fernex, "Essais nucléaires en Algérie," 1.
32. Fernex, "Essais nucléaires en Algérie," 1–2.
33. Fernex, "Essais nucléaires en Algérie," 2.
34. Fernex, "Essais nucléaires en Algérie," 3–4.
35. See, for example, Barrillot, *Les irradiés de la république* and *Essais nucléaires français: L'héritage empoisonné*; Sébastien Philippe and Tomas Statius, *Toxique: Enquête sur les essais nucléaires français en Polynésie* (Paris: Presses Universitaires de France/ Humensis, 2021).
36. https://www.icanw.org/france.

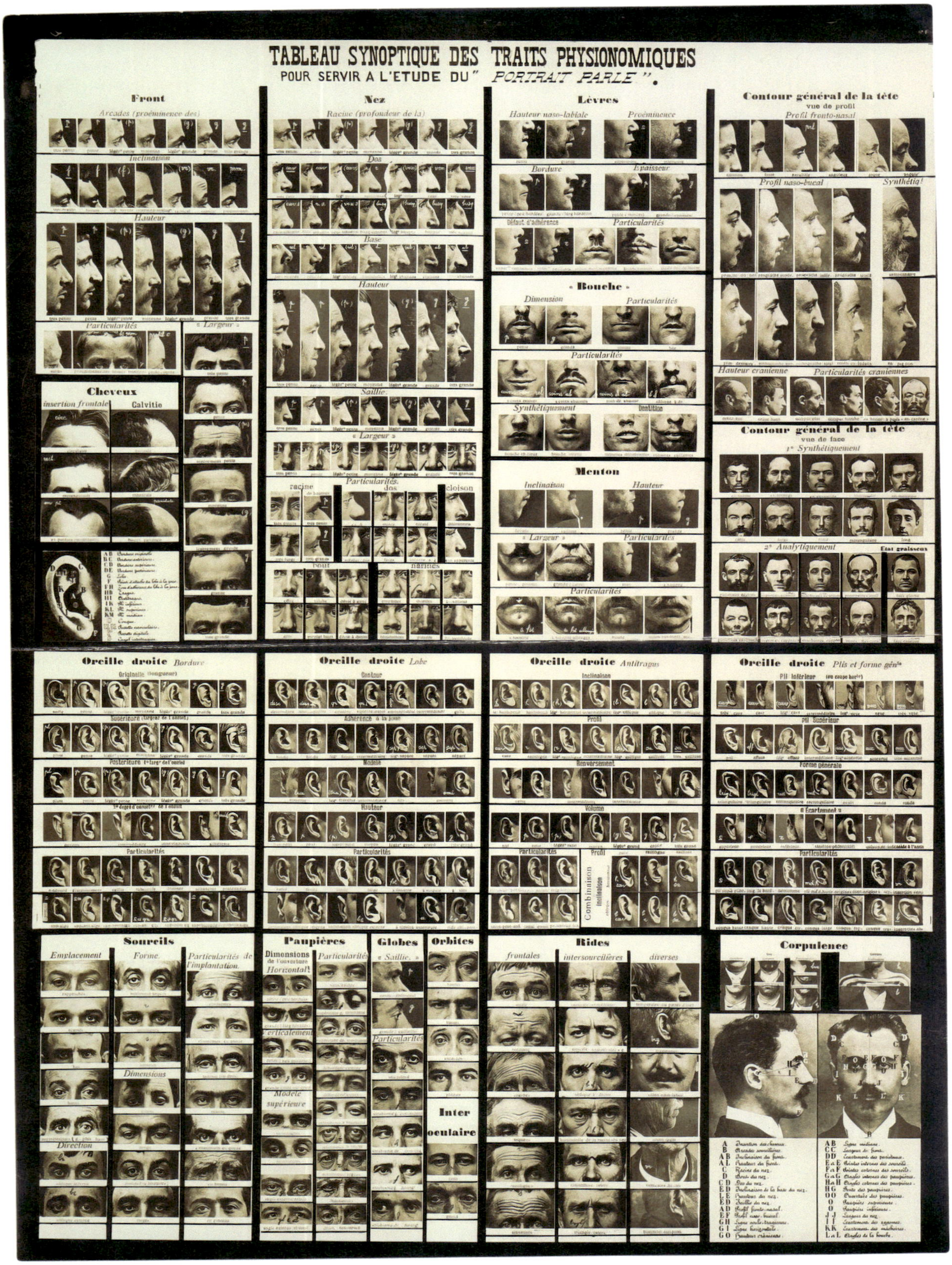

↑ Alphonse Bertillon, *Tableau synoptique des traits physionomiques: pour servir à l'étude du "portrait parlé,"* ca. 1909.

At the inauguration of the First Brazilian Congress of Eugenics in July of 1929, the physician and anthropologist Edgar Roquette-Pinto addressed an audience preoccupied with the question of how a country as vast as Brazil could best increase and improve its population. To accomplish this, Roquette-Pinto exalted "eugenia" as the new science that, together with medicine and hygiene, would guarantee the efficiency and perfection of the race.[1] With the following words, the Brazilian scientist underscored a positivist agenda that brought architecture to the very core of eugenics—the so-called science of race improvement: "It is critical to emphasize that the influence [on our race] does not stem from the natural environment but rather from the artificial environment, created by man."[2] With these opening remarks, Roquette-Pinto called attention to the crucial role played by the built environment in the "amelioration" of what he called "the biological patrimony" of Brazil's diverse population.[3] In an invitation to social engineering, Roquette-Pinto pointed to the environmental-genetic collusion that he hoped would bring with it the very possibility of progress.

This story begins at a global moment in which medical scientific discourses, first articulated in France, crossed the ocean and became intertwined with discourses of architecture, landscape, urban planning, and aesthetics in early twentieth-century Brazil. At the epicenter of this ideological encounter were two influential global movements, hygienics and eugenics, which became the dual vehicles for bringing architecture into active dialogue with social engineering. Conceived as a comprehensive program of reform for reconstituting and reorganizing human life, hygienics prescribed the control of human behavior, the abatement of harmful bacteria and diseases, the supply of clean water and air, and the provision of open space.[4] Eugenics, the social and biological movement that strove for nothing less than the improvement of a race, instrumentalized heredity and the environment. The form of eugenics adopted in France, and then in Brazil, was based on French naturalist Jean-Baptiste Lamarck's theory of the "inheritance of acquired characteristics," wherein evolution was driven by adaptation to environmental changes, in contrast to Mendelian eugenics, which viewed evolution as impervious to the environment and driven solely by genetics.[5] In fact, French ideas and practices of eugenics had taken root well before Francis Galton coined the very term "eugenics" (from the Greek εὐγενής, meaning "well-born") in 1883 to define the modern "science" that "deals with all influences that improve the inborn qualities of a race; also with those that develop them to the utmost advantage."[6] Fueled by increasingly urgent fears of degeneration, French physicians visualized medicine as the apparatus capable of regulating reproduction and disciplining society.

In modern Brazil, a region so culturally and scientifically influenced by France, and where medicine and the built environment were targeted as primary mechanisms of un-underdeveloping the population, it is no surprise that Lamarckian eugenics acted as a pervasive agent of modernity. The medicalization of bodies and spaces led to a normative program in which determinism—of race, gender, and the environment—contributed to a system of exclusion that was legitimized by science and materialized by architecture. The simultaneous construction of a white heterosexual society as the "normal" and desirable one, and of a healthy and modern environment that would contribute to it, consolidated the clinical agenda of architectural modernism.[7] Although this strategy was central to modernism at large, a specific transatlantic and interdisciplinary network of global actors, scientific theories, and spatial practices placed architecture at the center of eugenics' agenda of white supremacy in Brazil.[8]

Practicing Utopia

Influenced by the power of medical science and architecture's instrumentalization of nature, hygienic and eugenic practices became complicit in the process of constructing modern nations in the New World. In Brazil, the nation was seen as a sick organism, and reformers—including social scientists, architects, and urban planners—were tantamount to physicians with the responsibility of diagnosis and treatment. In the center of Rio de Janeiro, this mission brought together a diverse cast of characters: from the physicians and architects of the Parisian Musée Social, the early French think-tank that sought to undertake France's pressing "social question," to the physicians and architects of Rio de Janeiro who formulated the theories, practices, and ethos of Brazilian modernism, to Le Corbusier, who began consolidating a eugenicist ideology precisely during the months he spent in Brazil in the mid-1930s.[9]

In the early 1920s, a dramatic event occurred in Rio. The battle against bubonic plague, yellow fever, and other tropical diseases had led to sanitary and urban reform that reached its climax with the demolition of an entire populated mountain, the Morro do Castelo, in the center of the Brazilian capital.[10] This mountain was no ordinary mountain, however; it was the original site of the colonial city, where its historical buildings and institutions had first been established in 1567. But the idea of eliminating the mountain was not new. As far back as 1798, a medical report had argued for the mountain's demolition, since according to the author it acted as an enormous barrier that blocked the circulation of air from the sea, consequently facilitating the proliferation of diseases.[11] But it was not until the 1920s, when aesthetic and moral imperatives were added to sanitary ones, that the mountain came to be seen as the very

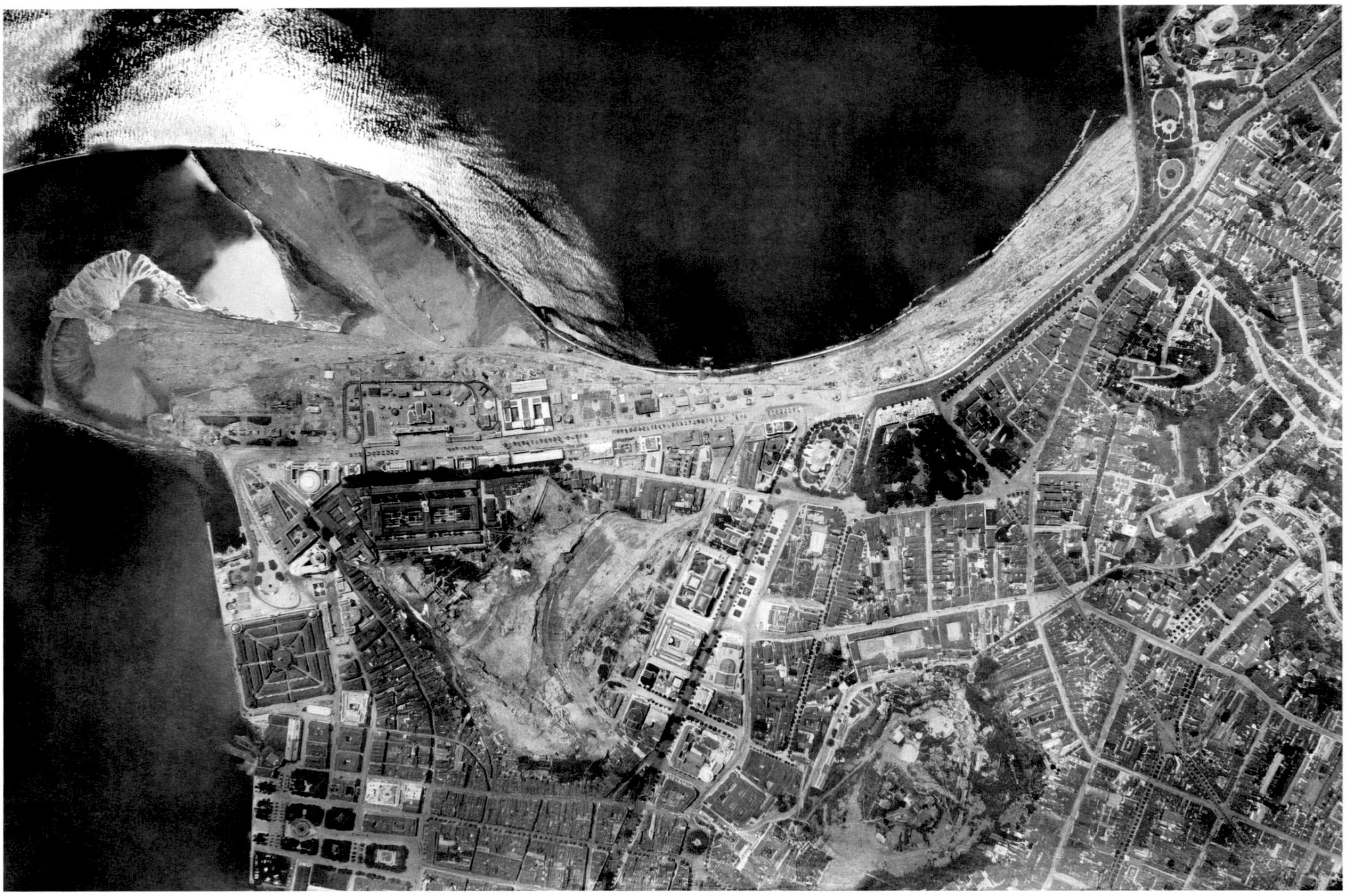

negation of modernity itself; a reservoir of vice and disease with a motley "marginal" population, including poor Blacks and formerly enslaved people who, according to the elites, invaded the center of the city "with their embarrassing practices of superstition and misery."[12] At that time, medicine was the principal tool used by the Brazilian government and scientific elites to study and then reconfigure the national population. It was only when hygiene—until then understood as personal or environmental—became social hygiene—an economic science concerned with the outputs of human capital (production and reproduction)—that the demolition of the Morro do Castelo became possible.

The demolition of Morro do Castelo represented the first and most radical action in the construction of a new national image, free of backward associations and racial exoticism. The extensive territory that resulted from this demolition was immediately occupied by the 1922 International Exhibition. Commemorating the hundredth anniversary of Brazil's independence, the exhibition was conceived as a self-portrait of a modern nation—a nation that undertook a self-remaking process, not only of its milieu but also of its population. Promoting this nation as a tabula rasa, the exhibition represented a literal "triumph" over the territory—a territory now cleansed of its history and unwanted inhabitants. Its more than 500-page catalog is striking in its complete elimination of all traces of the African and Indigenous components of Brazilian culture.[13] With the exception of one article briefly mentioning the abolition of slavery, the catalog presents Brazil as a white country. Its images demonstrate a new alliance between beauty, health, tropicality, and modernization that Brazilian elites adopted to represent themselves and their new nation. In most publicity materials, white men, women, and children of classic Greco-Roman appearance, wearing red or white robes and crowns, were arranged against European-looking hills and gardens to frame the architecture and machinery of modern factories.

Just as human beings were portrayed as icons of the ideal, so too were natural monuments released from their tropical fatality, politicized as new icons of collective identity and moralized as elements of transformation. Several advertisements in the catalog exalt the natural monuments of Rio de Janeiro, particularly those that were human-made or human-dominated. An advertisement for a medication, for instance, portrays the Pão de Açúcar as one of the Seven Wonders of the World.[14] The catalog also celebrates Corcovado, the extraordinary mountain at the center of the Tijuca Forest and the

← Centennial Exhibition of 1922, Esplanade Morro do Castelo, Rio de Janeiro.

→ Augusto Malta, Demolition of Morro do Castelo, Rio de Janeiro, June 1, 1922.

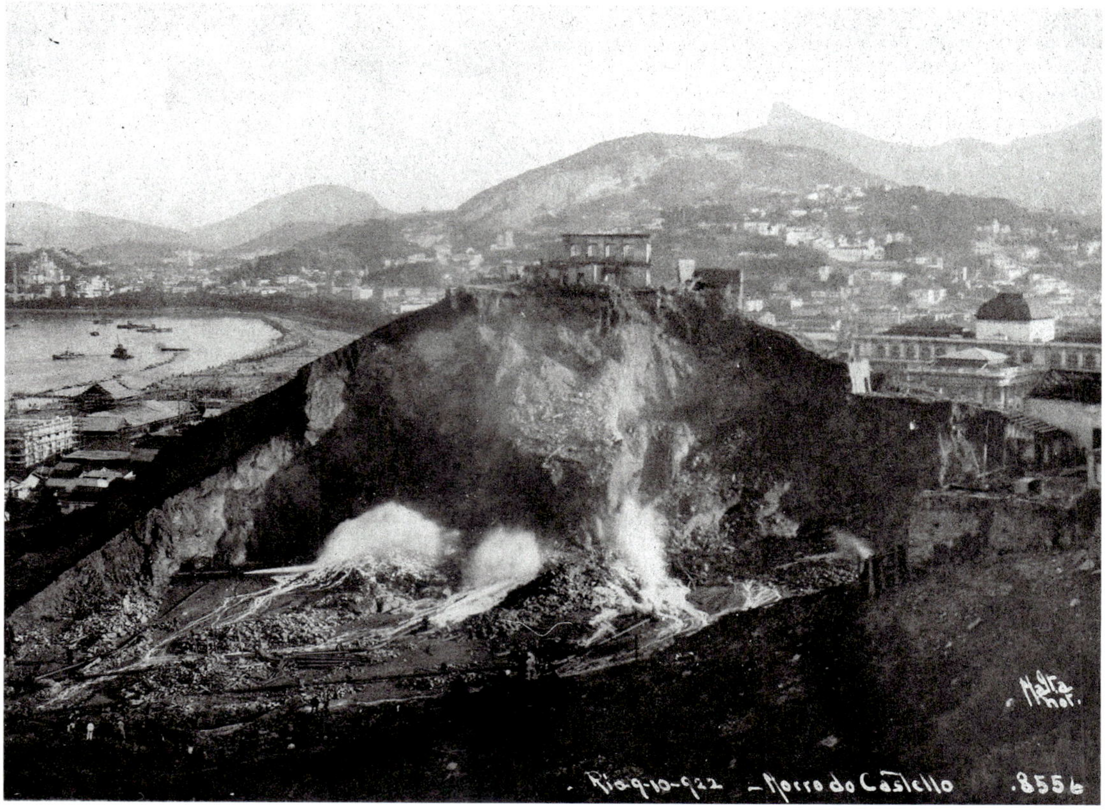

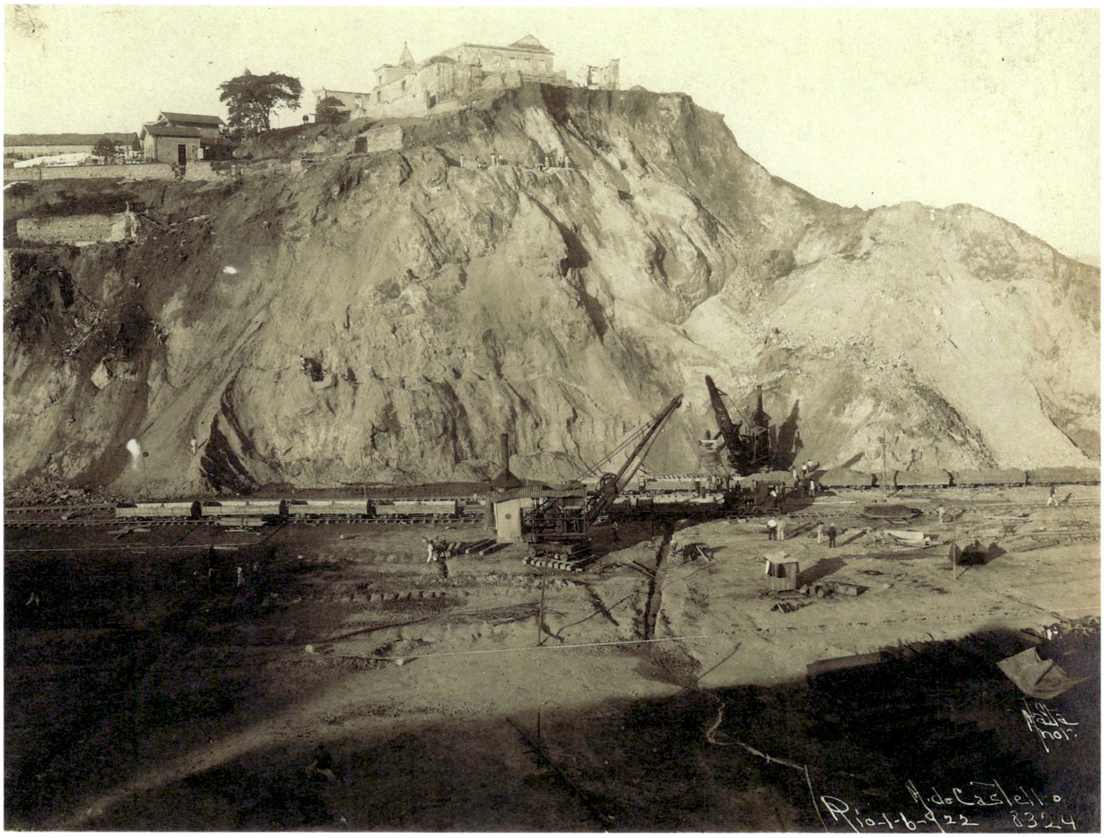

↓ Advertisements published in *O Livro de Ouro: Comemorativo do Centenário da Independência do Brasil e da Exposição Internacional do Rio de Janeiro* (Rio de Janeiro: Edição do Annuario do Brasil, 1923).

world's largest human-made urban rainforest which, only a few years later, would be crowned with the monumental forty-meter-tall statue of Christ the Redeemer.[15] By razing the Morro do Castelo while transforming these two other mountains within the city into sites of aesthetic pleasure, tropical nature—now monumentalized—is portrayed as a site of interplay between the body, labor, and technology.

The exhibition represented not only a triumph over nature, but a triumph over degeneration. The First Brazilian Congress for the Protection of Infants, an essential part of the exhibition, was an agent of Brazil's transformation of puericulture, the French faith-based science, into a neo-Lamarckian form of eugenics.[16] Debates in the congress focused on the importance of puericulture—the term that Adolphe Pinard, the French physician and member of the Parisian Musée Social, revitalized as a human analogue for agriculture, for the scientific cultivation of the mother-child unit.[17] Echoing Pinard, Brazilian physicians were convinced that "a child was the result of two forces in equilibrium: heredity and milieu," and that, consequently, puericulture was "one of the most accessible ways of conserving and perfecting the human species" while also whitening the population.[18]

While the exhibition catalog was overrun by Hellenic-looking people, the demolished mountain's footprint was suddenly overrun by neocolonial pavilions. Shortly after the exhibition in 1922, and lasting until 1938, neocolonial architecture was declared by the government to be the national style, mandatory for every building that would represent Brazil abroad.

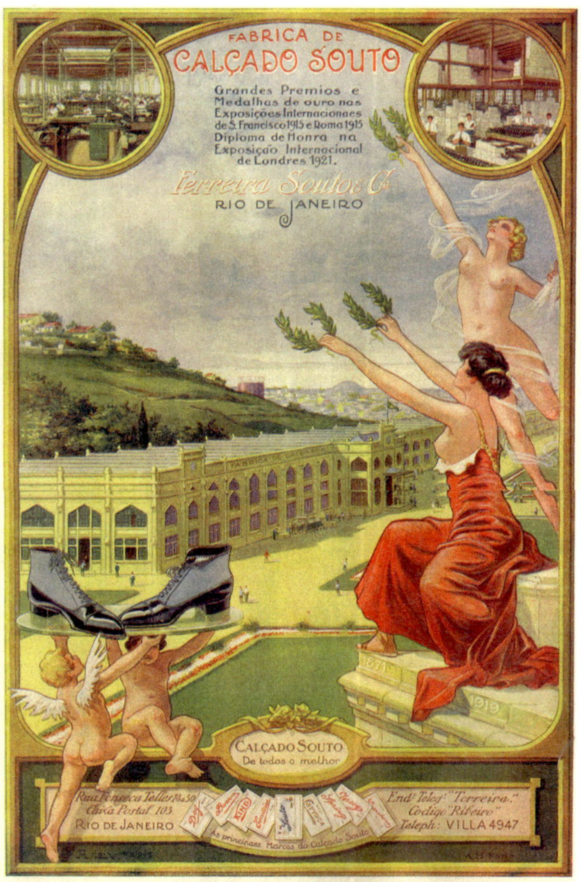

Fabrica de Calçado Souto — Rio de Janeiro.

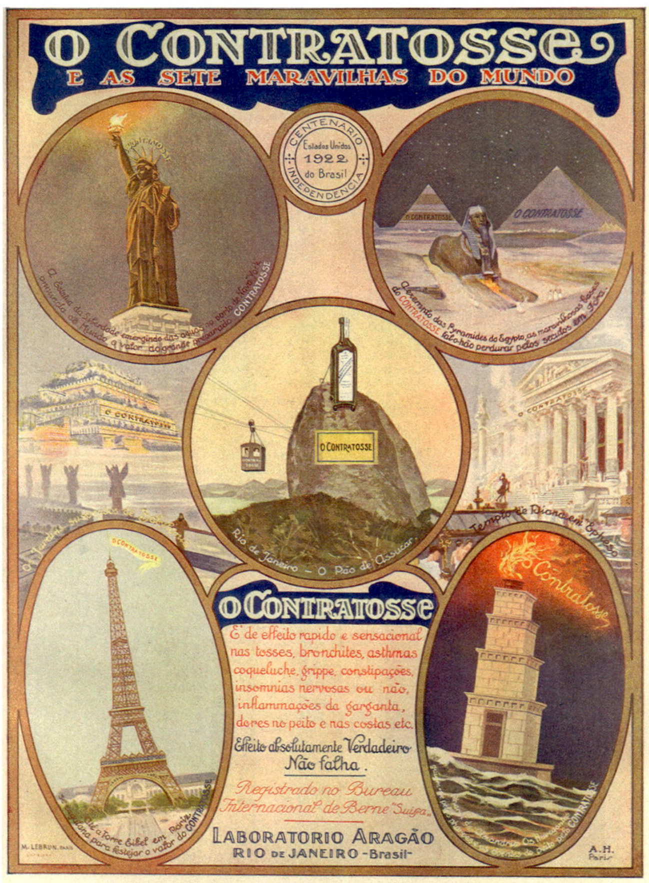

O CONTRATOSSE e as Sete Maravilhas do Mundo.

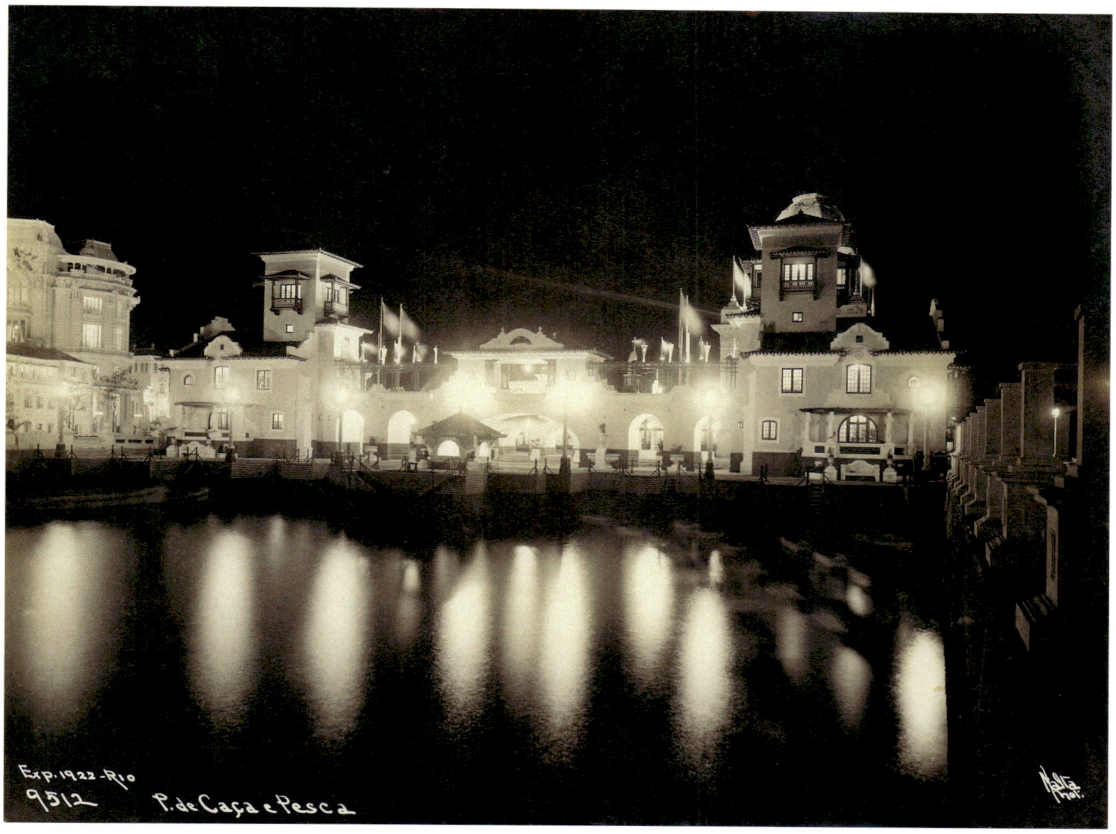

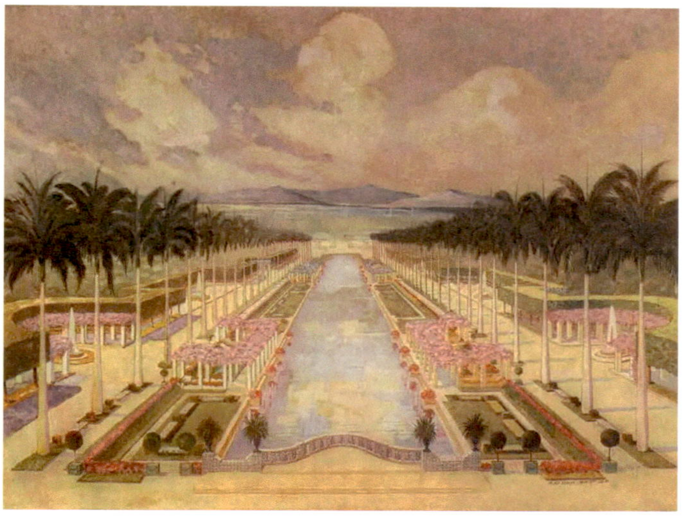

← Augusto Malta, Neocolonial Pavilion, Centennial Exhibition of 1922, Esplanade Morro do Castelo, Rio de Janeiro, 1922.

↙ Donat-Alfred Agache, Ponta do Calabouço, 1927–1930.

This requirement of presenting modern Brazil as a homogeneous white society needs to be seen alongside the omission of race as a demographic factor in every national census from 1890 to 1940, which was not the result of promoting a race-neutral society, but rather an explicit expression of the fantasy of a much-desired white Brazil.[19]

The adoption of neocolonial architecture was followed a few years later, in 1926, by an invitation to Donat-Alfred Agache, French Beaux-Arts architect and member of the Musée Social, to formulate an urban plan for the Morro do Castelo esplanade. Neocolonial and Beaux-Arts styles were interchangeable as representations of the visual ideology of the country, and Agache's invitation suggests a telling complicity between science and aesthetics in the practices of physicians and architects. Agache's proponents in Brazil were largely physicians who supported the neo-Lamarckian ideas proclaimed at the Musée Social, where both Pinard and Agache were active members.[20] Although Brazilian elites were not a homogeneous group, they seemed to agree on the image they wanted for their cities. Even Mário de Andrade, one of the main protagonists of the Semana de Arte Moderna in São Paulo, who celebrated Brazilian identity as a mixture of the European, Indigenous, and African, as well as Lúcio Costa, the architect of Brasilia, the modern capital ex-nihilo of Brazil, were both open supporters of José Mariano Filho, the Brazilian physician who became the most vehement promoter of neocolonial architecture and the main advocate for the appointment of Agache.

In 1928, in a series of articles published in *Diário Nacional*, Andrade celebrated the role of architects working for the "normalization" of the neocolonial as a Brazilian national style. In many ways, these "modern" attitudes sought to homogenize the city and its population by eradicating undesirable inhabitants and proclaiming the esplanade to be a political and economic altar to power, infused with white European forms. It was not a coincidence that the demolition of the mountain, the elimination of Rio de Janeiro's original urban nucleus, the displacement of its poor residents, and the construction of the exhibition pavilions were executed almost simultaneously with new policies and mandates such as the "white only" decree of 1921, which prohibited the immigration of Blacks to Brazil.

Why did the organizers of this exhibition select the neocolonial style to represent their new modern country in the centennial anniversary of its independence? In other words, what do these two images—white people and neocolonial architecture—have to do with one another? No one illustrates this connection between race and architecture better than Lúcio Costa—who, in 1928, made this link in a newspaper article:

> I am pessimistic about ... architecture and urbanism in general. All architecture is a question of race. When our nation is that exotic thing that we see on the streets, our architecture will inevitably be an exotic thing. It is not those half-dozen who travel and dress on Rue de la Paix, but that anonymous crowd that takes trains from Central [Station] and Leopoldina, people with sickly faces who shame us everywhere. What can we expect from people like this? Everything is a function of race. If the breed is good, and the government is good, the architecture will be good. Talk, discuss, gesticulate: our basic problem is selective immigration; the rest is secondary—it will change on its own.[21]

Neocolonial style, which was in a sense antimodernist, pro-Iberian, and "white," was thus appropriated as the emblem of progress and modernity. Costa intended for his eugenic syllogism of breed-begetting-good-government-begetting-good-architecture to also work in reverse.

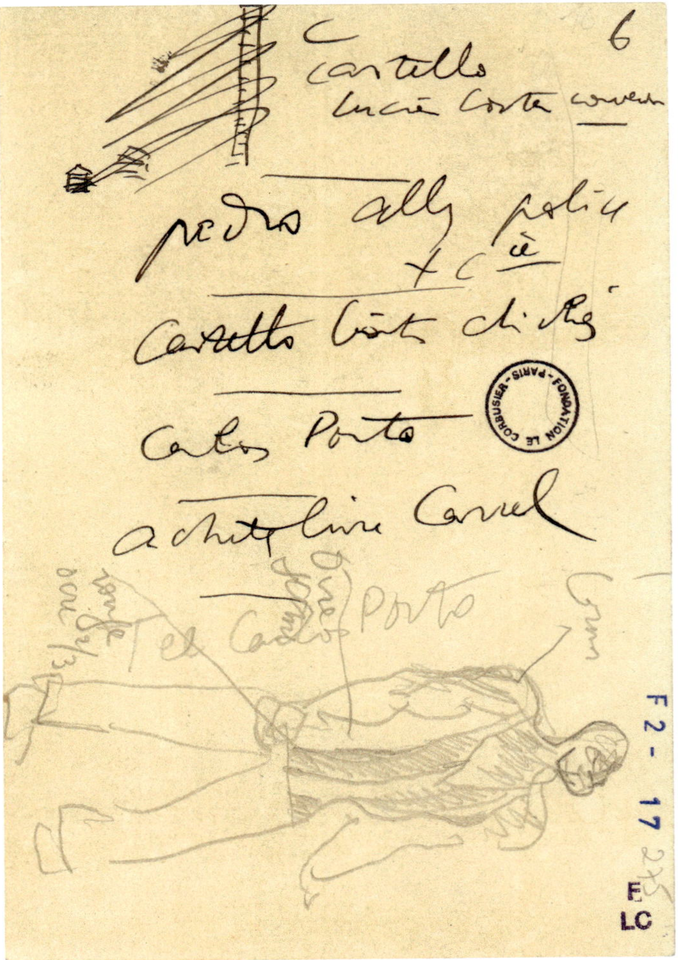

Built Biology When Le Corbusier traveled for the second time to Brazil in 1936, his discourses were centered on nature, death, and the racial and sexual "other." The fear of degeneration had haunted French society for decades, and a sense of impending death inhabited modernity.[22] For him, no other place represented this decay better than Rio de Janeiro, with its Black population and exotic tropical landscape. From the early 1930s, as an antidote to this irrevocable decay, Le Corbusier endorsed puericulture as a means of improving the quality of newborns and managing "defective" infants. As a Lamarckian of his time, he was convinced that the well-being of the child was linked to the mother's health and lineage, as well as to environmental influences. Le Corbusier intertwined pronatalist outlooks—which emphasized the traditional reproductive role of women in the family—with the built environment in which reproduction, maternity, and child rearing occurred. In a 1931 article published in the neosyndicalist journal *Plans*, he called for the establishment of special nurseries directly connected to every single dwelling, "run by qualified nurses and supervised by doctors: [to provide] security-selection-scientific child rearing—[in other words] puericulture."[23] A year later, he introduced the fourth section of an unpublished article with the conjoined term "eugénisme-puériculture."[24] This insistence on seeing eugenics and puericulture as inseparable continued for the next decade and ultimately led to his claim that "eugenics [and] puericulture will ensure a well-bred race."[25] Within this context, Le Corbusier came to believe not only that there was an intimate connection between architecture, health, and the perfection of the human race, but that he had been chosen as the primary agent to materialize this coalescence.

← Le Corbusier, notes and sketch, undated.

↓ Le Corbusier, adaptation of Lúcio Costa's sketch for the Ministry of Health and Education in Rio de Janeiro.

In 1936, while preparing a series of talks in Rio de Janeiro, Le Corbusier made a sketch on a piece of cardboard that distilled and concretized one of the most basic and accepted rationales of modernity: change the environment, change the man. Written at the top is the word "Castello," followed by the name "Lúcio Costa," the phrases "pedro aller police" and "Castello coûts clichés," the name of architect "Carlos Porto," the phrase "Acheter livre Carrel," and the sketch of a man.[26] The last phrase was a reminder for him to buy the new bestseller by the French Nobel Prize-winning physician Alexis Carrel, *Man, the Unknown* (1935), an unmistakable call for the implementation of eugenics and a manifesto for white supremacy.[27] What made Le Corbusier think of Carrel while in Rio de Janeiro? It is not a mere coincidence that Castelo, one of the most significant eugenic laboratories in Latin America, is the first word that appears on the cardboard. Castelo was not only the name of the pulverized mountain from which thousands of "undesirable" inhabitants had been displaced, or the stage for the 1922 International Exhibition with its neocolonial pavilions and its image of white Brazil, or the epicenter of the urban master plan that Agache had designed for Rio.[28] Castelo was also the name of the new building designed by Lúcio Costa for the Ministry of Health and Education, the institution charged with developing and enforcing

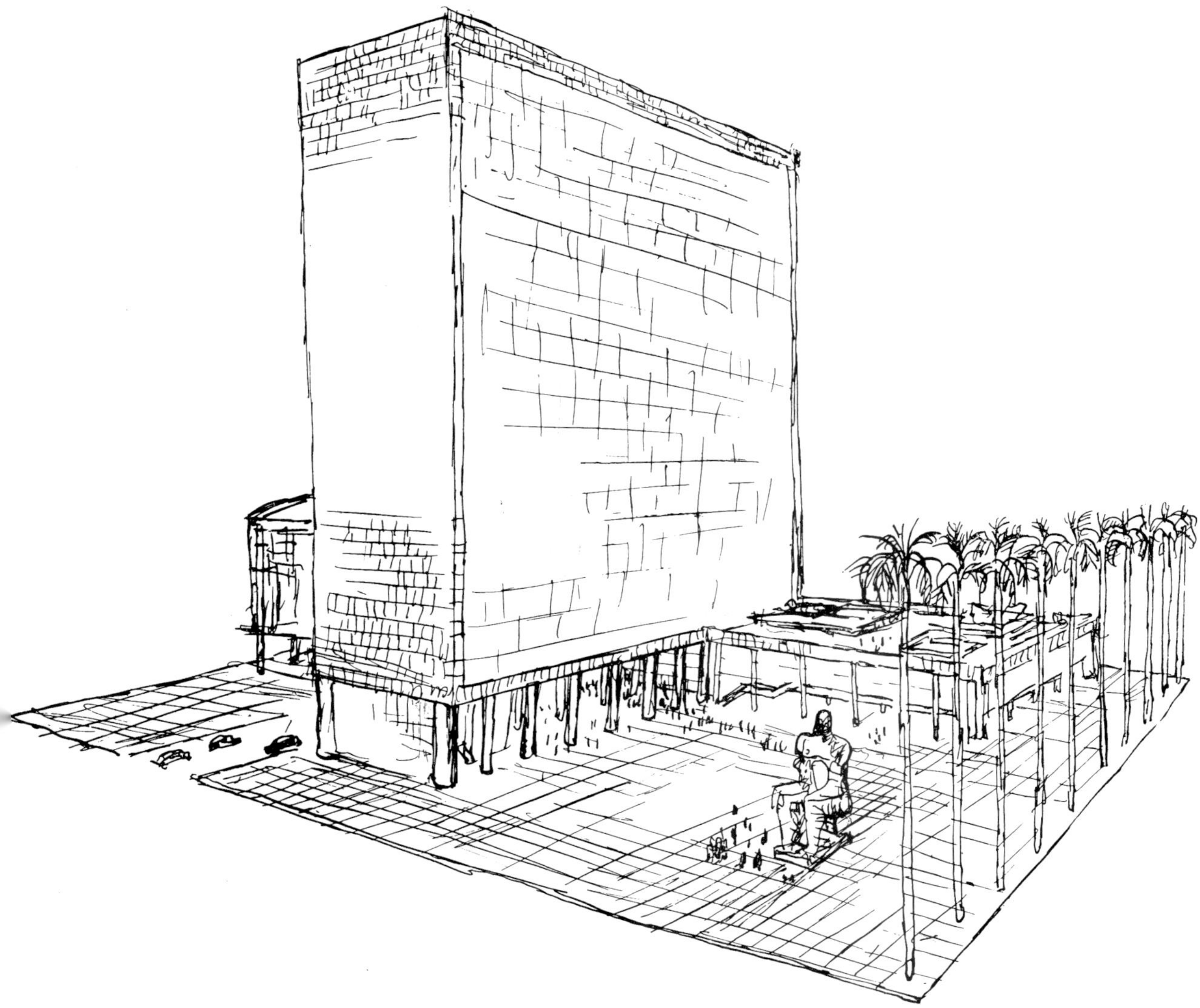

Brazil's eugenic policies under Getúlio Vargas's new authoritarian regime, for which Le Corbusier had been invited to be a design consultant. This sketch links the dramatic transformation of the urban territory of Rio de Janeiro to Lúcio Costa's project and to Carrel's vision for remaking society, along with the representation of a simple man, the ultimate object of transformation. For Le Corbusier, architecture was a tool for social engineering, an optimum medium for "the rebirth of the human body."[29]

The association between Carrel and the built environment would become the launching point for much of Le Corbusier's thinking over the next several years. But it was in Rio during that summer in 1936 that Le Corbusier directly aligned himself with Carrel's ideas. In his first talk, evoking Carrel's book, Le Corbusier commented to his audience:

> Plon, the editor who published my book [*When the Cathedrals Were White*] in North America, celebrates the success of his latest book: *Man, the Unknown* by Dr. Carrel. Write, [Plon] told me, a book that will be an echo of that one; I will do it with pleasure: the man and his shell, in other words, the habitus in which a man is obliged to pass a great portion of his life.[30]

This appears to be the very first time Le Corbusier made public reference to Carrel and his work. But the cardboard note, where he linked Carrel to Rio de Janeiro with the sketch of a man, was the spark for new theories that would become a viable doctrine for remaking man via nature, through which the built environment would be put to work.

Le Corbusier's book *La Maison des hommes* (*The House of Men*, 1942), coauthored with François de Pierrefeu and published by Plon during the Vichy regime, is this echo of Carrel's project for the remaking of society. The book begins with a stated connection between race and architecture: "It is over twenty years since, from every rostrum in France, the most authoritative voices raised the cry: 'We must build new houses, the future of our race depends on how it is housed.'" The book continues, claiming the redeeming power of the built domain "to create the necessary transformation of home life, or to infuse into it order, fecundity."[31] In the tone of a manifesto, the book emphasizes how remaking life is completely dependent on how humans are housed, whether in domestic dwellings, the workplace, the city at large, the countryside, or the metropole.

Remaking Man

In his *Oeuvre complète 1934–1938*, Le Corbusier included a sketch of Costa's Ministry of Health and Education building, depicting an open courtyard surrounded by pilotis and orderly tropical palms.[32] At its center is a colossal sculpture of a seated man with a strong, well-defined body and a tiny head.[33] Gustavo Capanema, the first Minister of Health and Education, had commissioned both the building, which he called the Ministry of Man and claimed was destined to "prepare, compose, and perfect the Brazilian man," and the sculpture, which he wanted to embody the ideal "Brazilian man" that the state itself would produce.[34] Personally invested in finding a tangible image for the ideal Brazilian genotype, Capanema pondered, "How will the body of the Brazilian man be, of the future Brazilian man, not the vulgar man or the inferior man but the best exemplar of the race? How will his head be? His color? The shape of his face? His physiognomy?"[35]

For Capanema, this sculpture would not simply be a work of art but rather a scientific tool to establish the Brazilian type: "the ideal figure that would be legitimate to imagine as representative of the future Brazilian human being."[36] To achieve this goal, Capanema looked to science. First, he turned to Francisco José de Oliveira Viana, one of the main voices of the "whitening" thesis, which argued that by mixing blacks and mulattos with whites, darker skin and "black" features would be "filtered."[37] Capanema also consulted with other scientists such as Juvenil da Rocha Vaz, Álvaro Fróes da Fonseca, and Edgar Roquette-Pinto, whose responses to Capanema's questions were extensively argued and supported by their own "scientific" studies, but who all agreed that the representation of the Brazilian man should be a white man. Roquette-Pinto in particular proposed the adoption of one of the "Leucodermos," an anthropological term he used to classify the predominant type of "whites" in Brazil. He suggested a white man with dark enough skin to look Mediterranean; "the white that would more easily 'acclimate' to Brazil."[38] According to Roquette-Pinto, the Leucodermo was the racial type toward which the "morphological evolution" of the Brazilian population was marching.[39]

Following Lúcio Costa and Le Corbusier's suggestion, Capanema asked the Brazilian artist Celso Antônio to produce the twelve-meter-high granite statue at the entrance of the Ministry building.[40] But Antônio objected to designing a figure like the one described by the scientists. He believed the Brazilian man should be the one he observed on the streets. In response, Capanema, "disgusted by the *mestizo* of rough feature ... that was taking shape in [Antônio's] atelier," invalidated their agreement and held a competition to select an artist who would take over the design of the statue.[41] The statue was never built, but the pressure to define the ideal "Brazilian man" remained on the Ministry's agenda, and the building itself, which had been created to transform a simple man into the Brazilian man, became the very embodiment of modernity.

When Le Corbusier returned to France and began collaborating with Alexis Carrel as members of Vichy committees on housing and urbanism, his vision of a clinically inspired habitat where all human needs could

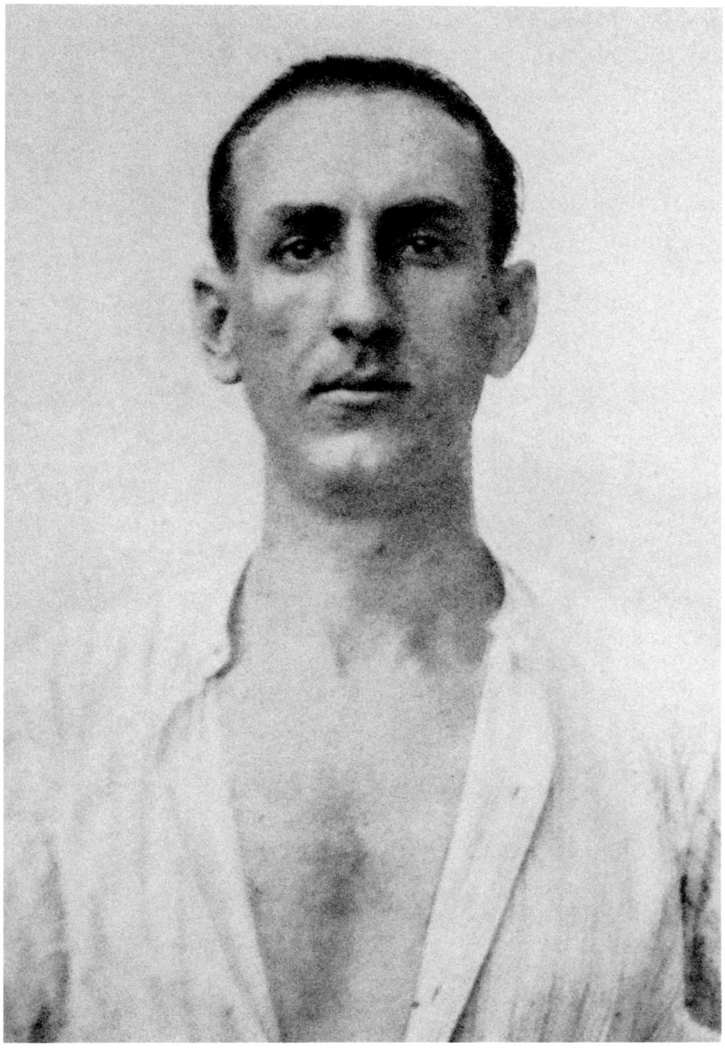

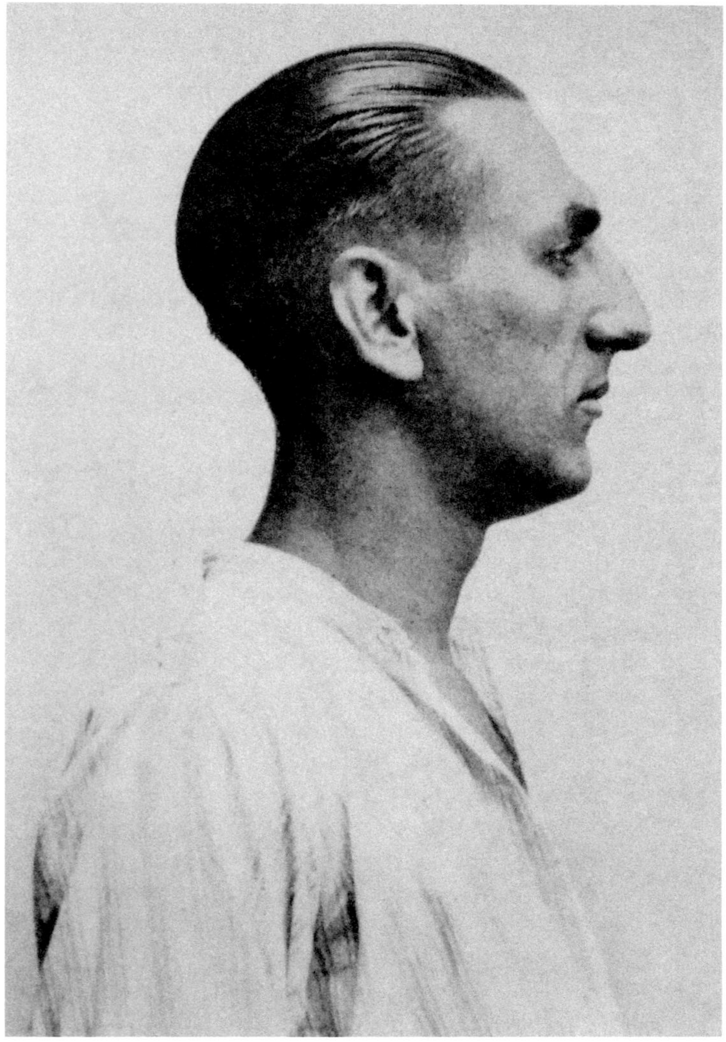

↑ "Leucodermo" type published in Edgar Roquette-Pinto's contribution to the proceedings of the First Brazilian Congress of Eugenics. "Nota sobre os typos antropológicos do Brasil," *Primeiro Congresso Brasileiro de Eugenia: Actas e Trabalhos* (Rio de Janeiro, 1929), 119–148.

be met reached a new level of specificity. For over a decade, he had looked for opportunities to assume the role of the "techno-social" international expert, a tradition initiated by the Musée Social's technocrats who, working for France and other nations, produced master plans for cities and villages in the so-called Latin world. He was convinced that the human body, the anatomo-politics of its productivity, and the built environment should be managed by the state. In a 1941 broadcast, he affirmed that "The housing problem ... is the key to both the family's regeneration and the spirit's regeneration, the key to the nation's regeneration." Collapsing milieu and heredity, he affirmed, "The degeneration of the house, the degeneration of the family, are one."[42]

For the remainder of that decade, Le Corbusier worked on universalizing the last and most blatant vestige of his modernist ideology. The Modulor—a term he invented from the word "module" and the notion of the golden section—came to life in 1946 as a way to epitomize the fruits of his doctrine.[43] Bridging both the metric and Anglo-Saxon systems, he conceived the Modulor as a six-foot-tall man with legs firmly rooted and an outstretched arm. Intended as a human model for scaling all aspects of architecture, Le Corbusier's Modulor became an antidote to disorder, an organizational scheme that infused regularity and normativity into architecture.[44] Its overly large hands and feet, so emblematic of primitivism in modern art, reference Le Corbusier's early sketches in Brazil. Representing a map of Le Corbusier's own history and his embrace of evolutionary theories, his pursuit of order, normativity, and purity, the Modulor is an enduring global symbol of architecture's past complicities with Lamarckian eugenics.

An earlier version of this essay was originally published by e-flux Architecture in 2022.

1. Edgar Roquette-Pinto, "Inaugural Session," in *Congresso Brasileiro de Eugenia, Actas e Trabalhos* (Rio de Janeiro, 1929), 12.
2. Edgar Roquette-Pinto, "Second Session," in *Congresso Brasileiro de Eugenia*, 16.
3. Roquette-Pinto, "Inaugural Session," 12.
4. Bruno Latour argues that within hygiene's ambition to reorganize society itself, there was "a mixture of urbanism, consumer protection, ecology (as we would say nowadays), defense of the environment, and moralization." Bruno Latour, *The Pasteurization of France* (Cambridge, MA: Harvard University Press, 1993), 17–23. See also Fabienne Chevallier, *Le Paris moderne: Histoire des politiques d'hygiène, 1855–1898* (Rennes: Presses universitaires de Rennes, 2010).
5. Jean-Baptiste Pierre Antoine de Monet de Lamarck, *Philosophie zoologique, ou Exposition des considérations relatives à l'histoire naturelle des animaux* (Paris, 1809).
6. Francis Galton, "Eugenics: Its Definition, Scope, and Aims," *American Journal of Sociology* 10, no.1 (1904): 1–25. This definition was first read at the London School of Economics, May 16, 1904.
7. Beatriz Colomina, in an interview with Anatxu Zabalbeascoa published in the Spanish newspaper *El País*, said that "architecture has been studied from every point of view except from the most obvious: the clinical one." Anatxu Zabalbeascoa, "Los Arquitectos buscamos Dioses para adorarlos," *El País*, April 20, 2009, http://elpais.com/diario/2009/04/20/ultima/1240178402_850215.html.
8. The core of these ideas draws from my book, Fabiola López-Durán, *Eugenics in the Garden: Transatlantic Architecture and the Crafting of Modernity* (Austin: University of Texas Press, 2018).
9. In France, the term "social question" refers to the bourgeoisie's haunting interrogation of a new form of poverty associated with the advent of industrialization, the crisis of philanthropic reform within the new liberal economy, and the impact of urban growth. At the turn of the twentieth century, the term also captured the fear of change itself, of workers and labor militancy. López-Durán, *Eugenics in the Garden*, 44.
10. The sanitary and urban reforms developed during the first decades of the century were not limited to sewage works and the opening of avenues; they also included medical policies that, among other actions, forced the population to be vaccinated for smallpox—a campaign widely rejected. Nicolau Sevcenko, *A Revolta da Vacina: Mentes insanas em corpos rebeldes* (São Paulo: Scipione, 2003); Jaime Benchimol, "Reforma urbana e revolta da vacina na cidade do Rio de Janeiro," in *O Brasil republicano: o tempo do liberalismo excludente—da Proclamação da República à Revolução de 1930*, ed. Jorge Ferreira and Lucilia de Almeida Neves Delgado (Rio de Janeiro: Civilização Brasileira, 2003); and Gilberto Hochman, *A era do saneamento: As bases da política de saúde pública no Brasil* (São Paulo: Hucitec/Ampocs, 1998).
11. In 1798, the city senate, preoccupied with the sanitary conditions of the city urban center, distributed an official questionnaire to determine the causes of endemic and epidemic diseases affecting Rio's population. In their responses, the physicians Manoel Joaquim Marreiros, Bernardino António Gomes, and António Joaquim de Medeiros judged the *morros*—the hills that emerged along the city's bays and valleys—as among the main causes of the bad circulation of air and the consequent proliferation of miasmas and other diseases. The physicians also considered that some nonnatural factors contributed to the proliferation of diseases, such as the architecture of most of the buildings that were too low-rise, humid, and poorly ventilated. They proposed the elimination of some of the hills and the construction of taller buildings. This questionnaire was first published in 1813, in the scientific and cultural newspaper *O Patriota*. See Luiz Otávio Ferreira, "Os periódicos médicos e a invenção de uma agenda sanitária para o Brasil (1827–1843)," *História, Ciências, Saúde-Manguinhos* 6, no. 2

(1999): 331–351.
12. José Antonio Nonato and Nubia Melhem Santos, *Era uma vez o Morro do Castelo* (Rio de Janeiro: IPHAN, 2000), 67.
13. *O Livro de Ouro: Comemorativo do Centenário da Independência do Brasil e da Exposição Internacional do Rio de Janeiro* (Rio de Janeiro: Edição do Annuario do Brasil, 1923), 77. Published in conjunction with the Exposição Internacional do Centenário do Brazil (Brazilian International Centennial Exhibition), held in Rio de Janeiro from September 7, 1922 to March 23, 1923.
14. *O Livro de Ouro*, 4–5.
15. The original Tijuca Forest, destroyed by the proliferation of coffee plantations, was replanted during the second half of the nineteenth century with the aim of protecting Rio de Janeiro's water resources. The Tijuca Forest in Rio covers thirty-two square kilometers, making it the largest urban forest in the world.
16. The First Brazilian Congress for the Protection of the Infants was held in Rio de Janeiro from August 27 to September 5, 1922.
17. I borrow the association between puericulture and agriculture from Jane Ellen Crisler, "Saving the Seed: The Scientific Preservation of Children in France during the Third Republic" (PhD diss., University of Wisconsin-Madison, 1984), 76. For Pinard the term puericulture refers to "the research and application of all knowledge relative to the reproduction, conservation, and improvement of the human species." Adolphe Pinard, "De la dépopulation de la France," *Revue Scientifique* (July 30, 1910): 30, quoted in Anne Carol, "Médecine et eugénisme en France, ou le rêve d'une prophylaxie parfait. XIXe–Première moitié du XXe siècle," *Revue d'histoire moderne et contemporaine* 43 (1996): 618–631.
18. Christovam Bezerra Dantas, "A Criança e a eugenía," published in the section on Sociology and Legislation in the Primeiro Congresso Brasileiro de Proteção *à* Infância, Boletim 7 (Rio de Janeiro: Imprensa Nacional, 1924), 175–179.
19. Thomas E. Skidmore, *Fact and Myth: Discovering a Racial Problem in Brazil* (São Paulo: Instituto de Estudos Avançados, 1992).
20. Lúcia Silva, "A trajetória de Alfred Agache no Brasil," in *Cidade, povo e nação: Gênese do urbanismo moderno*, ed. Luiz Cesar de Queiroz Ribeiro and Robert Pechman (Rio de Janeiro: Civilização Brasileira, 1996), 397–410; and Denise Cabral Stuckenbruck, *O Rio de Janeiro em questão: o Plano Agache e o ideário modernista dos anos 20* (Rio de Janeiro: IPPUR/FASE, 1996).
21. Lúcio Costa, "O arranha-céu e o Rio de Janeiro," *O País*, Rio de Janeiro, July 1, 1928.
22. M. Christine Boyer, *Le Corbusier: Homme de Lettres* (New York: Princeton Architectural Press, 2011), 457. See also Wendy Martin, "Remembering the Jungle: Josephine Baker and Modernist Parody," in *Prehistories of the Future: The Primitivist Project and the Culture of Modernism*, ed. Elazar Barkan and Roland Bush (Stanford: Stanford University Press, 1995), 310–325.
23. Le Corbusier, *The Radiant City* (New York: Orion Press, 1967), 115. In the original version in French, Le Corbusier uses the term *puériculture* later translated as "scientific child rearing." The original quote reads "sont confiées à des infirmières spécialisées surveillées par des médecins: sécurité—sélection—puériculture."
24. Le Corbusier, "Aménagement d'une journée équilibrée," unpublished article, dated May 1932. FLC.UE-5, 64-139.
25. In his 1945 book *Les Trois* établissements *humains*, Le Corbusier argues: "l'eugénisme, la puériculture, assurant l'élevage d'une race." Le Corbusier, *Les Trois* établissements *humains* (Paris: Les éditions de minuit, 1997), 116.
26. Le Corbusier, Notes and Sketch (n/d), Foundation Le Corbusier, document F2-17 No. 275.
27. Alexis Carrel's 1935 book was simultaneously published in French with the title *L'Homme cet inconnu*, by Plon in Paris, and in English with the title *Man, the Unknown*, by the American publisher Harper & Brothers, which also sold the rights to publish condensed chapters of the book in the popular American magazine *Reader's Digest* (which, by the mid-1930s, had a circulation of over 1.5 million copies), contributing to the book's commercial success. In this book, Carrel explicitly defends the elimination of defectives and criminals, and even recommends the use of gas chambers to accomplish this goal. See Andrés Horacio Reggiani, "Alexis Carrel, the Unknown: Eugenics and Population Research under Vichy," *French Historical Studies* 25 (2002): 331–356.
28. In June 1927, during his first lecture in Rio, Agache introduced himself as a physician, and "Mademoiselle Carioca" (the name he gave to Rio de Janeiro) as a single woman who required treatment and discipline. Clearly, he conceived his master plan as a medical treatment for a capital city cleansed of diseases and "undesirables," and therefore suitable for Europeans. Agache argued, "I want you to see me as a kind of doctor who has been consulted and who is more than pleased to bring his knowledge to bear and to be able to make use of it in his consideration of this pathological case submitted for examination. I say pathological case because Mademoiselle Carioca is certainly sick. But do not be afraid since her illness is not congenital: it is one that is curable, because it is an illness that consists of a growth crisis. ... What to do? A physician needs to prescribe a severe regime, a model of progress and discipline, and urgently provide her with a regulatory plan that allows her to blossom favorably." Donat-Alfred Agache, *Cidade do Rio de Janeiro. Extensão, remodelação, embellezamento* (Paris: Foyer Brésilien, 1930), 5, 21.
29. Le Corbusier, *The Radiant City*, 7.
30. Le Corbusier, Manuscript Lecture I, Rio de Janeiro, Brazil (07/1936–08/1936), FLC F2-17, Paris, 5.
31. Le Corbusier and François de Pierrefeu, *The Home of Man* (London: Architectural Press, 1948), 13.
32. Le Corbusier and Pierre Jeanneret, *Oeuvre complète 1934–1938* (Zurich: Editions Girsberger, 1953).
33. This sketch is an adaptation of the one Costa sent to Le Corbusier in July 1937. However, the colossal seated and naked man was already included in a report Le Corbusier submitted to Minister Capanema regarding the construction of the Ministry of Health and Education and the University City Campus for Rio de Janeiro. In this report, dated August 10, 1936, Le Corbusier argues that the ministry building should be located off the coast (at Praia Santa Luzia), rather than on the site of the esplanade proposed by Rio's Director of Public Works Marques Porto, the site where the Morro do Castelo once stood. Fundação Getulio Vargas, Arquivo Gustavo Capanema, Série F, 34.10.19, II-30, Rio de Janeiro.
34. Gustavo Capanema, letter to Getúlio Vargas, dated June 14, 1937. Arquivo Gustavo Capanema, Série F, 34.10.19, III-9, Fundação Getúlio Vargas, Rio de Janeiro.
35. Gustavo Capanema, letter to Oliveira Viana dated August 30, 1937, published in Mauricio Lissovsky and Paulo Sérgio Moraes de Sá, *Colunas da educação: A construção do Ministério da Educação e Saúde* (Rio de Janeiro: Fundação Getúlio Vargas CPDOC, 1996), 225.
36. Lissovsky and Moraes de Sá, *Colunas da educação*, 225–229.
37. Brazilians saw miscegenation not as a menace but as a solution—as the vehicle for "wiping out the black" and consequently "whitening" the country. Thomas E. Skidmore, *Fact and Myth: Discovering a Racial Problem in Brazil* (São Paulo: Instituto de Estudos Avançados, 1992).
38. Edgar Roquette-Pinto, letter to Gustavo Capanema dated August 30, 1937 published in Lissovsky and Moraes de Sá, *Colunas da educação,* 226.
39. Roquette-Pinto was the first anthropologist to create a system of classification of racial types in Brazil. In his paper "Note on the Anthropological Types of Brazil," Roquette-Pinto classifies the Brazilian population in four main groups: the "white type" or Leucodermo, representing fifty-one percent of the population; the "mulatto type" (descendants of mixing whites and Blacks) or Phaiodermo, representing the twenty-two percent; the "Caboclo type" (descendants of mixing whites and Indians) or Xanthodermo, representing the eleven percent; and the "Black type" or Melanodermo, representing fourteen percent of the population. As opposed to Oliveira Vianna, Roquette-Pinto rejected the idea that mixed races were degenerate or inferior types, although he accepted that they were, as well as the Blacks and the Indigenous, less beautiful than the Caucasian type. Roquette-Pinto, "Nota sobre os typos anthropológicos do Brasil," in *Primeiro Congresso Brasileiro de Eugenia: Actas e trabalhos*, vol. 1 (Rio de Janeiro: 1929), 119–148.
40. Celso Antônio was Costa's collaborator in his effort to reform the curriculum of the National School of Fine Arts in the early 1930s. In the 1920s he had been a disciple of the celebrated French sculptor Antoine Bourdelle. Costa and Bourdelle recommended Antônio as the project's sculptor, and in his letter to Capanema, Le Corbusier approved the selection of the Brazilian sculptor to model the "Brazilian Man." Le Corbusier, letter to Capanema dated December 30, 1937, published in Lissovsky and Moraes de Sá, *Colunas da educação*, 139–140.
41. M. Paulo Filho, "Homem Brasileiro," *Correio da Manhã*, September 23, 1938, 4.
42. Le Corbusier, *Destin de Paris* (Clermont-Ferrand: Fernand Sorlot, 1941), 60.
43. Le Corbusier, *The Modulor: A Harmonious Measure to the Human Scale Universally Applicable to Architecture and Mechanics* (London: Faber & Faber, 1956), 76–80.
44. Although this work began in the 1920s, it was not until the 1940s that it was codified under the influence of the Commissariat à la Normalisation, the committee for standards of the Order of Architects. Jean-Louis Cohen, "Le Corbusier's Modulor and the Debate on Proportion in France," *Architectural Histories* 2 (2014), http://doi.org/10.5334/ah.by.

ACKNOWLEDGMENTS

Many thanks to all the students, scholars, architects, and artists who have been vital to this ongoing project. In particular, Iván López Munuera, a teaching assistant of the first two seminars who also contributed to the editing of the students' papers for the first e-flux Architecture series. Nick Axel has been crucial to the project, bringing great energy and insight to both his editing of the series for e-flux Architecture and the essays that appear in this book. Guillermo S. Arsuaga has played a key role in the development of this volume, collaborating with authors in image research and shepherding grant applications together with Dante Furioso. Nikolaus Hirsch was an extraordinary partner in the e-flux Architecture series and as co-curator of the *Sick Architecture* exhibition at CIVA. Thanks also to Silvia Franceschini, curator of contemporary architecture at CIVA, for her vital participation in the exhibition, and Kersten Geers and Jelena Pančevac from OFFICE KGDVS for their unique exhibition design. All the CIVA staff, including Francis Carpentier and Stéphanie De Blieck, were remarkable.

Throughout this project, Monica Ponce de Leon, Dean of the School of Architecture at Princeton, has been unwaveringly supportive. We also want to express our deep gratitude to our colleagues within and beyond the university, particularly Sylvia Lavin, Francesca Hughes, James Graham, Dennis Pohl, and Mark Wigley.

Over the years, the project has been the recipient of financial support from many departments and centers at Princeton, including the Andlinger Center for Energy and Environment, the Center for Collaborative History, the Department of Art and Archeology, the Department of Comparative Literature, the East Asian Studies Program, the German Department, the Global Health Program at the School of Public and International Affairs, the Interdisciplinary Doctoral Program in the Humanities (IHUM), Princeton Institute for International and Regional Studies (PIIRS), the Program in Latin American Studies (PLAS), the Program in Media and Modernity (M+M), and the University Center for Human Values. In 2022, the Sick Architecture project received a Magic Grant from Princeton University's Humanities Council.

The publication of this book has been made possible by the generous support of the Barr Ferree Foundation Fund for Publications at Princeton University, the Graham Foundation for Advanced Studies in the Fine Arts, the Princeton University School of Architecture, and the Creative Industries Fund NL.

The editors are most grateful to Thomas Weaver and Victoria Hindley at the MIT Press for so thoughtfully guiding the material from draft to book, to Sarah Handelman and Matthew Abbate for their sensitive copyediting, and to Rosa Nussbaum for her inspiring design.

CONTRIBUTORS

Emily Apter is Julius Silver Professor of French and Comparative Literature at New York University and Chair of the Department of French Literature, Thought and Culture. Her books include *Unexceptional Politics: On Obstruction, Impasse and the Impolitic* (Verso, 2018); *Against World Literature: On the Politics of Untranslatability* (Verso, 2013); *Dictionary of Untranslatables: A Philosophical Lexicon* (Princeton, 2014), *coedited with Barbara Cassin, Jacques Lezra, and Michael Wood; and The Translation Zone: A New Comparative Literature* (Princeton, 2006). Her upcoming book, *What Is Just Translation?*, takes up questions of translation and justice across media.

Guillermo S. Arsuaga is an architect and PhD candidate in History and Theory of Architecture at Princeton University. He was a 2022–2023 Mellon-Marron Research Consortium Fellow at the Museum of Modern Art, New York. His research investigates how architecture and island territories shape spaces of exception and project imperial power, focusing on the late Francoist dictatorship in Spain.

Nick Axel is Deputy Editor of e-flux Architecture and the Head of the Architectural Design department at Gerrit Rietveld Academie.

Victoria Bergbauer is a PhD candidate in the Department of History at Princeton University. Her dissertation will offer the first transnational history of the formerly incarcerated.

Xhulio Binjaku is a PhD candidate in History and Theory of Architecture of Architecture at Princeton University. His research focuses on the interdisciplinary histories of geography and architecture.

Gideon Boie is an architect-philosopher, cofounder of the BAVO collective, and visiting professor at the KU Leuven Faculty of Architecture. His most recent edited volume is *Living in Monnikenheide: Care, Inclusion and Architecture* (Flanders Architecture Institute, 2023).

Edna Bonhomme is a historian of science and culture writer based in Berlin. She is the coeditor of *After Sex* (Silver Press, 2023) and the author of *A History of the World in Six Plagues* (Simon and Schuster, 2025) which explores the relationship between captivity and contagion. She holds a PhD in History of Science from Princeton University.

Ibiayi Briggs is a PhD candidate in History and Theory of Architecture at Princeton University. Her research follows the ways race and technology have worked together to shape the ideals and practices of modern architecture, particularly the role of blackness as a spectral presence in this history.

Angela H. Brown is a writer and editor based in Brooklyn. They are a PhD candidate in the Department of Art & Archaeology at Princeton University, focusing on textiles, modern craft practices, and anticolonial pedagogy, especially in the Caribbean and Latin America.

Holly Bushman is a PhD candidate in History and Theory of Architecture at Princeton University. She studies intellectual exchange and cultural diplomacy in twentieth-century Eastern and Central Europe.

Beatriz Colomina is the Howard Crosby Butler Professor of the History of Architecture at Princeton University. Her books include *X-Ray Architecture* (Lars Müller, 2019), *Are We Human? Notes on an Archaeology of Design* (Lars Müller, 2016) with Mark Wigley, *Domesticity at War* (Actar and MIT, 2007), *Privacy and Publicity: Modern Architecture as Mass Media* (MIT, 1994), and *Sexuality and Space* (Princeton Architectural Press, 1992). Her coedited volumes include *Radical Pedagogies* (MIT, 2022) and *Clip/Stamp/Fold* (Actar, 2010).

e-flux Architecture is an archive and editorial project founded by Nikolaus Hirsch and Anton Vidokle in 2016. e-flux Architecture describes strains of critical discourse surrounding contemporary architecture, culture, and theory internationally.

Clemens Finkelstein is a Research Associate at the Panel on Planetary Thinking of the University Giessen, a Fellow at the Princeton Institute for International and Regional Studies, and a PhD candidate in History and Theory of Architecture at Princeton University. His book *Planetary Forest* (DISTANZ, 2024) documents a recent art project with bioscientists and geoscientists.

Dante Furioso is an architect and PhD candidate in History and Theory of Architecture at Princeton University. His dissertation investigates the way plantations structured the nineteenth-century urbanization of Havana, focusing on the relationship between race and class with building materials and craft during the time of slavery and postslavery.

David Gissen is Professor of Architecture and Urban History at The New School in New York City. His books include *The Architecture of Disability* (Minnesota, 2023), *Manhattan Atmospheres* (Minnesota, 2014), and *Subnature: Architecture's Other Environments* (Princeton Architectural Press, 2009).

Samia Henni is a historian of the built, destroyed, and imagined environments. She is the author of *Architecture of Counterrevolution: The French Army in Northern Algeria* (gta, 2017) and *Colonial Toxicity: Rehearsing French Radioactive Architecture and Landscape in the Sahara* (fink, 2024), and the editor of *Deserts Are Not Empty* (Columbia, 2022) and *War Zones* (gta, 2018). She received her PhD in History and Theory of Architecture from ETH Zurich.

Brooke Holmes is the Susan Dod Brown Professor of Classics at Princeton University, where she is also Director of the Gauss Seminars in Criticism. She is the author of *The Symptom and the Subject: The Emergence of the Physical Body in Ancient Greece* (Princeton, 2010) and *Gender: Antiquity and Its*

Legacy (Bloomsbury, 2012). She is currently completing a book entitled *Sympathy and the Tissue of the World: Life, Community, and Nature in the Ancient Mediterranean.*

Patrick Jaojoco is a Filipino (Tagalog/Bisayan) American writer, organizer, musician, and PhD candidate in History and Theory of Architecture at Princeton University. His dissertation will explore Philippine experiments in civic and environmental development through the twentieth century as continuations of global empire.

Angelika Ellen Joseph is a dual-degree PhD Candidate in the History and Theory of Architecture and Humanistic Studies at Princeton University. She is a former Mellon Fellow in Democracy and Landscapes at Harvard University's Dumbarton Oaks, and is the incoming Charles Eastman Fellow in the Department of Native American and Indigenous Studies at Dartmouth College. Joseph's dissertation examines Native American activists' takeovers of colonial landscapes as a method of protest from 1969 to 1973.

Rebecca Kellawan is a historical archaeologist specializing in race, colonialism, infrastructure, and the built environment in the Americas. She is currently a PhD candidate in History and Theory of Architecture at Princeton University.

Johan Lagae is professor at Ghent University, where he teaches twentieth-century architectural history with a global focus. He holds a PhD on colonial architecture in the Democratic Republic of Congo and has published widely on the topic, as well as on urban history in Central Africa, on colonial built heritage, and on photography in (post)colonial Africa. Recently he coedited the volume *African Modernism and Its Afterlives* (Intellect, 2022).

Fabiola López-Durán is an associate professor of art and architectural history at Rice University. She is the author of *Eugenics in the Garden: Transatlantic Architecture and the Crafting of Modernity* (Texas, 2018), which received a SAH/Mellon Author Award in 2018 and the Robert Motherwell Book Prize in 2019. She earned her PhD in history, theory, and criticism of architecture from MIT.

Iván López Munuera is a New York-based scholar, critic, and curator working at the intersection of culture, technology, politics, and bodily practices in the modern period and on the global stage. He is an assistant professor at Bard College. He has exhibited his research widely and curated many exhibitions, including at La Casa Encendida (Madrid), Maat Lisbon, Museo Reina Sofía (Madrid), and CA2M (Mostoles).

Simon De Nys-Ketels is a postdoctoral researcher at the Université Libre de Bruxelles. He holds a PhD from Ghent University in which he questioned tenacious myths of Belgian Congo as a "medical model colony" by confronting bureaucratic procedures and ambitions behind medical architecture with the everyday realities of colonial hospitals.

Victoria Bugge Øye is Senior Curator of Architecture at the National Museum of Art, Architecture and Design in Oslo. Her research focuses on the intersections of post-1945 American and European architecture with the discourses of science, medicine, and psychology. She holds a PhD in the History and Theory of Architecture from Princeton University.

Kara Morgan Plaxa Arxa is a PhD candidate in the History and Theory of Architecture program at Princeton University, investigating the intersections of gender, sexualities, and queer leather communities in American urban landscapes.

Elizabeth A. Povinelli is Franz Boas Professor of Anthropology and Gender Studies, an affiliate of the Institute of Comparative Literature and Society, Australian Academy of the Humanities, Corresponding Fellow, and one of the founding members of the Karrabing Film Collective. Her books include *Routes/Worlds* (e-flux and Sternberg, 2022), *Between Gaia and Ground* (Duke, 2021), *The Inheritance* (Duke, 2021), *Geontologies* (Duke, 2016), *Economies of Abandonment* (Duke, 2011), *The Empire of Love* (Duke, 2006), and *The Cunning of Recognition* (Duke, 2002).

Karel Proot holds a master's degree in history from Ghent University. He is part of Breekijzer, a nonprofit bridging the environmental and spatial planning sectors. His research explores the deployment of new chemical technologies in colonial Congo.

Giuseppina Scavuzzo is an architect living in Venice. She is associate professor in Architectural and Urban Design at the University of Trieste where she serves as Director of the Master's Degree Course in Architecture. She holds a PhD in Architectural Design from the University Iuav of Venice. Her books include *Il Parco della guarigione infinita* (Letteraventidue, 2020).

Nicholas Shapiro is a multidisciplinary environmental researcher that studies, and designs interventions into, issues of chemical contamination and climate change. He is Assistant Professor at UCLA's Institute for Society & Genetics, and is the director of Carceral Ecologies, a lab focused on the environmental health conditions of carceral institutions.

Shivani Shedde is an architect and a PhD candidate in History and Theory of Architecture at Princeton University who specializes in histories of colonialism and anticolonialism across the Afro-Asian world.

Maxwell Smith-Holmes is a PhD candidate in History and Theory of Architecture at Princeton University who researches the economy and ecology of built environments and their representations.

Iason Stathatos is an architect and a PhD candidate in History and Theory of Architecture at Princeton University whose research focuses on the intertwined relationship between architecture and archaeology in colonized territories during the nineteenth and twentieth centuries.

An Tairan is a PhD candidate in History and Theory of Architecture at Princeton University. He is the recipient of a Citation of Special Recognition of the 2023 Graham Foundation Carter Manny Writing Award. His dissertation targets how a group of research institutions and field stations established for the scientific observation of nature in mid- to late nineteenth-century Italy incidentally mediated and redefined the natural world.

Meredith TenHoor is an architectural and urban historian and Professor in the School of Architecture at Pratt Institute. She is also editor, a founding board member, and former chair of the Aggregate Architectural History Collaborative. Her publications include *Toxics* (Aggregate, 2022), *Black Lives Matter* (Aggregate, 2015), *Street Value: Shopping, Planning and Politics at Fulton Mall* (Princeton, 2010), and a forthcoming book about the design history and political economies of French food systems.

Marie de Testa is an architect, a set designer for theater and performance, and a PhD candidate in History and Theory of Architecture at Princeton University rethinking the role of theater in the development of modern architecture.

Jessica Varner is an assistant professor at the University of Pennsylvania, Department of Landscape and Regional Planning, Stuart Weitzman School of Design. She works collectively on alternatives and repair in toxics with A People's EPA (cofounder), Environmental Data & Governance Initiative, and Coming Clean. She holds a PhD in the History of Art and Architecture from MIT, and is working with the University of Chicago Press on her forthcoming book *Chemical Desires: When the Chemical Industry Met Modern Design* (1870–1970).

Mark Wigley is Professor of Architecture and Dean Emeritus at Columbia University. He is a historian, theorist, and critic who explores the intersection of architecture, art, philosophy, culture, and technology. His books include *Konrad Wachsmann's Television: Post-Architectural Transmissions* (Sternberg, 2021); *Passing through Architecture: The 10 Years of Gordon Matta-Clark* (Power Station of Art, 2019); *Cutting Matta-Clark: The Anarchitecture Investigation* (Lars Müller, 2018); *Are We Human? Notes on an Archaeology of Design* (Lars Müller, 2016) with Beatriz Colomina; *Buckminster Fuller Inc.: Architecture in the Age of Radio* (Lars Müller, 2015); *Casa da Música / Porto* (Casa da Música, 2008); *Constant's New Babylon: The Hyper-Architecture of Desire* (010, 1998); *White Walls, Designer Dresses: The Fashioning of Modern Architecture* (MIT, 1995); and *Derrida's Haunt: The Architecture of Deconstruction* (MIT, 1993).

Jeremy Lee Wolin is a PhD candidate in History and Theory of Architecture at Princeton whose research explores the activists, designers, and policymakers who struggled to meet the Civil Rights Movement's demands for housing, education, and employment through Model Cities, the War on Poverty's primary urban development program.

Chenchen Yan is a PhD candidate in History and Theory of Architecture at Princeton University. Her dissertation examines the "becoming Chinese" of objects that were circulated around the turn of the twentieth century and how this resulted not only in the invention of Chinese architecture but also a shift in the epistemic structures of discourse on art and architecture in the US.

INDEX

Sick Architecture
Edited by Beatriz Colomina with Nick Axel, Guillermo S. Arsuaga, and e-flux Architecture

The MIT Press
Massachusetts Institute of Technology
77 Massachusetts Avenue, Cambridge, MA 02139
mitpress.mit.edu

This publication is made possible with support from the Barr Ferree Foundation Fund for Publications, Princeton University, the Graham Foundation, the Princeton University School of Architecture, and the Creative Industries Fund NL.

The MIT Press would like to thank the anonymous peer reviewers who provided comments on drafts of this book. The generous work of academic experts is essential for establishing the authority and quality of our publications. We acknowledge with gratitude the contributions of these otherwise uncredited readers.

Graphic design by Studio Christopher Victor
Typeset in ABC ROM by Seb McLauchlan (Dinamo)
Printed and bound in China

EU product safety and compliance information contact is:
mitp-eu-gpsr@mit.edu

Library of Congress Cataloging-in-Publication Data

Names: Colomina, Beatriz, editor.
Title: Sick architecture / edited by Beatriz Colomina with Nick Axel, Guillermo Sánchez Arsuaga, and e-flux Architecture.
Description: Cambridge, Massachusetts : The MIT Press, [2025] | Includes bibliographical references and index.
Identifiers: LCCN 2024059943 | ISBN 9780262049689 (hardcover)
Subjects: LCSH: Architecture and society. | Architecture--Health aspects.
Classification: LCC NA2543.S6 S555 2025 | DDC 720.1/03--dc23/eng/20241230
LC record available at https://lccn.loc.gov/2024059943

10 9 8 7 6 5 4 3 2 1